Comprehensive Clinical Plasma Medicine

Hans-Robert Metelmann
Thomas von Woedtke
Klaus-Dieter Weltmann
Editors

# Comprehensive Clinical Plasma Medicine

## Cold Physical Plasma for Medical Application

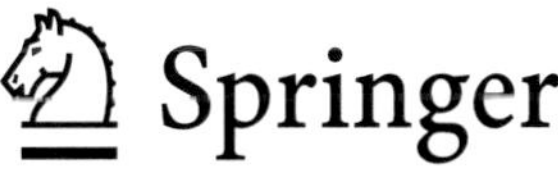

*Editors*
Hans-Robert Metelmann
University Medicine Greifswald
Department of Oral and Maxillofacial
Surgery/Plastic Surgery
Greifswald
Germany

Klaus-Dieter Weltmann
Leibniz Institute for Plasma Science
and Technology (INP Greifswald)
Greifswald
Germany

Thomas von Woedtke
Leibniz Institute for Plasma Science
and Technology (INP Greifswald) and
University Medicine Greifswald
Institute for Hygiene and
Environmental Medicine
Greifswald
Germany

The editors are members of National Centre of Plasma Medicine Berlin, Germany

Translation from the German language edition, revised and expanded: Plasmamedizin Kaltplasma in der medizinischen Anwendung edited by Hans-Robert Metelmann, Thomas von Woedtke and Klaus-Dieter Weltmann Copyright © Springer-Verlag Berlin Heidelberg 2016

ISBN 978-3-030-09806-3 ISBN 978-3-319-67627-2 (eBook)
https://doi.org/10.1007/978-3-319-67627-2


Softcover re-print of the Hardcover 1st edition 2018


Printed on acid-free paper

This Springer imprint is published by the registered company Springer International Publishing AG part of Springer Nature
The registered company address is: Gewerbestrasse 11, 6330 Cham, Switzerland

# Preface

Kind reader,

People usually do not read the preface. But in evidence some do so benevolently. As a sign of our gratitude we reveal only to you that you are holding a future collector's item in your hands, the first comprehensive textbook of a new specialized medical branch: clinical plasma medicine.

How it is actually created and what makes a new specialty in medicine? There is a substantial, significant, and proven evolution in medical technology and treatment concept, a meaningful contribution for the benefit of patients that is calling for natural scientists, engineers, and medical doctors to link their competences and build an innovative scientific community. There are health problems frequently encountered in daily medical practice that can be solved with the new concept and technology. There is an innovative area of scientific and medical expertise not covered by just one established discipline in medicine. There is a structure and concerted workflow that keeps the new specialty standing freely and growing, grounded on national and international organizational bodies, on coordinated research, consented development of treatment guidelines, standard educational courses and specialist training, on scientific journals and academic background, and not at least on books like these. Roaming the chapters of this textbook you will recognize that clinical plasma medicine truly meets the aforementioned criteria of a new medical discipline.

A book does not develop on its own. The existence of this book became possible under the auspices of the State Premier and Government of the north-eastern federal state of Germany, of Mecklenburg-Western Pomerania. Erwin Sellering as predecessor of Premier Manuela Schwesig set the goal, "by offering a common forum for global players of plasma medicine … [that] contributes to an even more effective cooperation and achievement of innovative objectives for the benefit of … patients all over the world." We very much appreciate the high honor and the privilege to see the international development of plasma medicine so much supported.

We are very grateful for the idea and initiation of the project by Sabine Springer, Lothar Kuntz, and Dr. Inga von Behrens from the publishing house. We extend our sincere thanks for excellent supporting, mentoring, and coaching to Kripa Guruprasad, Kerstin Boettger, Christina Rohde, and Christin Siedler. Our warm thanks go to Dr. Philine Metelmann for proofreading of the manuscripts before submission. As a matter of course our profound gratitude to all authors for their substantial contributions and professional cooperation!

And we are especially grateful for your personal getting involved with these reflections before starting to wander through the chapters. That looks like a keen and rewarding interest in clinical plasma medicine. We wish you success!

Hans-Robert Metelmann

Thomas von Woedtke

Klaus-Dieter Weltmann

# Contents

# Part I

# Understanding Physical Plasma: Background and Principles

# 1 Introduction to Plasma Medicine

Thomas von Woedtke, Anke Schmidt, Sander Bekeschus, and Kristian Wende

## 1.1 Preface

Plasma medicine is the name of a new field of medical research at the interface between plasma physics and life sciences that has been in development all over the world for more than 10 years. In this field, the term "plasma" does not mean the liquid part of the blood or the material within a living cell. Physical plasma is a special excited gas, sometimes named "the fourth state of matter."

Supply of energy to a gas by e.g., strong electric fields results in a partial or complete ionization of gas atoms or molecules respectively. Because of the resulting motile electrons and ions, plasmas are conductive. The energy supply and the resulting ionized atoms, molecules, or active states (gas metastables) lead to increased chemical reactivity of a plasma. Plasmas emit electromagnetic radiation, above all ultraviolet (UV) and visible light, and contain responsive ions, electrons and neutral reactive species like radicals.

The resulting characteristics of a plasma depend on a multitude of parameters, including type and composition of the gas or gas mixture used for plasma generation, applied energy or electrode configuration, pressure, and environment. This leads to very complex plasma characteristics. With regard to its application

T. von Woedtke (✉)
Leibniz Institute for Plasma Science and Technology (INP Greifswald)
and University Medicine Greifswald, Institute for Hygiene and Environmental Medicine, Greifswald, Germany
e-mail: woedtke@inp-greifswald.de

A. Schmidt
Leibniz Institute for Plasma Science and Technology (INP Greifswald), Greifswald, Germany
e-mail: anke.schmidt@inp-greifswald.de

S. Bekeschus • K. Wende
Center for Innovation Competence (ZIK) "plasmatis—plasma plus cell",
Leibniz Institute for Plasma Science and Technology (INP Greifswald), Greifswald, Germany
e-mail: sander.bekeschus@inp-greifswald.de; kristian.wende@inp-greifswald.de



H.-R. Metelmann et al. (eds.), *Comprehensive Clinical Plasma Medicine*,
https://doi.org/10.1007/978-3-319-67627-2_1

especially in the medical context, useful classifications are thermal *vs.* non-thermal plasmas and low pressure *vs.* atmospheric pressure plasmas.

The topic and aim of plasma medicine is the use of physical plasmas for medical applications.

When it comes to classifying biomedical applications of physical plasma, there are three main and partially overlapping fields (Fig. 1.1).

Plasma-based surface modification is frequently used in industry. For five decades, plasma has also been used to create and optimize bio-relevant surfaces to improve biocompatibility and biofunctionality of medical devices like implants. Laboratory materials and devices for e.g., cell cultivation and liquid analysis are often functionalized by using plasma treatment [1].

Another field of intensive research that started in the middle of the last century is the use of physical plasma to inactivate microorganisms. Established sterilization and disinfection procedures that are based on the application of high temperature, ionizing radiation, or highly reactive and usually toxic chemicals are not suitable for sensitive products and operational areas frequently used in medicine and hygiene. Here, plasma offers a promising alternative, particularly because it is well known that plasma is able not only to inactivate microorganisms or viruses, but also because it can be used to remove organic material completely. This opens completely new perspectives for plasma application in hygiene and infection control. Infection-transmitting proteins like prions that cannot be controlled using conventional sterilization or disinfection procedures are a potential target. Plasma is effective against multi-resistant pathogens, too [2–4]. Resistance of microorganisms to plasma has not yet been observed.

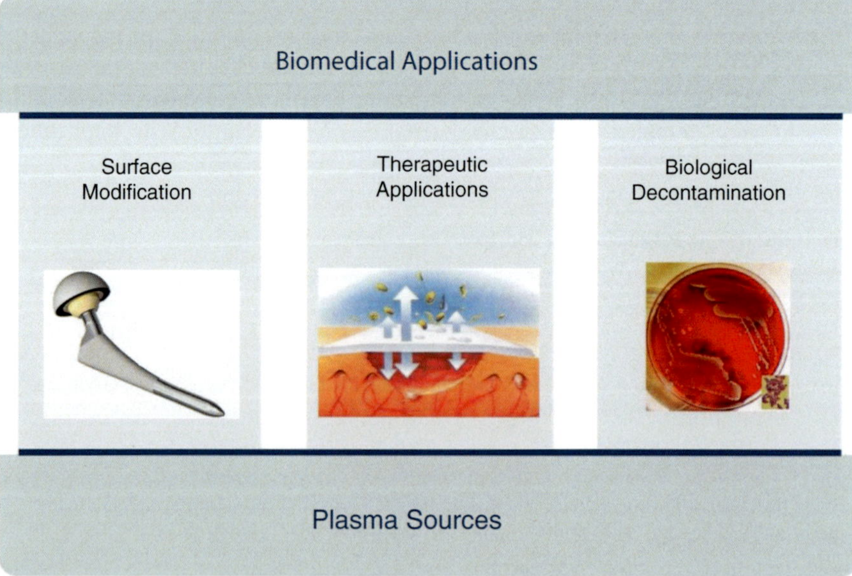


**Fig. 1.1** Fields of biomedical applications of physical plasma

Surface modification and biological decontamination can be categorized as indirect plasma applications because plasma is used to treat materials, surfaces, and devices that are subsequently applied for medical purposes. In both fields, low-pressure plasmas can be used i.e., plasmas that are ignited under well-defined conditions in closed chambers at near-vacuum pressure.

## 1.2 Plasma Medicine: A New Field of Research and Application in Medicine

The field of medical plasma application, plasma medicine, aims to achieve direct application of physical plasma on or in the human (or animal) body for therapeutic purposes.

The direct application of physical plasma on or in the human body is not really new. Historical examples are procedures like the application of so-called violet ray machines in the 1920s [5, 6], or the electro-therapeutic Zeileis method. These are obscure medical plasma applications that have no scientific basis and have always been judged with great skepticism [7].

Different techniques in the field of electro surgery based on thermal plasma use are firmly established in medicine, although they are not explicitly referred to as plasma medicine. Such techniques, like argon plasma coagulation (APC), rely on precisely targeted thermal necrotization of tissue to achieve hemostasis (cauterization), or to cut or remove tissue [8]. Furthermore, several plasma-based procedures in cosmetic and aesthetic surgery e.g., for wrinkle removal and skin regeneration, also rely on thermal plasma effects [9, 10].

The availability of technologies for stable and reproducible plasma generation at low temperature under atmospheric conditions—so-called cold atmospheric plasmas (CAP)—has improved considerably since the 1990s, and has led to considerable intensification of research in the field of therapeutic applications of physical plasma at tissue-compatible temperatures.

Cold atmospheric plasmas (CAP) are the most widespread plasmas in use or intended to be used for therapeutic applications in medicine.

The beginning of modern plasma medicine is associated with the experimental work of Eva Stoffels' group at University of Technology Eindhoven, Netherlands. Since the early 2000s, they have demonstrated that the *in vitro* treatment of cultivated cells with cold atmospheric plasma result in a reversible separation of cells out of a united cell structure, and away from the cultivation vessel base, without killing the cells. This was the first evidence of a selective, non-lethal manipulation of living cells by physical plasma [11, 12].

The main aim of research in plasma medicine is to refine the use of thermal plasmas associated with destructive effects to achieve selective non-thermal plasma effects for the manipulation of specific cell functions.

## 1.3 Scientific Basics of Plasma Medicine

Research in plasma medicine needs a consistent transdisciplinary approach. **Physics** describes the composition and activity of plasma and how it is influenced by technical parameters. **Life sciences** carry out basic research on plasma effects on cells, tissue, and organisms. **Medicine** explores biological plasma effects in a clinical context with a view to therapeutic applications. Interdependency of all three disciplines is the basis of the potential of plasma medicine and its application-oriented research approach **from bench to bedside**. In this context, the early investigation of possible unwanted side effects and risks of plasma application has been an important focus of research from the very beginning (Fig. 1.2) [13, 14].

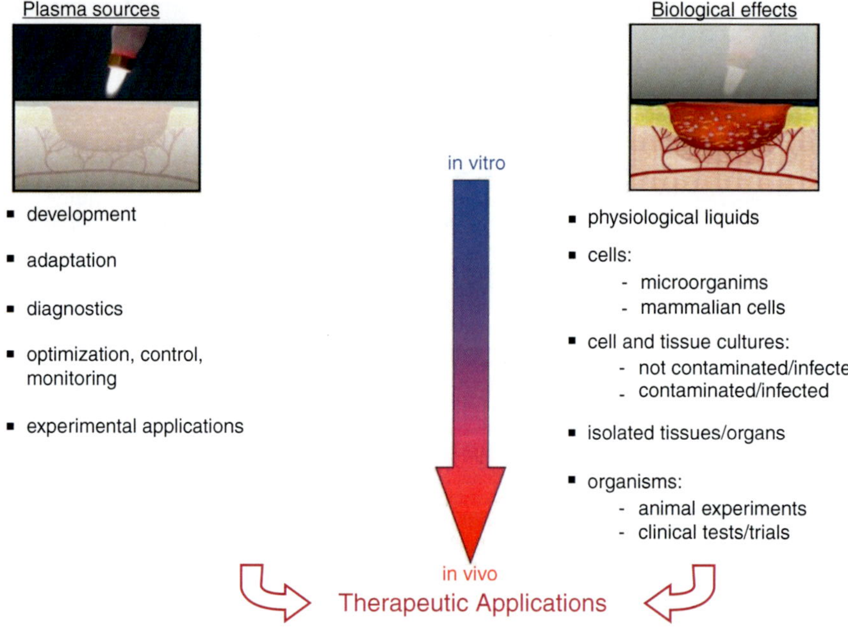


**Fig. 1.2** Research in plasma medicine: combined and coordinated research tasks in plasma physics and life sciences

Research in plasma medicine comprises both basic research on the mechanisms of biological plasma effects and application-oriented as well as clinical research to identify promising fields of implementation in medical practice.

### 1.3.1 Basic Mechanisms of Biological Plasma Effects

There is a large number of plasma sources potentially useful for medical application. These differ according to plasma generation technique, geometry, or working gases and, consequently, they vary in their application characteristics [6, 15–17].

Identification and quantification of active compounds of particular plasmas is key to meeting one of the most important current challenges of experimental plasma medicine, which is the detailed elucidation of mechanisms of biological effects caused by plasma in living systems, and the specific control of biological responses through plasma modification.

The initial point of all biological effects is the physical generation of plasma under atmospheric environmental conditions. To produce the different plasma compounds illustrated in Fig. 1.3, three basic processes can be outlined:

1. Ionization of atoms or molecules of a gas that itself is not directly biologically active (noble gases like argon or helium, gas mixtures containing oxygen, nitrogen and air, and air as working gas), preferably using electrical energy.
2. Interaction of ionized atoms/molecules and free electrons with other atoms or molecules in the plasma phase as well as with neighboring media (above all atmospheric air, but also liquids or surfaces), resulting in the generation of reactive species e.g., radicals.
3. Emission of electromagnetic radiation (UV/VUV, visible light, infrared/ thermal radiation, electromagnetic fields) as an additional result of ionization and excitation processes in the plasma.

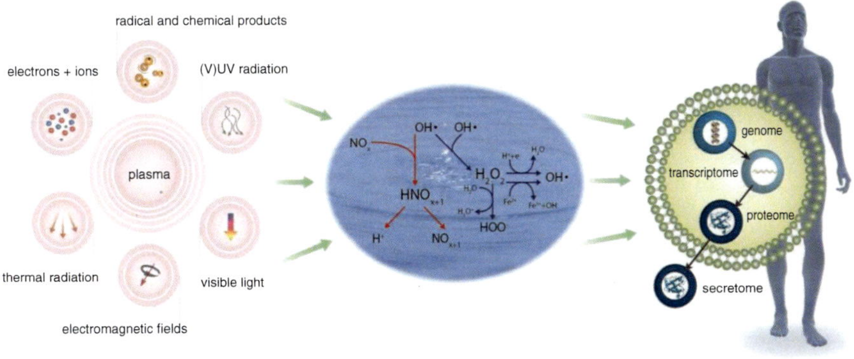


**Fig. 1.3** Cold atmospheric plasmas (CAP) are effective in liquid phases and redox-active species

Initially, the investigation of biological plasma effects was focused on microorganisms with the aim of characterizing and exploiting antimicrobial plasma activity. For a decade, basic research on specific effects on mammalian cells has broadened, as is documented by the growing number of publications in this field.

The following cellular effects in particular, which are seen *in vitro* and induced by cold atmospheric plasma, are described in the literature [18, 19]:

***Lethal effects of cold atmospheric plasma (CAP):***

- Inactivation/killing of microorganisms (prokaryotic cells) including antibiotic-resistant pathogens
- Inactivation or killing of mammalian cells (eukaryotic cells) including cancer cells mainly via induction of apoptosis depending on intensity (time) of plasma impact

***Non-lethal effects of cold atmospheric plasma (CAP)*:**

- Influence on/stimulation of metabolism of microorganisms (prokaryotic cells)
- Specific/selective effects on mammalian cells (eukaryotic cells):
  - Influence on cell migration
  - Influence on expression of surface proteins responsible for cell-cell and cell-matrix interactions
  - Influence on/stimulation of cell proliferation
  - Influence on/stimulation of angiogenesis
  - Reversible impact on DNA integrity, influence on cell cycle
  - Reversible permeabilization of cell membranes ("plasma poration")
  - Non-thermal blood coagulation

The nature and extent of these *in vitro* observations is dependent on various parameters e.g., cell type investigated; cellular environment (sort and composition of the surrounding liquid e.g., the cultivation medium); plasma source used and related plasma parameters; treatment time; and general experimental setup. Similar to microorganisms, mammalian cells show different sensitivities to physical plasma.

However, the fact that different plasma sources cause similar biological outcomes resulted in the basic assumption that biological plasma effects can be attributed to consistent basic mechanisms.

The current state of knowledge can be summarized in the following two fundamental insights about the mechanisms of the biological effects of cold atmospheric plasmas *in vitro* (see Fig. 1.3):

- Significant biological plasma effects are caused by plasma-induced changes to the liquid environment of cells.
- Reactive oxygen and nitrogen species (ROS, RNS/RONS) generated in or transferred into liquid phases play a dominant role in biological plasma effects.

Consequently, CAP influences cellular redox signaling through transiently or constantly increased concentrations of redox-active species (ROS, RNS/RONS; see Table 1.1) in the liquid cell environment [21, 22]. According to recent findings, this influence results from complex interactions between active (reactive) plasma compounds.

**Table 1.1** Important reactive oxygen and nitrogen species in biology; following [20]

| Reactive oxygen species (ROS) | Reactive nitrogen species (RNS/RONS) |
|---|---|
| Superoxide: $O_2^{-}\bullet$ | Nitric oxide: $\bullet NO$ |
| Hydrogen peroxide: $H_2O_2$ | Nitrogen dioxide: $\bullet NO_2$ |
| Hydroxyl radical: $\bullet OH$ | Peroxynitrite: $ONOO^-$ |
| Singlet oxygen: $^1O_2$ | |
| Ozone: $O_3$ | |
| Organic radicals: $RO\bullet$, $RO_2\bullet$ | |

It is of special significance that the modification of the cellular environment resulting from plasma is in most cases assumed to be caused by the same ROS and RNS/RONS as appear in regular cell metabolism in the body. These control and communicate physiological and pathological processes.

The impact of plasma on cellular functions is cell-type specific. In an exploratory study using cell culture models, Jurkat cells (T lymphocytes) were most sensitive to cold atmospheric plasma whereas other cells (human cell lines like MRC5 fibroblasts, HaCaT keratinocytes, THP1 monocytes) were remarkably robust [23]. Effects in skin cells are based on redox changes are caused mainly by oxygen-based radicals and hydrogen peroxide [24–28].

Important practical consequences result for the medical application of cold atmospheric plasmas (CAP) based on these insights from redox biology:

- Redox active species identified as active compounds of CAP play an important role in physiological wound-healing processes. This is the scientific basis of the concept of plasma-supported wound healing. Hence, plasma action supports the body's own functions that are pathologically impaired e.g., in the case of non-healing chronic wounds.
- Because of the physiological occurrence of these plasma-generated redox-active species, excess concentrations of these substances can be effectively antagonized by the body's own antioxidant defense systems. Consequently, under regular conditions, any input of these reactive oxygen and nitrogen species by local and time-limited plasma treatment will not cause increased risk of unwanted side effects.
- Different sensitivity of different cell types suggests the possibility of selective plasma effects.

To maintain the cellular redox balance, numerous antioxidants, redox sensors, redox enzymes, and repair mechanisms are involved. This has been proven experimentally using proteomics and transcriptomics. A low intensity of plasma impact stimulates cellular redox signaling, which results in increased anti-oxidative capacity as well as initiation of the repair processes if needed. This kinetics of biological effects is called hormesis, and is actually discussed in the field of redox biology as a general action principle of redox-active species [22, 29]. Generally, hormetic effects are characterized by low-dose stimulation and high-dose inhibition [30].

When exceeding the capacity of the cellular redox balance, an accumulation of harmful cellular effects will result in the initiation of programmed cell death (apoptosis) if the counter regulation processes of the cells are overburdened.

The transcription factor Nrf2 has a central regulatory function in the maintenance of the cellular redox balance [31, 32]. Via activation of the antioxidant response element (ARE) on DNA, Nrf2 is responsible for the upregulation of genes for transcription of protective proteins. Typically, cytosolic Nrf2 is bound to a complex containing the protein Keap1 among others. Through oxidation of Keap1 via reactive oxygen species (ROS), Nrf2 becomes detached from the protein complex and can diffuse into the nucleus of the cell to bind together with an additional regulatory protein (Maf) at ARE on DNA. In an experimental study, it could be demonstrated using human keratinocytes that this translocation of Nrf2 from cytosol to the nucleus occurs as a consequence of plasma treatment [28]. The result of such activation of the Nrf2 signal pathway is the protection of the affected cell from the damaging effects of redox active species.

Generally, the amount and activity of antioxidant systems as well as a cell's ability to repair modifications of DNA and proteins determines the response to plasma impact. Furthermore, plasma sensitivity depends on cell division rate: cells with high duplication rates are more sensitive compared to cells with slow reproduction metrics.

Translating these insights from redox biology to biological effects induced by cold atmospheric plasma means:

- Low treatment intensities (short treatment times) result in cell-stimulating effects.
- Higher treatment intensities (longer treatment times) result in inactivation/killing of cells.

Such interdependency has been demonstrated repeatedly by experimental studies. With an *in vitro* wound healing model using upper airway S9 epithelial cells, a plasma treatment time-dependent stimulation of cell proliferation and acceleration of wound closure was demonstrated up to an optimum level. A further prolongation of plasma treatment resulted in reduction up to complete stop of wound closure [33]. After *ex vivo* plasma treatment of human skin biopsies, a growing number of proliferating cells was detected. However, a further prolongation of plasma treatment time resulted in a decreasing number of proliferating cells, but an increasing number of apoptotic cells [34]. These results were corroborated in a murine wound model where accelerated wound healing was observed after short treatment times [35].

This state of basic research is the source for further detailed investigation of intracellular reaction cascades and mechanisms. Above all, the use of modern methods of bio analytics like genomics, proteomics and transcriptomics will support the progress of scientific knowledge. In extracellular analytics, detection of reactive species, particularly radicals in the plasma and gas phase as well as in the liquid cell environment, is a remaining challenge. Specific recording is hard to achieve because of high reactivity and the resultant ephemerality of the reactive species.

### 1.3.2 Risk Estimation

Because of the novelty of the technology and the strong focus on medical applications, questions of risk estimation have always played a central role in plasma medicine research [13]. As multi-component systems, plasmas potentially pose chemical and physical threats of different levels to the human organism. The risk potential is biased dominantly by the design of the plasma source and its operation strategy on the one hand, and the intended application field and operator on the other. Accordingly, a specific risk assessment protocol needs to be filed for any plasma source, and must be updated with any change of operation procedure e.g., alterations to working gas composition, distance, driving power or the application itself. The stage of development also affects the risk potential.

Essentially, the components of the physical plasma need to be taken into account: radiation and heat emission, chemical species produced (including free electrons), and electromagnetic fields surrounding the discharge. Additionally, the ability of plasmas to conduct electric currents, which can imply electrical hazards, must be considered. These aspects all vary with the plasma source, the target treated, and ambient conditions.

The basic finding that biological plasma effects are mainly meditated by reactive oxygen and nitrogen species (ROS, RNS/RONS) that are at least partially the same as those in regular cell physiology, leads to the general assumption that cellular antioxidative protection mechanisms [36] should be effective against plasma impact, too.

Investigation of the genotoxic effects of cold atmospheric plasma by *in vitro* standard procedures for mutagenicity testing of chemical substances demonstrated no extended mutation rate of plasma treated cells [37–39]. This was confirmed by an animal study using hairless immunocompetent mice [40].

These experimental results corroborated studies of skin biopsies after cold atmospheric plasma treatment [34, 41] as well as clinical follow-up investigations after plasma applications in wound treatment [42, 43]. Even if the risk assessment of CAP application is a work in progress, all these findings confirm that there is no genotoxic risk caused by the medical application of cold atmospheric plasma.

### 1.3.3 Cell-Biology Basics of Plasma-Supplemented Wound Healing

A starting point for the search for possible medical applications for cold atmospheric plasma was its well-known ability to inactivate microorganisms. This led very early on to the idea of using plasma for antiseptics e.g., in non-healing chronic wounds.

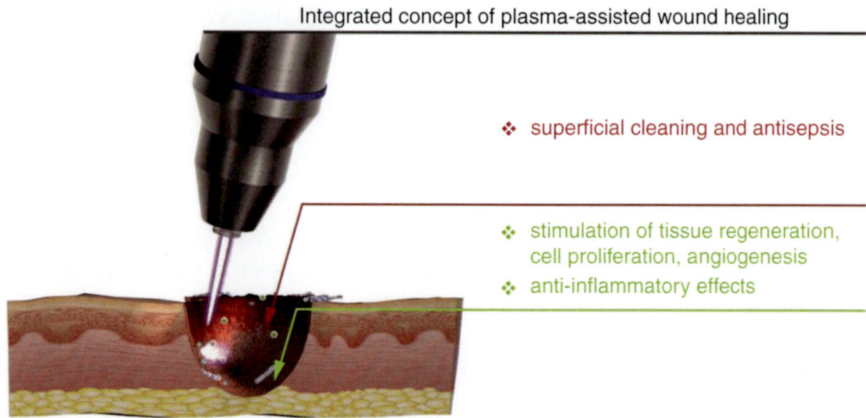


**Fig. 1.4** Basic concept of plasma-supported wound healing

The results of basic research gave rise to the early hypothesis that plasma-supported wound healing may be based not only on the reduction of bacterial colonization or elimination of wound infection, but also by direct stimulation of regeneration of damaged tissue. Based on this hypothesis, the concept of plasma-supported wound healing was developed. This is based on a combination of cleaning and antisepsis on the wound surface, with a stimulation of tissue regeneration in deeper wound areas (Fig. 1.4) [44–46].

Impeded wound healing is a big challenge for both patients and clinics. Despite different etiologies, this kind of wound is frequently characterized by disturbed synchronicity of the different processes of wound healing, wound infections, accumulation of liquid, necrosis of the wound edge, excessive tissue neogenesis, and increased release of proteinases and cytokines [47]. Proteinases disturb the generation of the extracellular matrix and inhibit the migration of fibroblasts and keratinocytes that is essential for successful re-epithelialization in later phases of wound healing. Besides a resulting deceleration and inhibition of wound closure, an increased number of immune cells is detected [48].

Usually, immune cells are attracted from the blood and the surrounding tissue fluid to the wound, which prolongs the inflammatory phase of wound healing. Persistence of immune cells is also given in low-germ chronic wounds. It is not yet completely clear whether this is the cause or the result of disturbance to wound healing. There are several signs that a misguided cellular redox signaling will hold the balance of wound inflammation. The concept of redox balance describes homeostasis of the oxidative and reductive processes in cells and tissues. Reactive oxygen and nitrogen species (ROS, RNS/RONS) or radicals, which are normally generated by the respiratory chain or in conjunction with inflammations, are eliminated by enzymatic and non-enzymatic defense mechanisms [49]. It was supposed for a long time that such reactive species alone cause cell-damaging effects. Nowadays, their necessity for cellular processes beyond pathophysiological effects is well known [50, 51].

Under physiological conditions, low concentrations of reactive species are present that are strictly controlled and are an important part of intracellular signal cascades with central functions in cell-cell communication, cell adhesion, cell proliferation, and cell differentiation. Above all, the innate immune system is associated with these molecules serving both as anti-pathogen compound and key controller of the signaling network.

Using cold atmospheric plasma treatment, redox active species (ROS, RNS/RONS) can be administered directly and locally into the tissue to modulate redox processes in a specific manner. It is known from the literature that redox processes are involved in the coordination of all cells in the wound environment [52, 53].

The concept of redox-control in wound healing is the most important scientific basis of plasma-supported wound healing.

Immune mediators, which are cytokines as well as growth factors, orchestrate the phases of wound healing [54]. In cultivated cells, plasma application results in increased gene expression of factors relevant for wound healing like oxidoreductases and matrix metalloproteases, along with several cytokines and growth factors [28, 55–57]. Low plasma treatment intensities (treatment times) induce cell proliferation that is stimulated by ROS-mediated excretion of the fibroblast growth factor FGF2 [24, 57–60].

In chronic wounds, a pro-inflammatory environment is dominated by increased concentrations of interleukins and cytokines [61]. Cold atmospheric plasma decreases the production of cytokines in activated human leucocytes. Simultaneously, an increased formation of anti-inflammatory mediators like IL-10 and TGFβ was found in T-lymphocytes, which are both associated with sufficient healing of wounds [62]. This is accompanied by an increased secretion of the highly inflammatory IL-8, which attracts mainly granulocytes.

Consequently, cold atmospheric plasma does not induce a simple pro-inflammatory or anti-inflammatory signature of cytokines, but modulates the quality of the inflammatory reaction. Such a graduation seems to be important because, by topical application of anti-inflammatory cytokines like TGFβ, less promising results than expected were achieved in chronic wound healing [63].

For wound healing processes, communication between cell populations via cell-cell contact is of great importance, because changes in migration, proliferation and inflammation are mediated by such communication processes [64]. Plasma is able to influence the expression of a multitude of cell adhesion and migration molecules [65–67].

Even if only a few studies on plasma treatment of immune cells have been completed up to now, promising results have been achieved. Relatively short-duration plasma treatment induces apoptosis in isolated human peripheral blood lymphocytes. A similar effect has been found in cytotoxic and T-helper cells, in B-lymphocytes, and in natural killer (NKT) cells that were described as negative regulators of wound healing [24]. On the other hand, only few γδ-T-cells were apoptotic compared to other lymphocytes. These cells are attributed to supporting wound healing [68].

In wounds, CAP can stimulate skin cells by directed application of redox active species, whereas regulatory monocytes would be just slightly affected. Infected chronic inflammations require activation of the adaptive immune system to support medium-term combat pathogens by highly specific antibodies. Cold atmospheric plasma induced apoptosis in a fraction of T-helper cells, but did not block amitosis in the remaining vital cells, which is important for immune reaction [69]. Additionally, proliferation of plasma-treated but non-mitogen-stimulated cells was found i.e., there was no non-specific stimulation of immune response by cold atmospheric plasma.

Even if there is further research needed on detailed mechanisms of plasma action in wound healing, previous experimental studies have proven the high potential of cold atmospheric plasma for therapeutic applications.

## 1.4 Perspectives and Challenges of Plasma Medicine

In a workshop in April 2012 in Greifswald, all German medical professionals at that time working in the field of pre-clinical and clinical research in plasma medicine prepared a consensus paper on the state and perspective of clinical plasma medicine. Based on the state of research it was stated that plasma application in dermatology as well as plastic and aesthetic surgery would have the best prospects for success [70]. In general, this assessment is as appropriate now as before, and is even confirmed by increasing clinical experience.

Therapeutic application of cold atmospheric plasma in wound healing has dominated research in plasma medicine for several years. Meanwhile, another large field of fundamental research in plasma medicine has opened: the investigation of possibilities of plasma application in **cancer treatment**. This is based on the widely published finding that cold atmospheric plasma is able to induce apoptosis in cancer cells [71, 72]. Again, redox active species transferred into the liquid cell environment by plasma treatment play an important role in this process [73]. Using an *in vivo* tumor model, it was demonstrated that treatment with cold atmospheric plasma resulted in inactivation of upper cell layers of solid tumors via induction of apoptosis [74]. Furthermore, in animal studies with subcutaneously induced solid tumors, a transcutaneous cold plasma treatment resulted in the reduction of tumor growth as well as in prolongation of survival of treated mice compared to non-treated controls [75, 76]. These research results led to new and promising options for future plasma application in cancer therapy. Inactivation of single layers of cancer cells might open up the possibility of supportive plasma application in combination with surgical tumor resections in cases where a large-scale tumor removal is impossible [77]. Any direct plasma use for reduction or complete removal of solid tumors as demonstrated in initial animal studies requires further research.

Another highly exciting field of research is the application of **plasma-treated liquids**. It was found that plasma-treatment of liquids may result in an at least temporary biological activity of the liquids. This was demonstrated using the example of antibacterial activity of plasma-treated water or physiological saline [78–80]. Meanwhile it was shown that plasma-treated cell culture medium could be used to induce apoptosis in cancer cells, opening up options to treat disseminated tumors in the abdominal cavity [81, 82]. This field of plasma-based generation, optimization and stabilization of liquids containing active agents called "plasma pharmacy" [83, 84] is still in the basic stages of research.

Application of plasma in **dentistry** has been part of research in plasma medicine for several years. Here, antimicrobial plasma activity including inactivation and removal of biofilm as well as plasma-assisted cleaning and optimization of tooth and implant surfaces to improve bone integration and ingrowth is at the center of medical interest [85]. Large-scale clinical applications in dentistry are not yet documented.

Up to now, there has been little research on cold atmospheric plasma application in **ophthalmology**. Nevertheless, it might be a promising field to exploit the antimicrobial plasma effects for infection treatment [86–88].

**Endoscopic** cold atmospheric plasma applications will open additional fields of plasma use in medicine. While this has already been achieved in electrosurgical applications like argon plasma coagulation [89], there are also promising concepts for endoscopic CAP devices under development [90–92]. Besides applications in gastroenterology, pneumology is a promising area.

Altogether, plasma medicine is well on the way to effective clinical use. Application of cold atmospheric plasma to improve wound healing is already a reality. **New questions** arise from clinical application e.g., appropriate intensity and duration of single plasma treatment, or duration and frequency of plasma-treatment cycles. Here, fundamental research and application-related clinical research must work together to find adequate answers.

Based on the observation of the biological effects of plasma treatment in deeper layers of the skin as well as in solid tumors, it would be interesting to see if such distant or systemic effects really occur as a result of local and superficial plasma treatment, what the mechanisms of such effects are, and how to use them.

According to the current state of knowledge, the medically useful effects of cold atmospheric plasma result from complex interactions of different plasma compounds with the liquid environment of cells and tissue. This represents the special quality and uniqueness of plasma medicine. On the other hand, one of the greatest challenges of plasma medicine results from this complexity. This is the identification of a parameter or set of parameters to monitor and control plasma activity in terms of a "dose" as it is known from phototherapy or radiotherapy. At present, the only means of control is treatment time. Because the specific treatment time to generate a certain biological effect may differ substantially between different cold plasma devices, any comparability of research as well as treatment results is limited. Moreover, any device-independent declaration of treatment intensities ("treatment doses") for clinical application has not yet been possible.

## 1.5 Summary and Conclusions

Use of cold atmospheric plasmas to support wound healing is already a clinical reality. This is a result of solid fundamental research and application-oriented research including technology transfer to industry. According to the latest findings, the therapeutic application of cold atmospheric plasmas is safe. Medical application in cancer therapy is the latest stage of clinical implementation.

The special and unique quality of cold atmospheric plasma in medicine can be summarized in the following three statements:

1. Active plasma components are generated locally and only for the required duration of the application by energy transfer to a biologically inactive gas (argon, helium, oxygen, nitrogen, air, or mixtures of it).
2. Biologically active (redox-active) plasma components that are transferred into the liquid cell environment or are generated there by plasma treatment are the same as those that occur in regular physiological and biochemical processes. Because of high reactivity, their stability is limited. Therefore, these plasma components cannot be applied adequately in drug form etc., but can be delivered *in statu nascendi* by plasma generation.
3. Because of localized and short-term generation by local plasma treatment, these substances can be metabolized through regular cell metabolism processes. Hence, the risk of plasma application is low, assessable and manageable.

Due to the amount of research in plasma medicine in recent years resulting in increased visibility in the media, physicians and patients have high expectations that plasma medicine will solve clinical problems that have so far been addressed unsatisfactorily or not at all. Even if the field is new, there has been a considerable economic impact, and increased interest and awareness.

Therefore, researchers, clinicians and manufacturers active in the field of plasma medicine are being forced to live up to such expectations, while not raising false hopes with hasty promises. They must be careful not to use insufficiently tested plasma sources that may discredit plasma medicine in general [70].

## References

1. d'Agostino R, Favia P, Oehr C, Wertheimer MR. Low-temperature plasma processing of materials: past, present, and future. Plasma Process Polym. 2005;2:7–15.
2. Daeschlein G, Scholz S, Emmert S, von Podewils S, Haase H, von Woedtke T, Jünger M. Plasma medicine in dermatology: basic antimicrobial efficacy testing as prerequisite to clinical plasma therapy. Plasma Med. 2012;2:33–69.

3. Daeschlein G, Napp M, von Podewils S, Lutze S, Emmert S, Lange A, Klare I, Haase H, Gümbel D, von Woedtke T, Jünger M. In vitro susceptibility of multidrug resistant skin and wound pathogens against low temperature atmospheric pressure plasma jet (APPJ) and dielectric barrier discharge plasma (DBD). Plasma Process Polym. 2014;11:175–83.
4. Moreau M, Orange N, Feuilloley MGJ. Non-thermal plasma technologies: new tools for biodecontamination. Biotechnol Adv. 2008;26:610–7.
5. Bauer A, Faulhaber J, Kober P. Der Hochfrequenzstrahlapparat, sein Wesen und seine Anwendung. Verlag Dr. H. Stock; cited in: Weltmann K-D, Polak M, Masur K, von Woedtke T, Winter J, Reuter S (2012) Plasma Processes and Plasma Sources in Medicine. Contrib Plasma Physics 1928;52:644–54.
6. Weltmann KD, Polak M, Masur K, von Woedtke T, Winter J, Reuter S. Plasma processes and plasma sources in medicine. Contrib Plasma Physics. 2012;52:644–54.
7. Burger H. The doctor, the quack and the appetite of the public for magic in medicine. P Roy Soc Med. 1933;27:171–6.
8. Raiser J, Zenker M. Argon plasma coagulation for open surgical and endoscopic applications: state of the art. J Phys D Appl Phys. 2006;39:3520–3.
9. Bentkover SH. Plasma skin resurfacing: personal experience and long-term results. Facial Plast Surg Clin North Am. 2012;20:145–62.
10. Foster KW, Moy RL, Fincher EF. Advances in plasma skin regeneration. J Cosmet Dermatol. 2008;7:169–79.
11. Stoffels E, Kieft IE, Sladek REJ. Superficial treatment of mammalian cells using plasma needle. J Phys D Appl Phys. 2003;36:2908–13.
12. Stoffels E. "Tissue Processing" with atmospheric plasmas. Contrib Plasma Physics. 2007; 47:40–8.
13. Fridman G, Friedman G, Gutsol A, Shekhter AB, Vasilets VN, Fridman A. Applied plasma medicine. Plasma Process Polym. 2008;5:503–33.
14. Weltmann KD, von Woedtke T. Campus PlasmaMed—from basic research to clinical proof. IEEE Trans Plasma Sci. 2011;39:1015–25.
15. Park GY, Park SJ, Choi MY, Koo IG, Byun JH, Hong JW, Sim JY, Collins GJ, Lee JK. Atmospheric-pressure plasma sources for biomedical applications. Plasma Sources Sci Technol. 2012;21:043001.
16. Weltmann KD, von Woedtke T. Basic requirements for plasma sources in medicine. The. Eur Phys J Appl Phys. 2011;55:13807.
17. Weltmann KD, Kindel E, von Woedtke T, Hähnel M, Stieber M, Brandenburg R. Atmospheric-pressure plasma sources: prospective tools for plasma medicine. Pure Appl Chem. 2010; 82:1223–37.
18. von Woedtke T, Reuter S, Masur K, Weltmann K-D. Plasmas for medicine. Phys Rep. 2013;530:291–320.
19. von Woedtke T, Metelmann HR, Weltmann KD. Clinical plasma medicine: state and perspectives of in vivo application of cold atmospheric plasma. Contrib Plasma Physics. 2014; 54:104–17.
20. Fang FC. Antimicrobial reactive oxygen and nitrogen species: concepts and controversies. Nat Rev Microbiol. 2004;2:820–32.
21. Graves DB. The emerging role of reactive oxygen and nitrogen species in redox biology and some implications for plasma applications to medicine and biology. J Phys D Appl Phys. 2012;45:263001.
22. Graves DB. Oxy-nitroso shielding burst model of cold atmospheric plasma therapeutics. Clin Plasma Med. 2014;2:38–49.
23. Wende K, Reuter S, von Woedtke T, Weltmann KD, Masur K. Redox-based assay for assessment of biological impact of plasma treatment. Plasma Process Polym. 2014;11:655–63.
24. Bekeschus S, von Woedtke T, Kramer A, Weltmann K-D, Masur K. Cold physical plasma treatment alters redox balance in human immune cells. Plasma Med. 2013;3:267–78.
25. Bekeschus S, Kolata J, Winterbourn C, Kramer A, Turner R, Weltmann K-D, Bröker B, Masur K. Hydrogen peroxide: a central player in physical plasma-induced oxidative stress in human blood cells. Free Radic Res. 2014;48:542–9.

26. Bekeschus S, Iséni S, Reuter S, Masur K, Weltmann K-D. Nitrogen shielding of argon plasma jet and its effects on human immune cells. IEEE Trans Plasma Sci. 2015;43:776–81.
27. Schmidt A, Wende K, Bekeschus S, Bundscherer L, Barton A, Ottmüller K, Weltmann K-D, Masur K. Non-thermal plasma treatment is associated with changes in transcriptome of human epithelial skin cells. Free Radic Res. 2013;47:577–92.
28. Schmidt A, Dietrich S, Steuer A, Weltmann KD, von Woedtke T, Masur K, Wende K. Non-thermal plasma activates human keratinocytes by stimulation of antioxidant and phase II pathways. J Biol Chem. 2015;290:6731–50.
29. Ristow M, Schmeisser K. Mitohormesis: promoting health and lifespan by increased levels of rective oxygen species (ROS). Dose Response. 2014;12:288–341.
30. Calabrese EJ, Baldwin LA. Hormesis: the dose-response revolution. Annu Rev Pharmacol Toxicol. 2003;43:175–97.
31. Bryan HK, Olayanju A, Goldring CE, Park BK. The Nrf2 cell defence pathway: Keap1-dependent and -independent mechanisms of regulation. Biochem Pharmacol. 2013;85:705–17.
32. Ma Q. Role of Nrf2 in oxidative stress and toxicity. Annu Rev Pharmacol Toxicol. 2013; 53:401–26.
33. Lendeckel D, Eymann C, Emicke P, Daeschlein G, Darm K, O'Neil S, Beule AG, von Woedtke T, Völker U, Weltmann K-D, Jünger M, Hosemann W, Scharf C. Proteomic changes of tissue-tolerable plasma treated airway epithelial cells and their relation to wound healing. BioMed Res Int. 2015;2015:06059.
34. Hasse S, Tran T, Hahn O, Kindler S, Metelmann HR, von Woedtke T, Masur K. Induction of proliferation of basal epidermal keratinocytes by cold atmospheric pressure plasma. Clin Exp Dermatol. 2015;41:202–9.
35. Schmidt A, Bekeschus S, Wende K, Vollmar B, von Woedtke T. A cold plasma jet accelerates wound healing in a murine model of full-thickness skin wounds. Exp Dermatol. 2017; 26:156–62.
36. Dröge W. Free radicals in the physiological control of cell function. Physiol Rev. 2002;82:47–95.
37. Boxhammer V, Li YF, Köritzer J, Shimizu T, Maisch T, Thomas HM, Schlegel J, Morfill GE, Zimmermann JL. Investigation of the mutagenic potential of cold atmospheric plasma at bactericidal dosages. Mutat Res Gen Tox En. 2013;753:23–8.
38. Kluge S, Bekeschus S, Bender C, Benkhai H, Sckell A, Below H, Stope MB, Kramer A. Investigating the mutagenicity of a cold argon-plasma jet in an HET-MN model. PLoS One. 2016;11:e0160667.
39. Wende K, Bekeschus S, Schmidt A, Jatsch L, Hasse S, Weltmann KD, Masur K, von Woedtke T. Risk assessment of a cold argon plasma jet in respect to its mutagenicity. Mutat Res-Gen Tox En. 2016;798:48–54.
40. Schmidt A, von Woedtke T, Stenzel J, Lindner T, Polei S, Vollmar B, Bekeschus S. One year follow up risk assessment in SKH-1 mice and wounds treated with an argon plasma jet. Int J Mol Sci. 2017;18:868.
41. Hasse S, Hahn O, Kindler S, von Woedtke T, Metelmann HR, Masur K. Atmospheric pressure plasma jet application on human oral mucosa modulates tissue regeneration. Plasma Med. 2014;4:117–1129.
42. Heinlin J, Isbary G, Stolz W, Morfill G, Landthaler M, Shimizu T, Steffes B, Nosenko T, Zimmermann JL, Karrer S. Plasma applications in medicine with a special focus on dermatology. J Eur Acad Dermatol. 2011;25:1–11.
43. Metelmann HR, TT V, Do HT, Le TNB, Hoang THA, Phi TTT, Luong TML, Doan VT, Nguyen TTH, Nguyen THM, Le DQ, Le TKX, von Woedtke T, Bussiahn R, Weltmann KD, Khalili R, Podmelle F. Scar formation of laser skin lesions after cold atmospheric pressure plasma (CAP) treatment: a clinical long term observation. Clin Plasma Med. 2013;1:30–5.
44. Kramer A, Hübner NO, Weltmann KD, Lademann J, Ekkernkamp A, Hinz P, Assadian O. Polypragmasia in the therapy of infected wounds—conclusions drawn from the perspectives of low temperature plasma technology for plasma wound therapy. GMS Krankenhaushyg Interdiszip. 2008;3:Doc13.

45. Lloyd G, Friedman G, Jafri S, Schultz G, Fridman A, Harding K. Gas plasma. Medical uses and developments in wound care. Plasma Process Polym. 2010;7:194–211.
46. Plasmatis Initiative Group. Declaration of the 1st International Workshop on Plasma Tissue Interactions. GMS Krankenhaushyg Interdiszip. 2008;3:Doc01.
47. Pastar I, Stojadinovic O, Yin NC, Ramirez H, Nusbaum AG, Sawaya A, Patel SB, Khalid L, Isseroff RR, Tomic-Canic M. Epithelialization in wound healing: a comprehensive review. Adv Wound Care. 2014;3:445–64.
48. Portou MJ, Baker D, Abraham D, Tsui J. The innate immune system, toll-like receptors and dermal wound healing: a review. Vasc Pharmacol. 2015;71:31–6.
49. Giorgio M. Oxidative stress and the unfulfilled promises of antioxidant agents. Ecancermedicalscience. 2015;9:556.
50. Circu ML, Aw TY. Reactive oxygen species, cellular redox systems, and apoptosis. Free Radical Biol Med. 2010;48:749–62.
51. Ray PD, Huang BW, Tsuji Y. Reactive oxygen species (ROS) homeostasis and redox regulation in cellular signaling. Cell Signal. 2012;24:981–90.
52. Sen CK, Roy S. Redox signals in wound healing. Biochim Biophys Acta. 2008;1780:1348–61.
53. Sen CK. Wound healing essentials: let there be oxygen. Wound Repair Regen. 2009;17:1–18.
54. Werner S, Grose R. Regulation of wound healing by growth factors and cytokines. Physiol Rev. 2003;83:835–70.
55. Barton A, Wende K, Bundscherer L, Hasse S, Schmidt A, Bekeschus S, Weltmann K-D, Lindequist U, Masur K. Nonthermal plasma increases expression of wound healing related genes in a keratinocyte cell line. Plasma Med. 2013;3:125–36.
56. Schmidt A, von Woedtke T, Weltmann KD, Masur K. Identification of the molecular basis of non-thermal plasma-induced changes in human keratinocytes. Plasma Med. 2013;3:15–25.
57. Schmidt A, Bekeschus S, Jablonowski H, Barton A, Weltmann K-D, Wende K. Role of ambient gas composition on cold physical plasma-elicited cell signaling in keratinocytes. Biophys J. 2017;112:2397–407.
58. Bundscherer L, Bekeschus S, Tresp H, Hasse S, Reuter S, Weltmann KD, Lindequist U, Masur K. Viability of human blood leukocytes compared with their respective cell lines after plasma treatment. Plasma Med. 2013;3:71–80.
59. Bundscherer L, Wende K, Ottmüller K, Barton A, Schmidt A, Bekeschus S, Hasse S, Weltmann KD, Masur K, Lindequist U. Impact of non-thermal plasma treatment on MAPK signaling pathways of human immune cell lines. Immunobiology. 2013;218:1248–55.
60. Kalghatgi S, Friedman G, Fridman A, Morss Clyne A. Endothelial cell proliferation is enhanced by low dose non-thermal plasma through fibroblast growth Factor-2 release. Ann Biomed Eng. 2010;38:748–57.
61. Mast BA, Schultz GS. Interactions of cytokines, growth factors, and proteases in acute and chronic wounds. Wound Repair Regen. 1996;4:411–20.
62. Bekeschus S. Effects of cold physical plasma on human leukocytes, PhD thesis, Mathematisch-Naturwissenschaftliche Fakultät der Ernst-Moritz-Arndt Universität Greifswald, 2015.
63. Barrientos S, Stojadinovic O, Golinko MS, Brem H, Tomic-Canic M. Growth factors and cytokines in wound healing. Wound Rep Regen. 2008;16:585–601.
64. Brandner JM, Houdek P, Hüsing B, Kaiser C, Moll I. Connexins 26, 30, and 43: differences among spontaneous, chronic, and accelerated human wound healing. J Invest Dermatol. 2004;122:1310–20.
65. Haertel B, Hähnel M, Blackert S, Wende K, von Woedtke T, Lindequist U. Surface molecules on HaCaT keratinocytes after interaction with non-thermal atmospheric pressure plasma. Cell Biol Int. 2012;36:1217–22.
66. Haertel B, von Woedtke T, Weltmann KD, Lindequist U. Physical plasma—possible application in wound healing. Biomol Ther. 2014,22:477–90.
67. Schmidt A, Bekeschus S, von Woedtke T, Hasse S. Cell migration and adhesion of a human melanoma cell line is decreased by cold plasma treatment. Clin Plasma Med. 2015;3:24–31.

68. Jameson JM, Sharp LL, Witherden DA, Havran WL. Regulation of skin cell homeostasis by gamma delta T cells. Front Biosci. 2004;9:2640–51.
69. Bekeschus S, Masur K, Kolata J, Wende K, Schmidt A, Bundscherer L, Barton A, Kramer A, Bröker B, Weltmann K-D. Human mononuclear cell survival and proliferation is modulated by cold atmospheric plasma jet. Plasma Process Polym. 2013;10:706–13.
70. Emmert S, Isbary G, Klutschke F, Lademann J, Westermann U, Podmelle F, Metelmann H-R, Daeschlein G, Masur K, von Woedtke T, Weltmann K-D. Clinical plasma medicine—position and perspectives. Clin Plasma Med. 2013;1:3–4.
71. Ratovitski EA, Cheng X, Yan D, Sherman JH, Canady J, Trink B, Keidar M. Anti-cancer therapies of 21st century: novel approach to treat human cancers using cold atmospheric plasma. Plasma Process Polym. 2014;11:1128–37.
72. Schlegel J, Köritzer J, Boxhammer V. Plasma in cancer treatment. Clin Plasma Med. 2013;1(2):2–7.
73. Graves DB. Reactive species from cold atmospheric plasma: implications for cancer therapy. Plasma Process Polym. 2014;11:1120–7.
74. Partecke LI, Evert K, Haugk J, Doering F, Normann L, Diedrich S, Weiss FU, Evert M, Hübner NO, Guenther C, Heidecke CD, Kramer A, Bussiahn R, Weltmann KD, Pati O, Bender C, von Bernstorff W. Tissue tolerable plasma (TTP) induces apoptosis in pancreatic cancer cells in vitro and in vivo. BMC Cancer. 2012;12:473.
75. Keidar M, Walk R, Shashurin A, Srinivasan P, Sandler A, Dasgupta S, Ravi R, Guerrero-Preston R, Trink B. Cold plasma selectivity and the possibility of a paradigm shift in cancer therapy. Br J Cancer. 2011;105:1295–301.
76. Vandamme M, Robert E, Lerondel S, Sarron V, Ries D, Dozias S, Sobilo J, Gosset D, Kieda C, Legrain B, Pouvesle JM, Le Pape A. ROS implication in a new antitumor strategy based on non-thermal plasma. Int J Cancer. 2012;130:2185–94.
77. von Woedtke T, Metelmann H-R. Editorial. Clin Plasma Med. 2014;2:37.
78. Julák J, Scholtz V, Kotúčová S, Janoušková O. The persistent microbicidal effect in water exposed to the corona discharge. Phys Med. 2012;28:230–9.
79. Naïtali M, Kamgang-Youbi G, Herry J-M, Bellon-Fontaine M-N, Brisset J-L. Combined effects of long-living chemical species during microbial inactivation using atmospheric plasma-treated water. Appl Environ Microbiol. 2010;76:7662–4.
80. Oehmigen K, Winter J, Hähnel M, Wilke C, Brandenburg R, Weltmann KD, von Woedtke T. Estimation of possible mechanisms of Escherichia coli inactivation by plasma treated sodium chloride solution. Plasma Process Polym. 2011;8:904–13.
81. Tanaka H, Mizuno M, Ishikawa K, Kondo H, Takeda K, Hashizume H, Nakamura K, Utsumi F, Kajiyama H, Kano H, Okazaki Y, Toyokuni S, Akiyama S, Maruyama S, Yamada S, Kodera Y, Kaneko H, Terasaki H, Hara H, Adachi T, Iida M, Yajima I, Kato M, Kikkawa F, Hori M. Plasma with high electron density and plasma-activated medium for cancer treatment. Clin Plasma Med. 2015;3:72–6.
82. Utsumi F, Kajiyama H, Nakamura K, Tanaka H, Mizuno M, Ishikawa K, Kondo H, Kano H, Hori M, Kikkawa F. Effect of indirect nonequilibrium atmospheric pressure plasma on anti-proliferative activity against chronic chemo-resistant ovarian cancer cells in vitro and in vivo. PLoS One. 2013;8:e81576.
83. Joslin JM, McCall JR, Bzdek JP, Johnson DC, Hybertson BM. Aqueous plasma pharmacy: preparation methods, chemistry, and therapeutic applications. Plasma Med. 2016;6:135–77.
84. von Woedtke T, Haertel B, Weltmann KD, Lindequist U. Plasma pharmacy—physical plasma in pharmaceutical applications. Pharmazie. 2013;68:492–8.
85. Cha S, Park Y-S. Plasma in dentistry. Clin Plasma Med. 2014;2:4–10.
86. Alekseev O, Donovan K, Limonnik V, Azizkhan-Clifford J. Nonthermal dielectric barrier discharge (DBD) plasma suppresses herpes simplex virus type 1 (HSV-1) replication in corneal epithelium. Trans Vis Sci Tech. 2014;3:2.
87. Hammann A, Huebner N-O, Bender C, Ekkernkamp A, Hartmann B, Hinz P, Kindel E, Koban I, Koch S, Kohlmann T, Lademann J, Matthes R, Müller G, Titze R, Weltmann K-D, Kramer A. Antiseptic efficacy and tolerance of tissue-tolerable plasma compared with two wound

antiseptics on artificially bacterially contaminated eyes from commercially slaughtered pigs. Skin Pharmacol Physiol. 2010;23:328–32.
88. Martines E, Brun P, Brun P, Cavazzana R, Deligianni V, Leonardi A, Tarricone E, Zuin M. Towards a plasma treatment of corneal infections. Clin Plasma Med. 2013;1(2):17–24.
89. Manner H, May A, Faerber M, Rabenstein T, Ell C. Safety and efficacy of a new high power argon plasma coagulation system (hp-APC) in lesions of the upper gastrointestinal tract. Digest Liver Dis. 2006;38:471–8.
90. Polak M, Winter J, Schnabel U, Ehlbeck J, Weltmann K-D. Innovative plasma generation in flexible biopsy channels for inner-tube decontamination and medical applications. Plasma Process Polym. 2012;9:67–76.
91. Weltmann K-D, von Woedtke T. Plasma medicine—current state of research and medical application. Plasma Phys Control Fusion. 2017;59:014031.
92. Robert E, Vandamme M, Brullé L, Lerondel S, Le Pape A, Sarron V, Riès D, Darny T, Dozias S, Collet G, Kieda C, Pouvesle JM. Perspectives of endoscopic plasma applications. Clin Plasma Med. 2013;1(2):8–61.

# 2 Plasma Sources for Biomedical Applications

Andreas Helmke, Torsten Gerling,
and Klaus-Dieter Weltmann

## 2.1 Plasma Characteristics

The term plasma describes the liquid, cell-free component of the blood in the medical linguistic usage since the late nineteenth century. In physics, however, plasma denotes an energetically excited gas state, which is sometimes referred to as the 4th state of matter. The expression "plasma" on the physical phenomenon of an electric gas discharge took place in 1928 by the US Nobel laureate Irving Langmuir [1]. An employee remembers the story that is connected with this name selection as follows: "… the discharge acted as a sort of substratum carrying particles of special kinds […] This reminded him of the way blood plasma carries around red and white corpuscles and germs. So he proposed to call our 'uniform discharge' a 'plasma'. Of course we all agreed" [2].

By energy supply, a solid—in Fig. 2.1 exemplarily shown for ice—can be converted into a liquid (water) and further into a gas (vapor). These transformations of the states of matter from solid to liquid to gaseous and the associated phase transitions go hand in hand with an increase in the mobility of the constituents—the atoms and molecules. Finally, the free mobility of all particles is achieved in the gas state.

Plasmas are also referred to as a non-classical state of matter. If further energy is added to a gas by heat or strong electromagnetic fields, the neutral gas particles are

A. Helmke (✉)
Application Center for Plasma und Photonics, Fraunhofer Institute for Surface Engineering and Thin Films IST, Göttingen, Germany
Faculty of Natural Sciences and Technology, HAWK University of Applied Sciences and Arts Göttingen, Germany
e-mail: andreas.helmke@ist.fraunhofer.de; andreas.helmke@hawk.de

T. Gerling • K.-D. Weltmann
Leibniz Institute for Plasma Science and Technology e.V., Greifswald, Germany
e-mail: gerling@inp-greifswald.de; weltmann@inp-greifswald.de



H.-R. Metelmann et al. (eds.), *Comprehensive Clinical Plasma Medicine*,
https://doi.org/10.1007/978-3-319-67627-2_2

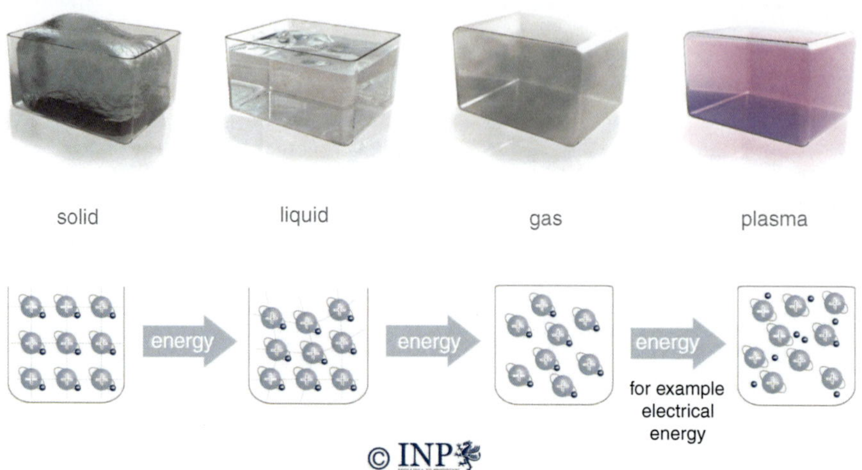


Fig. 2.1 Plasma—the 4th state of matter, INP Greifswald e.V

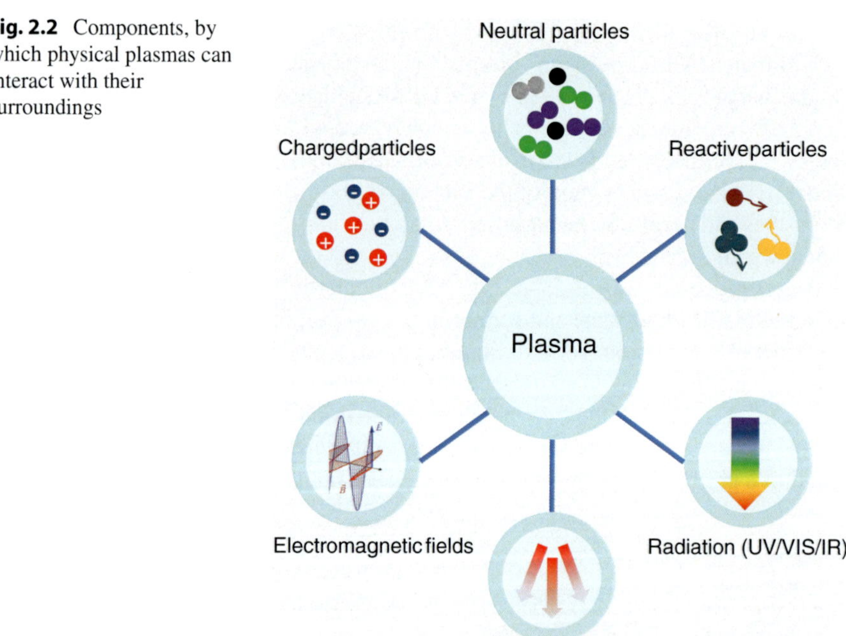


Fig. 2.2 Components, by which physical plasmas can interact with their surroundings

split into their electrically charged components (ionization). In this process, negatively charged electrons are split off from the previously electrically neutral particles, producing free electrons and positively charged particles (ions). In addition, the free electrons can adhere to neutral particles and thus form negative ions. As a result, a partially or completely ionized gas, a plasma, emerges.

According to Fig. 2.2, plasmas are composed of components such as neutral particles, charged particles and reactive particles, especially so-called radicals, resulting from chemical gas phase reactions, inter alia, from the decomposition of molecular gas particles into their atomic, reactive components (dissociation). In addition, plasmas are sources of electromagnetic radiation since some particles emit their previously absorbed energy as defined light quanta. Furthermore, significant gas heating can be associated with plasma generation whereby heat transfer can be relevant. As a consequence, increased chemical reactivity, electrical conductivity, emission of radiation as well as susceptibility to magnetic forces of a plasma compared to a gas is associated.

More than 95% of the visible matter of the entire universe is in the plasma state. On the universe scale, plasmas extend over approximately 10 magnitudes in temperature and approximately 30 magnitudes in density. One of the best known extraterrestrial plasma phenomena is the sun that makes our life on earth possible. Natural plasma phenomena occur in the atmosphere of our earth in the form of lightning and polar lights (*aurora borealis* and *aurora australis*, respectively).

The resulting properties of a plasma are determined by its parameters. For technical purposes, among the most important are the gas composition, the energy supply as well as the pressure conditions. Due to the extraordinary reactivity that can be controlled within wide limits, technological plasma applications as enabling technologies are omnipresent in production engineering as well as in everyday life—even if this is often hardly obvious to the public. On the other hand the attempts to use the core fusion technology "to bring the sun to earth" and thus to solve the energy problems of mankind are plasma technologies that are pursued with public interest. The generation of light in fluorescent tubes and energy-saving lamps is likewise carried out with the aid of plasma technology as the production of moving pictures by plasma display panels for television. Plasmas are an indispensable tool especially when processing surfaces and materials. Durable and abrasion-resistant printing of plastic surfaces, e.g., in the case of bank cards or shopping bags, is not possible without the use of plasma based pretreatment. The hardening and refinement of surfaces in machine and automotive manufacturing, the generation of versatile electromagnetic radiation, the production of microelectronic components, the air and water treatment and the coating of glass in various fields are only a few examples of the wide-spread industrial plasma applications depicted in Fig. 2.3.

## 2.2 Basics of Cold Physical Plasma

While heat is always a form of energy, energy does not necessarily mean heat. This differentiation is essential for understanding an exceptional plasma property: in addition to the thermodynamic equilibrium state (typical for solids, liquids and gases and common in everyday life), plasmas can also exist outside this equilibrium. In fact, plasmas can be tailored to be in non-equilibrium state. This additional degree of freedom originates from the fact that plasmas naturally exhibit more than one particle group. In principle, the electron temperatures $T_e$ are comparable to ion temperature $T_i$ and neutral particle (gas) temperature $T_g$ in equilibrium plasmas, whereas in non-equilibrium plasmas their temperature is significantly higher (see Sect. 2.3). This is due to significant differences in mass and charge of the particles involved.

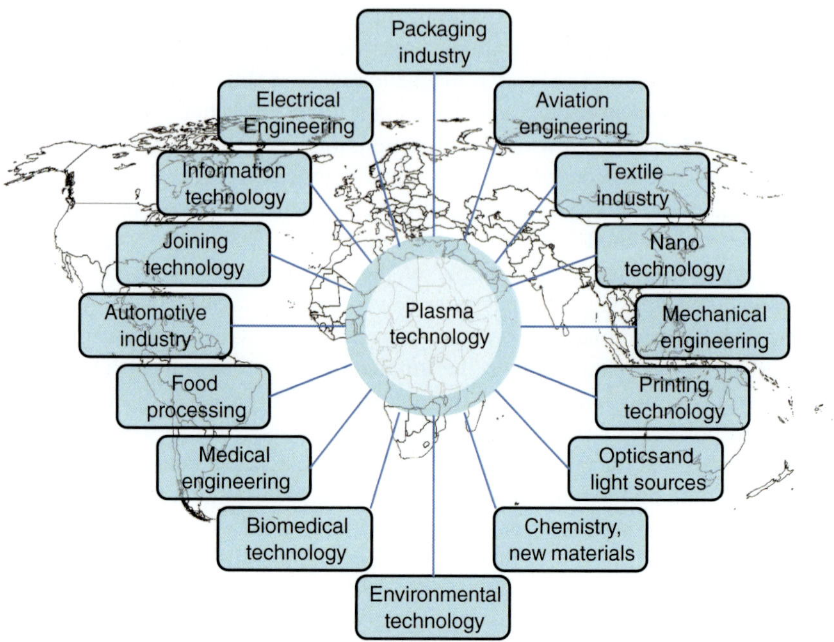


**Fig. 2.3** Industrial application fields of plasma technology

In technical plasmas, typically strong electromagnetic fields serve as sources of energy. Here, light electrons gain energy more efficiently than the comparatively heavy ions. Neutral particles cannot gain energy from the fields directly due to the lack of electrical charge.

Particles can transfer their energy via collisions. Yet, it is important to note, that energy transfer efficiency is highest when the particle masses of the collision partners match. Therefore, heat transfer between electrons and heavy particles (gaseous, liquid, solid) is very inefficient per se.

Electrons in non-equilibrium plasmas have typical mean temperatures of 10,000–100,000 K (corresponding to energies of about 1–10 eV). The temperature of the ions and neutral particles, however, is of the order of 300 K (room temperature) to 1000 K.

It is this feature that makes non-equilibrium plasmas interesting for a broad range of applications, the reduced thermal impact on matter while maintaining high reactivity during plasma processing. In low pressure regimes, the statistical collision frequency between particles is low thus impeding the formation of a thermodynamic equilibrium. Therefore low-pressure plasmas have been technologically utilized for decades. At atmospheric pressure, on the other hand, the collision frequencies are markedly higher than in the low-pressure regime. Together with sufficient and continuous energy supply this would support the formation of a thermodynamic equilibrium. For this reason, non-equilibrium plasma conditions at atmospheric pressure are more challenging to achieve and dependent on technological measures. Amongst the most important are specific electrode concepts, controlled energy supply and convective cooling.

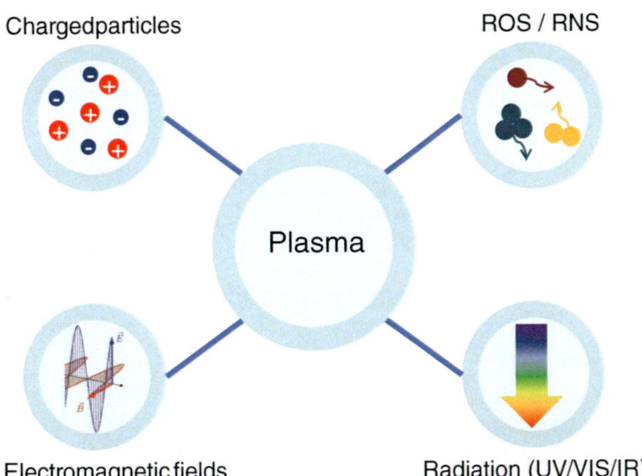


**Fig. 2.4** Principal components of cold atmospheric plasma (CAP)

Plasma medicine has been a powerful driver for cold plasma technologies at atmospheric pressure since the turn of the century [3]. Characteristics of cold atmospheric (pressure) plasma (CAP) (sometimes referred to as "tissue tolerable plasma (TTP)") include [4, 5]:

- operation at atmospheric pressure,
- mean electron temperatures sufficient or electron impact dissociation, excitation and ionization (>1 eV),
- mean gas temperatures of <40 °C,
- heat energy transfer to the target below an impairing level,
- (creeping) current to the target below significant induction of joule heating.

Plasmas with the above mentioned properties have expanded the field of application with organic substrates and surfaces. According to Fig. 2.4, these plasmas interact predominantly through a series of particle and radiation fluxes. Besides ions and electrons, the most important are reactive particles, which comprise reactive oxygen species (ROS) and reactive nitrogen species (RNS) depending on the gas composition, (vacuum) ultraviolet radiation (100–380 nm), visible light (380–780 nm), near infrared radiation (up to 1000 nm) as well as electromagnetic fields.

## 2.3 Technology

Technically, plasmas are gas discharges. The arrangement of a gas discharge consists of at least two electrically conductive electrodes, between which an electrical potential (voltage) is built up thus inducing an electromagnetic field. In order to ignite a plasma, which can be described as the maintenance of the continuity of ionization processes in the gas space, high field strength is required. The absolute value of the field strength is dependent on the type of gas as well as on the gas density. In general, it can be estimated using the so-called Paschen curve and is of the order of a few kV/mm [6].

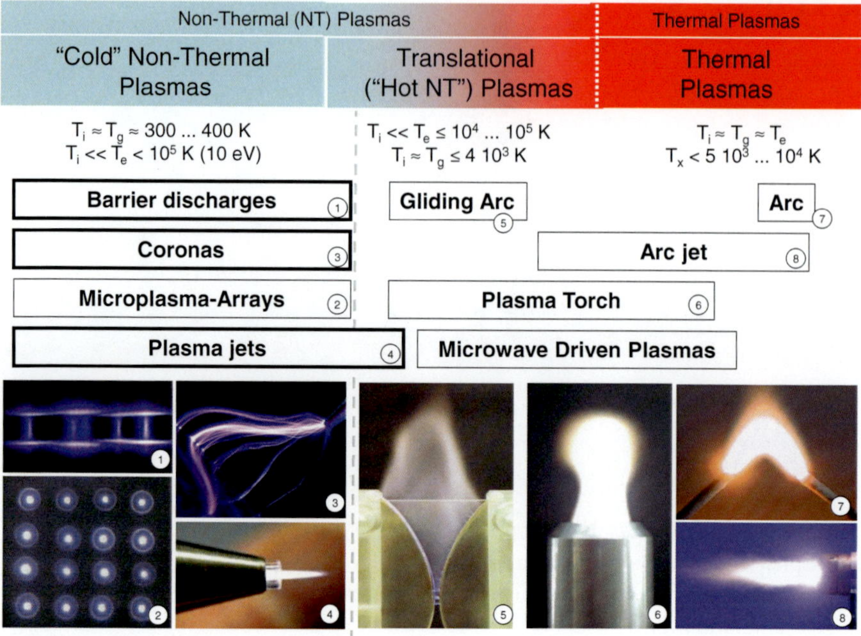


**Fig. 2.5** Toolbox of atmospheric pressure plasma techniques and their classification within the thermal regime (©EDP Science) [8]

## 2.3.1 Plasma Source Concepts

For the generation of atmospheric pressure plasmas, a toolbox of source concepts depicted in Fig. 2.5 is available. Plasma dimensions typically are of the order of a few $mm^3$ to $cm^3$. Depending on the concept, electrical powers from a few 10 mW to a few 10 W are converted. In the literature on plasma medical research the techniques of plasma jet as well as dielectric barrier discharge are in the focus [7–11].

A classification of the source concepts by means of their electrical configuration and interaction characteristics with objects facilitates the general distinction between direct and indirect plasma sources. However, technical solutions are versatile, so that hybrid concepts are prominent and briefly discussed.

### 2.3.1.1 Direct Plasma Sources

In direct plasma sources, the object to be treated plays the role of one of the electrodes and is therefore part of the electrical circuit of the device. This may induce current flow through the object in the form of displacement or conductive current [12]. The plasma physics and energy dissipation into the plasma are dependent on the electrical properties (e.g., conductivity, stray capacities) of the object as well as its geometry to some extent.

Direct plasma sources can be operated with all available technical gases. However, they are often used in such a way that they convert the ambient air (or surrounding gas) in close vicinity to the object surface into a plasma and are operated without separate gas flow. Thus, a gas-phase chemistry dominated by nitrogen and oxygen species is formed. The species fluxes and composition depend inter alia on the power density, the electrode area, the electrode spacing and the gas humidity. In a first approximation, ozone is predominantly generated at low power densities in the air plasmas, while at higher power densities not only the particle densities increase but also the formation of nitrogen oxides in the plasma is favored [13].

Apart from fluxes of charges (ions and electrons) and strong electromagnetic fields, plasma-induced short-lived neutral gaseous particles (e.g., atoms, radicals) may interact with the object's surface as a result of the direct contact to the plasma. In addition, fluxes of long-lived species (e.g., ozone, nitrogen oxides, hydrogen peroxide) produced in gas phase reactions as well as photons (UV/VIS/NIR) act upon the object's surface.

The **Corona** discharge concept in Fig. 2.6a is based on a point-to-plane arrangement where, due to the geometry, local excessive increase of electric field strength occurs at the pointed electrode. By operating with DC voltage, characteristic positive and/or negative coronas occur. The plasma forms filiform with a diameter of typically 200 μm [14]. Electric resistors are applied to limit the discharge current and thus also the gas temperature. Similar to volume DBD, the corona can be operated in a configuration, where the object's surface (e.g., tissue) acts as the second electrode.

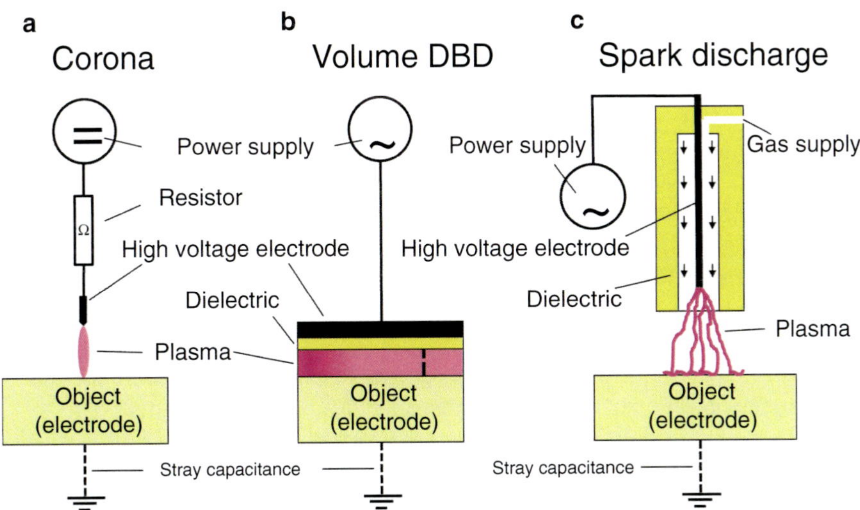


**Fig. 2.6** Schematic of Corona discharge (**a**) and volume DBD (**b**) as prominent concepts of direct plasma sources generating cold physical plasma. Spark discharges (**c**) are also direct plasma sources but are often associated with significant heat transfer to the object

**Dielectric Barrier Discharge (DBD)** is sometimes referred to as silent discharge or barrier discharge and describes a specific electrode arrangement characterized by in minimum one isolating layer—typically a dielectric—that is shielding at least one electrode from the other. The plasma typically manifests in the form of micro discharges (filaments) with diameters up to 200 μm. However, those can propagate stochastically distributed over the entire electrode surface, depending on the excitation voltage and frequency. Uniform (diffuse) discharge forms are also known [15]. The electric charges transported by the micro discharges accumulate on the dielectric surface which leads to quick self-termination of the gas discharge within $10^{-8}$–$10^{-7}$ s. This effect limits the maximum current flow thus preventing effective gas heating. As a consequence, for continuous operation alternating voltage is mandatory. DBD can optionally be operated with a special working gas or ignited in ambient air. In order to keep the gas temperatures sufficiently low (less than 40 °C), the electrical energy has to be controlled and minimized.

In general, the DBD can be divided into two classes, volume DBD and surface DBD. For details on surface DBD refer to Sect. 2.3.1.2., as this class can be considered as indirect plasma source. For **Volume DBD**, according to Fig. 2.6b the discharge takes place in the volume between two electrodes. The grounded electrode can in either case be at ground potential or optionally "float" at a relative potential. In a typical configuration in plasma medicine, tissue or liquid may act as the electrode. Hereby, the concept of volume DBD offers the possibility to treat large areas of up to a few 10 $cm^2$ at the same time [16].

The **Spark** discharge is depicted in Fig. 2.6c with a special cavity-based arrangement featuring a guided stream of working gas. Typically, pure noble gases such as argon or helium are used. In this configuration, the object to be treated serves as counter electrode. Centered in the cavity is the high voltage electrode that ignites a transient spark discharge developing into a streamer and operating also in glow discharge mode depending on polarity of the driven electrode [17]. Heat transfer is a dominant mode-of-action thus the plasma cannot be classified as cold physical plasma. Yet, especially in surgery, devices based on this concept are successfully marketed for the purpose of tissue cutting and blood coagulation since decades [18].

#### 2.3.1.2 Indirect Plasma Sources

The electrical circuit of indirect plasma sources is self-contained so that the electromagnetic field and thus the plasma physics are not strongly dependent on object or environmental properties. The chemical species generated in the plasma are transported to the object's surface via convection and diffusion mechanisms.

Operating indirect plasma sources at a separate and controlled gas flow is widely spread. Even though inert gases are prominent, at atmospheric pressure the plasma species inevitably interact with the ambient air thus inducing comparable air chemistry gas phase reactions as briefly described for direct plasma sources (Sect. 2.3.1.1).

In contrast to direct plasma, indirect plasma induces only minor, if any, fluxes of charged species to the object's surface [12]. Furthermore, typical electrode configurations do not induce electromagnetic field vectors onto the object's surface whereby the effective field strength at the object's surface is way smaller. Finally, short-lived neutral gaseous species (e.g., atoms, radicals) generated in the plasma may be consumed in gas phase reactions prior to reaching the object's surface. As a consequence, fluxes of long-lived species as well as photons (UV/VIS/NIR) predominantly determine the interaction with the object's surface. As soon as a gas flow is involved, dynamic pressure may also play a role.

For **Surface Dielectric Barrier Discharges (DBD)** the propagation of the plasma is limited by the structural specification of the electric field propagation to a thin layer at the dielectric surface according to Fig. 2.7a. The electrode design, which is structured on the surface or consists of several layers, comprises at least two electrodes. The grounded electrode can in either case be at ground potential or optionally "float" at a relative potential. For more details on DBD properties, refer to the general part on DBD in Sect. 2.3.1.1.

**Plasma jets** are cavity-based arrangements featuring a guided stream of working gas as depicted in Fig. 2.7b. Typically pure or mixtures of noble gases such as argon or helium are used. Within a cavity inside the device the plasma is ignited between first and second electrode. A combination of gas flow and electric field geometry then drives the plasma out of the cavity and into the ambient air, where it interacts to form reactive species in gas phase reactions. The emerging plume is referred to as "effluent" and is directed towards the surface to be treated. The effluent typically features diameters of 1–5 mm and lengths of up to a few cm. By parallel arrangement of multiple jets also large area treatment (several 10 $cm^2$) is possible. Besides potential-free jets, also concepts that induce a "creeping current" (like the DBD) exist, i.e., the surface can act as second or third electrode, which may lead to a more direct interaction mechanism with the treated object [19, 20].

According to Fig. 2.7c, a **Plasma torch** is generated in a cylindrical cavity and ejected at noble gas conditions. A characteristic feature in the distinction to the plasma jet is the significantly larger effluent diameter of up to 35 mm, which can be realized with an electrode and excitation concept applying high frequency to up to six electrodes and a matched resonator [21]. Even though the core plasma is typically too hot for biomedical applications, convective cooling can lead to biocompatible effluent temperatures at some distance to the nozzle.

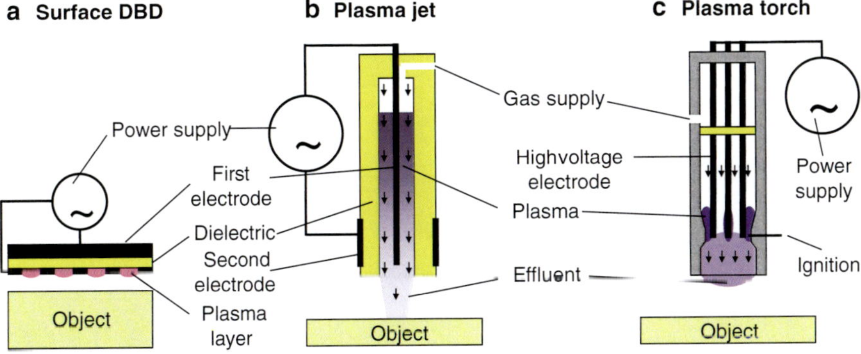


**Fig. 2.7** Schematic of surface DBD (**a**), plasma jet (**b**) and plasma torch (**c**) as prominent concepts of indirect plasma sources

#### 2.3.1.3 Hybrid Plasma Sources

Hybrid plasma sources combine properties of direct and indirect plasma sources.

**Barrier coronal discharge** is a configuration close to surface barrier discharges comprising two electrodes. As depicted in Fig. 2.8, the object to be treated is in direct contact with a planar mesh electrode that needs to be operated on ground potential in order to prevent current flow through the body. The high voltage electrode is covered by a dielectric and induces the formation of a thin plasma layer within the blanks of the mesh electrode [4, 22]. As a consequence of the close vicinity of the plasma layer to the object, also short-lived gas species may interact with the object surface.

**Plasma bullet Jets** feature an electrode configuration that introduces a significant electromagnetic field vector into the direction of the guided gas flow. This enables the generation and ultra-fast emission of ionization wave packages (often referred to as "bullets"), that according to Fig. 2.9 travel at velocities of up to some $10^5$ m/s into the ambient air [23, 24]. As a consequence, production of short-lived

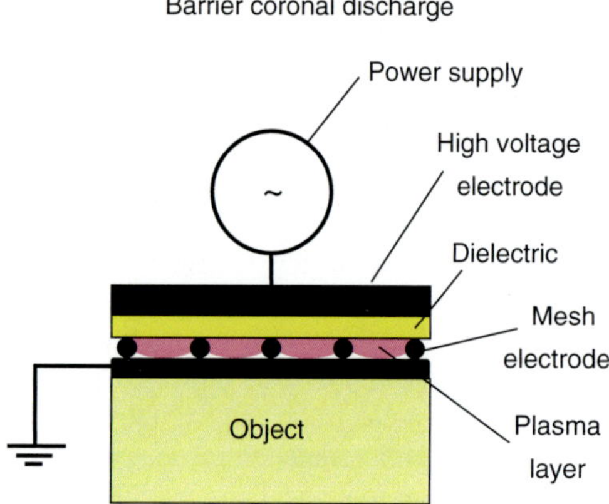


**Fig. 2.8** Schematic of the barrier coronal discharge

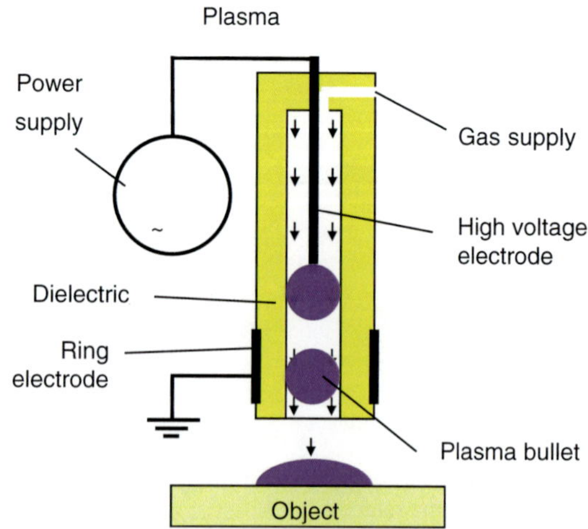


**Fig. 2.9** Schematic of the plasma bullet jet

species as well as significant local electromagnetic fields may be realized outside the cavity thus adding additional components for interaction with the object's surface compared to plasma jets [25, 26].

### 2.3.2 Control Units

Modern plasma sources for plasma medicine are predominantly designed in such a way, that they comprise a hand-held, cable-connected or mechanically guided head for the application of the plasma to the patient. This head module is connected to a control unit. The latter together with the power supply is accommodated in a housing providing a display for user feedback and optional control of process parameters such as start/stop, the treatment duration, the gas flow and the power input. The power supply of the control unit delivers the electrical signals which, in conjunction with the high voltage circuits and electrodes housed in the head module, provide sufficient electric field strength for plasma generation.

The power supply for corona plasma sources is usually based on a DC voltage of up to ±15 kV. The polarity of the voltage affects the propagation behavior of the filaments and, under certain conditions, a self-pulsation of the plasma by space charge effects can be observed despite DC operation [27].

Dielectric barrier discharges, on the other hand, are operated exclusively with alternating voltages of up to 20 kV. In addition to sinusoidal excitation, mainly pulsed operation is used to reduce the average power input thus limiting gas heating. High-frequency pulses with durations from a few 10 ns to a few 10 μs are used at repetition rates between 100 Hz and several kHz [10, 28, 29]. The total power consumption of such a control unit is less than 10 W.

Pulses at durations <1 μs with repetition rates of up to 10 kHz and amplitudes of up to 10 kV are also used to supply energy to the plasma jets [30]. In addition, sinusoidal excitations with frequencies of up to 1.1 MHz and amplitudes of 1–3 kV are used. In order to reduce the power input and avoid excessive gas heating, the sinusoidal signal can be operated at defined ratio of on-off times, which is often referred to as burst mode. The total power consumption of typical single jet systems is approximately 8 W [7].

The energy coupling in the torch arrangement is realized by microwaves with a prominent frequency of 2.45 GHz and amplitudes of typically only a few hundred Volts. In this concept, resonance effects form a standing wave between the electrodes and the walls of the housing (resonator). Resonance effects finally build up the field strength required for the generation of plasma. The power consumption is approximately 85 W [21].

### 2.3.3 Challenges and Solutions

A particular challenge for plasma source development arises as soon as large area treatment is required. Applications such as the treatment of burns often require the supply of areas up to some 10 $cm^2$ in as short a time as possible. With DBD, it is possible to achieve a high scaling of the basic configuration. However, this results in increased demands on dielectric strength of the applied materials, temperature resistance and power supply. If this is secured, DBD can be customized in a wide range. First prototypes of silica based and textile based wound patches are under development actually in Germany, The Netherlands and Japan. For plasma jets, a high scaling at atmospheric pressure is possible via an array arrangement of several individual jets. While temperature and dielectric strength remain essentially the same, the challenges are particularly in the case of an intelligent and cost-effective solution for the gas and power supply.

Another challenge, particularly relevant for volume DBD, is the demand for defined gaps between electrodes and tissues in scales of 1–2 mm. Technical solutions include the use of appropriate plastic spacers, the structuring of the dielectric surface pointing towards the object as well as a curved dielectric design.

Finally and particularly relevant for plasma jets and plasma torches is the challenge of temperature gradients that needs to be addressed. As gas temperatures of the effluent feature a physiologically harmless level only at distances of a few mm to cm to the nozzle, plastic spacers are mandatory to prevent thermal impact on tissue.

## 2.4 Medical Products

The development of plasma sources for biomedical applications dates back to the beginning of the twentieth century. Back then, the inventor Nikola Tesla developed the **Violet wand** (sometimes referred to as Violet Ray), copied by many suppliers and marketed within the framework of high-frequency therapy. Furthermore, the **Biogun** is marketed since 1989 by Dentron Limited, Clynderwen, United Kingdom. The device operates at direct current with amplitude of 10 kV and comprises a classical corona arrangement. The manufacturer claims antibacterial efficacy of the device for applications in dentistry, podiatry, and veterinary [31]. The **Plason** device is based on a DC arc configuration. It produces significant amounts of nitric oxide, which is cooled down and supplied via a gas stream to the wound site [32, 33]. For non-destructive biomedical applications, however, the plasma itself is not in direct contact with the tissue, whereas this technique is not in the focus of this book. The helium-based multi-jet arrangement **BioWeld1™** is CE cleared for surgical incision closure incorporating the use of a special chitosan plaster [34]. Yet, currently systematic clinical and publically available data with scientific quality assurance (peer-review) on the above mentioned devices are sparse.

It was the global scientific-driven independent research activities on cold atmospheric plasmas (CAP) for biomedical applications since the beginning of the millennium, which led to deeper insights into the biomedical potential of plasma technology and extensive publicly available data. On the basis of genuine data, two German manufacturers were able to declare conformity of their devices with Directive 93/42/EEC on medical products class IIa in 2013. A Japanese-English

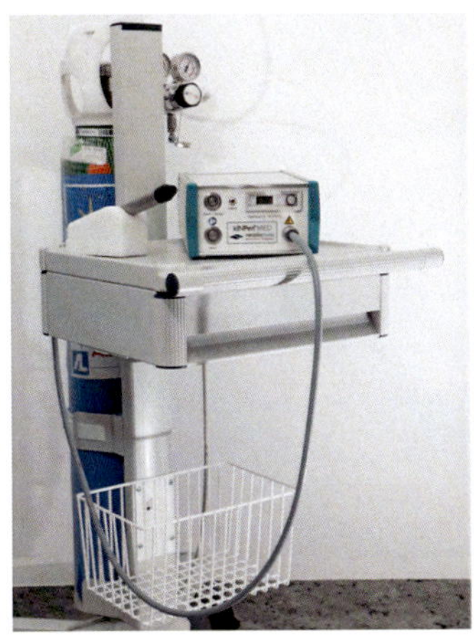
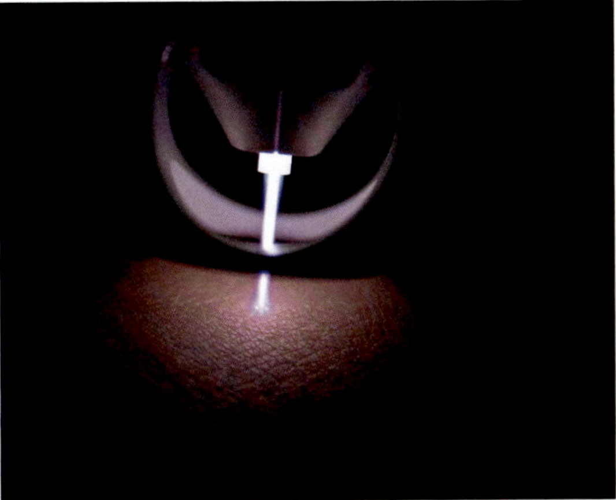

**Fig. 2.10** Photograph of the medical product kINPen® MED by neoplas tools GmbH (Greifswald, Germany) (left) and its application on tissue (right)

manufacturer followed in 2015. As the FDA approval for the devices explained in more detail below is still pending, they are currently only available on the European market.

The most intensively studied plasma source for medical use is the **kINPen® MED**, which was researched at INP Greifswald, University Medicine Greifswald and Charité Berlin and developed jointly with neoplas tools GmbH, Greifswald, Germany. It is a medical product (class IIa) approved in 2013 according to Directive 93/42/EEC. The device is shown in Fig. 2.10 and corresponds to a plasma jet arrangement. A needle electrode is centered in a cylindrical arrangement. While the cylindrical jacket is at ground potential, the needle electrode is at high voltage potential. The needle electrode is surrounded by a capillary and is thus shielded dielectrically against ground. The control unit supplies the hand-held head with a constant argon gas flow of about 5 standard liters per minute (slm) and a DC power of maximum 8 VA (110/230 V, 50/60 Hz). By means of the electric field geometry, the plasma generated between the needle electrode and mass is expelled as a so-called "effluent." The feed gas argon with mixtures such as oxygen and nitrogen mixes with the ambient air. By means of the energetic electrons and further components of the plasma, the generation of the effective "cocktail" is thus produced. By moving the hand-held head, it is also possible to place the plasma locally at the site of the treatment. Various measurements were carried out on the device to characterize the effectiveness and safety for possible applications [35].

A direct plasma source designed by the HAWK in Göttingen, then extensively studied in cooperation with the Ruhr-University Bochum, the Fraunhofer IST, the University Medical Center Göttingen as well as the Greifswald University Hospital and finally developed by CINOGY GmbH, Duderstadt, Germany to marketability, is the **PlasmaDerm®**. In 2013, the manufacturer declared the conformity of its devices with Directive 93/42/EEC on medical products of class IIa. The PlasmaDerm®

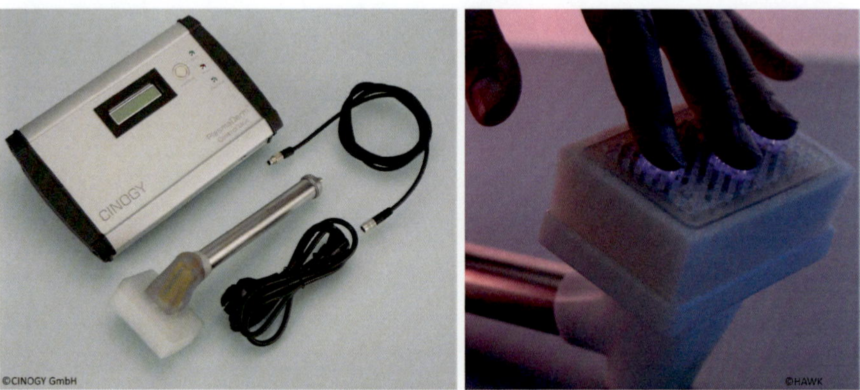


**Fig. 2.11** Components of the PlasmaDerm® FLEX 9060 by the CINOGY GmbH (Duderstadt, Germany) comprising one-button control unit, hand-held head with attached electrode and connection cables (left). Structured electrode for plasma generation directly on the skin surface (right)

operates according to the principle of volume DBD and is depicted in its third development stage in Fig. 2.11. The source is technically designed as a one-electrode system—a plane electrical conductor is encased in a high-voltage-resistant plastic. The counter electrode is the human body. Therefore, plasma generation starts not before the electrode is placed close to or on the tissue. The plastic is flexible and adapts to curvatures of the human body at gentle mechanical pressure. The surface of the electrode features a structure facilitating a steady air gap of approximately 2 mm to the tissue surface. This ambient air layer is then converted into cold physical plasma on an area of up to 27 $cm^2$. A separate gas supply is not required. The easily exchangeable electrodes are delivered in sterile packaging and are designed as disposables. Thus, cross-contamination between patients can be prevented. At the control unit, a treatment period of 1990 s is pre-programmed for reproducible treatment modalities. The entire system has a maximum power consumption of less than 10 VA (110/230 V, 50/60 Hz) and requires only a standard socket to be ready for action.

For first clinical trials in Germany, the MicroPlaSter® device of the Japanese manufacturer Adtec Plasma Technology Co. Ltd. was used and intensively studied by the Max Planck Institute for extraterrestrial physics, Munich, Germany. Such sources have been marketed since summer 2015 under the product name **SteriPlas** by Adtec Healthcare, London, United Kingdom as a wound management system. The SteriPlas is basically a plasma torch operated at microwave excitation. The argon gas flow is of the order of 2–3 slpm [36]. Continuous monitoring of gas temperature enhances safe treatment. At a distance of 2 cm from the nozzle, plasma gas temperature is <40 °C. In order to position the plasma head in the desired position, it is mounted to a balanced treatment arm according to Fig. 2.12. Operating time can be adjusted from 20 s to 9.5 min. The entire system has a maximum power consumption of 1500 VA (110/220 V, 50/60 Hz).

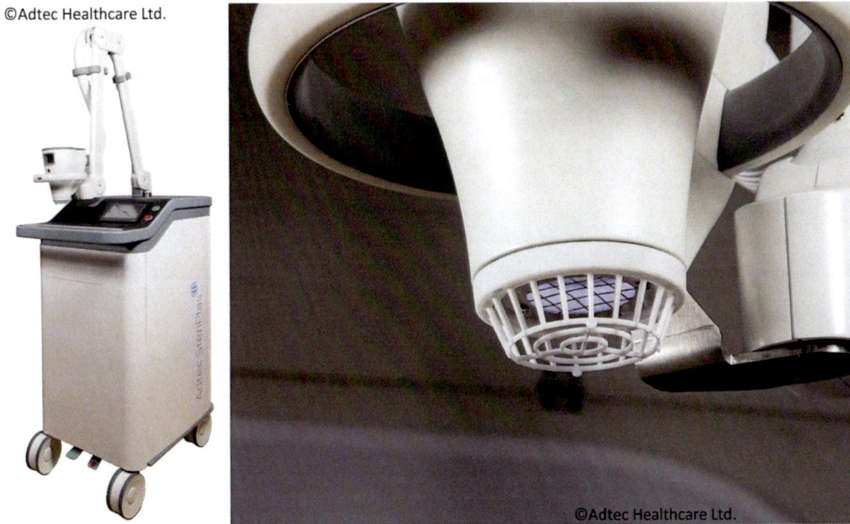


**Fig. 2.12** The Steriplas wound management system (London, United Kingdom) (left) is based on a plasma torch producing an argon plasma. The effluent is brought in contact with the tissue at some cm distance to the nozzle (right)

## 2.5 Conclusion

The availability of appropriate plasma sources is crucial for the success of biomedical plasma applications. At present, as a result of the worldwide activities on plasma medical research, three main devices of the cold plasma application are on the market as approved medical devices: kINPen® MED, PlasmaDerm® and SteriPlas supported by clinical trials. The comprehensive scientific background behind the devices is specific and the research is still proceeding rapidly. As part of the further development work, it has proved to be very helpful to consider individual aspects of standardization at intermediate stages in the development process. For example, the process of high-scaling of plasma sources is associated, among other things, with increased ozone production, which must be taken into account and reduced by adjustments. Despite the previously reported success in the use of plasma sources, a further intensification of clinical studies is necessary to argue and establish the use of atmospheric pressure plasma sources in daily clinical practice.

## 2.6 Outlook

In addition to the plasma sources described here, which have already undergone a long developmental path, new approaches for plasma sources are constantly being developed, based on the specific requirements, as well as through growing know-how and continuous material development. A prospect of potentially new sources of

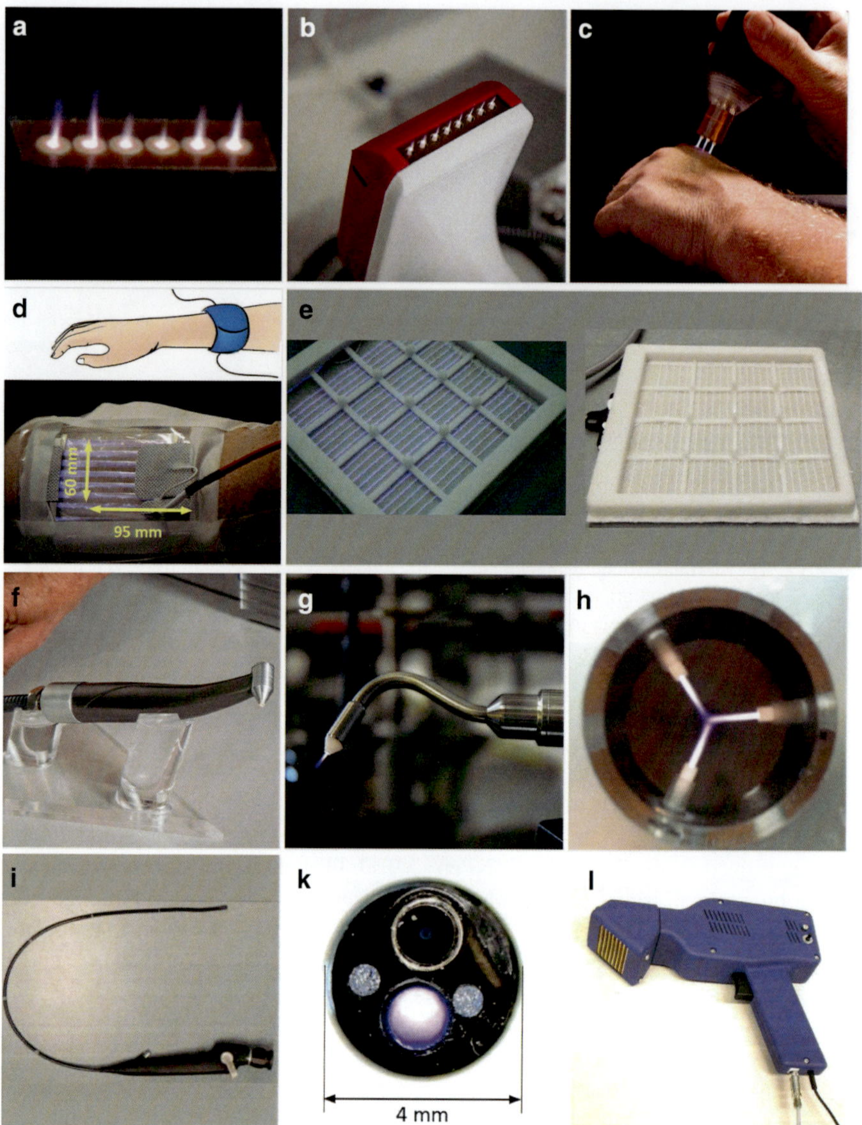


**Fig. 2.13** Selected prototypes in development at INP Greifswald (**a–c**) multi-Jet arrays for large area treatment, (**d–f**) flexible DBD devices using silicon or textile as electrode material for large area treatment, (**f**, **g**) devices optimized and intended to use for large area treatment, (**f**, **g**) devices optimized and intended to use for dental applications, (**h**) device for pre-treatment of dental abutments, (**i**, **k**) prototype of endoscope for treatment of hollow bodies, (**l**) large size DBD for surface treatment

the INP Greifswald is shown in Fig. 2.13. Larger area treatments in shorter time are a necessary extension of the present devices. This can be achieved either by multi—jet devices (Fig. 2.13a–c) or flexible DBD's (Fig. 2.13d,e) especially latter offer a wide range of applications from plasma plaster to the large area wound dressing.

Further battery-driven plasma sources will increase mobility of the patients allowing the treatments outside the hospital.

The intensive efforts of the CAP source development for biomedical applications and the resulting research show a leverage effect for other fields of the plasma application, such as clean air, clean water and clean surface and clean food. The newly developed plasma sources and the resulting experience in these areas can ensure the development of new plasma sources for individual problems. Examples are shown in Fig. 2.13f–h. For implant technology, dental implants could be treated with multiple plasma jets all around with the device shown. For this purpose, the implant is placed on a turntable and the jets installed at different heights clean the implant all round and could thus simultaneously optimize the ingrowth into the bone (see also Chap. 18 for further details). The treatment of hollow bodies or the use of plasma for minimal invasive technologies opens up a new field of medical applications, such as the use of endoscopes providing CAP, so called "plasmoscope" depicted in Fig. 2.13i,k. A mobile, air-operated hand-held device (Fig. 2.13l) generates a DBD at the site of application and can thus treat surfaces of germs or increase wettability.

Future devices will additionally be equipped with optical sensors and imaging techniques for automatic control of the treatment and detailed investigation of the treated area regarding contamination, blood circulation and temperature. Therewith an individual, optimized and standardized wound treatment will become possible.

**Acknowledgement** The authors Gerling and Weltmann thank the internal and external cooperation partners of the projects "Campus PlasmaMed I and II," funded by the German Federal Ministry of Education and Research (13 N9779 and 13 N11188); "Plasmamedizinische Forschung—neue pharmazeutische und medizinische Anwendungsfelder," funded by the Ministry for Research, Development and Culture of the State of Mecklenburg-Vorpommern and the European Union by the European Social Fund (AU 11 038, ESF/IV-BM-B35-0010/13); "Entwicklung eines neuartigen Wundbehandlungssystems auf Basis von Plasmatechnologien und dem Einsatz flächiger textiler Plasmaquellen für den mobilen und stationären Einsatz—PlasmaWundTex," funded by Zentrales Innovationsprogramm Mittelstand of the German Federal Ministry for Economic Affairs and Energy (KF2046509AK3); "Erweiterung der medizinischen Anwendungsmöglichkeiten kalter Atmosphärendruckplasmajets (MEDKAP)," funded by the German Ministry of Education; "Plasmamedizin—Anwendungsorientierte Grundlagenforschung zu physikalischem Plasma in der Medizin" funded by the Ministry of Education, Science and Culture of the State of Mecklenburg-Vorpommern (grant: AU 15 001).

The author Helmke thanks all cooperation partners of the research group "BioLiP", funded by the German Federal Ministry of Education and Research (BMBF, grant no. 13 N9089), the associated partners in the project "PlaStraKomb," funded by the BMBF (grant no. PNT51501), the partners of the research group "Campus PlasmaMed II," funded by the BMBF (grant no. 13 N11190), as well as the partners of the joint research project "WuPlaKo," funded by the BMBF (grant no. 13GW0041D) and "KonchaWu," funded by the Ministry of economics of the State of Niedersachsen and the European Regional Development Fund ERDF (grant no. ZW 3-85006987).

## References

1. Langmuir I. Oscillations in ionized gases. Proc Natl Acad Sci USA. 1928;14:627–37.
2. Mott-Smith HM. History of "plasmas". Nature. 1971;233:219.
3. von Woedtke T, Reuter S, Masur K, et al. Plasmas for medicine. Phys Rep. 2013;530:291–320.

4. Kong MG, Kroesen G, Morfill G, et al. Plasma medicine: an introductory review. New J Phys. 2009;11:115012.
5. Partecke LI, Evert K, Haugk J, et al. Tissue tolerable plasma (TTP) induces apoptosis in pancreatic cancer cells in vitro and in vivo. BMC Cancer. 2012;12:473.
6. Kuechler A. High voltage engineering. 1st ed. Heidelberg: Springer; 2018.
7. Weltmann K-D, Kindel E, von Woedtke T, et al. Atmospheric-pressure plasma sources: prospective tools for plasma medicine. Pure Appl Chem. 2010;82:1223–37.
8. Weltmann K-D, von Woedtke T. Basic requirements for plasma sources in medicine. Eur Phys J Appl Phys. 2011;55:13807.
9. Lu X, Laroussi M, Puech V. On atmospheric-pressure non-equilibrium plasma jets and plasma bullets. Plasma Sources Sci Technol. 2012;21:034005.
10. Kuchenbecker M, Bibinov N, Kaemling A, et al. Characterization of DBD plasma source for biomedical applications. J Phys D Appl Phys. 2009;42:045212.
11. Helmke A, Hoffmeister D, Berge F, et al. Physical and microbiological characterisation of Staphylococcus epidermidis inactivation by dielectric barrier discharge plasma. Plasma Process Polym. 2011;8:278–86.
12. Fridman G, Friedman G, Gutsol A, et al. Applied plasma medicine. Plasma Process Polym. 2008;5:503–33.
13. Eliasson B, Kogelschatz U. Modeling and applications of silent discharge plasmas. IEEE Trans Plasma Sci. 1991;19:309–23.
14. van Veldhuizen EM, Rutgers WR. Pulsed positive corona streamer propagation and branching. J Phys D Appl Phys. 2002;35:2169–79.
15. Kogelschatz U. Filamentary, patterned, and diffuse barrier discharges. IEEE Trans Plasma Sci. 2002;30:1400–8.
16. Helmke A, Franck M, Wandke D, Vioel W. Tempo-spatially resolved ozone characteristics during single-electrode dielectric barrier discharge (SE-DBD) operation against metal and porcine skin surfaces. Plasma Med. 2014;4:67–77.
17. Keller S, Bibinov N, Neugebauer A, et al. Electrical and spectroscopic characterization of a surgical argon plasma discharge. J Phys D Appl Phys. 2013;46:025402.
18. Zenker M. Argon plasma coagulation. GMS Krankenhaushyg Interdiszip. 2008;3:Doc15.
19. Laroussi M, Akan T. Arc-free atmospheric pressure cold plasma jets: a review. Plasma Process Polym. 2007;4:777–88.
20. Winter J, Brandenburg R, Weltmann K-D. Atmospheric pressure plasma jets: an overview of devices and new directions. Plasma Sources Sci Technol. 2015;24:064001.
21. Shimizu T, Steffes B, Pompl R, et al. Characterization of microwave plasma torch for decontamination. Plasma Process Polym. 2008;5:577–82.
22. Morfill GE, Kong MG, Zimmermann JL. Focus on plasma medicine. New J Phys. 2009;11:115011,8pp
23. Teschke M, Kedzierski J, Finantu-Dinu EG, et al. High-speed photographs of a dielectric barrier atmospheric pressure plasma jet. IEEE Trans Plasma Sci. 2005;33:310–1.
24. Reuter S, Winter J, Iseni S, Peters S, Schmidt-Bleker A, Duennbier M, Schaefer J, Foest R, Weltmann KD. Detection of ozone in a MHz argon plasma bullet jet. Plasma Sources Sci Technol. 2012;21:034015.
25. Lu X, Naidis GV, Laroussi M, et al. Reactive species in non-equilibrium atmospheric-pressure plasmas: generation, transport, and biological effects. Phys Rep. 2016;630:1–84.
26. Darny T, Pouvesle J-M, Puech V, et al. Analysis of conductive target influence in plasma jet experiments through helium metastable and electric field measurements. Plasma Sources Sci Technol. 2017;26:45008.
27. Bussiahn R, Brandenburg R, Gerling T, et al. The hairline plasma: an intermittent negative dc-corona discharge at atmospheric pressure for plasma medical applications. Appl Phys Lett. 2010;96:143701.
28. Fridman G, Peddinghaus M, Balasubramanian M, Ayan H, Fridman A, Gutsol A, Brooks A. Blood coagulation and living tissue sterilization by floating-electrode dielectric barrier discharge in air. Plasma Chem Plasma Process. 2006;26:425–42.

29. Helmke A, Mahmoodzada M, Wandke D, Weltmann KD, Viöl W. Impact of electrode design, supply voltage and interelectrode distance on safety aspects of a medical DBD plasma source. Contrib Plasma Phys. 2013;53:623–38.
30. Laroussi M, Lu X. Room-temperature atmospheric pressure plasma plume for biomedical applications. Appl Phys Lett. 2005;87:113902–3.
31. Dang CN, Anwar R, Thomas G, et al. The biogun: a novel way of eradicating MRSA colonization in diabetic foot ulcers. Diabetes Care. 2006;29:1176–7.
32. Shekhter AB, Kabisov RK, Pekshev AV, et al. Experimental and clinical validation of Plasmadynamic therapy of wounds with nitric oxide. Bull Exp Biol Med. 1998;126:829–34.
33. Pekshev AV, Shekhter AB, Vagapov AB, et al. Study of plasma-chemical NO-containing gas flow for treatment of wounds and inflammatory processes. Nitric Oxide. 2017; In press.
34. Hants Y, Kabiri D, Drukker L, et al. Preliminary evaluation of novel skin closure of Pfannenstiel incisions using cold helium plasma and chitosan films. J Matern Fetal Neonatal Med. 2014;27:1637–42.
35. Bekeschus S, Schmidt A, Weltmann K-D, et al. The plasma jet kINPen—a powerful tool for wound healing. Clin Plasma Med. 2016;4:19–28.
36. Isbary G, Morfill G, Schmidt H, et al. A first prospective randomized controlled trial to decrease bacterial load using cold atmospheric argon plasma on chronic wounds in patients. Br J Dermatol. 2010;163:78–82.

# Relevant Plasma Parameters for Certification

# 3

Torsten Gerling, Andreas Helmke, and Klaus-Dieter Weltmann

## 3.1 From Research to Hospital

The promising potential of cold atmospheric pressure plasma (CAP) technology for biomedical applications can only be lifted if appropriate sources are ready for clinical applications. For this purpose, the sources must acquire the status of a medical device. The general technical workflow for this usually several years-long process is visualized in Fig. 3.1. Once CAP sources are functional, they are characterized over a wide range of process parameters—technically as well as on potential biomedical efficacy and toxicity. As soon as results indicate suitability and safety for applications in human studies, pilot or case studies can be performed on the basis of positive ethic votes. When further operational safety can be assured and the manufacturers fulfill regulatory guidelines, they can declare conformity of their devices and CAP sources are ready to be applied in therapies.

In Europe, CAP sources for biomedical applications are currently covered by Directive 93/42/EEC. In the US, Title 21 of the Code of Federal Regulations covers the regulation of medical devices. In this chapter, we focus on the preclinical characterization of technical process parameters and the available diagnostics.

T. Gerling (✉) • K.-D. Weltmann
Leibniz Institute for Plasma Science and Technology e.V, Greifswald, Germany
e-mail: gerling@inp-greifswald.de; weltmann@inp-greifswald.de

A. Helmke
Fraunhofer Institute for Surface Engineering and Thin Films IST, Application Center for Plasma und Photonics, Göttingen, Germany

Faculty of Natural Sciences and Technology, HAWK University of Applied Sciences and Arts, Göttingen, Germany
e-mail: andreas.helmke@ist.fraunhofer.de; andreas.helmke@hawk.de



H.-R. Metelmann et al. (eds.), *Comprehensive Clinical Plasma Medicine*,
https://doi.org/10.1007/978-3-319-67627-2_3

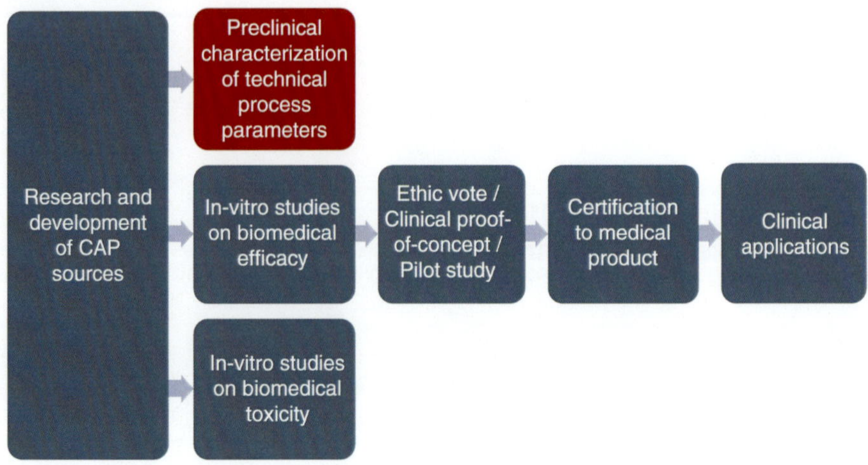


**Fig. 3.1** General workflow from plasma source development to clinical applications

## 3.2 Plasma Components and Their Relevant Biomedical Impact

In general, the term plasma describes a quasi-neutral gaseous mixture of charge carriers that are subject to external (electromagnetic) forces thereby exhibiting collective behavior. In addition to these free-moving electrons and ions, plasmas contain a variety of further physical and chemical components. This includes radiation from the (vacuum) ultraviolet to the near infrared range, a complex variety of gaseous species and radicals including reactive oxygen species (ROS) and reactive nitrogen species (RNS), optional heat transfer and electric fields [1].

Each particular component depicted in Fig. 3.2 is described as having a potential effect on living organisms. For instance, UV radiation is applied in the photo therapy of skin diseases such as psoriasis or atopic dermatitis [2, 3]. The general physiological function of ROS and RNS and their dual role as both deleterious and beneficial species is well known [4–6]. Electromagnetic fields and electrical currents are applied, e.g., for electrical muscle stimulation (EMS) and transcutaneous electrical nerve stimulation (TENS) [7, 8].

However, the specialty about the use of cold atmospheric plasmas (CAP) is that all of these components are effective at the same time and can even excite synergetic effectivity in the form of a so-called “cocktail”. Even short-lived chemical gas species can contribute at the site of the treatment. While this is very encouraging with regard to biomedical efficacy, specific challenges in the measurement of particular process parameters arise from the synchronized appearance of all components in time and space. In order to evaluate operational safety and furthermore to gain inside into the mechanisms of plasma interaction with living tissue, each component needs to be characterized as precise as possible.

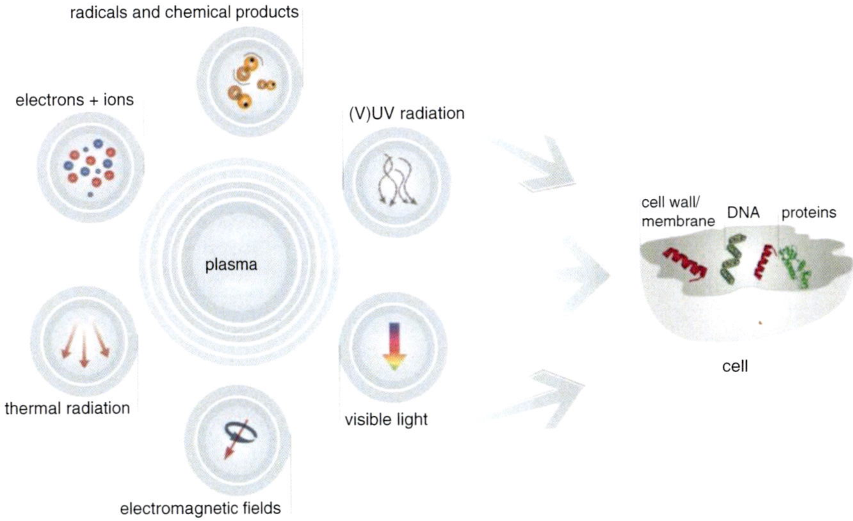


**Fig. 3.2** Components of CAP relevant for interaction with cells and tissue [1]

### 3.2.1 Antimicrobial Activity

Research groups from all over the world were able to observe a pronounced antimicrobial effect induced by CAP. Both gram-negative and gram-positive bacteria in adherent, planktonic or vegetative form as well as yeasts and fungi have been successfully inactivation [9–12]. Even the inactivation of biofilms of the methicillin-resistant *Staphylococcus aureus* or the extremophile genus *Deinococcus radiodurans* has been reported [13, 14]. According to current knowledge, no resistance buildup against CAP has been observed so far [15]. A detailed discussion on individual antimicrobial activity of the components from Fig. 3.2 is presented in Chap. 1.

### 3.2.2 Impact on Eukaryotic Cells

An important finding with regard to applications in wound care is the in vitro observation that proliferation of endothelial cells can be enhanced by controlled plasma exposure [16]. Likewise in vitro, a plasma impact on mammalian cells in liquid medium, which reached from the stimulation of cell proliferation up to the introduction of apoptotic events depending on process parameters, was observed. The effects were attributed to the formation of intracellular reactive oxygen species, but further studies suggest that ozone has no dominant impact [17, 18]. Instead, it was found that hydrogen peroxide mediates proliferation and differentiation of human fibroblasts [19].

### 3.2.3 Impact on Liquids

CAP operated partially or completely in air are sources of gas phase species such as, e.g., the hydroxyl radical (OH•), nitrogen oxides (NO·, $NO_2$•, $ONOO^-$), hydrogen peroxide ($H_2O_2$) or superoxide or hyperoxide ($O_2^-$), which can react with water to form acids. This can lead to a significant reduction of the pH value [20, 21]. As a result, pH-dependent biochemical reactions in the wound area should be sensitive to plasma exposure. Furthermore, blood coagulation was significantly accelerated by the use of a volume DBD in air with a power density of about 1 W/cm$^2$, however timescales need to be considered for clinical applications [22, 23].

### 3.2.4 Clinical Data

During the last years, different CAP sources have been applied in clinical practice. The following paragraphs give a short overview, yet, more details can be found in Part 2.

In 2010, interim results for clinical use (Phase II, proof-of-concept) of a CAP source (MicroPlaSter®) for wound care on 36 patients were published for the first time. It was demonstrated in vivo that the bacterial colonization of chronic wounds could be significantly reduced by 34% by the daily embedding of a 5-min plasma exposure into the therapy plan. In addition, no side effects were observed [24]. In a further study, the study design was modified in such a way that the treatment period was reduced to 2 min and a comparative study path was added using a further developed device version, the MicroPlaSter® β. The MicroPlaSter® β has the same plasma process parameters and differs only from its predecessor with a more compact design and more flexible mechanics. In both studies, significant reductions of the bacterial populations of 40% by the MicroPlaSter® and 23.5% by the MicroPlaSter® β were also demonstrated without side effects [25]. In a study on pruritus reduction, the effect of CAP as produced by the MicroPlaSter® was not superior of an argon gas stream after exposure for 2 min [26]. Applying the device to a group of 70 patients suffering from chronic infected wounds in order to evaluate the plasma effect on wound healing, no significant benefit was found. Yet, in a subgroup of 27 patients with chronic venous ulcers, a significant reduction of wound width but not wound length was observed [27]. On 40 patients, one half of the uninfected split-skin graft donor sites was treated with plasma for 2 min/5 cm$^2$, whereas the other half served as control. The examiners observed positive impact of the intervention on wound healing indicated by faster epithelization as well as less fibrin coating and scabs [28]. More details on clinical data on this plasma source, meanwhile renamed to SteriPlas, can be found in Part 5, Chap. 34.

Further investigations with seven healthy volunteers using a jet plasma source operated with argon as working gas observed a decrease in the beta-carotene concentration in the outer skin layer (stratum corneum) and an increase in transepidermal water loss (TEWL). This impact on the skin physiology was without obvious damage to the skin tissue [29]. In the in vivo inactivation of a physiological and an artificially contaminated skin flora a significant reduction of the bacterial load (log reduction factor of up to 1.7 after 90 s treatment period) was demonstrated for the kINPen® 09 as well as a volume DBD. At the same time, the treatment by both plasma sources was well tolerated by the subjects [30].

Clinical data on the use of kINPen® MED in wound healing were published in 2012. At controlled conditions, four artificial wounds were added to the forearms of five subjects, each of which was then treated with argon plasma in various samples (control, 10 s exposure, 30 s exposure and 10 s exposure on three consecutive days). After 10 days, the healing progress was evaluated in a blinded study layout from the aesthetic point of view focusing on the color and structure of the wound compared to healthy tissue. The best regenerative advances were achieved by the repeated plasma application for 10 s [31]. An evaluation of the healing outcome was performed again after 6 and 12 months, respectively, by 17 independent observers using a more sophisticated scheme. In addition to the fact that the plasma treatment appears to be most effective on the early inflammatory phase of wound healing (after 10 days), it could be shown as an important result that no precancerous changes of the skin tissue can be detected up to 12 months after exposure [32]. In a total of 34 patients suffering from venous ulcers, the antibacterial efficacy of kINPen® 09 was compared with the effect of an established liquid antiseptic (Octenidine). A significant antibacterial effect was documented in each case at a plasma treatment time of 1 min/cm compared to a dose of 0.2 mL/cm$^2$ Octenidine (0.1% octenidine dihydrochloride and 2% 2-phenoxyethanol) [33]. In assessing wound size, a 56% reduction was observed by the kINPen® and a 19% reduction by the use of Octenisept [34]. In the treatment of three plaques of six psoriatic patients, the argon plasma jet did not show significant advantage over conventional therapies [35]. More details on clinical data on this plasma source can be found in Part 5, Chap. 34.

With the volume DBD-based device PlasmaDerm®, a pilot study on safety and efficacy has been carried out from 2011 to 2012 on the indication venous ulcer at an exposure of 45 s/cm$^2$. The plasma treatment was classified as safe and resulted in a significant reduction in the bacterial loading of the wounds as well as a non-significant reduction in the wound size. Still, the only wound that closed after 7 weeks of treatment was assigned to the plasma group [36]. In a study applying a volume DBD in the working gas air for 90 s, acidification of skin specimen as well as substantial increase about a factor of four in dermal microcirculation parameters of four volunteers for up to 1 h after the intervention could be observed [37]. This general health-promoting effect was also demonstrated in 20 healthy subjects for the PlasmaDerm® [38]. Furthermore, it was shown that a repeated intervention of 90 s for three times in total further increased the perfusion until finally a saturation effect occurs at upregulated microcirculation [39]. More details on clinical data on this plasma source can be found in Part 5, Chap. 35.

## 3.3 Plasma Process Parameters Relevant for Medical Regulations (Safety)

While the plasma cocktail motivates the medical application of cold atmospheric plasmas (CAP), it simultaneously implies upcoming challenges. The field of medical technology and even the common people on summer vacation are well familiar with the side effect of e.g. UV overexposure. Hence an essential task for the development of plasma devices for medical application is the control and verification of regulatory limits to ensure safety of the application. Known regulatory limits concern the production of potentially toxic radicals such as ozone or nitrogen oxides, the UV radiation, thermal impact on skin as well as the patient leakage current. Furthermore, as long as a global plasma `dose' is not defined, a certain proof of antimicrobial and biological effectivity is required to verify functionality beside the safety aspects. Recently, a recommendation for a safe qualification of such CAP devices applicable during the research and development phase was presented. Herein, core criteria for the field of biomedical applications known in regulatory affairs are recapitulated. A compendium on legal regulation was summerized under DIN SPEC 91315 [40].

The literature discusses many plasma sources still under development and also the potential application in plasma medicine [41]. In order to ensure a certain level of comparability of plasma devices designed for application in plasma medical research, these devices need at least to be characterized concerning safety aspects for the patient and the attending staff. Figure 3.3 summarizes potential risks associated with plasma components such as electromagnetic fields, heat, radiation as well as reactive and charged particles. Process parameters of each individual plasma source need to be carefully balanced in order to prevent potential adverse events.

In the following sections we will describe the potential risks in more detail, refer to relevant regulatory literature and briefly discuss available diagnostics to ensure a throughout qualification of safety when applying CAP sources, even when still in development stage.

### 3.3.1 Operation at High-Voltage

CAP is generated using predominantly oscillating electromagnetic fields with amplitudes up to $10^6$ V/m. Therefore, application of high electric potentials (up to $10^4$ V) at elevated frequencies (up to $10^9$ Hz) and small distances (down to $10^{-3}$ m) is common. The handling of devices operated by high voltage requires a basic understanding of the associated risk potentials.

An immediate danger to human health might arise, when parts of the human body get in close vicinity or direct contact with high-voltage components thus inducing an electrical current flow through the body (see Sects. 3.4.2 and 3.4.3). In contrast to low-voltage applications, current flow might even be induced at

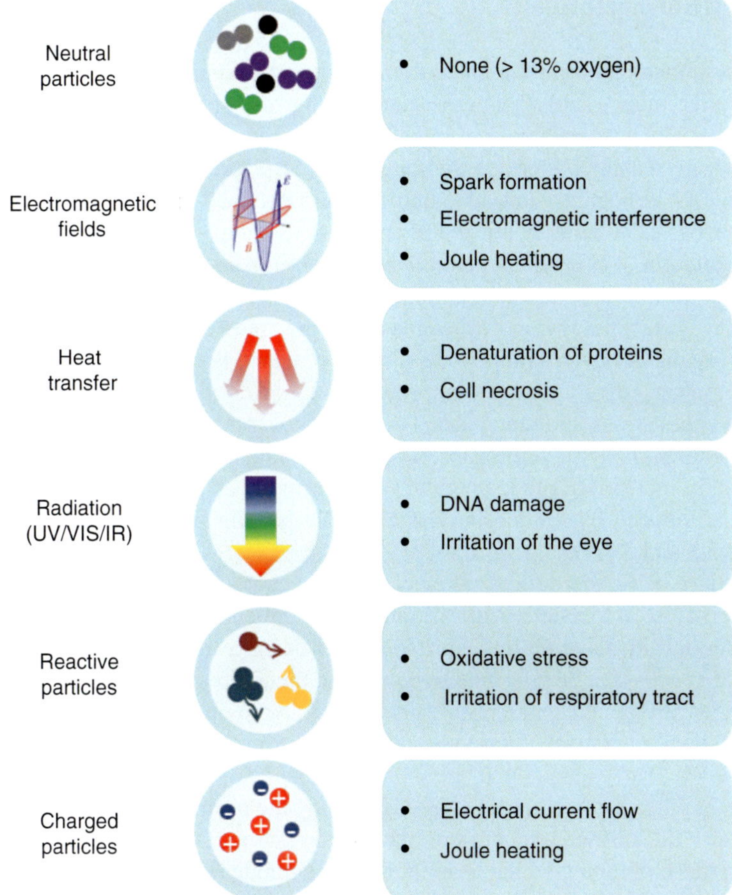


**Fig. 3.3** Components of CAP and their associated potential risks if process parameters are not carefully balanced

distances of some mm to cm (depending on the electric potential) to the electrodes due to the formation of an electrical spark. To avoid this risk, in all medical products for CAP generation, the direct access to high-voltage components is restricted construction-wise by embedding relevant components in an appropriate dielectric material or behind electrically grounded components. In individual cases, this protection can be particularly sensitive to mechanical damage of the components.

Furthermore, as sources of electromagnetic energy, plasma devices may potentially cause unwanted effects such as electromagnetic interference or even physical damage to technical equipment in their immediate environment or couple interferences into the electrical power network they are connected to. For medical products, it is up to the manufacturer to declare the conformity of their devices with the regulations of IEC 60601-1 and their national implementations [42].

### 3.3.2 Thermal Impact

It is well known, that heat can induce denaturation of biomolecules such as proteins or deoxyribonucleic acid (DNA) associated with a loss of biological activity. In this process, breaking of intramolecular bonds leads to reversible or permanent modification of the secondary, tertiary and quaternary structure of the biomolecule [43]. Excessive tissue heating can lead to tissue burns associated with cell necrosis. While denaturation is deliberately utilized in applications such as heat sterilization or tissue coagulation, it is generally accepted, that for humans the temperature must not exceed 40 °C in order to sustain biological activity.

In plasma technology, electromagnetic energy transfer leads to heating of the gaseous media or device components the rate of which is dependent on the applied thermal power, distribution mechanisms as well as cooling mechanisms. In biomedical applications applying plasma devices, heat transfer from the gas or device components to the tissue by means of thermal conduction, convection or radiation may locally increase tissue temperature. Furthermore, as soon as a patient leakage current is induced by the plasma device, Joule heating may also contribute (see Sects. 3.3.3 and 3.4.3).

A variety of standard methods is available to characterize the specific thermal characteristics associated with biomedical applications of plasma devices. Applying non-invasive optical emission spectroscopy, the rotational structure of emission spectra can be analyzed to determine the temperature of gaseous neutral gas species at typical accuracies of some ±10 K. Applying fibre optic temperature sensors, the temperature of gaseous and liquid media can be measured at an accuracy of ±1 K. Yet, especially at small plasma dimensions this method may lead to significant disturbance of plasma propagation by the probe. A non-contact method to measure the surface temperature of solids in a single spot is pyrometry. Alike infrared thermography, which is an imaging technique, pyrometry is based on the detection of black body radiation. Typical accuracies of marketable devices amount to ±1–5 K and are strongly dependent on the chosen emission coefficient.

For the determination of the thermal power output of a plasma source, a calorimetric method can be applied. Hereby, a metal substrate with defined mass and given specific heat connected to a fibre optic temperature probe can be positioned in the point of interest relative to the plasma source. From the heating rate ($\Delta T/\Delta t$), the thermal output power can be calculated [44]. This method is especially suitable for free-jet device configurations.

It has been demonstrated for many plasma sources based on a variety of technical concepts such as DBD, corona, jet and torch, that gas temperatures below 40 °C (corresponding to 313 K) can be realized in CAP and that these sources have minimal impact on tissue heating [45–48]. As in some jet-like configurations the gas temperature of the plasma enclosed in the cavity zone might exceed 40 °C, they need to be operated at an appropriate distance to the nozzle (technically realized by spacers) or have to be cooled to fulfill this criterion [44, 49].

### 3.3.3 Electrical Current Flow

Depending on the media in which an electrical current flows, either electrons or ions or both may act as charge carriers. Direct currents (DC) with continuous amplitude as wells as alternating currents (AC) with time varying amplitudes exist. Current flow in the human body is predominantly by ions solved in body liquids.

An important thermodynamic property of current flow is the induction of Joule heating in conductive media, e.g., prominent from incandescent light bulbs. The human body, from an electrical perspective, can be considered a combination of capacities and impedances. The power of Joule heating depends not only on the current but also on the impedance characteristics of the medium through which it flows. Thus, Joule heating may result in mild tissue heating but also in local burns. Furthermore, current flow through the body may lead to interference with nervous control, muscular contraction, ventricular fibrillation, and cardiac arrest depending on parameters such as current magnitude, voltage amplitude, frequency, current path through the body, and exposition duration.

Cold atmospheric plasma sources are operated by electrical energy and may induce an electric current flow as soon as they are applied on the human body. Thus, adequate medical products need to comply with international standards for medical electrical equipment published by the International Electrotechnical Commission (IEC). "IEC 60601-1: General requirements for basic safety and essential performance" applies to characteristics of medical electrical devices and medical electrical systems with one connection to a supply network intended for the diagnosis, treatment or monitoring of a patient according to the manufacturer's definition. These devices and systems transmit energy to or from the patient and are in physical or electrical contact with the patient. The patient leakage current is of central importance for plasma devices and it needs to be verified, that the induced effective current flow is well below the limits [40, 42].

### 3.3.4 Ultraviolet Radiation

In physics, electromagnetic radiation refers to waves of the electromagnetic field (also referred to as photons) characterized by amplitude and frequency $\nu$ or wavelength $\lambda$ and travelling through a medium. In terms of radiometry, the irradiance $E$ is the radiant flux received by a surface per unit area and is given in SI units of $W/m^2$. The irradiance is also referred to as intensity.

Relevant for the context of CAP are the wavelengths from approx. 10–1000 nm. According to ISO-21348, this radiation can be classified as bands of vacuum ultraviolet (VUV, 10–200 nm), ultraviolet C (UV-C, 200–280 nm), ultraviolet B (UV-B, 280–315 nm), ultraviolet A (UV-A, 315–400 nm), visible light (VIS, 380–760 nm), and near infrared (NIR, 760–1400 nm) [50].

For biomedical applications of CAP, ultraviolet radiation is of particular interest due to its mutagenic and cytotoxic potential. DNA is certainly one of the key targets of UV-induced damage in a variety of organisms. DNA lesions such as cyclobutane-pyrimidine dimers (CPDs) and 6-4 photoproducts (6-4PPs) and their Dewar valence Isomers can be induced by UV radiation [51]. Both the acute skin response to UV in the form of erythema as well as the long term risk of skin cancer seem to be related to these pathways. However, the physiological impact of UV is strongly dependent on the photon energy and thus to the wavelength of the UV radiation. To account for this dependency, the International Commission on Non-Ionizing Radiation Protection (ICNIRP) has proposed a spectral weighting function $S\lambda$ for non-therapeutic and non-elective ultraviolet exposure of the unprotected skin in the range 180–400 nm. Moreover, the ICNIRP has recommended not to exceed an effective exposure of $D_{max} = 30\ J/m^2$ or $3\ mJ/cm^2$ per day. This value should be applied for the most sensitive, non-pathologic, skin phototype (known as "melano-compromised") and should be considered a desirable goal to minimize the long-term risk [52]. It is worth noting, that $D_{max}$ is exceeded by a number of times in current UV-A and UV-B therapies targeting skin diseases [2, 53].

Depending primarily on working gas composition, physical plasmas emit radiation at specific spectral characteristics often including components in the UV range. As soon as rare gases such as argon or helium are employed, the generation and transport of radiation in the VUV also becomes relevant, while with significant admixtures of air VUV radiation can be efficiently absorbed by the neutral gas components $O_2$ (below 200 nm) and $N_2$ (below 100 nm) [54–57]. As a consequence, the UV emission characteristics of CAP devices need to be evaluated carefully - preferably at conditions as close as possible to the indicated clinical conditions. This can be particularly challenging for direct plasma sources (see Sect. 2.3.1.1) but also for indirect sources (see Sect. 2.3.1.2) individual experimental strategies need to be adapted.

An essential method for non-invasive investigation of plasmas is optical emission spectroscopy (OES). OES refers to the acquisition and analysis of the spectrally resolved emission of a radiation source. It is a powerful and widely spread method in order to gain insights into molecular processes. Thus, OES has long been prominent in plasma physics, e.g., to identify radiative particles from line emissions or calculate particle energies and temperatures from relative intensities as wells as electron densities based on broadening mechanisms of line profiles [58, 59]. Applying spectrographs based on refractive and/or diffractive optical components, electromagnetic radiation can be decomposed to intensity per unit of spectral bandwidth $E\lambda$. Experimental acquisition of VUV spectra is technically more demanding, whereas UV/VIS/NIR can be assessed quite comfortable by compact devices. Prior to spectrum acquisition, all spectrographs need to be calibrated in wavelength and relative (a.u.) or absolute (e.g. photons/m$^2$/s/nm, mW/m$^2$/nm) intensity, respectively [60]. Yet, in a post-processing workflow, spectral data in units of a.u. can be combined with experimental results on irradiances applying absolutely calibrated radiometers (W/m$^2$) in order to achieve absolute spectral data.

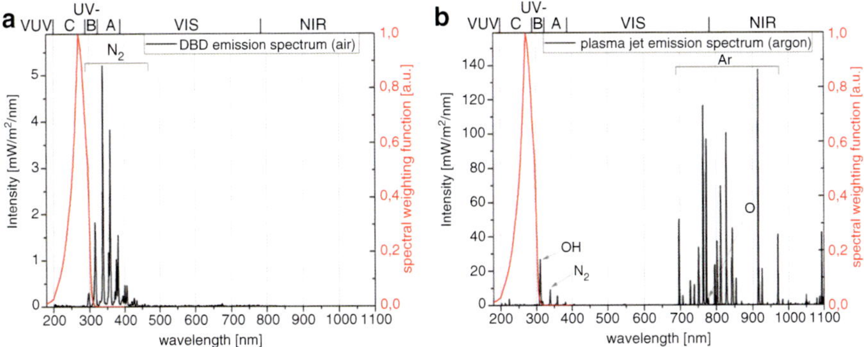


**Fig. 3.4** Typical emission spectra and intensities of CAP generated by a DBD operated with air (**a**) and a plasma jet operated with argon (**b**). In red, the spectral weighting function $S\lambda$ according to [52] is highlighted

In this section, we demonstrate a method for evaluating the UV characteristics of a direct plasma source (volume DBD) and an indirect plasma source (plasma jet) [44, 61]. For both source types, clearly diverse emission spectra as well as the spectral weighting function $S\lambda$ are given in Fig. 3.4.

In order to access the UV characteristics of the volume DBD, one has to put up with the task that the tissue acts as the counter electrode. Thus, the relevant plasma-induced irradiance is not accessible by measurement technology in the relevant tissue plane. For a plasma jet device, the propagation and thus emission characteristics of a free-jet configuration may differ from the real application conditions in which the effluent may be spatially expanded by interaction with the tissue surface. Consequently, an artificial counter electrode needs to be adapted for direct sources, whereas it is optional for indirect sources. The counter electrode can be any object of sufficient conductivity combined with optical transparency of defined transmittance $T\lambda$, e.g., a mesh electrode or a fused silica covered by a thin indium tin oxide (ITO) layer connected to ground potential. Connecting the counter electrode to ground potential resembles a worst-case scenario suitable for operational safety evaluation as the effective electric potential difference is maximized.

Yet, in contrast to the indicated clinical condition, applying an artificial counter electrode introduces an additional absorbing medium. As a result, only an absorption-reduced irradiance $I_{abs}$ can be detected experimentally—either by an absolutely calibrated spectrograph or an absolutely calibrated radiometer both in the position inferior to the counter electrode. As soon as the spectrograph is not absolutely calibrated, the plasma emission spectrum $E\lambda$ is recorded in a.u. applying a fibre based spectrograph at relevant positioning. Options for experimental set-ups featuring a radiometer configuration are shown in Fig. 3.5.

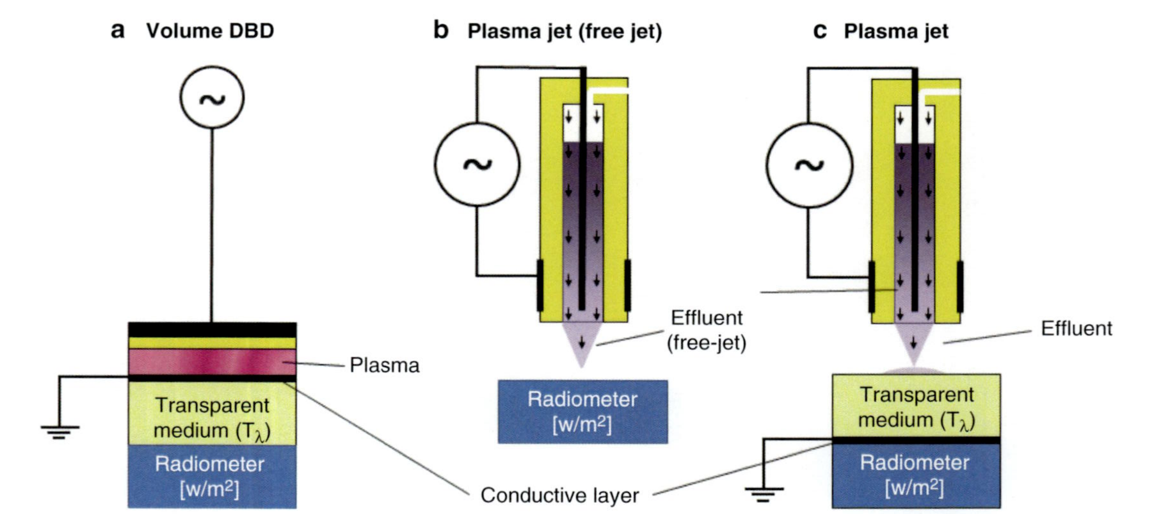


**Fig. 3.5** Options on experimental set-ups for determination of relevant irradiances induced by volume DBD (**a**), plasma jet in free-jet mode (**b**) and plasma jet inducing glide discharges on a dielectric surface (**c**)

Absolute values of $I_{abs}$ as recorded by the radiometer correlate with the integral of the plasma emission spectrum $E\lambda$ multiplied with the transmittance spectrum $T\lambda$ of the counter electrode within the sensitivity limits of the detector. Thus, the spectrally resolved irradiance distribution $I\lambda$ in units of mW/m$^2$/nm can be calculated according to eq. (3.1):

$$I_{\lambda} = E_{\lambda} \cdot \frac{|I_{abs}|}{\left|\int E_{\lambda} \cdot T_{\lambda} d\lambda\right|} \tag{3.1}$$

An effective irradiance $I_{eff}$ can be calculated by normalizing the spectrum to a monochromatic source at 270 nm via the spectral weighting function $S\lambda$ illustrated in Fig. 3.4 by eq. (3.2):

$$I_{eff} = \int_{180nm}^{400nm} I_{\lambda} \cdot S_{\lambda} d\lambda \tag{3.2}$$

Taking into account the effective exposure limit of $D_{max}$ = 30 J/m$^2$, a maximum daily treatment duration $T_{max}$ specific for the process parameters of the studied plasma source can be calculated by eq. (3.3) and be applied in order to ensure safe treatment conditions on human skin:

$$T_{\max} = \frac{D_{\max}}{I_{eff}} \tag{3.3}$$

Typical values $T_{max}$ for CAP devices are of the order of 30 min to some hours per day [40, 61].

### 3.3.5 Reactive Species Production

The application of CAP devices in an open surrounding implies the presence of reactive oxygen and nitrogen species (RONS) in close proximity. When operating either argon or air discharges, the energy put into reactive species production will at some point result in the exchange of energy with the ambient air and thus in the formation of ozone and nitric oxides (amongst many other species). These species themselves are crucial for antimicrobial effects of CAP but at the same time an overexposure of patients or attending staff may result in side effects ranging from small headache to irritation of the respiratory tract. As a consequence, threshold limits for save operation have been established, e.g. by the WHO, in order to prevent harm from befalling users. These byproducts are also known to occur, e.g., during the printing process of laser printers. General information and guidelines for the measurement of the formation of toxic gases are given in DIN EN ISO 12100 [62].

The first safety tests are always performed with mobile sensors to ensure safety even under laboratory conditions. In order to quantify the production of ozone and nitric oxide by the discharge, quick tests employing tubes with chemicals compound are used. The chemical compound is fabricated depending on the respective radical to be detected and reacts by a change in color and depending upon the length of color change inside the tube, quantification can be applied. This method was patented in 1919 and since then further developed towards the product today [63]. These measurements allow a first quantification of the emission of these products to ensure safety for a possible user of a device. For further investigations on the impact of each individual reactive species onto biomedical effects, more advanced techniques are necessary. These techniques are presented in Sect. 3.4.

## 3.4 Plasma Cocktail of Active Agents

Besides the quantification of atmospheric pressure plasma devices with respect to safety aspects, the fundamental understanding of these devices towards the core plasma and the cocktail of agents they create is required to understand the individual qualification for plasma medical research. This has to be performed under consideration of present diagnostic possibilities and limitations (Fig. 3.6).

In order to understand the effect of selected agents from the cocktail, a separation within the plasma is necessary. Some studies succeeded in separating excited species and radiation and showed individual biomedical efficacy [64–66]. But for a throughout understanding, the effect of all six components individually would be necessary. Yet, the measurement access and the separation possibilities are limited.

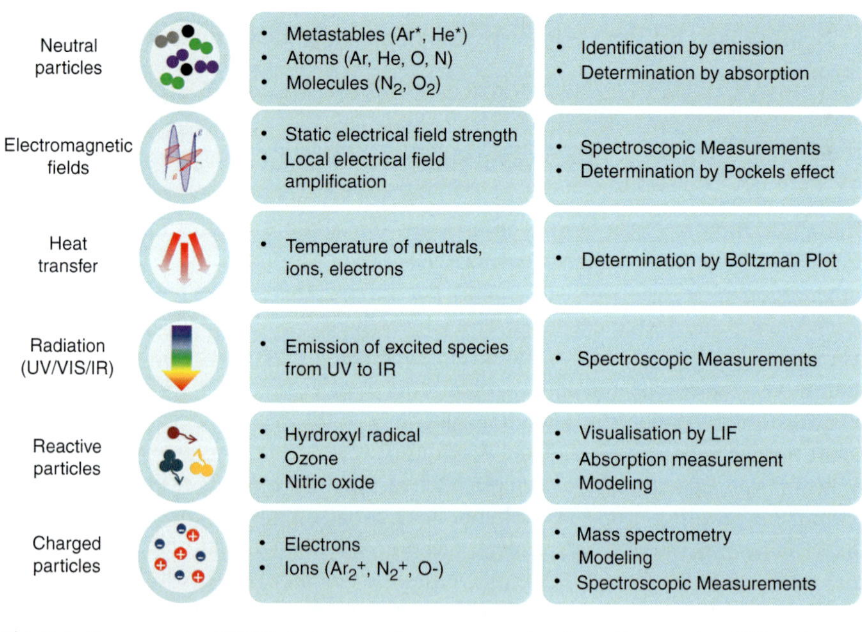


**Fig. 3.6** Components of CAP, their respective representative depending on the CAP under use and reported methods to access them

The current state of experimental and theoretical investigations is addressed in the following subchapters to reveal current holdbacks.

It has to be considered that the temporal resolution of each method depends on the investigated agent. A higher requirement on temporal resolution results typically in a more advanced diagnostic. When considering the range of timescales in plasma dynamic, a total of ten orders of magnitude are involved [67]. Projecting these timescales, e.g., on the hydroxyl radical (OH), the processes of water dissociation (0.1–10 ns), OH excitation (0.1–10 ns) and radical chemistry (0.1–500 μs) to form hydrogen peroxide ($H_2O_2$) are relevant and hence diagnostics from sub-nanosecond up to millisecond timescales are necessary. Typically, multiple diagnostics have to be combined to trace these cycles. Likewise, the spatial requirements range from sub-micrometer (plasma dynamic effects) up to millimeter (treatment distance).

Thus, plasma characterization is a challenging task with still many "blind spots" left. Consequently, scientists continuously develop new methods to gain more insights into the complex plasma dynamics for a diversity of plasma discharges, including CAPs.

### 3.4.1 Basic Electrical Characterization

For many studies the acquisition of the voltage and current signals is performed to evaluate plasma stability and reproducibility [67]. Furthermore, the electrical characterization of devices operating at frequencies below 1 MHz depicts the plasma dynamic with a sufficient temporal resolution. Even a first qualification of discharge type can be concluded.

In some cases, the electrical power is evaluated as well [68, 69]. By quantifying the plasma input power, an important reference value is acquired to compare the application of different devices of the same type. It is worth noting, that total power consumption of plasma devices does not scale with biomedical efficiency.

For basic electrical characterization, a digital oscilloscope is applied in combination with voltage and current probes. Depending on the stage of development of the respective plasma source, the metrological access to the operating voltage might not be possible due to construction and safety reasons. The current at the target, however, can generally be accessed.

### 3.4.2 Charged Species

The existence of a minimal number of charged species in a small volume is a characteristic of the fourth state of matter. For biomedical applications, electrons and ions were not yet found to individually affect the efficiency of the treatment. Nonetheless they have the key role inside a plasma discharge. All other active agents are somehow related to the electrons and ions. The interlinkage includes mainly collisions with electrons to excite, ionize or dissociate neutral species.

Accessing the electron density in atmospheric pressure plasma discharges requires advanced diagnostic methods. Typically, these discharges expand only over a limited dimension with low spatial stability and fast dynamics. One common method to access the electron density is to evaluate the stark broadening of the hydrogen lines (e.g. α-line at 656.28 nm or β-line at 486.13 nm) [70–72]. Due to the presence of a high electric field in the vicinity induced by nearby charged particles, the emission line profile is broadened and the broadening width correlates with the electron density. The experimental challenge arises from the high spectral resolution required to resolve the line broadening considering the low electron densities. Furthermore, a certain hydrogen content is needed to observe the intended line.

Other optical techniques to determine the electron densities are based on evaluation of the line ratio for argon discharges [73], on measuring the Thomson scattering [74] or on evaluating phase resolved imaging together with electrical parameters [75, 76]. All these methods have their own experimental challenges and need a sophisticated time before they can be applied to investigate the desired plasma source.

Beside the optical techniques, some atmospheric pressure plasma discharges were investigated towards electron density by electrical measurements [72] and several models are applied, characterizing electron dynamics together with the effect on the plasma chemistry [77–82].

The measurement of the ions (positive and negative) in the discharge is not well documented and difficult to perform. Besides modeling results [82–86], mass spectrometry is applied with special and expensive devices [87, 88]. First results applying customized electrical diagnostics [89] are also published. The Pockels effect was successfully applied by few groups to quantify at least the impact of the ions onto a surface by successfully determining the surface charge densities (Figs 3.7 and 3.8) [90–94]. And finally, by observing the emission signals via phase resolved optical emission spectroscopy, the temporal and spatial resolved trace of the ion movement is observed [95–99].

Aside from modeling results, no sophisticated access of ion densities is available so far and hence a quantification of the ions and their individual contribution is still an open topic. Additionally, the technological challenges remain to access these quantities.

### 3.4.3 Excited Species

In plasmas and especially in CAP, three body collisions are frequent and energy is distributed rapidly through the electrons into electronic, vibrational and rotational states of atoms and molecules. Furthermore, radicals are created by collisions and dissociation in the plasma and similarly excited into higher states. By applying optical emission spectroscopy, the existence of a few such species can be verified, but a previous excitation is required. The emission range depends on the applied equipment. A quantification of species concentration is dependent on a complex accompanying theoretical model. Hence, for an absolute measurement of excited species,

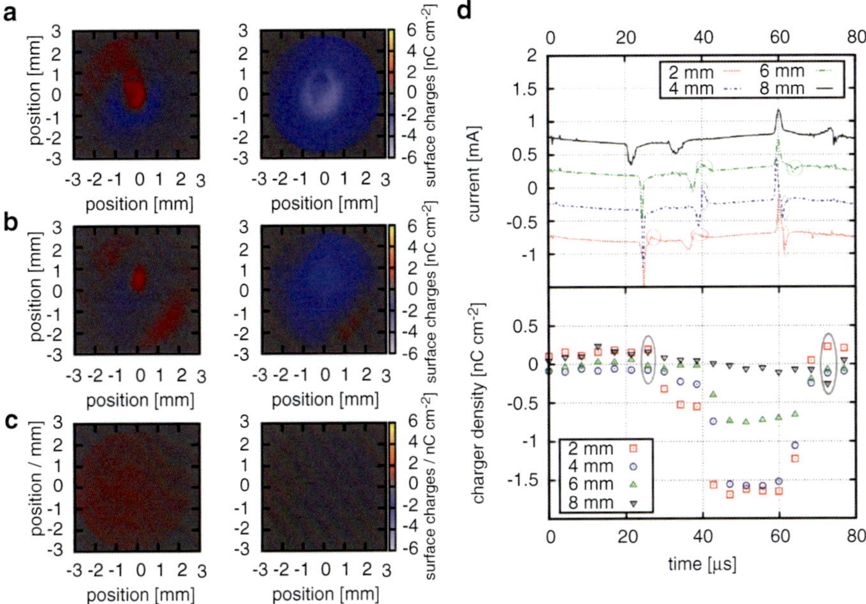


**Fig. 3.7** (**a–c**) Distribution of charges over the discharge phase deposited onto the surface by a helium CAP for three distances ((**a**) at 4 mm, (**b**) at 6 mm, (**c**) at 8 mm). Positive charges (positive ions) are colored red, negative charges (electrons and negative ions) are colored blue and (**d**) correlation of the temporal charge exchange with the electrical signals of the discharge [92]

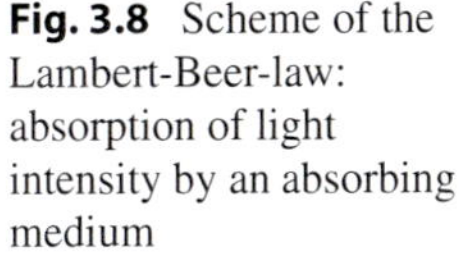

**Fig. 3.8** Scheme of the Lambert-Beer-law: absorption of light intensity by an absorbing medium

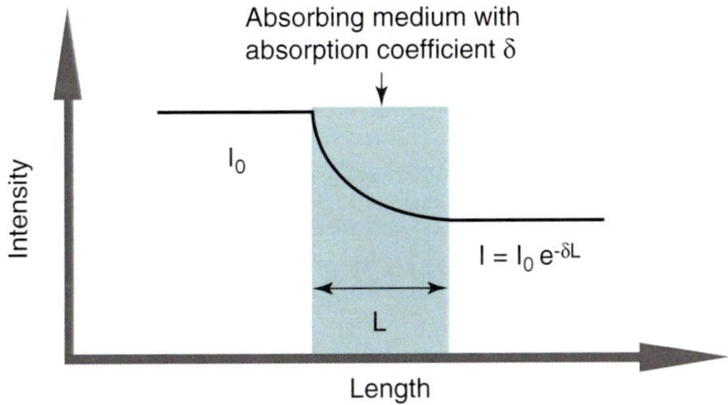


additional methods are investigated in the physical research on CAP [100]. A brief overview of recent results on quantifying reactive species with different methods and the literature focusing on it will be presented here.

A wide-spread method to measure absolute species densities is absorption spectroscopy. In general, the absorbed light intensity after passing an absorbing medium is measured, whereas the Lambert-Beer law facilitates quantification (Fig. 3.8). Among the large variety of absorption techniques, the most frequently used setups are the laser absorption spectroscopy due to the high temporal and spectral flexibility although a spatial reproducibility is necessary. Absolut densities were acquired for metastable argon atoms, metastable helium atoms and nitrogen oxide [84, 101–105]. Furthermore, infrared absorption, ultraviolet absorption and cavity ringdown spectroscopy were applied to measure absolute densities of nitric oxides, hydroxyl radicals and ozone [106–110].

A spectroscopic method that uses the birefringent nature of an absorbing transition was applied recently to investigate atmospheric pressure plasma devices. By providing a broad band background emission at the absorbing transition and by combining it with an interferometer and a grating, the change of dispersion near the absorbing transition is observed. The spectral distance between each point of change in dispersion either side of the absorbing transition then correlates with the density of the respective level with

$$N_i = \frac{\pi K \Delta^2}{r_0 f_{ik} \lambda_0^3 l} \tag{3.4}$$

with $\pi$ as pi, $K$ the setup constant, $r_0$ the electron radii, $f_{ik}$ the oscillator strength, $\lambda_0$ the wavelength of the absorbing transition and $l$ the absorption length. This method is the so called "hook" method, which was successfully applied to measure the hydroxyl radical density in an atmospheric pressure plasma [111, 112].

Further advanced diagnostics are based on laser induced fluorescence (LIF) inside a defined space volume of the discharge. By evaluating the induced fluorescence and considering quenching effects, the absolute concentrations of hydroxyl radicals and atomic oxygen could be measured [109, 113–115]. Also Fourier transformed infrared spectroscopy (FTIR) is utilized for quantification of gas phase species like ozone or hydrogen peroxide. In liquids, electron paramagnetic resonance spectroscopy (EPR) was applied to detect hydroxyl radical and superoxide radical [66, 82, 100, 116]. Lastly, computational approaches on the basis of, e.g., particle-in-a-cell (PIC) or fluid models can be utilized to quantify excited species production in CAPs [82, 85].

### 3.4.4 Plasma Emission

Due to the intense investigations of plasma emission during the fluorescent lamp development, a broad variety of diagnostic methods and devices is available for the investigation and quantification of plasma emission. Also the database for identification of species from atomic towards molecular is well established [117]. A detailed description of the most important quantification of emission in the UV range for medical purpose is given in Sect. 3.3.4. Other advanced diagnostics applying optical emission spectroscopy (OES) are discussed all through Sect. 3.4 for the identification, quantification or visualization of other active agents in cold atmospheric plasmas.

### 3.4.5 Plasma Temperatures

The plasma discharges at atmospheric pressure that are of interest for medical application are generally cold (below 40 °C) and the measurement of the neutral gas temperature, so of the heat that is transferred to a treated surface, is described already in Sect. 3.3.2.

Here the focus will be on more detailed temperature description of the discharge to understand and control the plasma in an advanced fashion. It is important to note that CAP cannot be described by just one temperature. In order to describe this non-equilibrium phenomenon, the knowledge of the temperature of each species as well as their available degree of freedom is necessary. In simple terms, a distinction between electron temperature $T_e$ (or excitation temperature $T_{ext}$), ion temperature $T_i$ (correlated with the vibrational temperature $T_{vib}$) and neutral species temperature $T_g$ (correlated with the rotational temperature $T_{rot}$) is applied. This correlation is only valid for CAP, as described in Sect. 2.3.1 (Fig. 2.5).

A first approach for an estimation of electron, ion or gas temperature alike is to apply the Boltzmann plot [118]. By measuring the spectral emission intensity for a respective transition (electronic, vibrational or rotational) and considering respective transition constants, the underlying Maxwellian energy distribution function is revealed and hence the respective temperature is resolved [71, 108, 118, 119]. Other possibilities to measure the temperature are by modeling, spectral line resolution and advanced techniques like the laser Schlieren deflectometry (LSD) [68, 82, 85, 118, 120, 121].

### 3.4.6 Electromagnetic Field Strength

Measurement of the electromagnetic field strength is currently in the focus of investigations when characterizing CAP devices. The existence of the research field of electroporation alone motivates a further understanding of the electrical field component within the plasma treatment [122, 123]. Here we will present the current approaches to distinguish the electrical field strength.

Meanwhile, commercial devices attract attention for measuring electrical field strength in CAPs [103, 124]. By utilizing the Pockels effect of a birefringent crystal and evaluating a shift in polarization, the electrical field strength is measured with a high temporal resolution. The Pockels effect is used by other groups as well [90, 92, 93, 125, 126] and even for electrical field measurement [127]. However, the introduction of additional surfaces into the plasma region is an invasive method and can result in changes of the plasma characteristics like ignition voltage or spatial propagation [92]. Further approaches to acquire electrical field values base on advanced spectroscopic methods [98, 128] or on computational modeling (Fig. 3.9) [77, 82, 129].

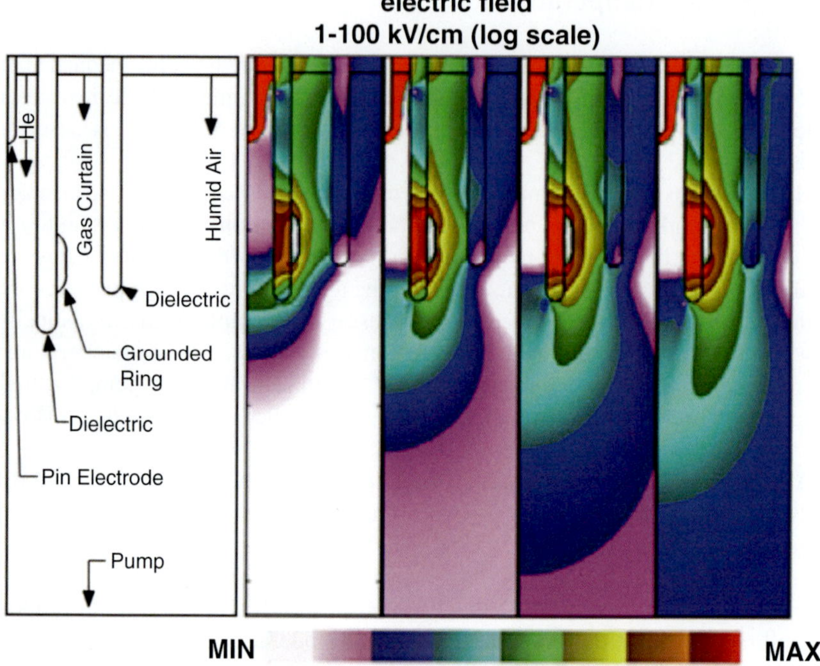


**Fig. 3.9** Modeling results on the electrical field development for the kINPen device operated with helium (geometry shown left) at different times after onset of the voltage (20 ns, 40 ns, 60 ns, 80 ns) [82]

**Conclusion**

When considering plasma medical research and further down the road biomedical applications in clinical environments, the minimum requirement is the availability of appropriate plasma devices. The INP Greifswald, the HAWK and the Fraunhofer IST in close collaboration with industrial partners each accompanied a device from the state of a "wired hedgehog" (pre-laboratory prototype state) towards a medical product class IIa. While many groups have developed individual devices for basic research on medical effects, the modern research landscape barely finances the step in between basic research and commercial development towards a medical product. Hence we find that even at the stage of laboratory research stage, a general evaluation of safety aspects should be performed in order to avoid overselling of the field before it is mature enough to meet the necessary challenges. A proposal for a minimal set of safety and effectivity measurements is hence summarized in DIN SPEC 91315 [130].

After first successful investigations in vitro and meanwhile in vivo, the application of CAP in medical research attracts a great deal of attention. One of the most important factors to raise the biomedical potential of CAP technology by bringing it into clinical routine is clinical evidence. Yet, up to now randomized controlled trials featuring significant sample sizes are sparse. It is therefore desirable to force and intensify clinical trials in the future. The findings and experiences gained in these studies can not only provide a wider understanding for fundamental research, but also serve as essential input for the development of the next generation of CAP medical products.

With the present chapter, the authors aim to make the reader aware of the complexity of plasma components, the up to now identified effects they have and the approach to measure them. Cold atmospheric plasma contributes a cocktail of six agents to the biomedical application and is shown to be antimicrobial active over a wide range of bacteria, enhance proliferation of eukaryotic cells and even acts through liquid films by a chemical cascade of aqueous species generation. A set of clinical trials with medical plasma products proofs the operation to be effective and safe even over a long timeframe after plasma treatment.

In order to thoroughly understand the induced effects and to trace the desired cocktail composition, a complex characterization of the plasma device is necessary. Such a characterization has two aims: first to verify the safety of operation of the device and second to measure the detailed composition of the plasma cocktail with an individual strategy. The safety considerations include handling of high voltage, thermal impact, patient leakage current, UV radiation and reactive species production. Respective safety considerations are summarized and a measurement access is described.

Accessing all active plasma agents of a discharge requires a wide range of diagnostic tools, detailed knowledge of multiple physical measurement methods and a spatial and temporal stable discharge. Since these requirements are hardly manageable, each device is currently investigated by an individual selection of agents to follow up on. An overview of the common and promising future diagnostics is reviewed with respective literature references.

Most diagnostic methods for CAPs still require a deep understanding of the experimental setup. Therefore, the way for an overall characterization to allow the individual tuning of a plasma device is still ongoing. Until the time of a complete diagnostic access, the plasma medical research will focus on finding tracers for plasma efficacy for single components rather than understanding the whole "cocktail".

**Acknowledgement** The authors Gerling and Weltmann thank the internal and external cooperation partners of the projects "Campus PlasmaMed I and II", funded by the German Federal Ministry of Education and Research (13 N9779 and 13 N11188); "Plasmamedizinische Forschung – neue pharmazeutische und medizinische Anwendungsfelder", funded by the Ministry for Research, Development and Culture of the State of Mecklenburg-Vorpommern and the European Union by the European Social Fund (AU 11 038, ESF/IV-BM-B35-0010/13); "Entwicklung eines neuartigen Wundbehandlungssystems auf Basis von Plasmatechnologien und dem Einsatz flächiger textiler Plasmaquellen für den mobilen und stationären Einsatz – PlasmaWundTex", funded by Zentrales Innovationsprogramm Mittelstand of the German Federal Ministry for Economic Affairs and Energy (KF2046509AK3); "Erweiterung der medizinischen Anwendungsmöglichkeiten kalter Atmosphärendruckplasmajets (MEDKAP)", funded by the German Ministry of Education;

"Plasmamedizin—Anwendungsorientierte Grundlagenforschung zu physikalischem Plasma in der Medizin" funded by the Ministry of Education, Science and Culture of the State of Mecklenburg-Vorpommern (grant: AU 15 001).

The author Helmke thanks all cooperation partners of the research group "BioLiP", funded by the German Federal Ministry of Education and Research (BMBF, grant no. 13 N9089), the associated partners in the project "PlaStraKomb", funded by the BMBF (grant no. PNT51501), the partners of the research group "Campus PlasmaMed II", funded by the BMBF (grant no. 13 N11190), as well as the partners of the joint research project "WuPlaKo", funded by the BMBF (grant no. 13GW0041D) and "KonchaWu", funded by the Ministry of economics of the State of Niedersachsen and the European Regional Development Fund ERDF (grant no. ZW 3-85006987).

## References

1. von Woedtke T, Reuter S, Masur K, et al. Plasmas for medicine. Phys Rep. 2013;530:291–320.
2. Grundmann-Kollmann M, Ludwig R, Zollner TM, et al. Narrowband UVB and cream psoralen-UVA combination therapy for plaque-type psoriasis. J Am Acad Dermatol. 2004;50:734–9.
3. Krutmann J, Czech W, Diepgen T, et al. High-dose UVA1 therapy in the treatment of patients with atopic dermatitis. J Am Acad Dermatol. 1992;26:225–30.
4. Valko M, Leibfritz D, Moncol J, et al. Free radicals and antioxidants in normal physiological functions and human disease. Int J Biochem Cell Biol. 2007;39:44–84.
5. Martinez-Sanchez G, Al-Dalain SM, Menendez S, et al. Therapeutic efficacy of ozone in patients with diabetic foot. Eur J Pharmacol. 2005;523:151–61.
6. Re L, Mawsouf MN, Menendez S, et al. Ozone therapy: clinical and basic evidence of its therapeutic potential. Arch Med Res. 2008;39:17–26.
7. Maffiuletti NA, Minetto MA, Farina D, et al. Electrical stimulation for neuromuscular testing and training: state-of-the art and unresolved issues. Eur J Appl Physiol. 2011;111:2391–7.
8. Kara M, Oezcakar L, Goekcay D, et al. Quantification of the effects of transcutaneous electrical nerve stimulation with functional magnetic resonance imaging: a double-blind randomized placebo-controlled study. Arch Phys Med Rehabil. 2010;91:1160–5.
9. Ehlbeck J, Schnabel U, Polak M, et al. Low temperature atmospheric pressure plasma sources for microbial decontamination. J Phys D Appl Phys. 2011;44:13002.
10. Daeschlein G, Scholz S, von Woedtke T, et al. In vitro killing of clinical fungal strains by low-temperature atmospheric-pressure plasma jet. IEEE Trans Plasma Sci. 2011;39:815–21.
11. Daeschlein G, Scholz S, Arnold A, et al. In vitro susceptibility of important skin and wound pathogens against low temperature atmospheric pressure plasma jet (APPJ) and dielectric barrier discharge plasma (DBD). Plasma Process Polym. 2012;9:380–9.
12. Helmke A, Gruenig P, Fritz U-M, et al. Low temperature plasma—a prospective microbicidal tool. Recent Pat Antiinfect Drug Discov. 2012;7:223–30.
13. Cooper M, Fridman G, Staack D, et al. Decontamination of surfaces from extremophile organisms using nonthermal atmospheric-pressure plasmas. IEEE Trans Plasma Sci. 2009;37:866–71.
14. Joshi SG, Paff M, Friedman G, et al. Control of methicillin-resistant Staphylococcus aureus in planktonic form and biofilms: A biocidal efficacy study of nonthermal dielectric-barrier discharge plasma. Am J Infect Control. 2010;38:293–301.
15. Zimmermann JL, Shimizu T, Schmidt H-U, et al. Test for bacterial resistance build-up against plasma treatment. New J Phys. 2012;14:73037.
16. Kalghatgi S, Friedman G, Fridman A, et al. Endothelial cell proliferation is enhanced by low dose non-thermal plasma through fibroblast growth factor-2 release. Ann Biomed Eng. 2010;38:748–57.
17. Kalghatgi S, Kelly CM, Cerchar E, et al. Effects of non-thermal plasma on mammalian cells. PLoS One. 2011;6:e16270.

18. Kalghatgi S, Fridman A, Azizkhan-Clifford J, et al. DNA damage in mammalian cells by non-thermal atmospheric pressure microsecond pulsed dielectric barrier discharge plasma is not mediated by ozone. Plasma Process Polym. 2012;9:726–32.
19. Balzer J, Heuer K, Demir E, et al. Non-Thermal Dielectric Barrier Discharge (DBD) effects on proliferation and differentiation of human fibroblasts are primary mediated by hydrogen peroxide. PLoS One. 2015;10:1–18.
20. Helmke A, Hoffmeister D, Mertens N, et al. The acidification of lipid film surfaces by non-thermal DBD at atmospheric pressure in air. New J Phys. 2009;11:115025.
21. Oehmigen K, Haehnel M, Brandenburg R, et al. The role of acidification for antimicrobial activity of atmospheric pressure plasma in liquids. Plasma Process Polym. 2010;7:250–7.
22. Fridman G, Peddinghaus M, Balasubramanian M, et al. Blood coagulation and living tissue sterilization by floating-electrode dielectric barrier discharge in air. Plasma Chem Plasma Process. 2006;26:425–42.
23. Kalghatgi SU, Fridman G, Cooper M, et al. Mechanism of blood coagulation by nonthermal atmospheric pressure dielectric barrier discharge plasma. IEEE Trans Plasma Sci. 2007;35:1559–66.
24. Isbary G, Morfill G, Schmidt H, et al. A first prospective randomized controlled trial to decrease bacterial load using cold atmospheric argon plasma on chronic wounds in patients. Br J Dermatol. 2010;163:78–82.
25. Isbary G, Heinlin J, Shimizu T, et al. Successful and safe use of 2 min cold atmospheric argon plasma in chronic wounds: results of a randomized controlled trial. Br J Dermatol. 2012;167:404–10.
26. Heinlin J, Isbary G, Stolz W, et al. A randomized two-sided placebo-controlled study on the efficacy and safety of atmospheric non-thermal argon plasma for pruritus. J Eur Acad Dermatol Venereol. 2013;27:324–31.
27. Isbary G, Stolz W, Shimizu T, et al. Cold atmospheric argon plasma treatment may accelerate wound healing in chronic wounds: results of an open retrospective randomized controlled study in vivo. J Clin Plasma Med. 2013;1:25–30.
28. Heinlin J, Zimmermann JL, Zeman F, et al. Randomized placebo-controlled human pilot study of cold atmospheric argon plasma on skin graft donor sites. Wound Repair Regen. 2013;21:800–7.
29. Fluhr JW, Sassning S, Lademann O, et al. In vivo skin treatment with tissue-tolerable plasma influences skin physiology and antioxidant profile in human stratum corneum. Exp Dermatol. 2012;21:130–4.
30. Daeschlein G, Scholz S, Ahmed R, et al. Skin decontamination by low-temperature atmospheric pressure plasma jet and dielectric barrier discharge plasma. J Hosp Infect. 2012;81:177–83.
31. Metelmann H-R, von Woedtke T, Bussiahn R, et al. Experimental recovery of CO2-laser skin lesions by plasma stimulation. Am J Cosmet Surg. 2012;29:52–6.
32. Metelmann H-R, Vu TT, Do HT, et al. Scar formation of laser skin lesions after cold atmospheric pressure plasma (CAP) treatment: a clinical long term observation. Clin Plasma Med. 2013;1:30–5.
33. Klebes M, Ulrich C, Kluschke F, et al. Combined antibacterial effects of tissue-tolerable plasma and a modern conventional liquid antiseptic on chronic wound treatment. J Biophotonics. 2015;8:382–91.
34. Bekeschus S, Schmidt A, Weltmann K-D, et al. The plasma jet kINPen—a powerful tool for wound healing. Clin Plasma Med. 2016;4:19–28.
35. Klebes M, Lademann J, Philipp S, et al. Effects of tissue-tolerable plasma on psoriasis vulgaris treatment compared to conventional local treatment: a pilot study. Clin Plasma Med. 2014;2:22–7.
36. Brehmer F, Haenssle HA, Daeschlein G, et al. Alleviation of chronic venous leg ulcers with a hand-held dielectric barrier discharge plasma generator (PlasmaDerm VU-2010): results of a monocentric, two-armed, open, prospective, randomized and controlled trial (NCT01415622). J Eur Acad Dermatol Venereol. 2015;29:148–55.

37. Heuer K, Hoffmanns MA, Demir E, et al. The topical use of non-thermal dielectric barrier discharge (DBD): Nitric oxide related effects on human skin. Nitric Oxide. 2015;44:52–60.
38. Kisch T, Helmke A, Schleusser S, et al. Improvement of cutaneous microcirculation by cold atmospheric plasma (CAP): results of a controlled, prospective cohort study. Microvasc Res. 2016;104:55–62.
39. Kisch T, Schleusser S, Helmke A, et al. The repetitive use of non-thermal dielectric barrier discharge plasma boosts cutaneous microcirculatory effects. Microvasc Res. 2016;106:8–13.
40. Mann MS, Tiede R, Gavenis K, et al. Introduction to DIN-specification 91315 based on the characterization of the plasma jet kINPen® MED. Clin Plasma Med. 2016;4:35–45.
41. Winter J, Brandenburg R, Weltmann K-D. Atmospheric pressure plasma jets: an overview of devices and new directions. Plasma Sources Sci Technol. 2015;24:64001.
42. DIN EN 60601-1-6:2010: Medical electrical equipment—Part 1–6: General requirements for basic safety and essential performance—Collateral standard: Usability (IEC 60601-1-6:2010); German version EN 60601-1-6:2010, Beuth-Verlag.
43. Thomsen S, Pearce JA. Termal damage and rate processes in biological tissues. In: Welch AJ, van Gemert MJC, editors. Optical-thermal response of laser-irradiated tissue. 2nd ed. Dordrecht: Springer; 2011. p. 487–549.
44. Weltmann K-D, Kindel E, Brandenburg R, et al. Atmospheric pressure plasma jet for medical therapy: plasma parameters and risk estimation. Contrib Plasma Physics. 2009;49:631–40.
45. Tuemmel S, Mertens N, Wang J, et al. Low temperature plasma treatment of living human cells. Plasma Process Polym. 2007;4:465–9.
46. Kuchenbecker M, Bibinov N, Kaemling A, et al. Characterization of DBD plasma source for biomedical applications. J Phys D Appl Phys. 2009;42:45212.
47. Bussiahn R, Brandenburg R, Gerling T, et al. The hairline plasma: an intermittent negative dc-corona discharge at atmospheric pressure for plasma medical applications. Appl Phys Lett. 2010;96:143701.
48. Helmke A, Franck M, Wandke D, et al. Tempo-spatially resolved ozone characteristics during single-electrode dielectric barrier discharge (SE-DBD) operation against metal and porcine skin surfaces. Plasma Med. 2014;4:67–77.
49. Shimizu T, Steffes B, Pompl R, et al. Characterization of microwave plasma torch for decontamination. Plasma Process Polym. 2008;5:577–82.
50. ISO 21348:2007(en). Space environment (natural and artificial)—process for determining solar irradiances. Definitions of Solar Irradiance Spectral Categories.
51. Sinha RP, Haeder DP. UV-induced DNA damage and repair: a review. Photochem Photobiol Sci. 2002;1:225–36.
52. The International Commission on Non-Ionizing Radiation Protection. Guidelines on limits of exposure to ultraviolet radiation of wavelengths between 180nm and 400nm (Incoherent optical radiation). Health Phys. 2004;87:171–86.
53. Kreuter A, Hyun J, Stuecker M, et al. A randomized controlled study of low-dose UVA1, medium-dose UVA1, and narrowband UVB phototherapy in the treatment of localized scleroderma. J Am Acad Dermatol. 2006;54:440–7.
54. Masoud N, Martus K, Becker K. VUV emission from a cylindrical dielectric barrier discharge in Ar and in Ar/N 2 and Ar/air mixtures. J Phys D Appl Phys. 2005;38:1674.
55. Foest R, Bindemann T, Brandenburg R, et al. On the vacuum ultraviolet radiation of a miniaturized non-thermal atmospheric pressure plasma jet. Plasma Process Polym. 2007;4:460–4.
56. Yoshino K, Parkinson WH, Ito K, et al. Absolute absorption cross-section measurements of Schumann-Runge continuum of O2 at 90 and 295 K. J Mol Spectrosc. 2005;229:238–43.
57. Chan WF, Cooper G, Sodhi RNS, et al. Absolute optical oscillator strengths for discrete and continuum photoabsorption of molecular nitrogen (11-200 eV). Chem Phys. 1993;170:81–97.
58. Kim JH, Choi YH, Hwang YS. Electron density and temperature measurement method by using emission spectroscopy in atmospheric pressure nonequilibrium nitrogen plasmas. Phys Plasma. 2006;13:93501.

59. Nikiforov AY, Leys C, Gonzalez MA, et al. Electron density measurement in atmospheric pressure plasma jets: Stark broadening of hydrogenated and non-hydrogenated lines. Plasma Sources Sci Technol. 2015;24:34001.
60. Bibinov N, Halfmann H, Awakowicz P, et al. Relative and absolute intensity calibrations of a modern broadband echelle spectrometer. Meas Sci Technol. 2007;18:1327–37.
61. Helmke A, Mahmoodzada M, Wandke D, et al. Impact of electrode design, supply voltage and interelectrode distance on safety aspects of a medical DBD plasma source. Contrib Plasma Phys. 2013;53:623–38.
62. DIN EN ISO 12100: Safety of machinery—general principles for design—risk assessment and risk reduction (ISO 12100:2010); German version EN ISO 12100:2011, Beuth-Verlag.
63. Lamb AB, Hoover CR, inventors. Gas-detector. United States patent 1321062. 4 Nov 1919.
64. Lackmann JW, Schneider S, Edengeiser E, et al. Photons and particles emitted from cold atmospheric-pressure plasma inactivate bacteria and biomolecules independently and synergistically. J R Soc Interface. 2013;10:20130591.
65. Brandenburg R, Lange H, von Woedtke T, et al. Antimicrobial effects of UV and VUV radiation of nonthermal plasma jets. IEEE Trans Plasma Sci. 2009;37:877–83.
66. Winter J, Tresp H, Hammer MU, et al. Tracking plasma generated $H_2O_2$ from gas into liquid phase and revealing its dominant impact on human skin cells. J Phys D Appl Phys. 2014;47:285401.
67. Bruggeman P, Brandenburg R. Atmospheric pressure discharge filaments and microplasmas: physics, chemistry and diagnostics. J Phys D Appl Phys. 2013;46:464001.
68. Hofmann S, van Gessel AFH, Verreycken T, et al. Power dissipation, gas temperatures and electron densities of cold atmospheric pressure helium and argon RF plasma jets. Plasma Sources Sci Technol. 2011;20:65010.
69. Gerling T, Brandenburg R, Wilke C, et al. Power measurement for an atmospheric pressure plasma jet at different frequencies: distribution in the core plasma and the effluent. Eur Phys J Appl Phys. 2017;78:10801.
70. Qian M, Ren C, Wang D, et al. Stark broadening measurement of the electron density in an atmospheric pressure argon plasma jet with double-power electrodes. J Appl Phys. 2010;107:63303–1.
71. Nikiforov A, Xiong Q, Britun N, et al. Absolute concentration of OH radicals in atmospheric pressure glow discharges with a liquid electrode measured by laser-induced fluorescence spectroscopy. Appl Phys Express. 2011;4:26102–1.
72. Janda M, Martišovitš V, Hensel K, et al. Measurement of the electron density in Transient Spark discharge. Plasma Sources Sci Technol. 2014;23:65016.
73. Zhu X-M, Pu Y-K, Balcon N, et al. Measurement of the electron density in atmospheric-pressure low-temperature argon discharges by line-ratio method of optical emission spectroscopy. J Phys D Appl Phys. 2009;42:142003.
74. Huebner S, Sousa JS, Puech V, et al. Electron properties in an atmospheric helium plasma jet determined by Thomson scattering. J Phys D Appl Phys. 2014;47:432001.
75. Karakas E, Akman MA, Laroussi M. The evolution of atmospheric-pressure low-temperature plasma jets: jet current measurements. Plasma Sources Sci Technol. 2012;21:34016.
76. Gerling T, Nastuta AV, Bussiahn R, et al. Back and forth directed plasma bullets in a helium atmospheric pressure needle-to-plane discharge with oxygen admixtures. Plasma Sources Sci Technol. 2012;21:34012.
77. Naidis GV. Modelling of streamer propagation in atmospheric-pressure helium plasma jets. J Phys D Appl Phys. 2010;43:402001.
78. Lee HW, Park GY, Seo YS, et al. Modelling of atmospheric pressure plasmas for biomedical applications. J Phys D Appl Phys. 2011;44:53001.
79. Breden D, Miki K, Raja LL. Computational study of cold atmospheric nanosecond pulsed helium plasma jet in air. Appl Phys Lett. 2011;99:111501.
80. Boeuf J-P, Yang LL, Pitchford LC. Dynamics of a guided streamer ("plasma bullet") in a helium jet in air at atmospheric pressure. J Phys D Appl Phys. 2013;46:15201.

81. Norberg SA, Tian W, Johnsen E, et al. Atmospheric pressure plasma jets interacting with liquid covered tissue: touching and not-touching the liquid. J Phys D Appl Phys. 2014;47:475203.
82. Schmidt-Bleker A, Norberg SA, Winter J, et al. Propagation mechanisms of guided streamers in plasma jets: the influence of electronegativity of the surrounding gas. Plasma Sources Sci Technol. 2015;24:35022.
83. Xu XP, Kushner MJ. Multiple microdischarge dynamics in dielectric barrier discharges. J Appl Phys. 1998;84:4153–60.
84. Schmidt-Bleker A, Winter J, Bösel A, et al. On the plasma chemistry of a cold atmospheric argon plasma jet with shielding gas device. Plasma Sources Sci Technol. 2016;25:15005.
85. Norberg SA, Johnsen E, Kushner MJ. Formation of reactive oxygen and nitrogen species by repetitive negatively pulsed helium atmospheric pressure plasma jets propagating into humid air. Plasma Sources Sci Technol. 2015;24:35026.
86. Wen Y, Fu-Cheng L, Chao-Feng S, et al. Two-dimensional numerical study of an atmospheric pressure helium plasma jet with dual-power electrode. Chin Phys B. 2015;24:65203.
87. Oh J-S, Aranda-Gonzalvo Y, Bradley JW. Time-resolved mass spectroscopic studies of an atmospheric-pressure helium microplasma jet. J Phys D Appl Phys. 2011;44:365202.
88. Dünnbier M, Schmidt-Bleker A, Winter J, et al. Ambient air particle transport into the effluent of a cold atmospheric-pressure argon plasma jet investigated by molecular beam mass spectrometry. J Phys D Appl Phys. 2013;46:435203.
89. Gerling T, Bussiahn R, Wilke C, et al. Time resolved ion density determination by electrical current measurements in an atmospheric pressure argon plasma. Europhys Lett. 2014;105:25001.
90. Stollenwerk L, Laven JG, Purwins H-G. Spatially resolved surface-charge measurement in a planar dielectric-barrier discharge system. Phys Rev Lett. 2007;98:255001.
91. Bogaczyk M, Nemschokmichal S, Wild R, et al. Development of barrier discharges: operation modes and structure formation. Contrib Plasma Phys. 2012;52:847–55.
92. Gerling T, Wild R, Nastuta AV, et al. Correlation of phase resolved current, emission and surface charge measurements in an atmospheric pressure helium jet. Eur Phys J Appl Phys. 2015;71:20808.
93. Wild R, Gerling T, Bussiahn R, et al. Phase-resolved measurement of electric charge deposited by an atmospheric pressure plasma jet on a dielectric surface. J Phys D Appl Phys. 2014;47:42001.
94. Szili EJ, Bradley JW, Short RD. A tissue model to study the plasma delivery of reactive oxygen species. J Phys D Appl Phys. 2014;47:152002.
95. Kozlov KV, Wagner H-E, Brandenburg R, et al. Spatio-temporally resolved spectroscopic diagnostics of the barrier discharge in air at atmospheric pressure. J Phys D Appl Phys. 2001;34:3164–76.
96. Grosch H, Hoder T, Weltmann K-D, et al. Spatio-temporal development of microdischarges in a surface barrier discharge arrangement in air at atmospheric pressure. Eur Phys J D. 2010;60:547–53.
97. Gerling T, Hoder T, Bussiahn R, et al. On the spatio-temporal dynamics of a self-pulsed nanosecond transient spark discharge: a spectroscopic and electrical analysis. Plasma Sources Sci Technol. 2013;22:65012.
98. Hoder T, Černák M, Paillol J, et al. High-resolution measurements of the electric field at the streamer arrival to the cathode: A unification of the streamer-initiated gas-breakdown mechanism. Phys Rev E. 2012;86:55401.
99. Tschiersch R, Bogaczyk M, Wagner H-E. Systematic investigation of the barrier discharge operation in helium, nitrogen, and mixtures: discharge development, formation and decay of surface charges. J Phys D Appl Phys. 2014;47:365204.
100. Lu X, Naidis GV, Laroussi M, et al. Reactive species in non-equilibrium atmospheric-pressure plasmas: generation, transport, and biological effects. Phys Rep. 2016;630:1–84.
101. Bussiahn R, Kindel E, Lange H, et al. Spatially and temporally resolved measurements of argon metastable atoms in the effluent of a cold atmospheric pressure plasma jet. J Phys D Appl Phys. 2010;43:165201.

102. Sands BL, Leiweke RJ, Ganguly BN. Spatiotemporally resolved Ar (1s 5 ) metastable measurements in a streamer-like He/Ar atmospheric pressure plasma jet. J Phys D Appl Phys. 2010;43:282001.
103. Darny T, Pouvesle J-M, Puech V, et al. Analysis of conductive target influence in plasma jet experiments through helium metastable and electric field measurements. Plasma Sources Sci Technol. 2017;26:45008.
104. Niermann B, Böke M, Sadeghi N, et al. Space resolved density measurements of argon and helium metastable atoms in radio-frequency generated He-Ar micro-plasmas. Eur Phys J D. 2010;60:489–95.
105. Pipa AV, Reuter S, Foest R, et al. Controlling the NO production of an atmospheric pressure plasma jet. J Phys D Appl Phys. 2012;45:85201.
106. Srivastava N, Wang C. Determination of OH radicals in an atmospheric pressure helium microwave plasma jet. IEEE Trans Plasma Sci. 2011;39:918–24.
107. Reuter S, Winter J, Iseni S, et al. Detection of ozone in a MHz argon plasma bullet jet. Plasma Sources Sci Technol. 2012;21:34015.
108. Bruggeman P, Cunge G, Sadeghi N. Absolute OH density measurements by broadband UV absorption in diffuse atmospheric-pressure He–$H_2O$ RF glow discharges. Plasma Sources Sci Technol. 2012;21:35019.
109. Verreycken T, Mensink R, van der Horst R, et al. Absolute OH density measurements in the effluent of a cold atmospheric-pressure Ar–$H_2O$ RF plasma jet in air. Plasma Sources Sci Technol. 2013;22:55014.
110. Iseni S, Zhang S, van Gessel AFH, et al. Nitric oxide density distributions in the effluent of an RF argon APPJ: effect of gas flow rate and substrate. N J Phys. 2014;16:123011.
111. Rozhdestvenski DS. Anomale Dispersion in Natriumdampf. Ann Phys. 1912;39:307.
112. Gerling T. Beiträge zur optischen und elektrischen Charakterisierung des dynamischen Verhaltens von Plasmaspezies in Atmosphärendruck-Plasmen. 2014.
113. Knake N, Niemi K, Reuter S, et al. Absolute atomic oxygen density profiles in the discharge core of a microscale atmospheric pressure plasma jet. Appl Phys Lett. 2008;93:131503.
114. Reuter S, Winter J, Schmidt-Bleker A, et al. Atomic oxygen in a cold argon plasma jet: TALIF spectroscopy in ambient air with modelling and measurements of ambient species diffusion. Plasma Sources Sci Technol. 2012;21:24005.
115. Voráč J, Dvořák P, Procházka V, et al. Measurement of hydroxyl radical (OH) concentration in an argon RF plasma jet by laser-induced fluorescence. Plasma Sources Sci Technol. 2013;22:25016.
116. Tresp H, Hammer MU, Winter J, et al. Quantitative detection of plasma-generated radicals in liquids by electron paramagnetic resonance spectroscopy. J Phys D Appl Phys. 2013;46:435401.
117. The National Institute of Standards and Technology: Atomic Spectra Database Version 5.
118. Fantz U. Basics of plasma spectroscopy. Plasma Sources Sci Technol. 2006;15:S137.
119. Schäfer J, Foest R, Ohl A, et al. Miniaturized non-thermal atmospheric pressure plasma jet - characterization of self-organized regimes. Plasma Phys Control Fusion. 2009;51:124045.
120. Schäfer J, Foest R, Reuter S, et al. Laser schlieren deflectometry for temperature analysis of filamentary non-thermal atmospheric pressure plasma. Rev Sci Instrum. 2012;83:103506.
121. Gaens WV, Bogaerts A. Kinetic modelling for an atmospheric pressure argon plasma jet in humid air. J Phys D Appl Phys. 2013;46:275201.
122. Barnett A, Weaver JC. Electroporation: A unified, quantitative theory of reversible electrical breakdown and mechanical rupture in artificial planar bilayer membranes. Bioelectrochem Bioenerg. 1991;25:163–82.
123. Beebe SJ, Fox PM, Rec LJ, et al. Nanosecond, high-intensity pulsed electric fields induce apoptosis in human cells. FASEB J. 2003;17:1493–5.
124. Gaborit G, Jarrige P, Lecoche F, et al. Single shot and vectorial characterization of intense electric field in various environments with pigtailed Electrooptic probe. IEEE Trans Plasma Sci. 2014;42:1265–73.

125. Bogaczyk M, Wild R, Stollenwerk L, et al. Surface charge accumulation and discharge development in diffuse and filamentary barrier discharges operating in He, $N_2$ and mixtures. J Phys D Appl Phys. 2012;45:465202.
126. Wild R, Benduhn J, Stollenwerk L. Surface charge transport and decay in dielectric barrier discharges. J Phys D Appl Phys. 2014;47:435204.
127. Sobota A, Guaitella O, Garcia-Caurel E. Experimentally obtained values of electric field of an atmospheric pressure plasma jet impinging on a dielectric surface. J Phys D Appl Phys. 2013;46:372001.
128. Sretenović GB, Krstić IB, Kovačević VV, et al. Spatio-temporally resolved electric field measurements in helium plasma jet. J Phys D Appl Phys. 2014;47:102001.
129. Xiong Z, Kushner MJ. Atmospheric pressure ionization waves propagating through a flexible high aspect ratio capillary channel and impinging upon a target. Plasma Sources Sci Technol. 2012;21:34001.
130. DIN-SPEC 91315: General requirements for medical plasma sources. Beuth-Verlag; 2014.

# Key Roles of Reactive Oxygen and Nitrogen Species

4

David B. Graves and Georg Bauer

## 4.1 Introduction

Biomedical aspects of cold atmospheric plasma (CAP) are known to generally include reactive oxygen and nitrogen species (RONS) as central players. Table 4.1 lists some of the RONS (in aqueous solution) of interest in biomedical applications of CAP. Biologically active RONS are created in air-associated CAP and many of the species created in these plasmas will dissolve in aqueous liquid phases, and this includes biological tissues. Rationalizing the effects of RONS created by CAP and delivered to cells and tissue relies in part on the growing understanding of how naturally-occurring RONS behave biologically. Reactive oxygen and nitrogen species generally react by exchanging electrons in a chemical process known as oxidation-reduction, or 'redox' reactions—and these reactions pervade biology. Study of biologically important redox phenomena is sometimes referred to as 'redox biology.' In plants, redox reactions are involved when sunlight, $CO_2$ and $H_2O$ are combined to create sugars (carbohydrates) and $O_2$. In these reactions, electrons making up the C-O and H-O bonds are converted to C-H and O-O bonds: C and H have thereby been 'reduced.' This process is energetically 'uphill,' using the leaf-collected sunlight's photon energy to create the products. In aerobic cellular respiratory metabolism, the reverse process takes place: carbohydrates and $O_2$ are ultimately converted back into $CO_2$ and $H_2O$. In this latter redox process, electrons in the C-H bonds are converted to C-O and C-H bonds. The C and H in the carbohydrates are thereby 'oxidized' by $O_2$ to form products, releasing chemical energy to be used by the cells

D. B. Graves (✉)
Department of Chemical and Biomolecular Engineering, University of California, Berkeley, CA, USA
e-mail: graves@berkeley.edu

G. Bauer
Institute of Virology, Medical Center and Faculty of Medicine, University of Freiburg, Freiburg, Germany
e-mail: georg.bauer@uniklinik-freiburg.de



H.-R. Metelmann et al. (eds.), *Comprehensive Clinical Plasma Medicine*,
https://doi.org/10.1007/978-3-319-67627-2_4

**Table 4.1** CAP-generated (aqueous) species

| |
|---|
| Oxygen atoms (O) |
| Ozone ($O_3$) |
| Superoxide anions/hydroperoxide ($O_2^{\cdot -}$/$HO_2$) |
| Hydrogen peroxide ($H_2O_2$) |
| Hydroxyl radical (·OH) |
| Nitric oxide (·NO) |
| Nitrogen dioxide (·$NO_2$) |
| Peroxynitrite/peroxynitrous acid ($ONOO^-$/ONOOH) |
| Nitrite/nitrous acid ($NO_2^-$/$HNO_2$) |
| Nitrate/nitric acid ($NO_3^-$/$HNO_3$) |
| Singlet delta oxygen ($^1O_2$) |
| Hypochlorite/hypochlorous acid ($OCl^-$/HOCl) |
| Dichloride anion radicals ($Cl_2^{\cdot -}$) |

for a variety of purposes, including building new cellular structures, making cellular repairs and conducting cellular defense, among others.

The importance and scope of redox biology is partly captured by the following recent observation [1]:

> Looking at life from the perspective of electron flow may be one of the most universal and fundamental approaches to Biology. This is because all known life forms depend on electrons that get stranded at the top of 'energy hills,' waiting to roll down the hill toward a low-energy resting place. This insight has been famously expressed in the words of Albert Szent-Gyorgyi: "Life is nothing but electrons looking for a place to rest" [2].

Redox biology connects cellular metabolism to many different cellular functions, including cell stress response and immunity; cell cycle control; cell development and differentiation; neuronal and vascular signaling; and other important functions. RONS created by CAP that are exposed to cells and tissue can certainly influence natural redox reactions, and this simple fact connects CAP and redox biology. Redox biochemistry can strongly influence cellular homeostasis—the maintenance of a near-constant set of cellular conditions in the face of constant environmental perturbations—that are necessary for health. In this way, CAP application can be therapeutic—or potentially damaging [3].

In the last decade or so, redox biology has grown into a large and increasingly sophisticated field. Ideally, CAP researchers interested in understanding the likely effects of RONS in aerobic biological systems need to read and understand this literature. The size, scope, sophistication and rapid growth of the field combine to make this study challenging, however. One goal of this chapter is to set out the broad outlines of the field, thereby helping researchers identify some of the key directions that are at the forefront of the field of RONS used for cold atmospheric plasma in biomedical applications. Figure 4.1 illustrates some of the key questions currently facing redox biology. Redox biologists want to know which RONS are present at what concentrations and in what cellular locations. Proteins are known to be affected by RONS—especially those that contain cysteine amino acids (with S-H 'thiol' groups), but which proteins are most affected is not fully known. Lackmann et al. [4] have

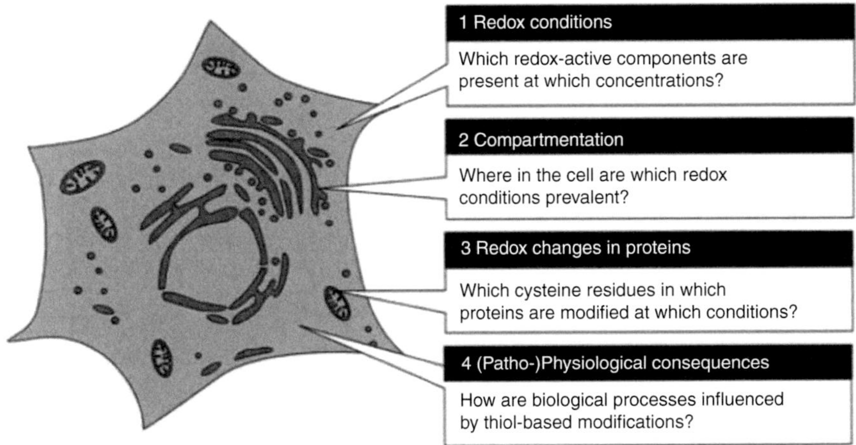


**Fig. 4.1** Some important questions currently facing redox biology (following [1])

shown that CAP (most likely through RONS) oxidizes sulfur-containing amino acids, but also may break disulfide bonds. Finally, the biological consequences—physiological or pathological—of these protein oxidative modifications are not known, except for some specific examples. Barcellos-Hoff and Dix [5] showed that the activation of TGF-beta1 can be mediated by reactive oxygen species. This finding is especially intriguing, as one of the many controlling functions of TGF-beta1 is related to the control of NOX1 activity [6]. Kim et al. [7] showed that singlet oxygen inactivates catalase and SOD through interaction with histidine residues at their active site. This reaction is the basis for singlet oxygen-mediated abrogation of tumor cell-specific control of their own extracellular RONS [8].

## 4.2 Classic and Tutorial References on RONS and Oxidation/Reduction Chemistry in Biology and Medicine

The multiple, complex biochemical effects of RONS have been seriously studied in biology and medicine for several decades at least. This short chapter cannot hope to summarize the entire field in any serious way, but it can at least identify some of the most important primary references and topics that a serious student can access to gain a deeper understanding of the field. Perhaps the single most influential book in this field (*Free Radicals in Biology and Medicine*) was originally published in 1985 by Halliwell and Gutteridge [9]. The latest edition (5th edition) was published in 2015 and a 6th edition is reportedly in preparation Nespolo [10]. The book does an admirable job of covering the field of reactive species, especially radicals, in biological systems with an eye towards the medical implications. The coverage is impressively broad and the authors make a serious attempt to make the book readable and useful to readers with a wide range of backgrounds, but the primary readers are assumed to be biologists and medical practitioners. Any serious researcher in the field of plasma medicine should have access to this book, preferably the latest edition. Halliwell published several other reviews over the years that summarize key ideas in a less formal way. These include the insightful papers entitled "Reactive species and antioxidants. Redox Biology is a Fundamental Theme of Aerobic Life," [11] and "Free radicals and antioxidants: updating a personal review" [12].

One complementary treatise to Halliwell and Gutteridge's book(s) is the classic review by Dröge: "Free Radicals in the Physiological Control of Cell Function" [13]. This paper is a relatively early attempt to summarize and categorize the redox effects of reactive species on cellular physiology. Dröge himself characterized the paper as a "...broad overview that summarizes the main principles of redox regulation" that "...describes the current knowledge and paradigms...but does not discuss future research directions, historical controversies or experimental methods.".

A useful and fairly complete tutorial of redox biochemistry is the book by I. Acworth, entitled "The Handbook of Redox Biochemistry" [14]. This reference situates itself more or less equally between chemistry and biology, with numerous helpful appendices on more specialized topics topics such as electrode potentials. Another, more recent tutorial reference is "Teaching the basics of redox biology to medical and graduate students: Oxidants, antioxidants and disease mechanisms," by B. Kalyanaraman [15]. Finally, the tutorial Khan Academy videos, available free online, are helpful initial introductions to basic ideas (e.g. for cellular respiration or redox biology), at essentially a high school or beginning university level.

Outstanding state-of-the-art reviews on redox biology include the previously mentioned mini-review by Herrmann and Dick: "Redox biology on the rise" [1]; "The redox code" by Jones and Sies [16]; "Cellular mechanisms and physiological consequences of redox- dependent signalling" by Holmstrom and Finkel [17]; and "Redox interplay between mitochondria and peroxisomes," by Lismont et al. [18].

The multifaceted set of roles of nitric oxide and its related compounds has prompted detailed study. Two of the many key papers on these compounds include [19] paper "Nitric oxide, superoxide, peroxynitrite: the good, the bad and the ugly." Nitric oxide (NO) is produced enzymatically by the various isoforms of nitric oxide synthase. As NO readily passes through biological membranes, it may find its reaction partner distant of the site of generation. Superoxide ($O_2^-$) is also produced enzymatically with NADPH oxidase and other enzymes. If a molecule of $O_2^-$ is near a molecule of NO, they react rapidly to form peroxynitrite ($ONOO^-$), a powerful and potentially damaging oxidizing agent. When peroxynitrite is generated close to membrane-associated protein pumps, the generation of peroxynitrous acid seems to be the favoured reaction [20]. Peroxynitrous acid spontaneously decomposes into $NO_2$ and hydroxyl radicals that may attack the membrane. Distant from the cell membrane, the reaction between peroxynitrite and $CO_2$ is favoured and leads to the formation of nitrosoperoxycarboxylate. This compound decomposes into $NO_2$ and carbonate radicals. Another comprehensive review on NO is "Nitric Oxide and Peroxynitrite in Health and Disease" by Pacher et al., published in [21]. The latter publication covers the history of the recognition of the importance of RNS in redox biology. The direct connections between these RNS species and CAP are detailed in subsequent sections.

Redox plant biology is admirably summarized in the 2009 review "Redox Regulation in Photosynthetic Organisms: Signaling, Acclimation and Practical Implications," by Foyer and Noctor [22]. Torres' [23] review "ROS in biotic interactions" emphasizes the role of reactive oxygen in the response of plants to pathogen attack.

## 4.3 The Role of RONS in Established Therapies: Cancer Therapy

The role of RONS, and especially ROS, in cancer initiation and progression has been a topic of intense debate for many years. The traditional view is that RONS are exclusively detrimental with respect to cancer. There is, for example, considerable evidence that continued exposure to elevated levels of RONS can lead to oncogenic DNA mutation. (e.g. [24]) Naturally, investigators thought of using antioxidants to prevent cancer occurrence and/or to treat existing tumors. However, multiple large scale clinical trials showed that antioxidants do not have the desired anti-cancer effects Gill et al. [24] summarize the current view in the literature in their conclusion:

> ROS promote cancer initiation by promoting mutagenesis and perhaps by activating signaling pathways that promote proliferation, survival, and stress resistance. However, ROS also limits cancer initiation and progression by causing oxidative stress that kills many cancer cells. For this reason, cancer cells depend on a variety of mechanisms to suppress ROS and to cope with oxidative stress. Antioxidants promote cancer initiation and progression in experimental mouse models as well as in clinical trials. Cancer may be more effectively treated with pro-oxidants that exacerbate the oxidative stress experienced by cancer cells or that prevent metabolic adaptations that confer oxidative stress resistance.

The situation is more complex than might be thought, however. For example, antioxidants like anthocyanidins have been shown to mediate a pro-oxidative effect selectively on tumor cells and cause their RONS-mediated apoptosis [25]. This apparent paradox is explained by the modulation of NO metabolism by the antioxidant, resulting finally in the generation of singlet oxygen and subsequent release of RONS from catalase-mediated control. It has been suggested that the antioxidant nature of anthocyanidins, i.e. their potential to donate electrons, interferes with the activity of NO dioxygenase [26].

Many groups have made similar points regarding the generally anti-tumor effects of pro-oxidant compounds, including Trachootham et al. [27, 28]; Schumaker [29, 30] and Gorrini et al. [31] among numerous others. Gorrini et al. [31] list over 20 treatments and drugs that either directly or indirectly act to therapeutically increase RONS levels in cancer treatment.

One of the most important cancer therapies is the use of ionizing radiation—either photons or energetic particles—that will both directly cause DNA double strand breaks and will also indirectly kill cells by creating radicals such as OH from interactions with cellular water. The indirect radical generation approach is thought to be responsible for more than half of the effects of ionizing radiation Baskar et al. [32]. The mechanisms by which radiation-generated radicals affect cells are therefore potentially relevant to CAP-generated RONS.

A relatively early paper highlighting the role of reactive oxygen and nitrogen in radiation biology and therapy was published by Mikkelson and Wardman, entitled "Biological chemistry of reactive oxygen and nitrogen and radiation induced signal transduction mechanisms" [33]. In this paper, the connection between the initial ionization events in cells exposed to therapeutic doses of ionizing radiation and subsequent creation of RONS that act as signaling agents, is emphasized. Ward had pointed out previously [34] that relatively few primary ionization events in cells exposed to therapeutic doses of radiation somehow result in a "...rapid and robust activation of cellular signal transduction pathways." It appears that RONS released in the initial burst of radiation are rapidly amplified by cellular cytoplasmic responses. RONS signaling must involve two steps in series, these authors concluded. Highly reactive oxygen species such as OH radicals, created following the initial cellular radiation, result in the generation of RONS as the actual "...effector/activators of the redox-dependent cellular signal transduction pathway." In line with these concepts, Temme and Bauer showed that low doses of gamma irradiation triggered a TGF-beta1-mediated bystander effect that resulted in substantial increase in NOX1-derived extracellular superoxide anions [6].

We would not necessarily expect CAP to behave exactly the same way as ionizing radiation in its effects on cells, if for no other reason than CAP acts primarily on the surface of tissue whereas radiation penetrates deeply into tissues. However, the fact that any non-superficial effects of CAP must be translated some distance into tissue suggests that an analogous signaling mechanism is likely to be involved. An important corollary of cell signaling induced by radiation is the so-called 'bystander effect' in which non-exposed cells near exposed cells experience the same or similar effects as directly exposed cells. A more general term for the cell-to-cell communication that can take place following ionizing radiation exposure is 'non-targeted effects' (NTE). Mavragani et al. [35] summarize current ideas about these processes. These authors note that oxidative mechanisms seem to be among the most important stressors inducing NTE. This topic is closely related to CAP-induced immune stimulation, a topic addressed later in this and subsequent chapters.

An alternative theory for CAP-dependent RONS signal transduction in cancer treatment has been recently proposed by Bauer and Graves [8] and Bauer [26, 36, 37]. These ideas focus on the notion of intercellular signaling rather than emphasizing intracellular phenomena. An important specie in these models of CAP in cancer treatment is the singlet delta oxygen molecule ($^1O_2$). It is known that this specie can be created in the gas phase by CAP, but it is less well known that it can be created by secondary aqueous phase reactions as well, starting with species that are well known to be created in CAP. This is summarized in a set of reactions listed in Table 4.2 and illustrated schematically in Fig. 4.2. Bauer [26, 36, 37] describes how these ideas are consistent with other recent CAP anti-cancer mechanisms. For example, Yan et al. (2016) [38] emphasize the role of cellular $H_2O_2$ generated following CAP exposure. Lin et al. (2016) [39] show evidence that CAP stimulates immune responses.

In addition to radiation-induced RONS anti-cancer activity, photodynamic therapy (PDT) is known to act through generation of reactive species. In PDT, a tumor-localizing photosensitizer compound is either systemically or locally given to the patient. The photosensitizer is then activated by exposure to red light, creating an electronically excited state that converts tissue-present ground state triplet $O_2$ to an

**Table 4.2** Aqueous reactions related to $^1O_2$ from CAP-generated species in solution (following [8, 36])

| |
|---|
| $H_2O_2 + ONOO^- \rightarrow {}^1O_2 + H_2O + NO_2^-$ (direct interaction suggested by Di Mascio et al. [53] |
| *Alternative mechanistic explanation # 1 ([8]):* |
| $ONOO^- + H^+ \rightarrow ONOOH$ |
| $ONOOH \rightarrow {}^\cdot NO_2 + {}^\cdot OH$ |
| ${}^\cdot OH + H_2O_2 \rightarrow HO_2^\cdot + H_2O$ |
| $HO_2^\cdot + O_2^{\cdot -} + H^+ \rightarrow H_2O_2 + {}^1O_2$ |
| $2\ HO_2^\cdot \rightarrow H_2O_2 + {}^1O_2$ |
| *Alternative mechanistic explanation # 2 ([26]):* |
| $ONOO^- + H^+ \rightarrow ONOOH$ |
| $ONOOH \rightarrow {}^\cdot NO_2 + {}^\cdot OH$ |
| ${}^\cdot OH + H_2O_2 \rightarrow HO_2^\cdot + H_2O$ |
| $HO_2^\cdot + {}^\cdot NO_2 \rightarrow O_2NOOH$ (peroxynitric acid) |
| $O_2NOOH \rightarrow O_2NOO^- + H^+$ (peroxynitrate) |
| $O_2NOO^- \rightarrow NO_2^- + {}^1O_2$ ( 50%) |
| $O_2NOO^- \rightarrow {}^\cdot NO_2 + O_2^{\cdot -}$ ( 50%) |
| *Consumption of peroxynitrite by $CO_2$:* |
| $ONOO^- + CO_2 \rightarrow ONOOCOO^-$ |
| $ONOOCOO^- \rightarrow {}^\cdot NO_2 + CO_3^{\cdot -}$ |

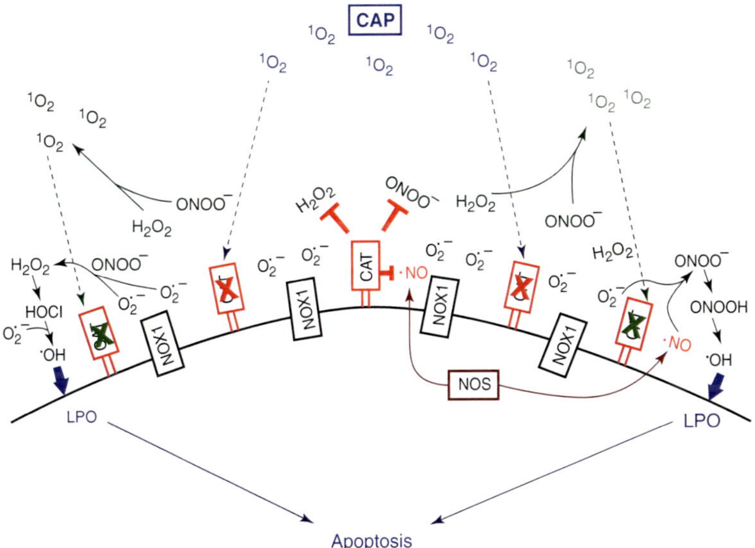


**Fig. 4.2** Summary of proposed model of CAP-generated $^1O_2$ leading to tumor cell apoptosis. Tumor cells create excess superoxide ($O_2^-$) in the vicinity of the cell membrane via enzyme NADPH oxidase (NOX1). Local $O_2^-$ can lead to tumor cell apoptosis either by forming peroxynitrite (via NO reaction) and/or hypochlorous acid via reaction with $H_2O_2$. The two major intercellular signalling processes involve ONOOH and HOCl that in turn lead to OH radical, but membrane-bound catalase (CAT) will abrogate this signalling. In order to selectively remove tumor cells, CAP must selectively eliminate CAT. Singlet delta $^1O_2$ is proposed to selectively inactivate membrane-bound catalase (CAT), leading ultimately to lipid peroxidation (LPO) and tumor cell apoptosis. This process is self-perpetuating, creating a wave of apoptotic tumor cells, as $^1O_2$ moves to adjacent cells and repeats the process (following [8]). The generation of $^1O_2$ through the interaction between $H_2O_2$ and peroxynitrite is more complex than the simplified direct interaction in the graph. This aspect is discussed in Bauer [26, 36]

excited state singlet delta $^1O_2$ (SDO). This ROS then reacts with various biomolecules in the adjacent tumor, inducing apoptotic or necrotic tumor cell death. It can also act against tumor vasculature and induce an immune response Dolmans et al. [40]. Although less well known and less widely used than radiation therapy, the modern use of PDT was developed for various therapeutic applications (e.g. for cancer and macular degeneration), starting in the 1970s [40].

CAP-mediated antitumor effects through singlet oxygen [8, 36] and PDT differ in the primary site of singlet oxygen action. Whereas CAP-derived singlet oxygen targets the control system of tumor cells on the outside of their membrane, singlet oxygen generation during PTD occurs intracellularly. Model experiments by Riethmüller et al. [41] have shown that intracellular singlet oxygen induces cell death in malignant and nonmalignant cells, whereas extracellular singlet oxygen causes a selective effect in malignant cells. Therefore, selectivity of PDT has to be achieved through enrichment of the photosensitizer in the tumor and site-specific illumination of the tumor to activate singlet oxygen generation, whereas CAP-derived singlet oxygen shows selective antitumor action per se, with an auto-amplificatory potential [8].

## 4.4 Nitric Oxide and Related Compounds

The fact that CAP can generate significant quantities of nitric oxide (NO) and related compounds such as $NO_2$, could be important in therapeutic applications of CAP [42]. NO is one of the few gaseous molecules that have been directly applied to tissue for proven therapeutic purposes. NO gas is currently used for delivery into the lungs of neonatal babies with pulmonary hypertension and severe hypoxic respiratory failure, although it is still considered experimental. NO acts as a pulmonary vasodilator in this application and has been used for adult respiratory distress syndrome as well as chronic obstructive pulmonary disease, although efficacy is not well established. Another area of intense investigation in the previous several decades is the use of NO donor drugs [43]. NO has also been extensively studied for its anti-cancer use. It has been identified as a compound that re-establish radiation- and chemotherapeutic-sensitivity to tumors [44].

The concentration of NO can be dramatically lowered through oxidation by compound I of catalase—a process that seems to take place at the surface of tumor cells. However, above a critical level, NO may turn the tables and inhibit catalase, thus opening novel RONS pathways [20, 26]. A related topic is the therapeutic use of aqueous nitrite ($NO_2^-$), a compound that has been widely observed in water adjacent to CAP in air (e.g. [45]). This water is sometimes referred to as 'plasma-activated water,' or PAW. In addition, $H_2O_2$ is commonly observed in PAW, and it has been shown that the well-known reaction between $H_2O_2$ and $NO_2^-$ under low pH conditions to form $ONOO^-$, a well-known biologically active molecule, as noted above [46]. Nitrite has been widely investigated for its ability to act, in part, as a source of biologically active nitric oxide (e.g. [47]). It also was suggested that peroxynitrite formed through the interaction between nitrite and $H_2O_2$ might interact with residual $H_2O_2$ and thus lead to the generation of singlet oxygen [37]. Though the concentration of singlet oxygen generated in this way can be expected to be relatively low, its specific interaction with tumor cells, leading to the generation of cell-derived extracellular singlet oxygen might cause sensitization of the tumor cells for RONS-mediated apoptosis induction.

## 4.5 Possible Mechanistic Models of RONS-Based CAP Therapies

One key concept regarding RONS-based therapies is that they can act only, or at least primarily, as triggers to longer time- and length-scale biological responses. This reasoning mimics that of Mikkelson and Wardman when they postulate highly reactive ionizing radiation-induced ROS (e.g. OH radicals) as the initiating factor in cellular signaling, but more stable RNS as the effectors of the cell signaling processes that lead to therapeutic effects. RONS that result from reactions following the biological creation of $O_2^-$ (e.g. by the enzyme NADPH oxidase, abbreviated NOX1) and NO (by enzyme nitric oxide synthase, abbreviated NOS) are illustrated in Fig. 4.3 [33].

RONS are applied at surfaces and have relatively short lifetimes. Any effect that occurs deeper in tissue must come from the biological responses of the system in its attempt to maintain homeostasis. This mechanistic argument is consistent with the knowledge that cells respond to stress by communicating to nearby cells. Stressed cells are also known to react by adapting or dying—they either become 'hardened' to additional stresses or they undergo some cell death process (e.g. apoptosis, necrosis,

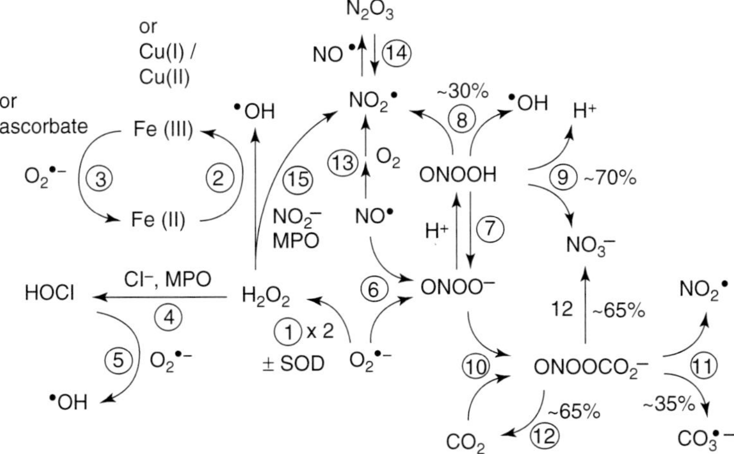


**Fig. 4.3** Main reactions following creation of $O_2^-$ and NO in biological systems. Superoxide and nitric oxide are also present in aqueous samples exposed to CAP (see Table 4.1), and it is expected that many of the illustrated reactions will also occur even in the absence of biologically created RONS (following [33])

autophagy, or some combination). Tissue has a way to engage in 'bystander signaling' or the 'bystander effect.' One example of cell adaptation to stress is physical exercise. Exercise is known to generate oxidative stress, but if the stress is not excessive, cells can adapt and become stronger. This is an example of the concept of 'hormesis' in which cells either adapt at relatively low levels of the applied stress or die if the stress becomes too great (e.g. [48]). One way to think of CAP and RONS-based therapies is to first recognize that cells normally respond to RONS signaling in their endogenous stress response. Thus a short (~1 min) CAP exposure to tissue might be similar in effect to an innate immune system oxidative (or respiratory) burst. In effect, the CAP treatment mimics an immune response to tissue damage, wounds or infection. This could initiate a natural healing response. This idea—modeling CAP therapy as an oxy-nitroso shielding burst—was previously described in detail [49].

## 4.6 CAP-Generated RONS and Immune Response

It is known that many different physico-chemical treatment protocols can stimulate immunogenic cell death (ICD) and a corresponding adaptive immune response. Methods that have been reported to be capable of stimulating an adaptive immune response include ionizing radiation, ultraviolet C light, photodynamic therapy, high hydrostatic pressure, hyperthermia and electrochemotherapy [50, 51]. CAP is reported to also have this capability and it is likely that CAP-generated RONS play some role in the triggering of ICD [39, 52]. As noted in Chap. 16, CAP can induce immunogenic cell death, with an accompanying T cell response at positions far from the site of CAP treatment. Bauer [36] describes in detail a model that couples what is known or suspected about inactivation of tumor membrane resident catalase, generation of secondary singlet oxygen, intercellular RONS signaling, $H_2O_2$/aquaporin mediated effects, and immune cell stimulation.

## References


1. Herrmann J, Dick T. Redox biology on the rise. Biol Chem. 2012;393(9):999–1004.
2. Trefil J, Morowitz H, Smith E. The origin of life: a case is made for the descent of electrons. Am Sci. 2009;97:206–13.
3. Graves DB. The emerging role of reactive oxygen and nitrogen species in redox biology and some implications for plasma applications to medicine and biology. J Phys D Appl Phys. 2012;45:263001.
4. Lackmann J-W, Baldus S, Steinborn E, Edengeiser E, Kogelheide F, Langklotz S, Schneider S, Leichert LIO, Benedikt J, Awakowicz P, Bandow JE. A dielectric barrier discharge terminally inactivates RNase A by oxidizing sulfur-containing amino acids and breaking structural disulfide bonds. J Phys D Appl Phys. 2015;48:494003. https://doi.org/10.1088/0022-3727/48/49/494003.
5. Barcellos-Hoff MH, Dix AT. Redox-mediated activation of latent transforming growth factor-beta-1. Mol Endocrinol. 1996;10:1077–83.
6. Temme J, Bauer G. Low-dose gamma irradiation enhances superoxide anion production by nonirradiated cells through TGF-β1-dependent bystander signaling. Radiat Res. 2013;179:422–32.

7. Kim YK, Kwon OJ, Park J-W. Inactivation of catalase and superoxide dismutase by singlet oxygen derived from photoactivated dye. Biochimie. 2001;83:437–44.
8. Bauer G, Graves DB. Mechanisms of selective antitumor action of cold atmospheric plasma-derived reactive oxygen and nitrogen species. Plasma Process Polym. 2016;13:1157–78. https://doi.org/10.1002/ppap.201600089.
9. Halliwell B, Gutteridge JMC. Free radicals in biology and medicine By Barry Halliwell and John M. C. Gutteridge. 5th ed. New York: Oxford University Press; 2015.
10. Nespolo M. Book review: free radicals in biology and medicine by Barry Halliwell and John M. C. Gutteridge. 5th ed. New York: Oxford University Press; 2015.
11. Halliwell B. Reactive species and antioxidants. Redox biology is a fundamental theme of aerobic life. Plant Physiol. 2006;141:312.
12. Halliwell B. Free radicals and antioxidants: updating a personal review. Nutr Rev. 2012; 70(5):257–65.
13. Droge W. Free radicals in the physiological control of cell function. Physiol Rev. 2002;82:47.
14. Acworth I. The handbook of redox biochemistry. Chelmsford: ESA Biosciences; 2003.
15. Kalyanaraman B. Teaching the basics of redox biology to medical and graduate students: oxidants, antioxidants and disease mechanisms. Redox Biol. 2013;1:244–57.
16. Jones D, Sies H. The redox code. Antioxid Redox Signal. 2015;23(9):734–46.
17. Holmstrom K, Finkel T. Cellular mechanisms and physiological consequences of redox-dependent signalling. Nat Rev Mol Cell Biol. 2014;15(6):411–21.
18. Lismont C, Nordgren M, Van Veldhoven PP, Fransen M. Redox interplay between mitochondria and peroxisomes. Front Cell Dev Biol. 2015;3:35.
19. Beckman J, Koppenol W. Nitric oxide, superoxide, peroxynitrite: the good, the bad and the ugly. Am J Physiol. 1996;271(5 Pt 1):C1424–37.
20. Bauer G. Increasing the endogenous NO level causes catalase inactivation and reactivation of intercellular apoptosis signaling specifically in tumor cells. Redox Biol. 2015;6:353–71.
21. Pacher P, Beckman JS, Liaudet L. Nitric oxide and peroxynitrite in health and disease. Physiol Rev. 2007;87:315.
22. Foyer CH, Noctor G. Redox regulation in photosynthetic organisms: signaling, acclimation, and practical implications. Antioxid Redox Signal. 2009;11:861–905.
23. Torres MA. ROS in biotic interactions. Physiol Plant. 2010;138:414–29.
24. Gill J, Piskounova E, Morrison SJ. Cancer, oxidative stress, and metastasis. Cold Spring Harb Symp Quant Biol. 2016;81:163–75.
25. Scheit K, Bauer G. Direct and indirect inactivation of tumor cell protective catalase by salicylic acid and anthocyanidins reactivates intercellular ROS signaling and allows for synergistic effects. Carcinogenesis. 2015;36:400–11.
26. Bauer G. Nitric oxide contributes to selective apoptosis induction in malignant cells through multiple reaction steps. Crit Rev Oncog. 2016;i21(5–6):365–98. DOI: 10.1615/CritRevOncog.2017021056.
27. Trachootham D, Zhou Y, Zhang H, Demizu Y, Chen Z, Pelicano H, Chiao PJ, Achanta G, Arlinghaus RB, Liu J, Huang P. Selective killing of oncogenically transformed cells through a ROS-mediated mechanism by beta-phenylethyl isothiocyanate. Cancer Cell. 2006;10(3): 241–52.
28. Trachootham D, Alexandre J, Huang P. Targeting cancer cells by ROS-mediated mechanisms: a radical therapeutic approach? Nat Rev Drug Discov. 2009;8:579–91.
29. Schumaker P. Reactive oxygen species in cancer cells: live by the sword, die by the sword. Cancer Cell. 2006;10(3):175–6.
30. Schumaker P. Reactive oxygen species in cancer: a dance with the devil. Cancer Cell. 2015;27(2):156–7.
31. Gorrini C, Harris I, Mak T. Modulation of oxidative stress as an anticancer strategy. Nat Rev Drug Discov. 2013;12:931–47.
32. Baskar R, Dai J, Wenlong N, Yeo R, Yeoh K-W. Biological response of cancer cells to radiation treatment. Front Mol Biosci. 2014;1(24).1–9.

33. Mikkelsen RB, Wardman P. Biological chemistry of reactive oxygen and nitrogen and radiation-induced signal transduction mechanisms. Oncogene. 2003;22:5734–54.
34. Ward JF. DNA damage as the cause of ionizing radiation-induced gene activation. Radiat Res. 1994;138:S85–8.
35. Mavragani I, et al. Key mechanisms involved in ionizing radiation-induced systemic effects. A current review. Toxicol Res. 2016;5:12–33.
36. Bauer G. Signal amplification by tumor cells: clue to the understanding of the antitumor effects of cold atmospheric plasma and plasma-activated medium. IEEE Transactions on Radiation and Plasma Medical Sciences. 2018;2: 87–98. DOI: 10.1109.TRPMS.2017.2742000.
37. Bauer G. Targeting the protective catalase of tumor cells with cold atmospheric plasma-treated medium (PAM). Anticancer Agents Med Chem. 2017. DOI: 10.2174/1871520617666170801103708. (in press).
38. Yan D, Xiao H, Zhu W, Nourmohammadi N, Zhang L, Bian K, Keidar M. The role of aquaporins in the anti-glioblastoma capacity of the cold plasma-stimulated medium. J Phys D Appl Phys. 2017;50(5):055401.
39. Lin A, Truong B, Pappas A, Kirifides L, Oubarri A, Chen S, Lin S, Dobrynin D, Fridman G, Fridman A, Sang N, Miller V. Uniform nanosecond pulsed dielectric barrier discharge plasma enhances anti-tumor effects by induction of immunogenic cell death in tumors and stimulation of macrophages. Plasma Process Polym. 2015;12:1392–9.
40. Dolmans D, Fukumura D, Jain RK. Photodynamic therapy for cancer. Nature. 2003;3:1–8.
41. Riethmüller M, Burger N, Bauer G. Singlet oxygen treatment of tumor cells triggers extracellular singlet oxygen generation, catalase inactivation and reactivation of intercellular apoptosis-inducing signaling. Redox Biol. 2015;6:157–68.
42. Suschek C, Opländer C. The application of cold atmospheric plasma in medicine: the potential role of nitric oxide in plasma-induced effects. Clin Plasma Med. 2016;4:1–8.
43. Wang P, Xian M, Tang X, Wu X, Wen Z, Cai T, Janczuk J. Nitric oxide donors: chemical activities and biological applications. Chem Rev. 2002;102(4):1091–134.
44. Coulter J, et al. Nitric oxide—a novel therapeutic for cancer. Nitric Oxide. 2008;19:192–8.
45. Kamgang-Youbi G, Herry JM, Meylheuc T, Brisset JL, Bellon-Fontaine MN, Doubla A, Naïtali M. Microbial inactivation using plasma-activated water obtained by gliding electric discharges. Lett Appl Microbiol. 2009;48(1):13–8.
46. Lukes P, Dolezalova E, Sisrova I, Clupek M. Aqueous-phase chemistry and bactericidal effects from an air discharge plasma in contact with water: evidence for the formation of peroxynitrite through a pseudo-second-order post-discharge reaction of $H_2O_2$ and $HNO_2$. Plasma Sources Sci Technol. 2014;23:015019.
47. Lundberg JO, Weitzberg E, Gladwin MT. The nitrate–nitrite–nitric oxide pathway in physiology and therapeutics. Nat Rev Drug Discov. 2008;7:15.
48. Graves DB. Reactive species from cold atmospheric plasma: implications for cancer therapy. Plasma Process Polym. 2014;11:1120.
49. Graves DB. Oxy-nitroso shielding burst model of cold atmospheric plasma therapeutics. Clin Plasma Med. 2014;2:38.
50. Adkins I, Fucikova J, Garg A, Agostinis P, Spisek R. Physical modalities inducing immunogenic tumor cell death for cancer immunotherapy. Oncoimmunology. 3(12):e968434. https://doi.org/10.4161/21624011.2014.968434.
51. Calvet C, Mir L. The promising alliance of anti-cancer electrochemotherapy with immunotherapy. Cancer Metastasis Rev. 2016;35:165–77.
52. Mizuno K, Yonetamari K, Shirakawa Y, Akiyama T, Ono R. Anti-tumor immune response induced by nanosecond pulsed streamer discharge in mice. J Phys D Appl Phys. 2017;50:12LT01. https://doi.org/10.1088/1361-6463/aa5dbb.
53. Di Mascio P, Bechara EJH, Medeiros MHG, Briviba K, Sies H. Singlet molecular oxygen production in the reaction of peroxynitrite with hydrogen peroxide. FEBS Lett. 1994;355:287–9.

# Safety Aspects of Non-Thermal Plasmas

5

Kristian Wende, Anke Schmidt, and Sander Bekeschus

## 5.1 Preface

Non-thermal plasmas potentially pose a number of chemical and physical threats of different levels to the human or animal organism. In order to increase safety and acceptance of this novel treatment strategy, they need to be addressed as broad as possible. Clearly, the risk potential is predetermined by the design of the plasma source and its operation strategy, e.g. if we compare a jet based source and volume dielectric barrier discharge, two source varying largely in electrode design and electrical powering. This and the working gas composition (e.g. ambient air, noble gases), the size of the active plasma zone and its position in the system all affect the reactive species and radiation output, and with that the potential impact created by the plasma. In addition, the intended application field influences the risk management: a plasma source intended for surface refinement of an implant and source to be used in the oral cavity will need to be treated differently. Further the assumed operator, e.g. a health care professional on one hand, a consumer or an engineer on the other, calls for a differentiated evaluation. Finally, the developmental stage of the plasma source affects the risk potential and must be considered.

K. Wende (✉) • S. Bekeschus
Center for Innovation Competence (ZIK),
Plasmatis—Plasma Plus Cell at Leibniz Institute for
Plasma Science and Technology (INP Greifswald),
Greifswald, Germany
e-mail: kristian.wende@inp-greifswald.de; sander.bekeschus@inp-greifswald.de

A. Schmidt
Leibniz Institute for Plasma Science and Technology (INP Greifswald),
Greifswald, Germany
e-mail: anke.schmidt@inp-greifswald.de



H.-R. Metelmann et al. (eds.), *Comprehensive Clinical Plasma Medicine*,
https://doi.org/10.1007/978-3-319-67627-2_5

## 5.2 Potential Physical Hazards of Non-Thermal Plasmas

Non-thermal atmospheric pressure plasmas, or cold plasmas, are multi-component gas-like systems. Upon energy input, a number of atoms or molecules of a gas are dissociated. The resulting excited or ionized gas particles (either atoms or molecules, depending on the gas) on one side and the free electrons on the other side may subsequently trigger further physicochemical reactions. In a cold plasma, the percentage of dissociated particles is low, and the discharge is not self-sustaining—permanent energy input is necessary (non-equilibrium plasmas). Therefore, we have a small amount of fast (energy-rich) electrons, ions or excited states within a dominant background of unaltered gas particles. With that, the energy of most particles is very low. Interspersed energy rich, fast particles (=hot) increase the mean energy only a little—so cold plasmas for biomedical applications are typically cool to the touch. However, not completely ionized gases are by definition cold plasmas, and temperatures can be as high as 10,000°K. Alongside with thermal energy, plasmas also emit energy at other wavelength of the electromagnetic spectrum. Especially excited states (=gas particles which absorbed energy, e.g. by being hit by an electron) can return to the ground state by emitting a photon. These photons are representatives for the plasma they have been created in and can be used for diagnostic purposes as number and wavelength differ with the plasma source. Especially photons belonging to the ultraviolet region of the light (Vacuum-UV, UV-C, UV-B, UV-A) contain enough energy to interact with biomolecules and needs to be taken into consideration for the risk assessment. In addition, electrical currents and electrical fields can be emitted by the plasma if electrode geometry and source design permits. This type of energy emission is least investigated, and due to the comparable low capability to interact with biomolecules, is assumed to play a smaller role.

Finally, beside the physical forms of energy emission, also chemical energy is spilling from cold plasmas (see Sect. 5.3 “Potential chemical hazards of non-thermal plasmas”). This and the interconnection of the described energy emission processes of a plasma make selective experimental approaches to substantiate or to reject the risk of a single entity very complex. Accordingly, experiments performed to assess the safety of medical plasma applications usually use a holistic approach.

### 5.2.1 Emission of Thermal Energy

Non-thermal plasmas for biomedical applications should be cool or cold to the touch in order to avoid thermal damage to the tissue (hyperthermia). This may occur, if the temperature exceeds 43 ° C. The damage relates to the thermal dose a tissue receives according to

$$CEM_{43} = DtR^{(43-T)},$$

where $CEM_{43}$ is the cumulative equivalent minutes at 43 °C, T the average temperature during the time interval tm, and R is a constant equal to 0.25 for $T < 43$ °C and 0.5 for $T > 43$ °C [1]. Local hyperthermia results in changes to the cell membrane and molecular structures, edema formation, time-dependent cell death (necrosis, apoptosis) and devitalization. Higher temperatures can cause protein and collagen denaturation as well as membrane destruction up to evaporation of cell liquid. For full human skin it has been shown, that 48 °C for 2 s results in no damage, and 6 s at 59 °C just starts to create a blister [2]. In contrast, when looking at the single cell level of *in vitro* experiments, cell necrosis can be observed for all temperatures above 42 °C [2].

All modern cold plasma sources are engineered to avoid excessive temperatures. For the argon jet kINPen09 several works related to this topic have been published [3–5] (Fig. 5.1).

While the effluent temperature may reach up to 62 °C [5], the temperature at 9–12 mm (= treatment distance) is just below to above 40 °C, depending on the power. Any thermal damage of the skin can be disregarded assuming a typical brush-type treatment regimen with a velocity of about 10 mm/s [3]. This result has been reproduced with the kINPen Med, which was optimized for medical applications (lower patient leakage current), and no damage could be found even for slower that typical treatment velocities (6–8 mm/s) using intravital confocal microscopy [4]. Several case studies in humans using various plasma sources did not observe any deterioration due to thermal effects [6–8]. In mice, using a dielectric barrier gun discharge, no thermal lesion were observed for up to 15 min treatment [9]. In recent wound healing studies in mice no thermal damage to the wound bed, or the intact epithelium around it have been observed for treatment times of up to 20 s for small wound areas about 3 mm$^2$ [10]. Similar results have been obtained for the SteriPlas [7, 11] and the PlasmaDerm [12].

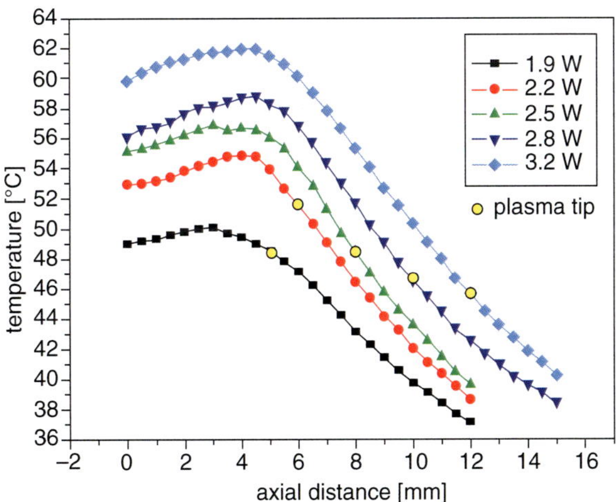


**Fig. 5.1** Thermal profile of the kINPen 09 using 3 standard liter/minute (slm) of argon gas flow [5]

**In summary:**
In approved plasma sources, thermal damage can be disregarded if recommendations for the application are followed.

### 5.2.2 Emission of Ultraviolet Radiation

Depending on geometric factors, energy input, electrode configuration, and working gas composition plasmas emit light of various wavelength [13, 14]. The sum intensity may reach relevant levels, especially in small and condensed geometries, like in jet-type plasma sources [15, 16].

Ultraviolet radiation is an interesting facet of light due to its ability to interact with biomolecules. Depending on the wavelength (vacuum UV 100–200 nm, UVC 201–280 nm, UVB 281–315 nm, UVA 316–400 nm), photon energies lie between 12.4 eV or 1200 kJ $mol^{-1}$ (100 nm) and 3.1 eV or 300 kJ $mol^{-1}$ (400 nm). Accordingly, the fission of chemical bonds is possible: many single bonds in organic molecules have bond energies starting from 305 kJ $mol^{-1}$ (C-N) and 347 kJ $mol^{-1}$ (C-C)[1]. Such, photochemical processes can be triggered, especially with large, heteroatom-rich biomolecules like proteins or DNA [17]. The penetration depth in biological systems correlates inversely with energy: light below 200 nm is absorbed by the ambient atmosphere and cannot penetrate water. UVC is blocked by ozone and oxygen but can penetrate water. UVB and UVA are only reduced, not blocked by the components of the atmosphere, especially ozone. In skin, some UVB can penetrate into the intact dermis whereas UVA penetrates even better and deeper. The highly energetic UVC is blocked, e.g. by urocaninic acid [18]. With damaged skin, situation changes. The keratohyalin forming the *stratum corneum* is missing, as is the coat of natural sun screens (e.g. urocaninic acid), increasing potentially the sensitivity towards UV light. Excessive UV radiation leads to erythema, early skin aging, and melanoma [19]. This is triggered by photoreaction with the DNA of sufficiently superficial cells, leading to dimerization of nucleotides (CPD, cyclobutane pyrimidine dimers or pyrimidine-(6–4)-pyrimidone dimers) or oxidation (8-oxoguanine) [17]. As a result, DNA damage repair of the cells is finally overridden and dermal fibroblast cells undergo senescence (UVA-related) or melanoma cells transform into cancer cells (UVB-driven) [20]. However, UV radiation is also a valuable medical tool and is used, typically in combination with sensitizers in the concept of photodynamic therapy (PDT), for the treatment of vitiligo [21, 22], psoriasis [23], and cancer [24, 25].

In plasma medicine, two contradictory concepts significantly influencing the impact of UV from the plasma source are used: direct treatment and indirect treatment [26–28]. In indirect treatment, interaction of the radiation with cellular DNA is shunned. Instead, photoproducts of the treated transfer liquid may occur, e.g. atomic hydrogen and hydroxyl radicals from water photolysis [29, 30]. Due to their short live time, it is unlikely that they will play a role in the clinical effects observable, even when reacting with dissolved oxygen $O_2$ forming hydroperoxide ($H_2O_2$). Alternatively, photochemical processes may modify organic components of complex liquids like cell culture medium, but information is scarce [31]. In contrast, direct plasma treatment of skin or cancer lesions can be performed and is the

[1] https://chem.libretexts.org/Core/Physical_and_Theoretical_Chemistry/Chemical_Bonding/Fundamentals_of_Chemical_Bonding/Bond_Energies.

mode of choice for many surgical clinicians [32]. Here, UV radiation may attribute to the effectivity. However, total photon fluxes are limited. It has been shown for the helium COST jet (e.g. Bochum) that the plasma generated UV light diminished the growth of microorganisms, but the combination of UV and plasma generated chemical entities was much more effective [15]. For the kINPen, a UV radiation in the UVB-range of 0.35 $W_{eff}$ $m^{-2}$ was measured [5]. Hence, if a one $cm^2$ areal is treated for the maximal recommend 60 s, only one $J_{eff}$ $m^{-2}$ UV is delivered which is well below the ICNIRP[2] recommendations (30 $J_{eff}$ $m^{-2}$). A possible transmission of vacuum UV along with the noble gas flow axis can be neglected as it is immediately quenched by oxygen or traces of water. Accordingly, observed clinical effects are mainly attributed to plasma generated reactive oxygen (ROS) and nitrogen species (RNS). Dielectric barrier discharges running in ambient atmosphere usually emit only very low fluxes of photons, limiting the impact of UV light on their *in vitro* and *in vivo* effectivity. A DBD (Cinogy GmbH) was found to produce 0.016 $W_{eff}$ $m^{-2}$ UV light [33]. However, UV emission of DBD can be increased under special conditions, e.g. by using a $N_2$-$N_2O$ atmosphere [34] or cascade of DBDs [35]. Photon fluxes are orders of magnitude higher in low pressure plasmas, especially if designed as light source [36]. Such devices must be considered separately, as here the impact of UV may dominate the observable effects/efficacies [37].

**In summary:**
Non-thermal plasmas can produce UV light if geometry and electrode configuration allow, with jets emitting usually higher photon fluxes than DBDs. Accordingly, UV radiation must be taken into account, both, for plasma source risk assessment and clinical effectivity. UVB and UVA dominate short wave UV light. As far as information is available, overall safety impact of UV light is limited.

### 5.2.3 Electrical Currents and Electrical Fields

Most plasma sources for biomedical application are powered by electricity. Depending on the type of discharge (plasma jet, dielectric barrier discharge, etc.), the electrode design and position, the driving frequencies of the electrical current, the general power deposition, electrical currents and electrical fields must be taken into account.

Plasmas, as ionized gases, possess free charge carriers like electrons and gas ions that allow electrical currents to be transported. This phenomenon is exploited in technical applications of plasmas, e.g. welding of metals ("light arcs") [38], or switching of very high electrical currents [39]. In plasmas for biomedical research or medical application, currents are orders of magnitude lower. However, as long a non-thermal plasma is used in direct mode, touching the treated surface (e.g. skin),

[2] http://www.icnirp.org/en/frequencies/uv/index.html.

a low current flowing into it cannot be avoided. This is especially true if a plasma source is designed in a way that the skin (or the treated object) acts as counter electrode (e.g. floating electrical barrier discharge). Additionally, jet plasma sources featuring a central electrode (surrounded by a dielectric barrier such as a kINPen jet) are prone to allow electrical currents to be dissipated to the treated object. Depending on distance between nozzle and object and its conductivity, the material acts as a second counter electrode, and allowing electrical currents to flow through the body. In compliance with the German Medicinal Devices Act, the IEC 60601, and the DIN SPEC 91315 [40], the patient leakage current must be limited to 100 μA to avoid electrical hazards [41]. Accordingly, the kINPen MED (Neoplas GmbH, Greifswald) has been specifically designed to meet this criterion, e.g. by reducing the plasma-on-time. Similar measures have been taken for the other two plasma sources which are currently recognized to be medical products in Germany (Cynogy GmbH, and Adtec Ltd.) and for experimental plasma sources [42].

In all plasma sources, charged particles move in space and electrical potentials on powered or counter electrodes change with time. Thereby, electrical fields arise and depending on the source design (e.g. presence of a Faraday shielding, dimension, and orientation of the electrodes), these fields can protrude into the ambient and potentially interact with living matter [43–45]. Strong, pulsed electric fields interact with polarized entities like cell membranes, potentiallyup to their breakage and the formation of pores [46–48]. If the electric fields created by non-thermal plasma sources are high enough to trigger biological effects such as pore formation is still under debate [49, 50]. Initial results indicate that a certain impact on cell performance, e.g. growth characteristics, cannot be neglected [51–53]. So far, no adverse effects have been attributed to electrical fields. Accordingly, this facet of plasmas needs future vigilance. In the meantime, readers are directed towards the large research field of pulsed electric fields.

**In summary:**
The patient leakage current created by plasma sources may pose a possible threat. Modern devices, which are approved as medical products, are designed to comply with regulations. The electrical properties of some plasmas sources allow the protrusion of electric fields into the treated tissue. While no adverse effects are reported, these fields may contribute to the clinical effects.

## 5.3 Potential Chemical Hazards of Non-Thermal Plasmas

Beside thermal energy, fields, and radiation, plasmas also emit chemical energy. This form of energy is very diverse, and mainly characterized by the ability of a particle (the reactant) to react with another. This can happen either within the plasma core, the plasma effluent or whatever the plasma has contact to, forming a new chemical bond or changing the excitation state of the counterpart. Many of the particles created in a plasma are very reactive, and they are typically short lived, they exist only during the plasma is ignited or briefly longer. Here, many of the well-known reactive oxygen and reactive nitrogen species belong to (ROS/RNS). They are created in the plasma, e.g. by the interaction of an electron or an excited particle with a gas particle, allowing a huge variety of small chemicals to be present in a time and location dependent manner. Additionally, gas phase reactions of the plasma may also lead to etching of components used for the plasma source, releasing potentially toxic compounds. Moreover, the working gases and stable gases created in the plasma and being released into the effluent can be toxic.

### 5.3.1 Impact of the Plasma Source Material

Typically, non-thermal plasma sources are designed from various materials. In contact with the active plasma core mainly inert materials are used: noble metals or alloys for the electrodes and mineral solids (glass, quartz, ceramics) as construction material and dielectric, respectively [54]. For these substances, no etching or corrosion has been observed and their usage in non-thermal plasma sources for clinical applications can be regarded as safe [55].

However, in modern, bendable plasma sources polymers may be an options due to their enormous flexibility [56, 57]. This is a trend, which also poses a threat and therefore should be subject to vigilance. Polymers are organic materials, typically involving carbon-carbon (C-C, C=C), carbon-oxygen (C-O, C=O), carbon-fluorine (C-F), and carbon-hydrogen (C-H) single or double bonds. Each of these bonds may be attacked by components of the active plasma core and even the effluent, leading to etching processes, and finally, to the loss of the polymeric material. In result, organic material will appear in the effluent, and, ultimately, in or at the plasma treated (biological) matter. Depending on the structure and composition of the polymer, these compounds can be potentially toxic. Especially fluorine containing polymers like polytetrafluoroethylene (PTFE, Teflon), polyvinylidene fluoride (PVDF), polyvinylfluoride (PVF) and many others. PTFE shows an excellent thermal stability, attributed to (1) the high carbon-fluorine bond strength (487 kJ/mole in $CF_4$ compared with 418 kJ/mole for C-H bonds in $CH_4$ and to (2) the shielding effect that the highly electronegative fluorine atoms have on the carbon backbone [58]. So far, no inadvertent corrosion of PTFE has been reported for non-thermal plasma sources composed of this material. In contrast, observations have been made that PVDF, although having excellent and desirable insulating properties, is not inert towards non-thermal plasmas. A strong leeching of fluorine (as $F^-$ ions) was detected in non-negliglible amounts in liquids treated with the respective plasma source (Fig. 5.2). While an essential micro nutrient, higher amounts of fluoride are toxic to the gastrointestinal tract and disturb bone formation [59, 60]. The exact mechanism of the PVDF corrosion has not been investigated, but is has been reported that PVDF when heated above 180 °C suffer from chain stripping reactions, leading to a massive production of hydrogen fluoride (HF) and residual C=C double bonds at the polymer backbone [61, 62]. Polyvinylchloride (PVC)

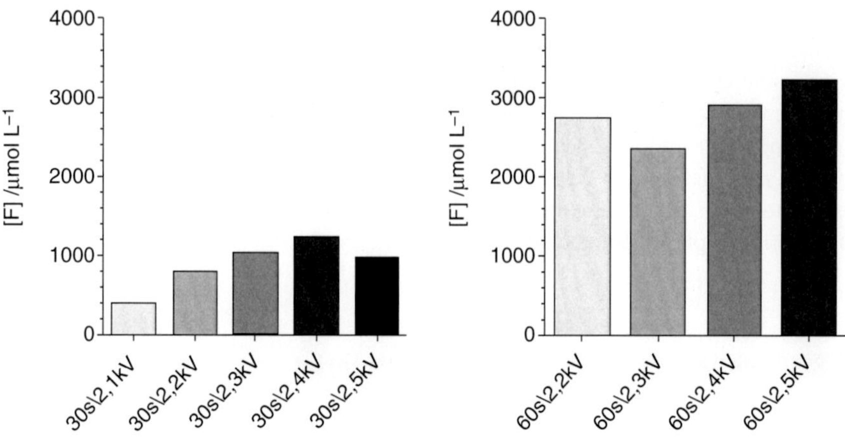


**Fig. 5.2** Treatment time and parameter (power) dependent critical fluoride deposition in tap water by a tissue-based dielectric barrier discharge in air. Electrodes were insulated with polyvinylidene fluoride (PVDF)

shows the same chemistry, yet the evolving chloride ion ($Cl^-$) is far less toxic [61]. In contrast, PTFE cannot undergo an identical reaction as the polymer is virtually free of hydrogen, rendering it more stable.

Other materials, e.g. polyether ether ketone (PEEK), contain only carbon, oxygen, and hydrogen, rendering them more biocompatible. PEEK shows an excellent thermal resilience (up 575 °C), making it a suitable candidate for non-thermal plasma sources. However, the compound contains unsaturated aromatic structures, which can be attacked by electrophiles or reactive radicals from the plasma. In the combination of heat and chemical entities, chain scission chemistry occurs, yielding aromatic alcohols and ethers with unknown biological properties [63]. Yet, only low etching rates have been reported, making PEEK a reasonable alternative to the fluoride polymers [64, 65]. For other polymers, e.g. polyethylene (PE), polypropylene (PP), polystryrene (PS) plasma etching was observed. Moreover, it is used to render the surface properties to facilitate technical applications (PS, PP) or biocompatibility (PS) [56, 66–68].

Further research will substantiate or disperse the concerns touched here in brief.

**In summary:**

Metals, ceramics, or mineral compounds are well suited materials for medical plasma sources and can be regarded as safe. In contrast, polymers, especially if they contain fluorine, need substantial consideration when designing a plasma source. Stability of the material under the intended working parameters must be observed. A release of toxic fluorine (as HF) must be avoided. PTFE seems to be sufficiently inert.

### 5.3.2 Impact of the Working Gas or Gases Emitted by Non-Thermal Plasma

For physical and engineering reasons (homogeneity of the discharge, temperature, etc.), plasma jets frequently use non-toxic noble gases like helium (He), argon (Ar), or neon (Ne) as bulk gas. For tuning of plasmas, small additions of more reactive gases or liquids (oxygen, nitrogen, water) are used. Gases of highest purity available and/or (if possible) of medical grade are advisable [69, 70]. All components within the gas will otherwise also be carried to the treated area and cause intoxications or adverse effects. The noble gases itself are no matter of toxicological concern in external applications of plasma as they do not form chemical products stable under the ambient conditions [71, 72]. Their ions or active states only occur in the active plasma core or parts of the effluent, and they are immediately quenched upon contact with air or biological matter. However, when using endoscopic plasma sources, consideration must be given to the removal of the inert noble gas from the cavity treated. Because of the weak solubility in water, noble gases are a potential risk [73, 74].

Beside the working gas, also gases produced by the discharge may accumulate. Among the gases investigated most are ozone ($O_3$) and nitric oxide (NO). NO is a strong vasodilator, and at concentrations above 2500 ppm acutely fatal (in mice 12 min).[3] The maximum permanently tolerable concentration is 0.5 ppm (MAK value). Current plasma sources for medical application do not create large amounts of the gas as its generation is endothermal and needs higher temperatures. In an argon radio frequency jet, up to 40 ppm NO were detected at the nozzle using laser induced fluorescence. However, values dropped to zero at 25 mm distance [75]. The kINPen is even colder, and NO formation is lower by factor 10 [76]. Ozone is a pale blue gas with a pungent smell. According to the NIOSH, 0.1 ppm is acceptable, which is also the odour threshold (100 ppb). In the EU, directive 2002/3/EG 0.055 ppm are listed as acceptable. Ozone is relatively stable and poorly soluble in aqueous liquids. Plasma sources, especially DBDs, operating in contact with ambient air or contain oxygen in the working gas can produce significant amounts [77, 78]. For the kINPen, 0.10 ppm to 0.13 ppm were detected in close vicinity (< 10 cm), at 30 cm distance values were below 0.1 ppm [79]. Because of short treatment times (max. 60 s), no direct danger is assumed for this plasma source. However, smell might be an undesired side effect. Ozone is hard to remove from the plasma generated species mixture, so information on $O_3$ contribution to *in vitro* or *in vivo* effects of plasmas in humans is scarce [80]. Accordingly, removal using charcoal filters or suction hoods can be useful. However, it contributes to microbial inactivation [81].

**In summary:**
Typical working gases for plasma sources for medical application pose no threat provided they are of suitable purity. Gases created by the plasma source during application can be potentially harmful, but due to limited treatment times and condensed treatment areas total amounts created are low. Additionally, they contribute to the desired effects.

[3] https://www.cdc.gov/niosh/idlh/10102439.html.

### 5.3.3 Reactive Oxygen and Nitrogen Species Deposition from Cold Plasmas

Beside light and electric fields, chemical species are emitted from the non-thermal plasma as an inevitable part of their existence. A plethora amount of data from *in vitro*, *ex vivo* and *in vivo* studies indicates, that ROS and RNS (often summarized as RONS) are major effectors in non-thermal plasmas [31, 70, 82–85].

Under the respective terms, ROS and RNS various small molecules are united (Fig. 5.3).

Although having a different structure, they share a common feature, i.e. an unstable electron configuration in either an atomic orbital (e.g. atomic oxygen, O; atomic nitrogen N) or a molecular orbital (e.g. hydroxyl radicals, OH; superoxide anion radical, $O_2^-$). This instability is very often a result of an unpaired electron in such a structure, a situation referred to as radical species. Also, a huge number of paired electrons (e.g. in peroxinitrite $ONOO^-$ or in peroxynitrate $OONOO^-$) leads to an unstable molecule, rendering them very reactive [86, 87]. According to thermodynamic laws, these chemicals seek a (more) stable configuration, thereby initiating fast and typically irreversible chemical reactions, often with a low reactant specificity [88]. This is best demonstrated by the hydroxyl radical (OH). The unpaired electron in its molecular orbital results in the molecules extreme fast reaction rates of $10^{-9}$ $M^{-1}$ $s^{-1}$ at virtually all pH-values and almost all chemical structures, both in gas and liquid phase [89]. Depending on the reactant and their chemical structure, reaction products are, e.g. organic radicals like alkyl radicals, dimeric structures, hydroxylated molecules, or in reaction with itself, hydrogen peroxide ($H_2O_2$) [90, 91]. The fast reaction translates into a diffusion rate controlled quenching of OH, thereby indicating a second common feature of RONS: short live- time. For OH in liquids, the live time lies around the nanosecond range, singlet oxygen ($\Delta^1O_2$) is stable for microseconds, and superoxide anion radical ($O^{2-}$) almost one second [89, 92]. Along with the short live time, a very limited activity range is connected which is determined by the diffusion rate and chemical composition of the environment to be travelled (Fig. 5.4) [87, 93]. Compared with the treatment times used in plasma medicine these lifetimes are very short, raising the question of effective treatment durations and in-depth effectivity of plasma (discussed elsewhere in this book) [94].

The reactivity of the ROS/RNS is boon and bane at the same time: they are effectors of non-thermal plasma—most effects observed were attributed to these small chemicals, and threat—they may be deleterious to the cells (macro-) molecules and especially, to its genetic code.

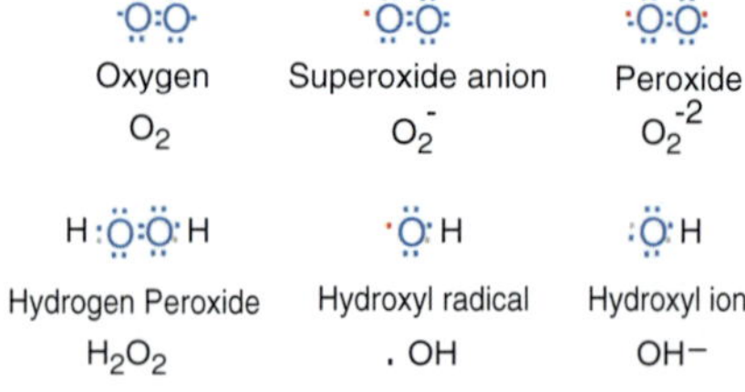


**Fig. 5.3** Structure and chemical composition of ROS relevant in plasma medicine

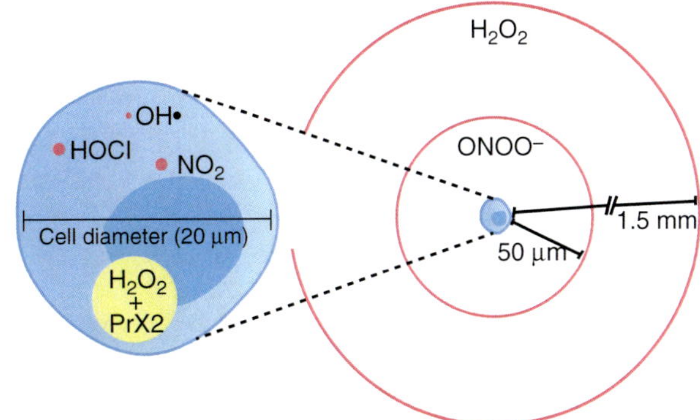


**Fig. 5.4** Activity range of ROS/RNS common in cell physiological processes [93]

Beside the nucleotides, forming the genetic code storage and transport forms, cells are made of sugars, fatty acids, and amino acids, all of whom can be components of larger molecules (carbohydrates, complex lipids, proteins). Knowledge on the direct interaction between plasma generated ROS/RNS and these components is limited, especially regarding the impact of potentially formed (toxic) products. For sugars/carbohydrates, literature suggests a good reactivity of glucose, mannose, and others with OH radicals and report reaction rates in the range of $10^{-9}$ $M^{-1}$ $s^{-1}$. Singlet oxygen is also reported to react with sugars, but at much lower rates ($1–2 \times 10^{-4}$ $M^{-1}$ $s^{-1}$) [95]. The resulting small carbonyl compounds (mainly ketones) have no reported impact on cell physiology. Fatty acids, consists of repetitive $–CH_2$- groups [96]. This hydrocarbon structure is also present in fuels used for combustion, and accordingly, a wealth of data exists on the respective gas-phase plasma chemistry (plasma-aided combustion) [97–99]. In liquids, like the cellular environment or cell culture medium, the reactivity between saturated lipids and plasma-generated species remains unclear. While simulations using a strictly defined chemical environment suggest the attack of OH to these structures, experimental evidence is lacking [100, 101]. In contrast, an impact on polar lipid head groups (e.g. phosphatidylcholines) was seen as well as a chain fissure at unsaturated double bond positions resulting in truncated lipids and small aldehydes [102–104]. It is known from lipid research, that the α-position to a double bond (allyl position) can easily be attacked by oxygen derivatives [105]. Reaction products vary broadly, e.g. hydroperoxides, hydroxylated fatty acids, short-chain fatty acids, aldehydes, and cyclic products, summarized as lipid peroxidation products [106]. In cells and tissues, lipid oxidation products are recognized as signaling molecules, stimulating a general anti-oxidant response via Nrf2-related signaling or inducing inflammatory alert effects via prostaglandin receptors [106–108]. Hence, interaction of plasma-generated species with unsaturated lipids may result in the production of important signal molecules (e.g. 4-hydroxynonenale, 4-HNE) which are connected to active cell responses. So far, only limited data are available to prove this scenario. However, several publications suggest the formation of pores in the cell membrane due to lipid peroxidation [109, 110], others report the activation of NRF2 and its downstream targets as an indirect proof of potential lipid peroxidation [111]. Reports on lipid oxidation by plasma treatment, using liposomes or similar models, are scarce [102, 104, 112].

Knowledge on plasma liquids chemistry to modulate amino acids is growing [113]. Depending on the amino acid structure, numerous covalent modifications are reported.

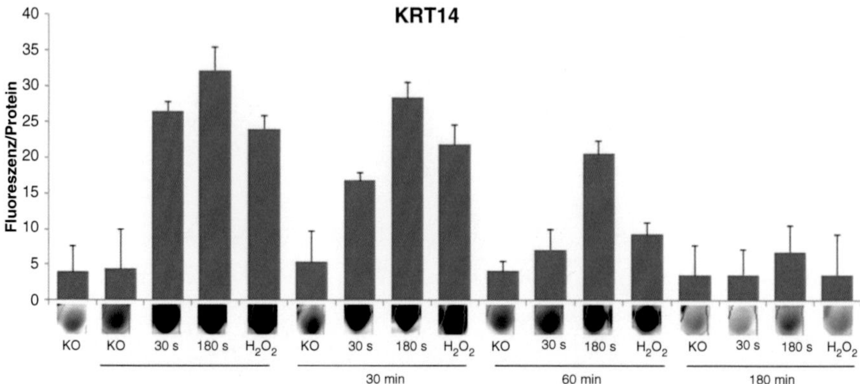


**Fig. 5.5** In situ oxidation level of keratin 14 in HaCaT cells by an argon plasma treatment. A treatment and incubation time-depending modulation of cysteine oxidation was observed after plasma challenge (2D–gel, densiometric measurement by Delta2D-Software)

Prominent targets are the aromatic structures of tyrosine, phenylalanine, or tryptophane, and the thiol groups of methionine and cysteine. So far, only negligible impact on cell vitality after treatment with modulated amino acids has been observed, probably because of the limited concentrations of chemically modified acids and the intracellular storage capable of sustaining a period of deprivation [114]. A chemical modification of amino acids within a complete protein by plasma has so far only been shown for cysteine residues [115]. When proteins featuring one or more cysteine moieties in their active centers and are treated singularly in dried state by plasma, a loss of function was reported (e.g. glyceraldehyde 3-phosphate dehydrogenase) [116]. RNA endonuclease A (RNAse A) was inactivated by a dielectric barrier discharge, but not by a helium plasma jet [115, 116]. In contrast, the treatment of dissolved catalase by an argon plasma jet in buffered systems (e.g. cell culture medium) does not result in its inactivation, even under prolonged treatment (unpublished own observations). In a cellular environment, a loss of function has not been demonstrated, yet 2D–gel based redox proteomics revealed changes in the redox state of several proteins (Fig. 5.5), which could both indicate an inactivation of the protein as well as its activation.

Accordingly, interpretation remains challenging and the impact of non-thermal plasma on cells or tissue may predominantly be related to signaling rather than bulk chemistry effects. So far, the available information on plasma—amino acid/protein interactions allow to draw an incomplete picture only. Data describing chemical modifications of proteins by different plasma sources quantitatively, preferentially in complex systems (cells, tissues), are needed.

**In summary:**
Non-thermal plasma liquid chemistry allows the chemical modification of all major cell components when present in controlled environments. Yet, no indications of a safety issue have been published for any of the three discussed cellular components (carbohydrates, lipids, proteins). Rather, the modification of lipids and proteins contribute to the observed effects in plasma medicine via signaling events.

## 5.4 Safety of Non-Thermal Plasma Application with Respect to Genetic Stability

The human genome consists of deoxyribonucleic acid, packed into 23 chromosome pairs and some small DNA molecules in the mitochondria [117]. With a few exceptions, it can be found in all somatic cells of the body. About 20,000 genes are encoded in the DNA, though the major part of roughly 6.5 billion base pairs is non-coding (98% ncDNA), having an unknown functionality hotly debated ("dark matter") [118–120]. There is a small inter-individual variance of less than 0.1%, whereas the DNA of our closest relatives (chimpanzees) differs by 4% [121]. Epigenetic processes (histone acetylation, DNA methylation, etc.) add additional levels of gene/gene product regulation [122]. An elaborated DNA replication machinery ensures highest fidelity, determined to be one error per $10^7$ nucleotides in baker's yeast for the initial synthesis. Further it increased by proof-reading [123] and mismatch repair mechanisms [124] to only one error in 250 cell replication cycles [125, 126]. This high precision ensures the ability of organisms to transfer genetic information safely from generation to generation, contributing to the diversity of life [127]. If disturbed, deleterious changes to the code, and accordingly to the gene products (proteins), may occur resulting in mutations or even abiosis.

Since the fatal thalidomide disaster, vigilance of clinicians and other health care professionals when approving a drug or treatment in humans massively increased, ensuring safety especially with regards to the genetic information [128]. Procedures violating this *conditio sine qua non* are only approved for the treatment of otherwise uncontrollable conditions as an *ultima ratio*, e.g. certain tumors, infections with multi-resistant microorganism, or orphan diseases, using strict guidelines.

As dealt with above, non-thermal plasma generates ROS/RNS that can react with chemical structures present in the DNA and related molecules (RNA). This would lead to DNA oxidation, e.g. 8-oxoguanine which results in mismatch pairing [129]. Additionally, the ultraviolet light emitted by most plasma sources can also interact with structures of the nucleotides, especially the aromatic rings (UVB light, see section above). This could result in photo lesions, such as CPD (cyclobutane pyrimidine dimers) or 6,4 PP (pyrimidine-(6–4)-pyrimidone dimers) [130]. However, it should be mentioned, that humans deliberately expose themselves to UV irradiation ("sun bathing"), and that UV light is used in clinics (e.g. photodynamic therapy: vitiligo, psoriasis, etc.). Such, care must be taken to observe radiation energies, exposure times, and exposed area when evaluating UV impact from plasmas and other sources.

Consequently, in the concept of plasma medicine, safety of use was focused early with a special emphasis on the absence of adverse effects, e.g. as reported by the following authors [11, 131–136]. Scarcely, damage of intensely treated skin was reported recently [137]. In all these works, no experiments to show the impact of the plasma treatment on the genetic information were included, but from the successful *in vivo* studies and the clinical follow-up, an absence of genotoxicity was concluded. Initial *in vitro* experiments focusing on genotoxicity were performed using well controllable systems, e.g. singular DNA plasmids in inorganic buffers or in dry state, and straightforward readout systems, e.g. molecule length, coiling, etc. Typically, authors reported a treatment time dependent decay of the DNA molecule

[138–140]. A decay of DNA was observed again more recently with an advanced model, but in this case naked DNA was treated by the plasma [12]. Although valuable to infer on plasma liquid chemistry or for the comparison of plasma sources or treatment parameters, such results are biologically irrelevant. The DNA is a reasonable stable molecule, but it is not designed to be specifically stable in the environment [141, 142]. Additionally, as random genetic information poses a threat to other organisms, DNA degrading enzymes (DNAes) are secreted from most living cells. In contrast, the DNA is stored in eukaryotic cells in a well-protected state: coiled and supercoiled on nucleosomes (histone proteins) and situated mainly in the cell's nucleus [143, 144]. Thus, direct reachability by short-lived plasma generated species is limited or impossible (see Fig. 5.4). Additionally, mammalian cells feature very extensive DNA repair mechanisms [145–147], which evolved during evolution to ensure high fidelity replication and to eliminate the spontaneously occurring $10^4$ DNA lesions per day and cell [148]. This situation is addressed in later experiments using complex set ups, e.g. cell lines, primary cells, *ex vivo* tissue, or animal studies which generally demonstrated the absence of genotoxic effects for the plasma sources studied with a few exceptions. In all cases when complete organisms were treated—animals (rodents, frog, zebra fish, pig), or humans, no signs of tumorigenicity were detected [4, 7, 8, 10, 28, 42, 54, 131, 136, 149–152].

This apparent discrepancy is expression of a very complex situation. The plasma generated ROS/RNS have lifetimes modulated by the chemical properties of the experimental system, in cell linemodels possess ROS handling enzymes and lipid membranes protecting the DNA, but lacks the bulk layers of proteins/proteoglycans the extracellular matrix in tissue models or complete animals is made off [153]. In the following paragraphs, the present knowledge on this topic will be discussed.

### 5.4.1 Genotoxicity Risk Assessment of Non-Thermal Plasma Sources

The absence of genotoxicity is a mandatory prerequisite for medical applications of non-thermal plasmas in humans, especially in non-palliative settings like wound healing. Accordingly, efforts to verify its safety using generally approved methods have been undertaken by several research groups.

In the DIN EN ISO 10993-3:2015-02, also adapted by the FDA (U.S.A.), the in vitro and in vivo micronucleus assay (MN assay) is recommended to proof genetic safety [154, 155]. Micronuclei appear during cell division if chromosomal aberrations occur (e.g. double strand breaks, loss of centromer) and genetic material is left behind during karyokinesis, indicating aberrations in the genetic information [156]. For the argon plasma jet kINPen two different research groups showed the absence of genotoxic effects using the MN assay either in normal human keratinocytes (HaCaT, in vitro) or in peripheral chicken's egg blood cells (in vivo. In cultivated HaCaT cells, using RPMI cell culture medium with fetal calf serum, up to 180 s of kINPen 09 plasma treatment did not result in an increase of micronuclei formation in cytochalasin-blocked cells above control levels (5%), while positive controls UVB (6%) and mitomycin C (12%) did [152]. This result was confirmed in vivo using chicken's egg peripheral erythrocytes (HET-MN). Briefly, the egg's chorioallantoic membrane was treated on day 8 for up to 10 min with the kINPen MED and after 3 days, presence of micronuclei in the chicken's erythrocytes was estimated after May-Grünwald Giemsa staining. Positive controls (methotrexate, cyclophosphamide) did result in strong micronucleus formation, while all plasma treatments did not yield any increase above control (0.03%) [150].

The mammalian gene mutation assay HRPT1 (encoding the protein Hypoxanthine-guanine phosphoribosyltransferase) exploits the presence of one singular gene in male cells (e.g. Chinese hamster lung cells V79, located on the Y chromosome). The assay has been adopted by the OECD for mutagenicity testing: upon DNA damage, the gene product is malfunctioning, allowing cells to grow in 6-thioguanine, a toxic nucleotide precursor. In control cells, when HRPT is working, the toxification of 6-TG leads to cell death. One DBD (MiniFlatPlaSter), a microwave exited argon jet (MicroPlaSter; both Adtec, UK), and a MHz driven argon plasma jet kINPen (Neoplas GmbH, Germany) was assayed for HRPT1 mutagenicity. Using the MiniFlatPlaSter, up to 240 s of plasma treatment in DMEM did not yield a significant increase in mutagenicity [149]. In a similar setup, up to 5 min treatment of V79 cells in PBS with the MicroPlaSter or untreated control yielded between 10 and 20 mutants per one million cells. In both cases, ethlymethanosulfonate or UVC yielded significantly higher number of mutants (≈ one order of magnitude). The kINPen was assayed in HRPT1 genotoxicity assay for up to 180 s indirect, 30 s direct, or mock treatment using complete RPMI. Between 10 and 20 mutants per one million cells were detected, with no detectable difference between treatment and control. Positive controls (UVB 40 $J_{eff}$ $m^{-2}$, ethlymethanosulfonate) yielded a 1 to 1.5 orders of magnitude higher mutation frequency [152]. In another approach, a high throughput micronuleus assay was established using THP1 cells and an imaging flow cytometer [94]. Results confirm the absence of mutagenic effects for the kINPen MED.

Clearly, these results show the absence of genotoxic effects for the plasma sources under test. However, care must be taken when generalizing the outcome: For a high voltage volume DBD, authors report the presence of epithelial cell CHO-K1 HRPT1 mutants after prolonged treatment (5–10 min, DMEM/F12 medium w/FBS) [157]. However, experimental issues may have influenced the result: an increased cell motility was observed, impeding correct colony estimation. This is in accordance with other reports on increased epithelial cell migration after plasma treatment in the concept of plasma aided wound healing [27].

Other not officially approved assays have been used to estimate genotoxicity of non-thermal plasmas (see Sect. 5.4). In contrast to the above, these assays do not account cell performance but rely on molecular analytics, detecting dedicated events such as DNA fragmentation or protein expression/activation. As discussed, the treatment of naked DNA cannot easily be used to confer on cell physiology, but changes detected in intracelluar proteins can be valuable tools for mechanistic insights into the background of plasma medicine. A frequently used reporter is the histone γH2AX, whose phosphorylation is one early signal of DNA double strand breaks [158]. A number of papers report such event after non-thermal plasma treatment [84, 159, 160], while others do not [161] or put it into another context [162]. Beside its role in DNA damage signaling, this protein also serves as redox state sensor, contributing in antioxidant defense [163, 164]. Such, overlapping signals may evolve impeding interpretation. Similarly, care must be taken evaluating data from the single cell gel electrophoresis assay (Comet Assay). This assay detects the lability of the DNA, either due to oxidation causing single strand breaks (alkaline comet assay) or double strand breaks (neutral comet assay) [165, 166]. However, during apoptosis which is well recognized cell death mechanism after suitable plasma treatment [165, 167], nucleases cut the cellular DNA which than leads to positive assay results mimicking DNA strand breaks [168].

**In summary:**
Non-thermal plasmas can have a strong impact on mammalian cells, including the triggering of cell death. Yet, for some plasma sources reports indicate the absence of genotoxicity, as could be shown by micronucleus assay and HRPT1 assay: either a potential damage can be repaired or cells undergo apoptosis. In animals or humans no sign of tumorigenicity have been detected. However, this statement cannot be generalized and safety needs to be tested for every new plasma source.

### 5.4.2 Risk Assessment of Murine Wounds Treated with an Argon Plasma Jet

For the atmospheric pressure argon plasma jet kINPen, first evidence pointed at a lack of genotoxic and/or mutagenic activity [150, 152]. However, studies on tissues as well as long-term observations are scarce [136]. Here, a murine model of dermal full-thickness wounds was used, which closely resembles wound healing in humans [169]. After anesthesia, full-thickness ear wounds with 3 $mm^2$ area were created on both ears. kINPen plasma treatment was carried out using the tip of the plasma effluent at a distance of eight mm using an autoclavable spacer. Wounds were treated daily with 20 s of plasma over 14 consecutive days, which seems advisable for toxicological investigations, or were left untreated. Quantitative analysis by microscopy demonstrated a significantly accelerated wound epithelialization, as indicated by faster wound closure beginning with day 3 until day 9 after wounding [27]. Consecutively, we investigated long-term side effects of the repetitive plasma treatment in this immunocompetent mouse model [28]. To monitor long-term effects and tumorigenicity plasma-treated mice were observed for 350 days and compared with untreated controls. Thereafter, skin, organs, and blood were collected, and different assays were performed as shown in Fig. 5.6.

We were able to conclude key aspects with regard to efficacy and safety of that device using non-invasive methods such as magnetic resonance imaging (MRI) and positron-emission tomography/computed tomography (PET/CT) using 18F–FDG tracer. Within the sensitivity and resolution limits, no apparent signs of tumor manifestation were found in any of the investigated structures and organs at the deliverable spatial resolution. Likewise, histological and immunohistochemical analysis

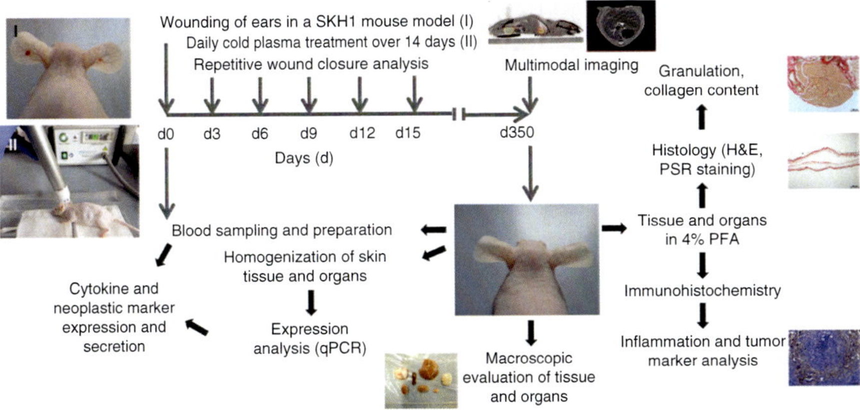


**Fig. 5.6** Study design of one-year follow-up risk assessment. Immunocompetent SKH1 mice were wounded on both ears and daily treated with an argon plasma jet over 14 consecutive days. After 350 days, any potential tumor formation was analyzed by non-invasive methods such as anatomical magnetic-resonance imaging (MRI) and positron emission tomography-computed tomography (PET/CT) as well as by histological (H&E and PSR staining), immune histochemical (IHC) and molecular biological analyses (quantitative PCR, ELISA) [28]

failed to detect abnormal morphological changes and presence of tumor markers such as neighbor of Punc 11 (NOPE), α-fetoprotein (AFP), β-microglobulin, (β2M) or carcinoembryonic antigen (CEA). In blood, systemic changes of the pro-inflammatory cytokines interleukin 1β (IL-1β) and tumor necrosis factor α (TNFα) were absent. Similarly, tumor marker levels of α-fetoprotein and calcitonin remained unchanged. Absence of neoplastic lesions was confirmed by quantitative PCR. mRNA expression levels of several cytokines and tumor markers in liver, lung, brain and skin were similar in the control and treatment group (Fig. 5.7).

Wounded skin tissue healed physiologically without excessive scar formation or abnormalities. The plasma treatment was safe as demonstrated by the absence of a wound-restricted tumor formation. No transformation of tissue was found in any other major organ including liver, lymph node, spleen, heart, lung, and brain. The lack of tumor markers in blood plasma suggested an absence of tumor tissue at other body sites not investigated. Moreover, the analysis of cytokines and immune cells indicated a physiological immune regulation without pathological enhanced inflammation. These results suggest that the beneficial effects of cold plasma in wound healing come without apparent side effects including tumor formation or chronic inflammation. Cold plasma applied topically is a safe adjuvant strategy in dermatology, which is in agreement with previous studies.

**In summary:**
In a long term observation of repeatedly argon plasma jet (kINPen) treated mice no adverse effects with regards to genotoxicity could be observed, neither locally nor systemically. The applied treatment can be regarded as safe.

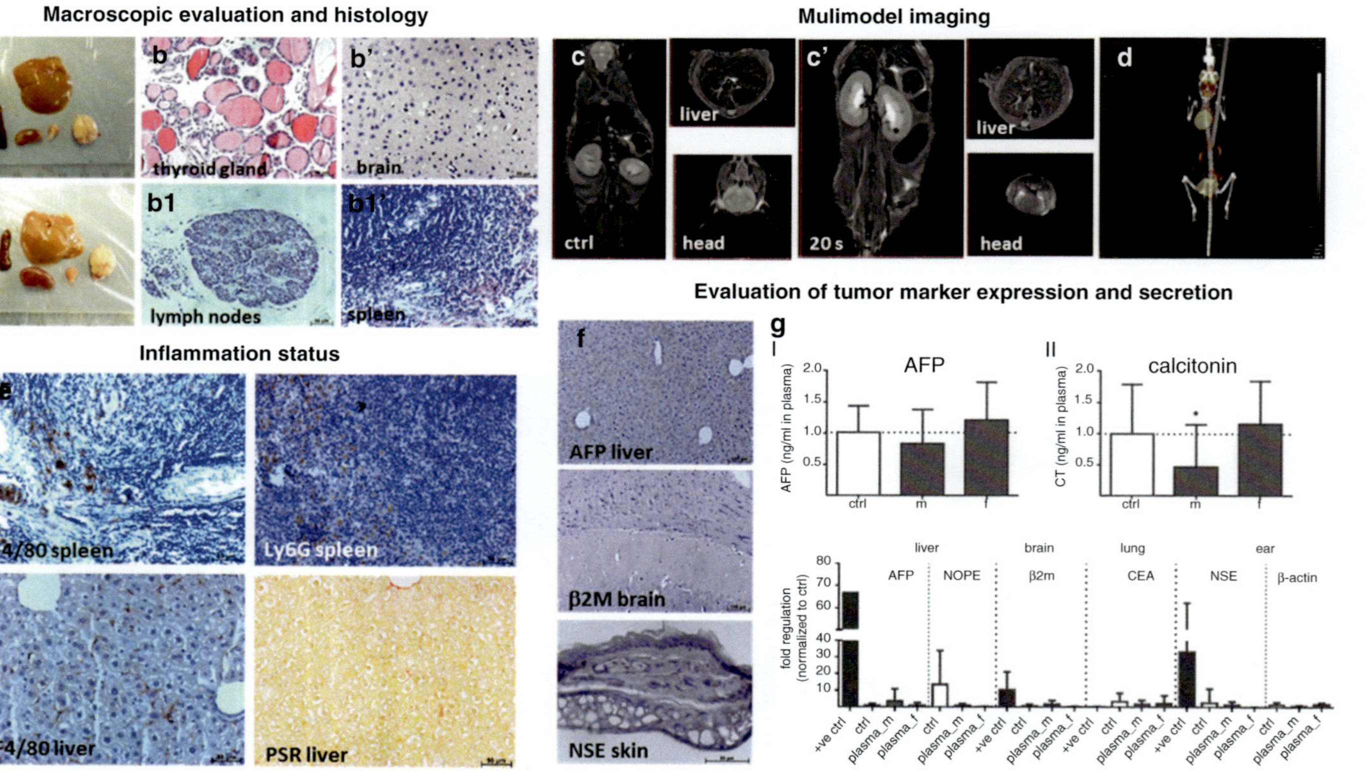


**Fig. 5.7** Evaluation of potential risk hazards of the kINPen plasma in mice. Animals were treated daily with 20 s of plasma over 14 days and tissue was removed after one year. Macroscopic evaluation (**a**) and hematoxylin and eosin (H&E) staining (**b**) of different organs (lung, spleen, liver, heart, kidney, thyroid glands, and brain) lacking visible tumor formation, Non-invasive imaging methods such as magnetic resonance imaging (MRI, **c**) or positron emission tomography-computed tomography (PET/CT, **d**) showed no signs of metastatic or primary tumor formation. Normal macrophage (f4/80) and granulocyte (Ly6G) distribution in spleens and normal hepatic architecture with ramified Kupffer cells (F4/80) and picrosirius red (PSR) staining were demonstrated using immunhistochemistry (IHC, **e**). Several tumor markers in different organs (liver, lung, brain, lymph nodes, thyroid glands) and tissue (ear skin) were analyzed using IHC (**f**), ELISA (**g**), and quantitative PCR (**h**) confirming no systemic long-term transformation after plasma application [28]

## 5.5 Summary and Conclusions

Modern non-thermal plasma sources for biomedical applications can be regarded as safe, if recommendations for use are followed and test according to the DIN SPEC and officially requested test have been performed. A chemically inert composition of the source, clean and safe gases for operation and a low heat and patient leakage current can be well designed and controlled. The biochemical safety of the discharge is influenced by the emission of UV light, the electrical fields, and the deposition of ROS and RNS. Together with the engineered plasma source design it determines the impact on the desired target and potentially adverse side effects. Due to a permanently growing knowledge on the fundamental basics of plasmas and the changing medical application fields, risk assessment is not a static but a highly kinetic field. Appropriate experiments need to be performed for any plasma source and application area specifically, and needs to be updated with any change of operation procedure, e.g. changes in working gas composition, distance, driving power or the application itself etc. Evidently, risk assessment and safety of the plasma treatment is permanently *work in progress* as plasma source and applications develop further from the prototype stage into clinical fields. Furthermore, *good clinical practice* procedures ask for the re-evaluation of the risk assessment/safety file at times, especially upon the finding of new insights related to the mentioned risks. To this end, it must be stated that a lot of work is still to be done—many plasma sources or applications are currently in a preliminary status. Even for the more established plasma sources, which are approved as a medical device like the kINPen (neoplas tools, Greifswald), the PlasmaDerm (Cinogy GmbH, Duderstadt), or the SteriPlas (Adtec Ltd., UK), further efforts will be necessary to keep step with improving knowledge and medical application foci.

## References

1. Yarmolenko PS, Moon EJ, Landon C, Manzoor A, Hochman DW, Viglianti BL, Dewhirst MW. Thresholds for thermal damage to normal tissues: An update. Int J Hyperthermia. 2011;27(4):320–43.
2. Dewhirst MW, Viglianti B, Lora-Michiels M, Hanson M, Hoopes P. Basic principles of thermal dosimetry and thermal thresholds for tissue damage from hyperthermia. Int J Hyperthermia. 2003;19(3):267–94.
3. Lademann J, Richter H, Alborova A, Humme D, Patzelt A, Kramer A, Weltmann KD, Hartmann B, Ottomann C, Fluhr JW, Hinz P, Hubner G, Lademann O. Risk assessment of the application of a plasma jet in dermatology. J Biomed Opt. 2009;14(5):054025.
4. Lademann J, Ulrich C, Patzelt A, Richter H, Kluschke F, Klebes M, Lademann O, Kramer A, Weltmann KD, Lange-Asschenfeldt B. Risk assessment of the application of tissue-tolerable plasma on human skin. Clin Plasma Med. 2013;1(1):5–10.
5. Weltmann KD, Kindel E, Brandenburg R, Meyer C, Bussiahn R, Wilke C, von Woedtke T. Atmospheric pressure plasma jet for medical therapy: plasma parameters and risk estimation. Contrib Plasma Phys. 2009;49(9):631–40.
6. Brehmer F, Haenssle H, Daeschlein G, Ahmed R, Pfeiffer S, Görlitz A, Simon D, Schön M, Wandke D, Emmert S. Alleviation of chronic venous leg ulcers with a hand-held dielectric barrier discharge plasma generator (PlasmaDerm® VU-2010): results of a monocentric, two-armed, open, prospective, randomized and controlled trial (NCT01415622). J Eur Acad Dermatol Venereol. 2015;29(1):148–55.

7. Isbary G, Heinlin J, Shimizu T, Zimmermann JL, Morfill G, Schmidt HU, Monetti R, Steffes B, Bunk W, Li Y, Klaempfl T, Karrer S, Landthaler M, Stolz W. Successful and safe use of 2 min cold atmospheric argon plasma in chronic wounds: results of a randomized controlled trial. Br J Dermatol. 2012;167(2):404–10.
8. Von Woedtke T, Metelmann HR, Weltmann KD. Clinical plasma medicine: state and perspectives of in vivo application of cold atmospheric plasma. Contrib Plasma Phys. 2014; 54(2):104–17.
9. Collet G, Robert E, Lenoir A, Vandamme M, Darny T, Dozias S, Kieda C, Pouvesle JM. Plasma jet-induced tissue oxygenation: potentialities for new therapeutic strategies. Plasma Sources Sci Technol. 2014;23(1):012005.
10. Schmidt A, von Woedtke T, Bekeschus S. Periodic exposure of keratinocytes to cold physical plasma: an in vitro model for redox-related diseases of the skin. Oxid Med Cell Longev. 2016;2016:9816072.
11. Isbary G, Heinlin J, Shimizu T, Zimmermann J, Morfill G, Schmidt HU, Monetti R, Steffes B, Bunk W, Li Y. Successful and safe use of 2 min cold atmospheric argon plasma in chronic wounds: results of a randomized controlled trial. Br J Dermatol. 2012;167(2):404–10.
12. Tiede R, Hirschberg J, Viöl W, Emmert S. A µs-pulsed dielectric barrier discharge source: physical characterization and biological effects on human skin fibroblasts. Plasma Process Polym. 2016;13(8):775–87.
13. Wattieaux G, Yousfi M, Merbahi N. Optical emission spectroscopy for quantification of ultraviolet radiations and biocide active species in microwave argon plasma jet at atmospheric pressure. Spectrochim Acta B At Spectrosc. 2013;89:66–76.
14. Winter J, Brandenburg R, Weltmann K. Atmospheric pressure plasma jets: an overview of devices and new directions. Plasma Sources Sci Technol. 2015;24(6):064001.
15. Lackmann J-W, Schneider S, Edengeiser E, Jarzina F, Brinckmann S, Steinborn E, Havenith M, Benedikt J, Bandow JE. Photons and particles emitted from cold atmospheric-pressure plasma inactivate bacteria and biomolecules independently and synergistically. J R Soc Interface. 2013;10(89):20130591.
16. Lange H, Foest R, Schafer J, Weltmann KD. Vacuum UV radiation of a plasma jet operated with rare gases at atmospheric pressure. IEEE Transact Plasma Sci. 2009;37(6):859–65.
17. Sinha RP, Häder D-P. UV-induced DNA damage and repair: a review. Photochem Photobiol Sci. 2002;1(4):225–36.
18. Anderson RR, Parrish JA. The optics of human skin. J Investig Dermatol. 1981;77(1):13–9.
19. Ichihashi M, Ueda M, Budiyanto A, Bito T, Oka M, Fukunaga M, Tsuru K, Horikawa T. UV-induced skin damage. Toxicology. 2003;189(1):21–39.
20. Diepgen T, Mahler V. The epidemiology of skin cancer. Br J Dermatol. 2002;146(s61):1–6.
21. Schallreuter K, Wood J, Lemke K, Levenig C. Treatment of vitiligo with a topical application of pseudocatalase and calcium in combination with short-term UVB exposure: a case study on 33 patients. Dermatology. 1995;190(3):223–9.
22. Scherschun L, Kim JJ, Lim HW. Narrow-band ultraviolet B is a useful and well-tolerated treatment for vitiligo. J Am Acad Dermatol. 2001;44(6):999–1003.
23. Weischer M, Blum A, Eberhard F, Röcken M, Berneburg M. No evidence for increased skin cancer risk in psoriasis patients treated with broadband or narrowband UVB phototherapy: a first retrospective study. Acta Derm Venereol. 2004;84(5).
24. Dolmans DE, Fukumura D, Jain RK. Photodynamic therapy for cancer. Nat Rev Cancer. 2003;3(5):380–7.
25. Ge J, Lan M, Zhou B, Liu W, Guo L, Wang H, Jia Q, Niu G, Huang X, Zhou H. A graphene quantum dot photodynamic therapy agent with high singlet oxygen generation. Nat Commun. 2014;5.
26. Adachi T, Tanaka H, Nonomura S, Hara H, Kondo S, Hori M. Plasma-activated medium induces A549 cell injury via a spiral apoptotic cascade involving the mitochondrial–nuclear network. Free Radic Biol Med. 2015;79:28–44.
27. Schmidt A, Bekeschus S, Wende K, Vollmar B, Woedtke T. A cold plasma jet accelerates wound healing in a murine model of full-thickness skin wounds. Exp Dermatol. 2017; 26(2):156–62.

28. Schmidt A, Woedtke TV, Stenzel J, Lindner T, Polei S, Vollmar B, Bekeschus S. One year follow-up risk assessment in SKH-1 mice and wounds treated with an argon plasma jet. Int J Mol Sci. 2017;18(4):868.
29. Attri P, Kim YH, Park DH, Park JH, Hong YJ, Uhm HS, Kim K-N, Fridman A, Choi EH. Generation mechanism of hydroxyl radical species and its lifetime prediction during the plasma-initiated ultraviolet (UV) photolysis. Sci Rep. 2015;5:9332.
30. Jablonowski H, Bussiahn R, Hammer M, Weltmann K-D, von Woedtke T, Reuter S. Impact of plasma jet vacuum ultraviolet radiation on reactive oxygen species generation in bio-relevant liquids. Phys Plasmas. 2015;22(12):122008.
31. Bruggeman P, Kushner MJ, Locke BR, Gardeniers J, Graham W, Graves DB, Hofman-Caris R, Maric D, Reid JP, Ceriani E. Plasma–liquid interactions: a review and roadmap. Plasma Sources Sci Technol. 2016;25(5):053002.
32. Metelmann H-R, Nedrelow DS, Seebauer C, Schuster M, von Woedtke T, Weltmann K-D, Kindler S, Metelmann PH, Finkelstein SE, Von Hoff DD. Head and neck cancer treatment and physical plasma. Clin Plasma Med. 2015;3(1):17–23.
33. Rajasekaran P, Opländer C, Hoffmeister D, Bibinov N, Suschek CV, Wandke D, Awakowicz P. Characterization of dielectric barrier discharge (DBD) on mouse and histological evaluation of the plasma-treated tissue. Plasma Process Polym. 2011;8(3):246–55.
34. Boudam M, Moisan M, Saoudi B, Popovici C, Gherardi N, Massines F. Bacterial spore inactivation by atmospheric-pressure plasmas in the presence or absence of UV photons as obtained with the same gas mixture. J Phys D Appl Phys. 2006;39(16):3494.
35. Heise M, Neff W, Franken O, Muranyi P, Wunderlich J. Sterilization of polymer foils with dielectric barrier discharges at atmospheric pressure. Plasmas Polym. 2004;9(1):23–33.
36. Vig JR. UV/ozone cleaning of surfaces. J Vac Sci Technol A. 1985;3(3):1027–34.
37. Lerouge S, Fozza A, Wertheimer M, Marchand R, Yahia LH. Sterilization by low-pressure plasma: the role of vacuum-ultraviolet radiation. Plasmas Polym. 2000;5(1):31–46.
38. Fan H, Kovacevic R. A unified model of transport phenomena in gas metal arc welding including electrode, arc plasma and molten pool. J Phys D Appl Phys. 2004;37(18):2531.
39. Khakpour A, Franke S, Uhrlandt D, Gorchakov S, Methling R-P. Electrical arc model based on physical parameters and power calculation. IEEE Transact Plasma Sci. 2015;43(8):2721–9.
40. Mann MS, Tiede R, Gavenis K, Daeschlein G, Bussiahn R, Weltmann K-D, Emmert S, von Woedtke T, Ahmed R. Introduction to DIN-specification 91315 based on the characterization of the plasma jet kINPen® MED. Clin Plasma Med. 2016;4(2):35–45.
41. IEC/VDE. Effects of current on human beings and livestock: part 1–general aspects. IEC/TS. 2005;60479:1.
42. Lehmann A, Pietag F, Arnold T. Human health risk evaluation of a microwave-driven atmospheric plasma jet as medical device. Clin Plasma Med. 2017;7-8:16–23.
43. Babaeva NY, Kushner MJ. Intracellular electric fields produced by dielectric barrier discharge treatment of skin. J Phys D Appl Phys. 2010;43(18):185206.
44. Guo A, Song B, Reid B, Gu Y, Forrester JV, Jahoda CA, Zhao M. Effects of physiological electric fields on migration of human dermal fibroblasts. J Investig Dermatol. 2010;130(9):2320–7.
45. Ignarro LJ, Bush PA, Buga GM, Wood KS, Fukuto JM, Rajfer J. Nitric oxide and cyclic GMP formation upon electrical field stimulation cause relaxation of corpus cavernosum smooth muscle. Biochem Biophys Res Commun. 1990;170(2):843–50.
46. Chen X, Kolb JF, Swanson RJ, Schoenbach KH, Beebe SJ. Apoptosis initiation and angiogenesis inhibition: melanoma targets for nanosecond pulsed electric fields. Pigment Cell Melanoma Res. 2010;23(4):554–63.
47. Jordan CA, Neumann E, Sowers AE. Electroporation and electrofusion in cell biology. New York: Springer Science & Business Media; 2013.
48. Steuer A, Schmidt A, Labohá P, Babica P, Kolb JF. Transient suppression of gap junctional intercellular communication after exposure to 100-nanosecond pulsed electric fields. Bioelectrochemistry. 2016;112:33–46.
49. Babaeva NY, Tian W, Kushner MJ. The interaction between plasma filaments in dielectric barrier discharges and liquid covered wounds: electric fields delivered to model platelets and cells. J Phys D Appl Phys. 2014;47(23):235201.

50. Neyts EC, Yusupov M, Verlackt CC, Bogaerts A. Computer simulations of plasma–biomolecule and plasma–tissue interactions for a better insight in plasma medicine. J Phys D Appl Phys. 2014;47(29):293001.
51. Emmert S, Brehmer F, Hänßle H, Helmke A, Mertens N, Ahmed R, Simon D, Wandke D, Maus-Friedrichs W, Däschlein G. Atmospheric pressure plasma in dermatology: Ulcus treatment and much more. Clin Plasma Med. 2013;1(1):24–9.
52. Norberg SA, Johnsen E, Kushner MJ. Helium atmospheric pressure plasma jets interacting with wet cells: delivery of electric fields. J Phys D Appl Phys. 2016;49(18):185201.
53. Vandamme M, Robert E, Pesnel S, Barbosa E, Dozias S, Sobilo J, Lerondel S, Le Pape A, Pouvesle JM. Antitumor effect of plasma treatment on U87 glioma xenografts: preliminary results. Plasma Process Polym. 2010;7(3–4):264–73.
54. Weltmann K, von Woedtke T. Plasma medicine—current state of research and medical application. Plasma Phys Control Fusion. 2016;59(1):014031.
55. Cao X, Vassen R, Stoever D. Ceramic materials for thermal barrier coatings. J Eur Ceram Soc. 2004;24(1):1–10.
56. Foerch R, McIntyre N, Sodhi R, Hunter D. Nitrogen plasma treatment of polyethylene and polystyrene in a remote plasma reactor. J Appl Polym Sci. 1990;40(11–12):1903–15.
57. Polak M, Winter J, Schnabel U, Ehlbeck J, Weltmann KD. Innovative plasma generation in flexible biopsy channels for inner-tube decontamination and medical applications. Plasma Process Polym. 2012;9(1):67–76.
58. Critchley J, Knight G, Wright W. Fluorine-containing polymers. In: Heat-resistant polymers. New York: Springer; 1983. p. 87–123.
59. Barbier O, Arreola-Mendoza L, Del Razo LM. Molecular mechanisms of fluoride toxicity. Chem Biol Interact. 2010;188(2):319–33.
60. Kohn WG, Maas WR, Malvitz DM, Presson SM, Shaddix KK. Recommendations for using fluoride to prevent and control dental caries in the United States. Morb Mortal Wkly Rep. 2001;50:1–42.
61. Beyler CL, Hirschler MM. Thermal decomposition of polymers. In: DiNenno PJ, editor. SFPE handbook of fire protection engineering, vol. 2. 3rd ed. Quincy: Protection Association; 2002. p. 111–31.
62. Stapler JT, Barnes WJ, Yelland WE. Thermal degradation of polyvinylidene fluoride and polyvinyl fluoride by oven pyrolysis, Army Natick Labs MA Clothing and Organic Materials Lab.; 1968.
63. Patel P, Hull TR, McCabe RW, Flath D, Grasmeder J, Percy M. Mechanism of thermal decomposition of poly (ether ether ketone)(PEEK) from a review of decomposition studies. Polym Degrad Stab. 2010;95(5):709–18.
64. Fricke K, Reuter S, Schroder D, Schulz-von der Gathen V, Weltmann K-D, von Woedtke T. Investigation of surface etching of poly (ether ether ketone) by atmospheric-pressure plasmas. IEEE Transact Plasma Sci. 2012;40(11):2900–11.
65. Fricke K, Steffen H, Von Woedtke T, Schröder K, Weltmann KD. High rate etching of polymers by means of an atmospheric pressure plasma jet. Plasma Process Polym. 2011;8(1):51–8.
66. Flamm DL, Auciello O. Plasma deposition, treatment, and etching of polymers: the treatment and etching of polymers. Amsterdam: Elsevier; 2012.
67. Oehrlein GS, Phaneuf RJ, Graves DB. Plasma-polymer interactions: a review of progress in understanding polymer resist mask durability during plasma etching for nanoscale fabrication. J Vac Sci Technol. 2011;29(1):010801.
68. Wende K, Schröder K, Lindequist U, Ohl A. Plasma-based modification of polystyrene surfaces for serum-free culture of osteoblastic cell lines. Plasma Process Polym. 2006;3(6–7):524–31.
69. Ohorodnik S, DeGendt S, Tong S, Harrison W. Consideration of the chemical reactivity of trace impurities present in a glow discharge. J Anal At Spectrom. 1993;8(6):859–65.
70. Winter J, Wende K, Masur K, Iseni S, Dünnbier M, Hammer M, Tresp H, Weltmann K, Reuter S. Feed gas humidity: a vital parameter affecting a cold atmospheric-pressure plasma jet and plasma-treated human skin cells. J Phys D Appl Phys. 2013;46(29):295401.

71. Frenking G, Koch W, Reichel F, Cremer D. Light noble gas chemistry: STRUCTURES, stabilities, and bonding of helium, neon, and argon compounds. J Am Chem Soc. 1990;112(11):4240–56.
72. Grochala W, Khriachtchev L, Räsänen M. Noble-gas chemistry. In: Khriachtchev F, editor. Physics and chemistry at low temperatures, vol. 13. Singapore: Pan Stanford; 2011. p. 419.
73. Eisenhauer D, Saunders C, Ho H, Wolfe B. Hemodynamic effects of argon pneumoperitoneum. Surg Endosc. 1994;8(4):315–21.
74. Leighton TA, Liu S-Y, Bongard FS. Comparative cardiopulmonary effects of carbon dioxide versus helium pneumoperitoneum. Surgery. 1993;113(5):527–31.
75. Van Gessel A, Alards K, Bruggeman P. NO production in an RF plasma jet at atmospheric pressure. J Phys D Appl Phys. 2013;46(26):265202.
76. Iseni S, Zhang S, van Gessel A, Hofmann S, van Ham B, Reuter S, Weltmann K, Bruggeman P. Nitric oxide density distributions in the effluent of an RF argon APPJ: effect of gas flow rate and substrate. New J Phys. 2014;16(12):123011.
77. Kogoma M, Okazaki S. Raising of ozone formation efficiency in a homogeneous glow discharge plasma at atmospheric pressure. J Phys D Appl Phys. 1994;27(9):1985.
78. Zhang S, van Gaens W, van Gessel B, Hofmann S, van Veldhuizen E, Bogaerts A, Bruggeman P. Spatially resolved ozone densities and gas temperatures in a time modulated RF driven atmospheric pressure plasma jet: an analysis of the production and destruction mechanisms. J Phys D Appl Phys. 2013;46(20):205202.
79. Bussiahn R, Lembke N, Gesche R, von Woedtke T, Weltmann KD. Plasmaquellen für biomedizinische Anwendungen. HygMed. 2013;38:216–21.
80. Kalghatgi S, Fridman A, Azizkhan-Clifford J, Friedman G. DNA damage in mammalian cells by non-thermal atmospheric pressure microsecond pulsed dielectric barrier discharge plasma is not mediated by ozone. Plasma Process Polym. 2012;9(7):726–32.
81. Ziuzina D, Patil S, Cullen P, Keener K, Bourke P. Atmospheric cold plasma inactivation of Escherichia coli in liquid media inside a sealed package. J Appl Microbiol. 2013;114(3):778–87.
82. Graves DB. The emerging role of reactive oxygen and nitrogen species in redox biology and some implications for plasma applications to medicine and biology. J Phys D Appl Phys. 2012;45(26):263001.
83. Reuter S, Tresp H, Wende K, Hammer MU, Winter J, Masur K, Schmidt-Bleker A, Weltmann K-D. From RONS to ROS: tailoring plasma jet treatment of skin cells. IEEE Transact Plasma Sci. 2012;40(11):2986–93.
84. Vandamme M, Robert E, Lerondel S, Sarron V, Ries D, Dozias S, Sobilo J, Gosset D, Kieda C, Legrain B. ROS implication in a new antitumor strategy based on non-thermal plasma. Int J Cancer. 2012;130(9):2185–94.
85. Wende K, Williams P, Dalluge J, Van Gaens W, Aboubakr H, Bischof J, von Woedtke T, Goyal SM, Weltmann K-D, Bogaerts A. Identification of the biologically active liquid chemistry induced by a nonthermal atmospheric pressure plasma jet. Biointerphases. 2015;10(2):029518.
86. Bielski BH, Cabelli DE, Arudi RL, Ross AB. Reactivity of HO2/O− 2 radicals in aqueous solution. J Phys Chem Ref Data Monogr. 1985;14(4):1041–100.
87. Hanschmann E-M, Godoy JR, Berndt C, Hudemann C, Lillig CH. Thioredoxins, glutaredoxins, and peroxiredoxins—molecular mechanisms and health significance: from cofactors to antioxidants to redox signaling. Antioxid Redox Signal. 2013;19(13):1539–605.
88. Neta P, Huie RE, Ross AB. Rate constants for reactions of inorganic radicals in aqueous solution. J Phys Chem Ref Data Monogr. 1988;17(3):1027–284.
89. Buxton GV, Greenstock CL, Helman WP, Ross AB. Critical review of rate constants for reactions of hydrated electrons, hydrogen atoms and hydroxyl radicals ( OH/· O− in aqueous solution). J Phys Chem Ref Data Monogr. 1988;17(2):513–886.
90. Joshi AA, Locke BR, Arce P, Finney WC. Formation of hydroxyl radicals, hydrogen peroxide and aqueous electrons by pulsed streamer corona discharge in aqueous solution. J Hazard Mater. 1995;41(1):3–30.

91. Winter J, Tresp H, Hammer M, Iseni S, Kupsch S, Schmidt-Bleker A, Wende K, Dünnbier M, Masur K, Weltmann K. Tracking plasma generated H2O2 from gas into liquid phase and revealing its dominant impact on human skin cells. J Phys D Appl Phys. 2014;47(28): 285401.
92. Buettner GR, Oberley LW. Considerations in the spin trapping of superoxide and hydroxyl radical in aqueous systems using 5, 5-dimethyl-1-pyrroline-1-oxide. Biochem Biophys Res Commun. 1978;83(1):69–74.
93. Winterbourn CC. Reconciling the chemistry and biology of reactive oxygen species. Nat Chem Biol. 2008;4(5):278–86.
94. Bekeschus S, Liedtke KR, von Woedtke T, Partecke LI. Pro-oxidant tumor therapy in murine melanoma and pancreatic cancer. Free Radic Biol Med. 2017;108:S76.
95. Choe E, Min DB. Chemistry and reactions of reactive oxygen species in foods. J Food Sci. 2005;70(9).
96. Fahy E, Subramaniam S, Brown HA, Glass CK, Merrill AH, Murphy RC, Raetz CR, Russell DW, Seyama Y, Shaw W. A comprehensive classification system for lipids. J Lipid Res. 2005;46(5):839–62.
97. Dorai R, Kushner MJ. A model for plasma modification of polypropylene using atmospheric pressure discharges. J Phys D Appl Phys. 2003;36(6):666.
98. Fridman A. Plasma chemistry. Cambridge: Cambridge University Press; 2008.
99. Reinke M, Mantzaras J, Bombach R, Schenker S, Inauen A. Gas phase chemistry in catalytic combustion of methane/air mixtures over platinum at pressures of 1 to 16 bar. Combust Flame. 2005;141(4):448–68.
100. Van der Paal J, Aernouts S, van Duin AC, Neyts EC, Bogaerts A. Interaction of O and OH radicals with a simple model system for lipids in the skin barrier: a reactive molecular dynamics investigation for plasma medicine. J Phys D Appl Phys. 2013;46(39):395201.
101. Van der Paal J, Neyts EC, Verlackt CC, Bogaerts A. Effect of lipid peroxidation on membrane permeability of cancer and normal cells subjected to oxidative stress. Chem Sci. 2016;7(1):489–98.
102. Maheux S, Frache G, Thomann J, Clément F, Penny C, Belmonte T, Duday D. Small unilamellar liposomes as a membrane model for cell inactivation by cold atmospheric plasma treatment. J Phys D Appl Phys. 2016;49(34):344001.
103. Svarnas P, Matrali S, Gazeli K, Aleiferis S, Clément F, Antimisiaris S. Atmospheric-pressure guided streamers for liposomal membrane disruption. Appl Phys Lett. 2012;101(26):264103.
104. Yusupov M, Wende K, Kupsch S, Neyts E, Reuter S, Bogaerts A. Effect of head group and lipid tail oxidation in the cell membrane revealed through integrated simulations and experiments. Sci Rep. 2017;7:5761.
105. Roehm JN, Hadley JG, Menzel DB. Oxidation of unsaturated fatty acids by ozone and nitrogen dioxide. Arch Environ Health. 1971;23(2):142–8.
106. Guéraud F, Atalay M, Bresgen N, Cipak A, Eckl PM, Huc L, Jouanin I, Siems W, Uchida K. Chemistry and biochemistry of lipid peroxidation products. Free Radic Res. 2010;44(10):1098–124.
107. Ayala A, Muñoz MF, Argüelles S. Lipid peroxidation: production, metabolism, and signaling mechanisms of malondialdehyde and 4-hydroxy-2-nonenal. Oxid Med Cell Longev. 2014;2014.
108. Kansanen E, Jyrkkänen H-K, Levonen A-L. Activation of stress signaling pathways by electrophilic oxidized and nitrated lipids. Free Radic Biol Med. 2012;52(6):973–82.
109. Hammer MU, Forbrig E, Kupsch S, Weltmann K-D, Reuter S. Influence of plasma treatment on the structure and function of lipids. Plasma Med. 2013;3(1–2):97–114.
110. Tero R, Yamashita R, Hashizume H, Suda Y, Takikawa H, Hori M, Ito M. Nanopore formation process in artificial cell membrane induced by plasma-generated reactive oxygen species. Arch Biochem Biophys. 2016;605:26–33.
111. Schmidt A, Dietrich S, Steuer A, Weltmann K-D, von Woedtke T, Masur K, Wende K. Non-thermal plasma activates human keratinocytes by stimulation of antioxidant and phase II pathways. J Biol Chem. 2015;290(11):6731–50.

112. Leduc M, Guay D, Coulombe S, Leask RL. Effects of non-thermal plasmas on DNA and mammalian cells. Plasma Process Polym. 2010;7(11):899–909.
113. Takai E, Kitamura T, Kuwabara J, Ikawa S, Yoshizawa S, Shiraki K, Kawasaki H, Arakawa R, Kitano K. Chemical modification of amino acids by atmospheric-pressure cold plasma in aqueous solution. J Phys D Appl Phys. 2014;47(28):285403.
114. Yan D, Talbot A, Nourmohammadi N, Cheng X, Canady J, Sherman J, Keidar M. Principles of using cold atmospheric plasma stimulated media for cancer treatment. Sci Rep. 2015;5:18339.
115. Lackmann J, Baldus S, Steinborn E, Edengeiser E, Kogelheide F, Langklotz S, Schneider S, Leichert L, Benedikt J, Awakowicz P. A dielectric barrier discharge terminally inactivates RNase A by oxidizing sulfur-containing amino acids and breaking structural disulfide bonds. J Phys D Appl Phys. 2015;48(49):494003.
116. Lackmann J-W, Bandow JE. Inactivation of microbes and macromolecules by atmospheric-pressure plasma jets. Appl Microbiol Biotechnol. 2014;98(14):6205–13.
117. Venter JC, Adams MD, Myers EW, Li PW, Mural RJ, Sutton GG, Smith HO, Yandell M, Evans CA, Holt RA. The sequence of the human genome. Science. 2001;291(5507):1304–51.
118. Fatica A, Bozzoni I. Long non-coding RNAs: new players in cell differentiation and development. Nat Rev Genet. 2014;15(1):7.
119. Frøkjær-Jensen C, Jain N, Hansen L, Davis MW, Li Y, Zhao D, Rebora K, Millet JR, Liu X, Kim SK. An abundant class of Non-coding DNA can prevent stochastic gene silencing in the C. elegans Germline. Cell. 2016;166(2):343–57.
120. Ling H, Vincent K, Pichler M, Fodde R, Berindan-Neagoe I, Slack FJ, Calin GA. Junk DNA and the long non-coding RNA twist in cancer genetics. Oncogene. 2015;34(39):5003–11.
121. Varki A, Altheide TK. Comparing the human and chimpanzee genomes: searching for needles in a haystack. Genome Res. 2005;15(12):1746–58.
122. Bernstein BE, Meissner A, Lander ES. The mammalian epigenome. Cell. 2007;128(4):669–81.
123. Reha-Krantz LJ. DNA polymerase proofreading: multiple roles maintain genome stability. Biochim Biophys Acta. 2010;1804(5):1049–63.
124. Kunkel TA, Erie DA. Eukaryotic mismatch repair in relation to DNA replication. Annu Rev Genet. 2015;49:291–313.
125. Lujan SA, Clausen AR, Clark AB, MacAlpine HK, MacAlpine DM, Malc EP, Mieczkowski PA, Burkholder AB, Fargo DC, Gordenin DA. Heterogeneous polymerase fidelity and mismatch repair bias genome variation and composition. Genome Res. 2014;24(11):1751–64.
126. St Charles JA, Liberti SE, Williams JS, Lujan SA, Kunkel TA. Quantifying the contributions of base selectivity, proofreading and mismatch repair to nuclear DNA replication in Saccharomyces cerevisiae. DNA Repair. 2015;31:41–51.
127. Ganai RA, Johansson E. DNA replication—a matter of fidelity. Mol Cell. 2016;62(5):745–55.
128. Ridings JE. The thalidomide disaster, lessons from the past. Methods Mol Biol. 2013;947:575–86.
129. Kanvah S, Joseph J, Schuster GB, Barnett RN, Cleveland CL, Landman U. Oxidation of DNA: damage to nucleobases. Acc Chem Res. 2009;43(2):280–7.
130. Marrot L, Meunier J-R. Skin DNA photodamage and its biological consequences. J Am Acad Dermatol. 2008;58(5):S139–48.
131. Bender CP, Hübner N-O, Weltmann K-D, Scharf C, Kramer A. Tissue tolerable plasma and polihexanide: are synergistic effects possible to promote healing of chronic wounds? In vivo and in vitro results. In: Machala Z, Hensen K, Akishev Y, editors. Plasma for bio-decontamination, medicine and food security. Heidelberg: Springer; 2012. p. 321–34.
132. Fluhr JW, Sassning S, Lademann O, Darvin ME, Schanzer S, Kramer A, Richter H, Sterry W, Lademann J. In vivo skin treatment with tissue-tolerable plasma influences skin physiology and antioxidant profile in human stratum corneum. Exp Dermatol. 2012;21(2):130–4.
133. Fridman G, Peddinghaus M, Balasubramanian M, Ayan H, Fridman A, Gutsol A, Brooks A. Blood coagulation and living tissue sterilization by floating-electrode dielectric barrier discharge in air. Plasma Chem Plasma Process. 2006;26(4):425–42.

134. Lademann J, Richter H, Alborova A, Humme D, Patzelt A, Kramer A, Weltmann K-D, Hartmann B, Ottomann C, Fluhr JW. Risk assessment of the application of a plasma jet in dermatology. J Biomed Opt. 2009;14(5):054025.
135. Lademann J, Ulrich C, Patzelt A, Richter H, Kluschke F, Klebes M, Lademann O, Kramer A, Weltmann K, Lange-Asschenfeldt B. Risk assessment of the application of tissue-tolerable plasma on human skin. Clin Plasma Med. 2013;1(1):5–10.
136. Metelmann H-R, von Woedtke T, Bussiahn R, Weltmann K-D, Rieck M, Khalili R, Podmelle F, Waite PD. Experimental recovery of CO2-laser skin lesions by plasma stimulation. Am J Cosmet Surg. 2012;29(1):52–6.
137. Kos S, Blagus T, Cemazar M, Filipic G, Sersa G, Cvelbar U. Safety aspects of atmospheric pressure helium plasma jet operation on skin: in vivo study on mouse skin. PLoS One. 2017;12(4):e0174966.
138. Kurita H, Nakajima T, Yasuda H, Takashima K, Mizuno A, Wilson JI, Cunningham S. Single-molecule measurement of strand breaks on large DNA induced by atmospheric pressure plasma jet. Appl Phys Lett. 2011;99(19):191504.
139. O'Connell D, Cox L, Hyland W, McMahon S, Reuter S, Graham W, Gans T, Currell F. Cold atmospheric pressure plasma jet interactions with plasmid DNA. Appl Phys Lett. 2011;98(4):043701.
140. Ptasińska S, Bahnev B, Stypczyńska A, Bowden M, Mason NJ, Braithwaite NSJ. DNA strand scission induced by a non-thermal atmospheric pressure plasma jet. Phys Chem Chem Phys. 2010;12(28):7779–81.
141. Lindahl T. Instability and decay of the primary structure of DNA. Nature. 1993;362(6422): 709–15.
142. Vijayaraghavan R, Izgorodin A, Ganesh V, Surianarayanan M, MacFarlane DR. Long-term structural and chemical stability of DNA in hydrated ionic liquids. Angew Chem Int Ed. 2010;49(9):1631–3.
143. Peterson CL, Laniel M-A. Histones and histone modifications. Curr Biol. 2004;14(14): R546–51.
144. Tessarz P, Kouzarides T. Histone core modifications regulating nucleosome structure and dynamics. Nat Rev Mol Cell Biol. 2014;15(11):703.
145. Hoeijmakers JH. Genome maintenance mechanisms for preventing cancer. Nature. 2001;411(6835):366.
146. Iyama T, Wilson DM. DNA repair mechanisms in dividing and non-dividing cells. DNA Repair. 2013;12(8):620–36.
147. Jackson SP, Bartek J. The DNA-damage response in human biology and disease. Nature. 2009;461(7267):1071.
148. Hoeijmakers JH. DNA damage, aging, and cancer. N Engl J Med. 2009;361(15):1475–85.
149. Boxhammer V, Li Y, Köritzer J, Shimizu T, Maisch T, Thomas H, Schlegel J, Morfill G, Zimmermann J. Investigation of the mutagenic potential of cold atmospheric plasma at bactericidal dosages. Mutat Res. 2013;753(1):23–8.
150. Kluge S, Bekeschus S, Bender C, Benkhai H, Sckell A, Below H, Stope MB, Kramer A. Investigating the mutagenicity of a cold argon-plasma jet in an HET-MN model. PLoS One. 2016;11(9):e0160667.
151. Maisch T, Bosserhoff A, Unger P, Heider J, Shimizu T, Zimmermann J, Morfill G, Landthaler M, Karrer S. Investigation of toxicity and mutagenicity of cold atmospheric argon plasma. Environ Mol Mutagen. 2017;58(3):172–7.
152. Wende K, Bekeschus S, Schmidt A, Jatsch L, Hasse S, Weltmann K, Masur K, von Woedtke T. Risk assessment of a cold argon plasma jet in respect to its mutagenicity. Mutat Res. 2016;798:48–54.
153. Hay ED. Cell biology of extracellular matrix. New York: Springer Science & Business Media; 2013.
154. Fenech M, Chang W, Kirsch-Volders M, Holland N, Bonassi S, Zeiger E. HUMN project: detailed description of the scoring criteria for the cytokinesis-block micronucleus assay using isolated human lymphocyte cultures. Mutat Res. 2003;534(1):65–75.

155. Fenech M. Cytokinesis-block micronucleus assay evolves into a "cytome" assay of chromosomal instability, mitotic dysfunction and cell death. Mutat Res. 2006;600(1):58–66.
156. Fenech M. Cytokinesis-block micronucleus cytome assay. Nat Protoc. 2007;2(5):1084–104.
157. Boehm D, Heslin C, Cullen PJ, Bourke P. Cytotoxic and mutagenic potential of solutions exposed to cold atmospheric plasma. Sci Rep. 2016;6:21464.
158. Burma S, Chen BP, Murphy M, Kurimasa A, Chen DJ. ATM phosphorylates histone H2AX in response to DNA double-strand breaks. J Biol Chem. 2001;276(45):42462–7.
159. Hirst AM, Frame FM, Maitland NJ, O'Connell D. Low temperature plasma causes double-strand break DNA damage in primary epithelial cells cultured from a human prostate tumor. IEEE Trans Plasma Sci. 2014;42(10):2740–1.
160. Kalghatgi S, Kelly CM, Cerchar E, Torabi B, Alekseev O, Fridman A, Friedman G, Azizkhan-Clifford J. Effects of non-thermal plasma on mammalian cells. PLoS One. 2011;6(1):e16270.
161. Schlegel J, Köritzer J, Boxhammer V. Plasma in cancer treatment. Clin Plasma Med. 2013; 1(2):2–7.
162. Schmidt A, Rödder K, Hasse S, Masur K, Toups L, Lillig CH, von Woedtke T, Wende K, Bekeschus S. Redox-regulation of activator protein 1 family members in blood cancer cell lines exposed to cold physical plasma-treated medium. Plasma Process Polym. 2016;13(12):1179–88.
163. Ahmed K, Tabuchi Y, Kondo T. Hyperthermia: an effective strategy to induce apoptosis in cancer cells. Apoptosis. 2015;20(11):1411–9.
164. Rybak P, Hoang A, Bujnowicz L, Bernas T, Berniak K, Zarębski M, Darzynkiewicz Z, Dobrucki J. Low level phosphorylation of histone H2AX on serine 139 (γH2AX) is not associated with DNA double-strand breaks. Oncotarget. 2016;7(31):49574.
165. Collins AR. The comet assay for DNA damage and repair. Mol Biotechnol. 2004;26(3):249.
166. Tice RR, Agurell E, Anderson D, Burlinson B, Hartmann A, Kobayashi H, Miyamae Y, Rojas E, Ryu JC, Sasaki Y. Single cell gel/comet assay: guidelines for in vitro and in vivo genetic toxicology testing. Environ Mol Mutagen. 2000;35(3):206–21.
167. Iseki S, Nakamura K, Hayashi M, Tanaka H, Kondo H, Kajiyama H, Kano H, Kikkawa F, Hori M. Selective killing of ovarian cancer cells through induction of apoptosis by nonequilibrium atmospheric pressure plasma. Appl Phys Lett. 2012;100(11):113702.
168. Nagata S. Apoptotic DNA fragmentation. Exp Cell Res. 2000;256(1):12–8.
169. Schmidt A, Bekeschus S, Wende K, Vollmar B, Woedtke T. A cold plasma jet accelerates wound healing in a murine model of full-thickness skin wounds. Exp Dermatol. 2016; 26(2):156–62.

# Part II

# Applying Physical Plasma: Clinical Use

# 6 Antimicrobial Activity of Plasma

Georg Daeschlein

## 6.1 Summary

Cold plasma is now available since a lot of years and since approval apart from a multitude of in vitro experiments many patients have undergone plasma therapy. Actually tumor and antimicrobial skin and wound treatment seem the most attractive treatment options with an urgent need for alternative therapies. This is also valid for recalcitrant ulcer wounds, whereby actually no valid multicenter studies but promising observations with good results of plasma therapy are available. Before general recommendations are to be made regarding use of "plasma antisepsis" and treatment of recalcitrant wounds evidence based studies must show the clinical suitability of the intervention. Own studies show excellent results of plasma in the treatment of nosocomial pathogens on skin and wounds as well as of dermal precancerosis. It must be emphasized to ever keep sight of ethical aspects of any use of new methods in medicine: Less marketing and more serious results of valid tolerability as well as efficacy studies should persuade the doctor in practice to assume responsibility for his patients and to let. This will be a mutual benefit for patients and public health as well.

## 6.2 Introduction

The new medical field plasma medicine is celebrating its decennial birthday [1, 2].

Beside multiple applications in technology and biology cold and plasmas are worldwide under investigation to create innovative applications.

This is possible since already known "hot" plasma could be domesticated to skin tolerated treatments.

G. Daeschlein
Department of Dermatology, University of Greifswald, Greifswald, Germany
e-mail: georg.daeschlein@uni-greifswald.de



H.-R. Metelmann et al. (eds.), *Comprehensive Clinical Plasma Medicine*,
https://doi.org/10.1007/978-3-319-67627-2_6

On the other hand "cold" plasmas were already sold about 100 years ago in USA and Europe as high-frequency therapy and at the moment still two companies offer "high-frequency" related plasma devices in Germany. The antimicrobial activity was one of the mostly claimed properties of these devices, and meanwhile could be approved in vitro for important pathogens of bacteria, fungi, viruses and parasites [3]. Even the background being not fully understood, it can be assumed that this activity of the plasma is responsible for the effectiveness of most clinical applications, except antitumor efficacy, which currently is under vigorous investigation.

## 6.3 Why Plasma

Physical treatments to defeat microbial challenges have a long-standing tradition and many medical applications focus on broad antimicrobial activity by distance. However up to date no device with pure physical antimicrobial efficacy has entered medical business and potential treatments with potent antimicrobial properties like UV photons are to be dropped out because of safety reasons.

In contrast to all kind of physical skin and wound treatments up to day in use now cold plasma offers a wide spectrum of effective species with potent antimicrobial properties allowing disinfection of skin and wounds.

CAP effects include

- reactive oxidative and nitrogen species (ROS and RNS),
- free radicals,
- ions,
- electric fields,
- electrons
- UV photons [4, 5],

These species justify antimicrobial applications of CAP inducing bacteriocidic effects based upon membrane oxidation, cell wall and DNA disintegration [6]. In comparison with other means like UV radiation the "cocktail" offered by CAP can be realized with far less energy dosage which enables safer clinical applicability. Not any of the mentioned reactive species alone could be applied without the danger of harmful skin effects because the need for much higher doses.

## 6.4 Worldwide Problems with Multi Drug Resistance

The actual situation regarding multi drug resistance is far from being desirable.

Despite some efforts fighting MRSA, these bugs still represent a relevant challenge up to day and in the US ambulant variants CA-MRSA (community-acquired) meanwhile have supplanted hospital-acquired MRSA (HA-MRSA) as first pathogen in patients with wound infections [7].

Coincident with worldwide decreasing MRSA incidence now another group of multi drug resistant pathogens, the MRGN (multi drug resistant gramnegative rods, mostly enterobacteriaceae) have entered the stage and pose significant problems in intensive care units [8].

Additionally regarding new antibiotic development the situation seems not optimistic. In parallel to lacking approvals of new therapeutics decreasing investments for antibiotic research can be noticed.

A way out could be realized by CAP, because its antimicrobial properties rely on completely different mechanisms compared with any conventional antimicrobial chemotherapeutic.

Therefore a benefit using CAP in the fight against multi drug resistance can be assumed, i.e. treating wound infections caused by MDR bugs but also decolonizing colonized skin in the hospital. Although full susceptibility of pathogens to CAP can be expected and was supported by first experiments we now can differentiate some distinct variations between species, which are further discussed in Chaps. 6.9–6.11.

## 6.5 Not Only Bacteria To Be Focused

Apart from bacteria many more microorganisms causing infections worldwide still pose substantial problems, thereof among others atypical mycobacteria, fungi (yeasts and also molds), chlamydia, mycoplasma and viruses like hepatitis virus and some parasites such as toxoplasma gondii, leishmania spp. and entamoeba histolyticum. A special case are cryptosporidia, which can cause important gastrointestinal diseases exhibiting important resistance towards disinfectants in the environment. Against Leishmania Fridman et al. could demonstrate CAP efficacy [9], our group was able to show potent CAP-efficacy against Demodex folliculorum [10]. In contrast to antibacterial efficacy with multidrug resistance as main problem, the problem with parasites means to find at all effective treatments with good tolerability.

## 6.6 Antimicrobial Applications

For CAP as for any other new treatment option a clear indication based upon evidence of efficacy is recommended and for clinical practice the treatment of choice is this one with best efficacy together with best tolerability. When both treatments fulfill these recommendations the product with best price will be advised.

Therefore before a treatment is planned alternatives and potential adverse effects and costs have to be weighted prior to use. As an example it makes no sense to use CAP as a disinfectant on surfaces where simple ethanol based disinfectants make the same job over 30 s exposure. CAP applications seem meaningful when conventional procedures are not (fully) successful, i.e. MRSA sanitization on human skin in case of recalcitrant colonization. Another purpose is CAP application for wound healing after successful elimination of those factors which were responsible for impaired healing capacity like chronic venous insufficiency or bacterial biofilms. At the moment CAP is clinically mainly used to improve healing in patients with chronic wounds.

## 6.7 Less Antimicrobial Susceptibility Under Cap-Treatment?

Since antimicrobial CAP activity is not related to the mechanisms described for chemotherapeutic drugs it can be assumed that the feared selection of resistant strains which are propagated throughout the world may be omitted. The mode of action by CAP which can be compared most likely with antiseptics and disinfectants is based upon biophysical attack together with strong oxidation and follows an overkill model. Only at low concentrations disinfectants do not work and allow survival of pahogens thus promoting spread situations in hospitals. At right concentrations not one cell can survive providing high confidence in routine disinfection procedures. This is the only condition highly recommended during CAP use treating i.e. biofilms and the lack of resistance development now is referenced by several groups. However, since up to day no standardized method for susceptibiity testing of CAP is available, implementation of such a test model and larger studies with species and strains from different regions are strongly warranted.

## 6.8 Susceptibility Testing of CAP In Vitro

Over decades standard tests exist to evaluate susceptibility of bacteria towards antibiotics with different methods following national and international proceeding guidelines. Over years microbouillon dilution methods were developed to gold standard in susceptibility testing resulting in minimal inhibitory concentrations (MIC), which are tested as break point values in routine testing. This test procedure has replaced the former used agar diffusion method (Agardiffusionstest nach Bauer und Kirby; [11]) which is much easier to perform but provides values that cannot be related to therapeutic serum levels as MIC. Nevertheless agar diffusion still is used for special questions like ESBL-testing and as orientating test for some difficult to test organisms. Both test methods refer on stringently chosen drug but also pathogen concentrations in suspensions. For MIC testing geometric dilutions of drugs are incubated with stable pathogen suspensions and resulting growth quantified after turbidimetric measurement in microvials. Our group has undertaken MIC testing of CAP in microtiterplates by adapting standard methods, resulting in doses by which complete killing of a known pathogen is achieved. This method seems valid but needs copious validation. The main problem is standardisation with exposure times of half a second changing significantly test results which causes larger experimental effort to gain stable data. Therefore most experimentators experience modifications of Bauer and Kirby's agar diffusion method which is much easier to perform. It has to be mentioned that both methods were worked out for solids but per se not for radiation testing and (see above) up to we still have no standard test for CAP susceptibility testing. Even when CAP is assumed as working by oxidizing species, the complexity of such mode of action (chemical reactions cannot be reduced to a simple calculable value) causes the described difficulties resulting from MIC testing in suspensions [12].

When CAP was tested on agar, we could show that CAP efficacy rapidly decreased with increasing concentrations but also with maturity of colonies, a phenomenon which may be related to physical density ("shadow effect") [12]. This has to be mentioned for better understanding and estimation of CAP effects in complex situations (biofilms, wound secretions) and underline the importance to correlate inhibition zones to clinical outcome in larger studies.

Up to now a multitude of species was tested against CAP including all kind of clinical relevant pathogens causing acute and chronic skin and wound infections and septcemia. With the important restriction that we can conclude that by no author CAP resistant strains or species were recorded (means no inhibition zone obtained after 1–60 s on solid media like agar) [13, 14]. Our group tested some thousands of strains and neither with the most in use CAP device, the Argon fed kINPen (INP Greifswald, Germany) nor different DBD (i.e. CINOGY, Duderstadt, Germany, TEFRA, Berlin, Germany, PMS, Bad Ems, Germany) showed resistant strains.

The lack of resistant strains does not mean that all strains show identic inhibition zones or MICs. We found significant and not significant differences between gram positive and negative species and also between strains with different susceptibility towards chemotherapeutic drugs. I.e. for some enterococci and also S. aureus the degree of drug resistance determined the susceptibility towards CAP, in detail VRE and HLGR were less susceptible to CAP (for more details see also the following chapters) [12].

Other authors published less CAP susceptibility of spore forming bacteria [15], what was explained by the envelope lacking water.

Also Lee et al. found differences in susceptibility between gram positive and gram negative bacteria with gram negative bacteria exhibiting better susceptibility to CAP [16], other authors could not verify these differences [17]. Our group found that the described differences depend on the CAP technique, with Argon fed jets we found no significant differences, but using DBD we did (see above, [18]).

## 6.9 Technique of CAP Treatment

Our group in Greifswald uses the following CAP devices

- APPJ, gepulsed and non-pulsed Modus (kINPen Med, INP Greifswald, Germany),
- DBD (PlasmaDerm®, CINOGY, Duderstadt, Germany)
- DBD with glass electrode (plasma MEDICAL SYSTEMS, Bad Ems, Germany), DBD with glass electrode (TEFRA, Berlin, Germany)
- Argonplasma-Jet (Maxium®-Beamer, KLS Martin, Tuttlingen, Germany)

The above mentioned CAP devices produced very similar antimicrobial efficacy as tested on semisolid media in vitro against all up to now tested clinical strains and species independently of the chemotherapeutic drug susceptibility and after 3–60 s of treatment in vitro [10, 18, 19]. Albeit principally susceptibility, some important differences could be noted [12, 18].

Except most relevant clinical bacterial species also clinical relevant fungi and molds were tested against CAP. As examples with excellent susceptibility to CAP here Trichophyton (interdigitale zoophil and anthropophil, rubrum and verrucosum), Microsporum canis, Candida (albicans, glabrata and krusei), Penicillium and Aspergillus should be mentioned.

In representative in vitro study we investigated the dependence of the degree of multi drug resistance of a strain on the susceptibility to CAP and tested 194 multi drug resistant wound isolates against two CAP sources (DBD and pulsed and non-pulsed Argon fed jet).

The following 13 species were tested: *Escherichia coli, Pseudomonas aeruginosa, Extended spectrum beta-lactamase* builder (ESBL), *Staphylococcus epidermidis, Staphylococcus aureus (Methicillin-susceptible, MSSA, Methicillin-resistant, MRSA, Methicillin-resistant Staphylococcus epidermidis, MRSE, Acinetobacter spp., Klebsiella group (Klebsiella pneumoniae ssp. pneumoniae, Klebsiella oxytoca), Enterococcus faecalis, Enterococcus faecium, Vancomycin resistant enterococci VRE and High level gentamycin resistant enterococci HLGR* [19]. In general we could show that the pulsed jet was less effective than the non-pulsed variant ($p < 0.001$) when the inhibition zones on growth agar were compared showing larger zones with the non pulsed jet and best susceptibility of the Gram negative species P. aeruginosa (Figs. 6.1 and 6.2)

Additionally we found gram positive species significantly more susceptible to DBD plasma than gram negative species ($p < 0.001$) (Fig. 6.1). Jet plasma showed

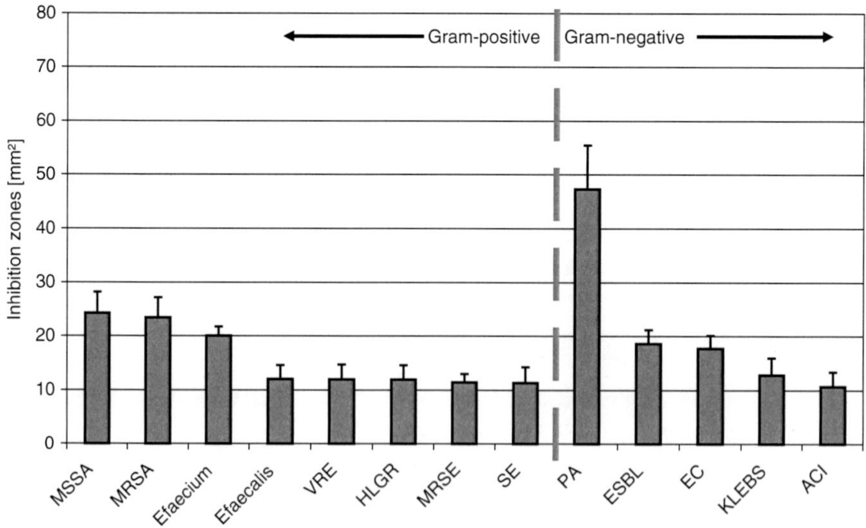


**Fig. 6.1** Ranked inhibition zones (mean and SD) obtained after 3s plasma treatment with non-pulsed APPJ for different Gram positive and Gram negative species

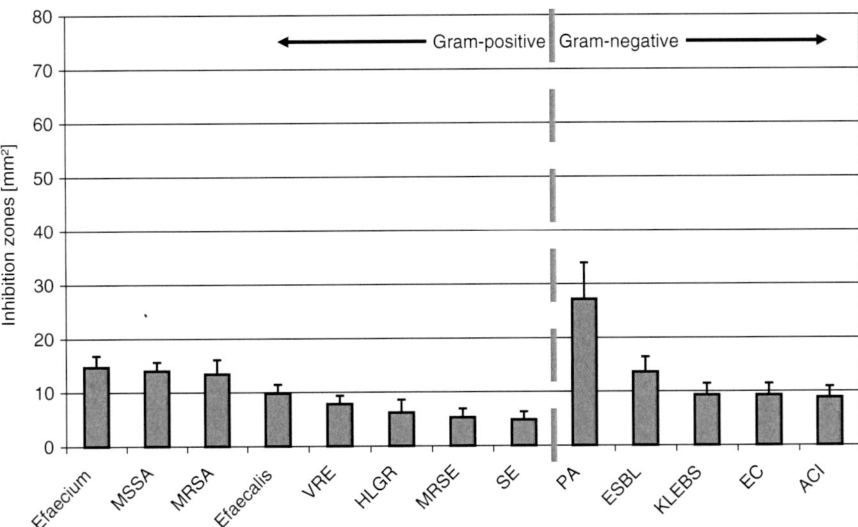


**Fig. 6.2** Ranked inhibition zones (mean and SD) obtained after 3s plasma treatment with pulsed APPJ for different Gram positive and Gram negative species

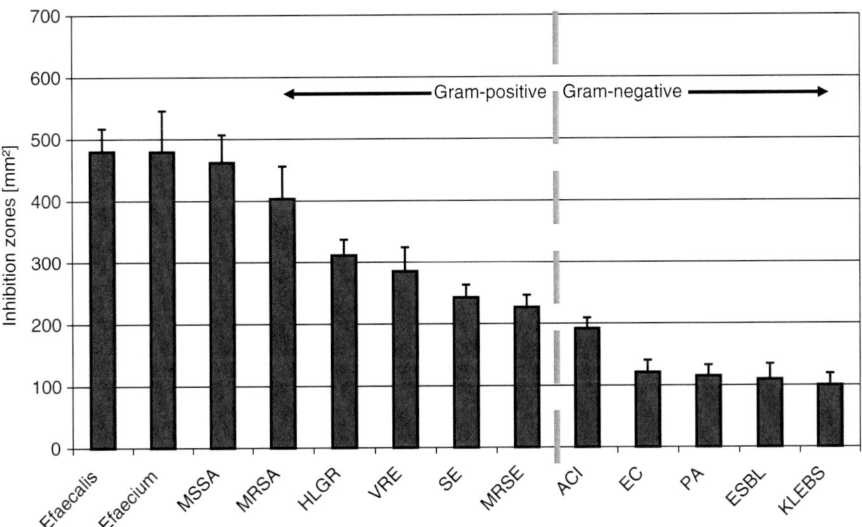


**Fig. 6.3** Ranked inhibition zones (mean and SD) obtained after 3s plasma treatment with DBD for different Gram positive and Gram negative species

another pattern with best susceptibility of the gram negative P. aeruginosa followed by the gram positive S.aureus (MSSA) for both sources (Fig. 6. 2 and 6.3). Interestingly with increasing multi drug resistance (number of classes of antibiotics showing resistance as obtained by conventional susceptibility testing) of a species, susceptibility to

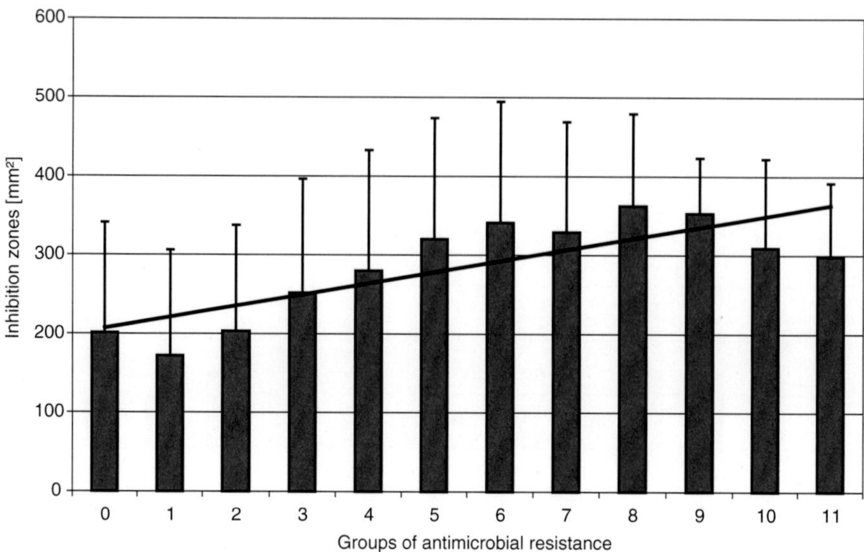


**Fig. 6.4** Increasing antimicrobial resistance against antibiotics (number of classes of antibiotics to which a species showed resistance, x axis) an related inhibition zones (y axis) obtained after 3 s of DBD plasma treatment and trendline (calculated via method of least squares). CAP susceptibility increased with degree of multi drug resistance

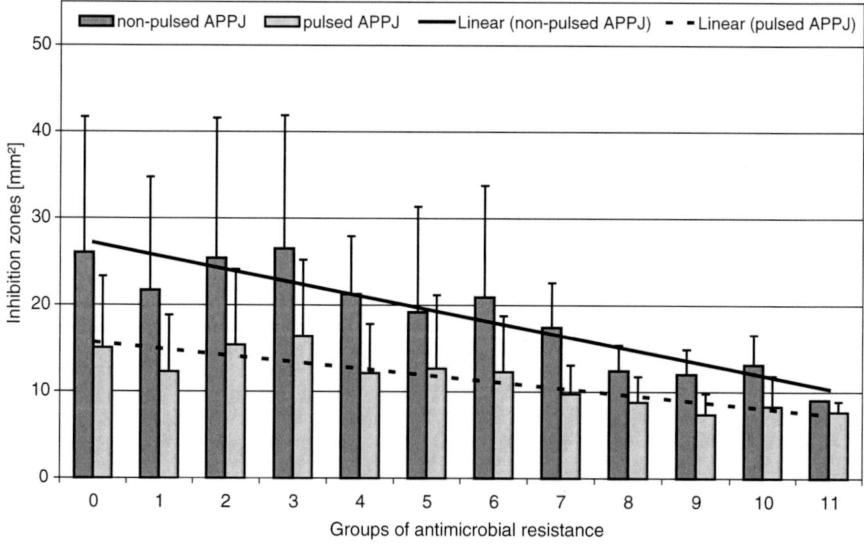


**Fig. 6.5** Increasing antimicrobial resistance against antibiotics (number of classes of antibiotics to which a species showed resistance, x axis) and related inhibition zones (y axis) obtained after 3 s of jet plasma (non pulsed and pulsed) treatment and trendline (calculated via method of least squares). CAP susceptibility decreased with degree of multi drug resistance

CAP decreased when DBD and increased when jets were used (Fig. 6.4 and 6.5) underlining the potential suitability of CAP (DBD) in case of multi drug resistant bacteria bacteria in wounds or elsewhere.

Additionally we found that gras were significantly more susceptible than gram positive ones, regardless the CAP jet source used ($p < 0.001$) (Fig. 6.2) and when DBD was compared with the jets, gram positive species showed more susceptibility to the DBD ($p < 0.001$) (Figs. 6.1, 6.2 and 6.3).

## 6.10 Efficacy Against MRSA In Vitro

Several authors report different CAP susceptibility of MRSA and MSSA in vitro testing some strains and species. In a larger collective of clinically defined strains we investigated 50 MRSA (48 HA-MRSA, 1 LA-MRSA, 1 CA-MRSA) and 168 MSSA [20]. Both bacterial groups MRSA and MSSA showed good susceptibility to CAP (all three sources) but some important differences could be noted. The DBD was the CAP source with the largest electrode surface and showed the largest inhibition zones, however the activity against MRSA was less pronounced in comparison with the jets, what cannot be explained up to now. One explanation could be the thicker cell wall of some strains of MRSA as described by Kawai et al. [21].

## 6.11 Efficacy Against Enterococci In Vitro

Having demonstrated important differences between Staphylococci we intended to investigate also the group of clinically most relevant gram positive cocci, the enterococci.

We further would correlate the influence of conventional drug susceptibility of these bacteria on CAP susceptibility.

As for MRSA and MSSA we could demonstrate different susceptibility to the CAP device in the tests. All tested 39 isolates (including VRE, HLGR) showed 100% susceptibility to any of the three CAP devices but with DBD the anti enterococcal efficacy against the more resistant strains was less strong compared with both jets [12]. In detail using DBD *Vancomycin-resistant enterocci* (VRE) were significantly more resistant than all other enterococci. Also HLGR-isolates showed significantly smaller inhibition areas than other enterococci when treated with the DBD. Surprisingly with both jets HLGR proved significantly more resistant compared with all other enterococci. When both jets were compared generally the non pulsed was more effective than the pulsed variant. With DBD it was shown for all enterocci that with increasing drug resistance (MIC as tested in routine susceptibility testing) the susceptibility to CAP decreased.

## 6.12 Efficacy In Vivo

Ex vivo Maisch et al. [22] could demonstrate a significant decolonization of MRSA by CAP, in vivo, Isbary et al. [23] and Brehmer et al. [24] found significant bacterial reduction (more than 30%) in patients with chronic wounds. Our group investigated antmicrobial CAP activity in chronic wounds with a CAP device used over decades in surgery (plasma knife, thermocoagulation) and which can be also used in a cold plasma mode (Maxium®-beamer, KLS Martin, Germany). Eighteen chronic wounds (included infected ones) from 11 patients were treated with CAP [14], the effect quantified evaluating the microbial load of wounds after swabbing using a modified Levine-technique [25]. In total 24 bacterial pathogens were recorded thereof 17 (71%) multi drug resistant. CAP exhibited strong antimicrobial effects reducing significantly or eliminating the pathogen load.

Differences of efficacy against different species with and without multi resistance were not found, however, most prominent effects were found regarding gram negative species, interestingly markedly against *Pseudomonas aeruginosa* and *Serratia marcescens*) [14]. Al referenced by other authors (Isbary et al. [23] Brehmer et al. [24]) we found excellent tolerability by patients.

## 6.13 Practical Points of View

In the context of a multimodal wound treatment concept CAP can provide important supportive benefit especially in chronic wounds colonized with multi drug resistant pathogens.

CAP treatment allows elimination or strong reduction of microbial load within seconds of treatment including highly resistant strains and species. This works using all CAP devices up to now certified as medical products following the referenced data an own experiences. However, different CAP variants can exhibit varying results regarding inhibition zones and killing kinetics using identical treatment times. Because up to now no practical measurements for comparable dosage (output power) are available it is very difficult and often impossible to adjust two CAP devices for comparing purpose. Since unexpectedly technically quite differing CAP sources and techniques (DBD, jets) in many experiments show very similar antimicrobial effects (same exposure time) we conclude robust and similar reaction products. All kind of clinical species seem highly susceptible to CAP, pointing at a working mechanism independent of biochemical acting like conventional drugs. Meanwhile we have found differences in CAP-susceptibility with better susceptibility of strains with low grade multi drug resistance challenging this supposition. In opposite to principally CAP susceptibility, this phenomenon was only observed for specific CAP techniques which now has to be further analyzed in detail. It is important to point at the good susceptibility of bacteria, which also can be experienced by treating bacteria with plasma activated solutions [25, 26]. These solutions (including buffer) were shown to have good effects in vitro and in vivo trials i.e. for antisepsis are promising.

For clinical practice CAP electrodes are important and determine the wound type to be treated. The jets predestinate for point treatment of smaller wounds, and the larger DBD electrodes for larger wound areas. When several $cm^2$ of a wound are to be treated by CAP-jets, with the need of about 60 s of treatment (beam contact to the wound surface) per $cm^2$ several minutes may be necessary for total wound treatment, with typical DBD (2–3 cm electrode diameter) this time will be shorter. However, this treatment time needs further shortening and electrodes with larger surfes (DBD dressing electrodes) are under investigation. Up to now plasma technology of jets is limited to a certain diameter thus larger treatment zones can be reached by completing two or more jets to bundle-jets ("revolver jet" actual under investigation).

### 6.13.1 Overview

Facts antimicrobial CAP treatment

- All common clinical species and strains highly CAP susceptible
- Also multi drug resistant strains susceptible
- Also effective against fungi, molds and parasites
- From 3 s treatment microbiocidal CAP-effects possible,
- Proteins (blood, secretions) can lower CAP efficacy
- Good biofilm activity, not yet in vivo fully satisfying
- No selection of resistant strains
- Treating staphylococci and enterococci less efficacy towards higher drug resistant strains (dependent on CAP source type)

## 6.14 Open Questions

The impressing antimicrobial properties of CAP are the base of treatment of colonized and infected skin and wounds. (▶ Abschn. 4.9, ▶ Abschn. 4.10) Most wounds show reduction to elimination of bacterial load thus supporting healing. Why some wounds do not respond well to CAP treatment has to be investigated in larger studies with stratification of the wound type.

No resistant strains or species but differences in susceptibility to CAP may occur, depend on the CAP type and can be compensated by longer treatment. The role of this phenomenon has to be further evaluated (Relations between cell wall robustness, escape mechanisms and peroxide effects).

Another important effect is the different susceptibility to CAP in dependence on Gram stain ability [27] which also has to be further analyzed questionnating the role of cell membrane and wall stability.

Mainstays of ongoing research are

- DBD more effective against gram positive pathogens?
- Jets more effective against gram negative pathogens?
- DBD less effective towards MRSA than MSSA?

Since CAP sources can exhibit quite different and unexpected antimicrobial effect variations in future all CAP devices should undergo as technical as well as biologic examination during the course of certification by authorities in order to better compare the suitness for the intended use in clinical practice. This analysis should include tests against defined panels of clinical pathogens including multi drug resistant strains like MRSA, VRE and ESBL. Before such a recommendation can be realized, the implementation for normative test methods is strongly warranted.

## References


1. Fridman G, Friedman G, Gutsol A, Shekhter AB, Vasilets VN, Fridman A. Applied plasma medicine. Plasma Process Polym. 2008;5:503–33.
2. Laroussi M. Low temperature plasmas for medicine? IEEE Trans Plasma Sci. 2009; 37(6):714–25.
3. Daeschlein G, Napp M, Lutze S, Arnold A, von Podewils S, Guembel D, Jünger M. Skin and wound decontamination of multidrug-resistant bacteria by cold atmospheric plasma coagulation. J Dtsch Dermatol Ges. 2015c;13(2):143–50.
4. Hury S, Vidal DR, Desor F, Pelletier J, Lagarde T. A parametric study of the destruction efficiency of Bacillus spores in low pressure oxygen-based plasmas. Lett Appl Microbiol. 1998; 26:417–21.
5. Lassen KS, Nordby B, Grün R. The dependence of the sporicidal effects on the power and pressure of RF-generated plasma processes. J Biomed Mater Res B Appl Biomater. 2005;74:553–9.
6. Lerouge S, Wertheimer MR, Marchand R, Tabrizian M, Yahia L. Effect of gas composition on spore mortality and etching during low-pressure plasma sterilization. J Biomed Mater Res. 2000;51:128–35.
7. Cosgrove SE, Sakoulas G, Perencevich EN, Schwaber MJ, Karchmer AW, Carmeli Y. Comparison of mortality associated with methicillin-resistant and methicillin-susceptible Staphylococcus aureus bacteremia: a meta-analysis. Clin Infect Dis. 2003;36:53–9.
8. Pasternack MS. Decontamination strategies for MRSA-colonized patients. Curr Infect Dis Rep. 2008;10(5):385–6.
9. Fridman G, Shereshevsky A, Peddinghaus M, Gutsol A, Vasilets V, Brooks A, Balasubramanian M, Friedman G, Fridman A. Bio-medical applications of non-thermal atmospheric pressure plasma. In: 37th AIAA plasmadynamics and lasers conference, fluid dynamics and co-located conferences, San Francisco, CA; 2006. https://doi.org/10.2514/6.2006-2902.
10. Daeschlein G, Scholz S, Arnold A, von Woedtke T, Kindel E, Niggemeier M, Weltmann KD, Jünger M. In vitro activity of atmospheric pressure plasma jet (APPJ) against clinical isolates of Demodex folliculorum. IEEE Trans Plasma Sci. 2010b;38(10):2969–73.
11. Bauer AW, Kirby WM, Sherris JC, Turck M. Antibiotic susceptibility testing by a standardized single disk method. Am J Clin Pathol. 1966;36:493–6.
12. Daeschlein G, Napp M, von Podewils S, Klare I, Haase H, Kasch R, Ekkernkamp A, Jünger M. Does antibiotic susceptibility impair plasma susceptibility of multi drug resistant enterococci in vitro? Gut Pathog. 2015b;8(1):41.
13. Daeschlein G, von Woedtke T, Kindel E, Brandenburg R, Weltmann KD, Jünger M. Antibacterial activity of an atmospheric pressure plasma jet against relevant wound pathogens in vitro on a simulated wound environment. Plasma Process Polym. 2010a;7(3–4):224–30.
14. Daeschlein G, Napp M, von Podewils S, Scholz S, Arnold A, Emmert S, Haase H, Napp J, Spitzmüller R, Gümbel D, Jünger M. Antimicrobial efficacy of a historical high-frequency plasma apparatus in comparison with 2 modern, cold atmospheric pressure plasma devices. Surg Innov. 2015a;22(4):394–400.
15. Hong YF, Kang JG, Lee HY, Uhm HS, Moon E, Park YH. Sterilization effect of atmospheric plasma on Escherichia coli and Bacillus subtilis endospores. Lett Appl Microbiol. 2009;48:33–7.
16. Lee K, Paek K, Ju W, Lee Y. Sterilization of bacteria, yeast, and bacterial endospores by atmospheric-pressure cold plasma using helium and oxygen. J Microbiol. 2006;44:269–75.
17. Kayes MM, Critzer FJ, Kelly-Wintenberg K, Roth JR, Montie T, Golden DA. Inactivation of foodborne pathogens using a one atmosphere uniform glow discharge plasma. Foodborne Pathog Dis. 2007;4:50–9.
18. Daeschlein G, Scholz S, Arnold A, von Podewils S, Haase H, Emmert S, von Woedtke T, Weltmann KD, Jünger M. In vitro susceptibility of important skin and wound pathogens against low temperature atmospheric pressure plasma jet (APPJ) and dielectric barrier discharge plasma (DBD). Plasma Process Polym. 2012;9(4):380–9.

19. Daeschlein G, Napp M, von Podewils M, Lutze S, Emmert S, Lange A, Klare I, Haase H, Gümbel D, von Woedtke T, Jünger M. In vitro susceptibility of multidrug resistant skin and wound pathogens against low temperature atmospheric pressure plasma jet (APPJ) and dielectric barrier disc harge plasma (DBD). Plasma Process Polym. 2014;11(2):175–83. https://doi.org/10.1002/ppap.201300070.
20. Napp M, Daeschlein G, von Podewils S, Hinz P, Emmert S, Haase H, Spitzmueller R, Gümbel D, Katsch R, Jünger M. In vitro susceptibility of methicillin-resistant and methicillin-sensitive strains of Staphylococcus aureus to two different cold atmospheric plasma sources. Infection. 2016;44(4):531–7.
21. Kawai M, Yamada S, Ishidoshiro A, et al. Cell-wall thickness: possible mechanism of acriflavine resistance in 05.16 – 17:59 Springer-book-ProfMed Seite 11 von 11 meticillin-resistant Staphylococcus aureus. J Med Microbiol. 2009;58(3):331–6.
22. Maisch T, Shimizu T, Li YF, Heinlin J, Karrer S, Morfill G, Zimmermann JL. Decolonisation of MRSA, S. aureus and E. coli by cold-atmospheric plasma using a porcine skin model in vitro. PLoS One. 2012;7(4):e34610.
23. Isbary G, Morfill G, Schmidt HU, Georgi M, Ramrath K, Heinlin J, Karrer S, Landthaler M, et al. A first prospective randomized controlled trial to decrease bacterial load using cold atmospheric argon plasma on chronic wounds in patients. Br J Dermatol. 2010;163(1):78–82.
24. Brehmer F, Haenssle HA, Daeschlein G, et al. Alleviation of chronic venous leg ulcers with a hand-held dielectric barrier discharge plasma generator (PlasmaDerm® VU-2010): results of a monocentric, two-armed, open, prospective, randomized and controlled trial (NCT01415622). J Eur Acad Dermatol Venereol. 2015;29(1):148–55. https://doi.org/10.1111/jdv.12490.
25. Daeschlein G, Kramer A. Microbiological sampling in chronic wounds. GMS Krankenhaushyg Interdiszip. 2006;1(1):Doc10.
26. Traylor MJ, Pavlovich MJ, Karim S, Hait P, Sakiyama Y, Clark DS, Graves DB. Long-term antibacterial efficacy of air plasma-activated water. J Phys D. 2011;44:1–4.
27. Ermolaeva SA, Varfolomeev AF, Chernukha MY, Yurov DS, Vasiliev MM, Kaminskaya AA, et al. Bactericidal effects of non-thermal argon plasma in vitro, in biofilms and in the animal model of infected wounds. J Med Microbiol. 2011;60:75–83.

# Treatment of Ulcerations and Wounds

7

Regina Tiede, Steffen Emmert, and Georg Isbary

## 7.1 Etiology of Chronic Wounds

In general, a wound can be defined as any tissue destruction which is accompanied by the loss of tissue. Thus, wounds comprise a very heterogeneous group, which is indicated by a plethora of wound classifications.

The consequence of this heterogeneity is that there is no uniform and clear wound definition; the classification rather depends on the specialist's perspective. The German guideline "wounds and wound treatment" e.g. defines chronic wounds as wounds that persist for more than 2–3 weeks [1]. The German guideline "local therapy of chronic wounds", however, defines chronic wounds as a loss of skin integrity including one or more subcutaneous structures and without healing signs within 8 weeks [2]. For this reason a variety of wound classifications exist (Table 7.1).

R. Tiede
Clinic for Dermatology, Venereology and Allergology, University Medical Center Göttingen, Göttingen, Germany

S. Emmert (✉)
Clinic for Dermatology, Venereology and Allergology, University Medical Center Göttingen, Göttingen, Germany

Clinic and Policlinic for Dermatology and Venereology, University Medical Center Rostock, Rostock, Germany
e-mail: steffen.emmert@med.uni-rostock.de

G. Isbary
Roche Pharma AG, Grenzach-Whylen, Germany



H.-R. Metelmann et al. (eds.), *Comprehensive Clinical Plasma Medicine*,
https://doi.org/10.1007/978-3-319-67627-2_7

**Table 7.1** Classification of wounds

| Classification of wounds |
|---|
| • Form/structure |
| • Open/closed wound |
| • Acute/chronic wound |
| • According to type: |
| – Scrape: tangential pressure (excoriation) |
| – Laceration: blunt force |
| – Contused wound: blunt force |
| – Lacerated wound: frayed wound edges |
| – Cut: sharp |
| – Stab wound: spiky |
| – Bite: often bacterially colonized |
| – Gun shot wound |
| • According to cause: |
| – Infected wound |
| – Mechanical pressure |
| – Thermal |
| – Chemical burn |
| – Radiation-induced |

Wounds can be classified according to their form or structure, as open or closed wounds, or according to their depth.

A skin erosion is a wound that only affects the epidermis and heals without any residues. An excoriation is defined as skin tissue damage down to the epidermal-dermal barrier where the papillary valleys are still present. From these reservoirs of kerationocytes re-epithelialization can occur resulting in a scar-free healing of excoriations. However, pigmentary changes with hyper- and hypo-pigmentations often remain as visible signs of former excoriations.

An ulcer or skin ulceration is defined as a deep skin tissue damage which goes down to at least the subcutaneous tissue and at which the healing is always entailed by scar formation due to the complete loss of basal keratinocytes.

There is no limitation to the depth of an ulceration; an ulcer can expose muscles, tendons, and even bone tissue [3]. Causes of such ulcers include circulation disorders, infections, immunological phenomena, and tumors or combinations of thereof.

Another wound categorization classifies acute and chronic wounds depending on the duration of the tissue damage.

Often, a combination of the above mentioned classifications is used: Acute wounds—according to their structure—can be classified as scrapes, lacerations, contused wounds, lacerated and bite wounds, stab wounds, bullet wounds, and others. Chronic wounds which persist for several weeks up to years are often classified in combination with their cause: mechanical, pressure, thermal, chemical burn, radiation-induced, or infectious [1, 2].

The most common causes of skin wounds are venous and/or arterial circulation disorders, diabetes, or constant tissue pressure.

In the following we will focus on skin wounds that result from malnutrition of skin cells and on the effects of cold atmospheric pressure plasma on those wounds.

Constant tissue pressure lead to an impaired perfusion of the papillary capillaries. This results in a malnutrition of skin cells; inter alia causes a reduced nutrient supply of epidermal keratinocytes by diffusion. Eventually, a decubital ulcers develops (Fig. 7.1).

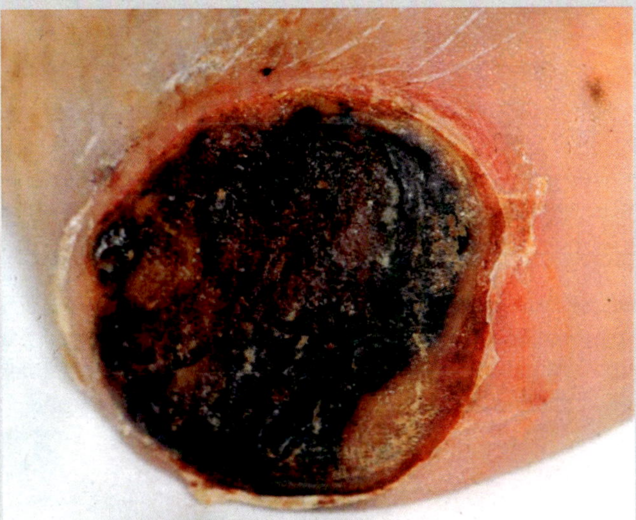

**Fig. 7.1** Decubitus at the heel due to constant tissue pressure

Constant tissue pressure can occur when someone is bedridden. Typical pressure points such as the buttocks or the heels then experience a reduced microcirculation in the papillary capillaries due to the body weight. Another cause of reduced

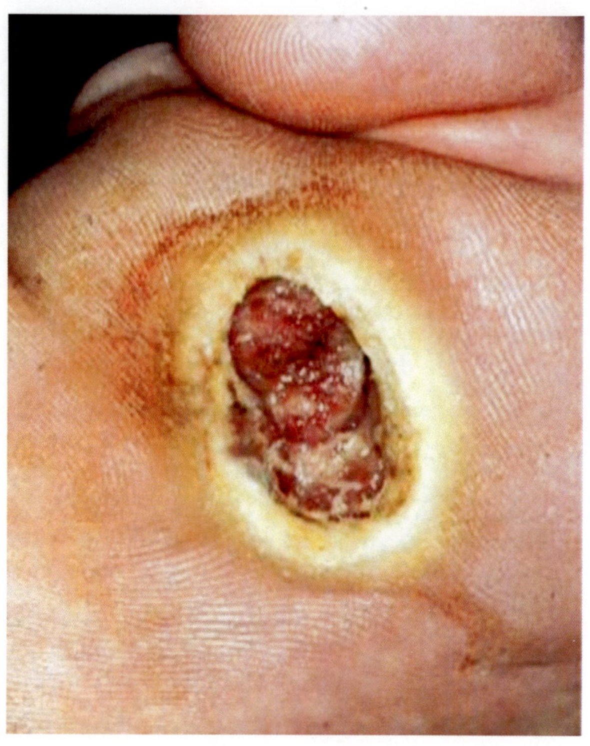

**Fig. 7.2** Plantar diabetic ulcer due to microangiopathy and diabetic neuropathy

microcirculation and malnutrition of the epidermis is the peripheral arterial occlusive disease. Here, occlusion of arteries that deliver oxygenized blood to the leg results in reduced perfusion of terminal vessels and malnutrition of the skin affecting the forefoot or the tip of the toes. This is also called the "principle of the last meadow" describing a necrosis when the oxygenized blood stream runs dry. The results are visible as typical skin ulcerations (Fig. 7.2).

The molecular causes of skin ulcerations due to diabetes are quite comparable to ulcers due to arterial occlusive diseases. Diabetes leads to neuropathic angiopathy, i.e. constriction of small arterial vessels (microangiopathy), also resulting in reduced perfusion of the papillary capillaries and therefore to skin ulcerations (Fig. 7.3). Varicose veins caused by dilated vessels also lead to venous ulcers at the lower leg caused by reduced perfusion (Fig. 7.4). In more detail, as a consequence of the venous stasis the bloodstream back to the trunk is impeded and a "backwater" of the blood down to the skin capillaries develops. This reduces the arterial afflux and, thus, impairs a sufficient nutrient supply to the epidermis [4].

A leg ulcer (ulcer cruris) defines a tissue defect in pathologically malnourished skin of the lower leg.

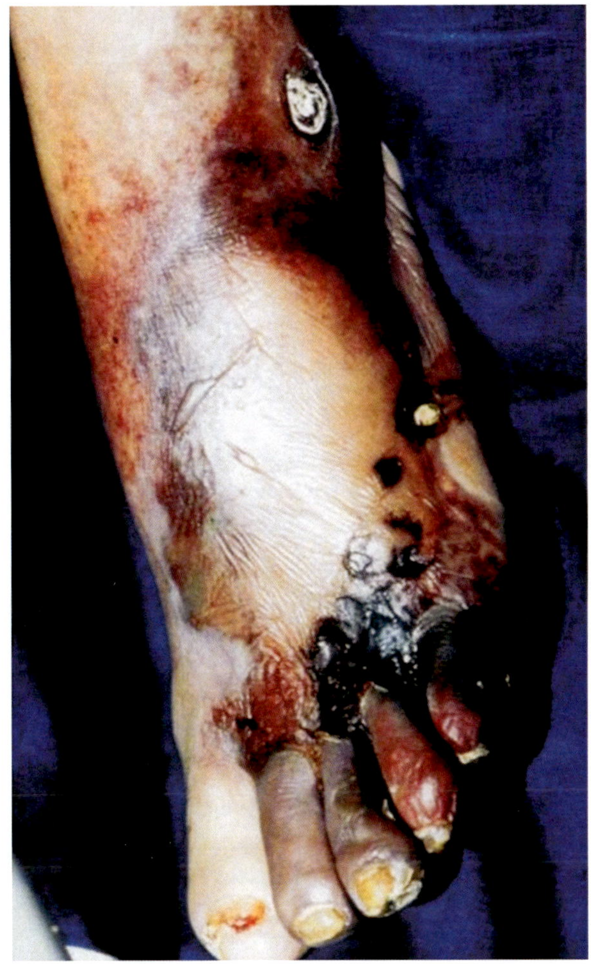

**Fig. 7.3** Arterial ulcer due to peripheral arterial occlusive vascular disease. Gangrene at the tip of the toe indicating the last grassland phenomenon

80% of lower leg ulcers develop due to venous diseases [5]. Reports on the prevalence of leg ulcers vary between 0.3 and 1%, i.e. between 240,000 and 800,000 patients in Germany [6, 7]. The prevalence of leg ulcers increases with increasing age and in most cases ulcers develop in 60–80 years-olds [8]. On average venous ulcers require about 24 weeks to heal. However, 15% of the ulcers never heal completely and after complete healing the recurrence rate is about 15–71% [9, 10]. The lifetime prevalence is up to 2% [5].

Depending on the definition the prevalence of peripheral arterial circulatory diseases is estimated at 3–10% of the population. The percentage of patients with arterial circulatory disorders among 70-years-olds and older people rises to 15–20% [11].

With respect to diabetic foot syndrome and diabetic ulcers the prevalence is estimated—according to country and study—at 2–6% of all diabetics. The annual

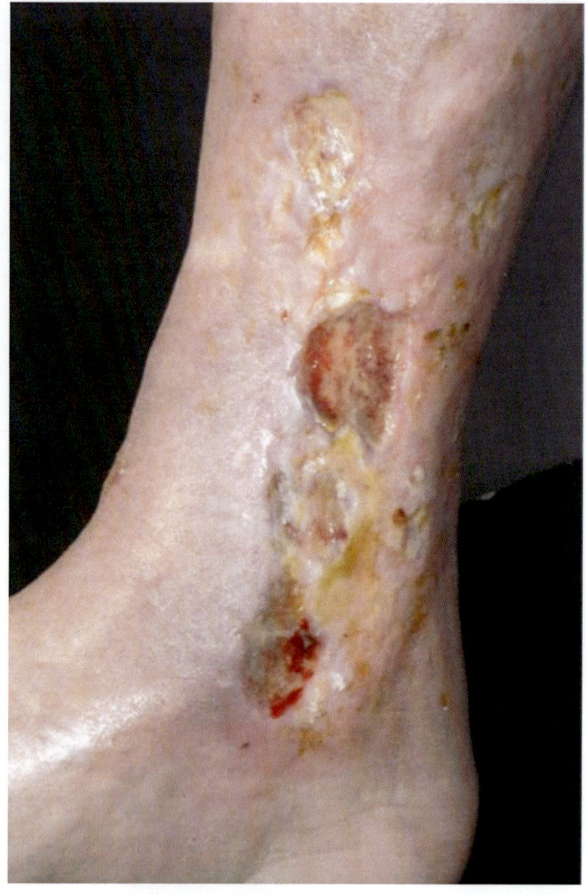

**Fig. 7.4** Venous ulcer at the typical location on the inner malleolus, the area of highest venous pressure due to insufficiency of the Vena saphena magna

incidence may also range between 2–6% of all diabetics [12]. The quality report 2009 of the disease management program diabetes mellitus type II of the Association of Statutory Health Insurance Physicians in Nordrhein-Westfalen/Germany reports that 3.4% of 424,000 diabetic patients suffer from diabetic foot syndrome and a foot amputation is necessary in 0.8% of these cases [13].

Venous ulcers comprise a considerable socio-economic burden for the health system.

Due to the high prevalence in the elderly population and the high treatment costs venous ulcers comprise a considerable socio-economic burden for the health system. In Europe, about 1–2% of the total health care budget is spend for treatments of venous diseases, which adds up to 600–900 million Euro for the Western European Countries [4, 6]. Mean costs of leg ulcer treatment are calculated to be

9560 Euro per patient per year [14]. In Germany, total costs for the treatment of decubital ulcers, diabetic foot syndrome, and leg ulcers are estimated above five billion Euro per year [7]. Indirect costs, such as fitness for employment or early retirement, which additionally hamper patients' quality of life, as well as the high risk for relapse worsen the situation even more. About 1.2% of all sick leave dependent nonproductive days are caused by venous diseases in Germany. And about 1% of all in-patients hospital costs relate to the treatment of venous leg ulcers [15]. In addition, the costs for the public health will rise in future as a consequence of the demographic development with an increase of the elderly population. Therefore, there is a great need for and high interest in developing novel and innovative therapeutic approaches to accelerate the wound healing process and optimize wound treatment.

## 7.2 Stages of Wound Healing

The human skin is one of the largest organs and serves as an important barrier to the exterior world. The skin protects our body from external environmental influences like ultraviolet (UV) radiation, chemical substances, and microorganisms. If the skin is damaged, almost immediately skin cells and immunological defense mechanisms are activated, which initiate the process of wound healing. Small and superficial wounds usually heal very quickly. Larger and deeper wounds may need some more time to heal but, in general, can be well coped by the body if it is not struggling with any other disease.

The normal process of wound healing is based on a variety of different mechanisms including coagulation, inflammation, matrix synthesis, and deposition as well as angiogenesis, fibrosis, and tissue remodeling [16].

> The physiological process of wound healing can be divided into three phases: Hemostasis and inflammation (cleaning phase), re-epithelialization, and remodeling.

In the following the biologic course and the main components of the three wound healing phases will be described in more detail.

### 7.2.1 Hemostasis and Inflammation

If blood vessels are injured thrombocytes are recruited to the damaged wound area. These thrombocytes then come in contact with connective tissue components as collagen and consequently activate blood coagulation, which stops the bleeding; this is also defined as hemostasis. The activated thrombocytes eventually release different signaling molecules like blood clotting factors or cytokines, the latter of which initiate the inflammatory process within the wound. Here, the signaling molecule platelet-derived growth factor (PDGF) plays an important role. Upon PDGF release from the thrombocytes neutrophils, macrophages, fibroblasts, and muscle cells are attracted and migrate into the wound milieu. Additional growth factors like transforming growth factor beta (TGF-β) lead to further chemotaxis of macrophages, fibroblasts, and muscle cells. TGF-β also activates macrophages, which then secrete additional signaling molecules like fibroblast growth factor (FGF), PDGF, tumor necrosis factor alpha (TNF-α), or interleukins (IL). TGF-β furthermore activates the expression of collagens and suppresses the collagenase activity [17]. During the later phases of this inflammatory process neutrophils become active, which clean the wounds from eliminating germs, destroyed tissue matrix, and dead cells by secreting matrix metalloproteinases (MMPs) and elastases [18–20]. Mast cells release amines and enzymes, which digest surrounding vessels to allow for an accelerated transport of additional cells into the wound milieu. This results in cellular and edematous swelling and the typical inflammatory symptoms as calor and rubor [17, 21]. In parallel, monocytes differentiate into special wound macrophages and support the cleaning process of the wound. They also release PDGF and TGF-β to intensify chemotaxis of fibroblasts and muscle cells [22].

### 7.2.2 Re-epithelialization

During the re-epithelialization phase keratinocytes play a dominant role in reconstituting the normal epidermal skin layers and the skin barrier to prevent transepidermal water loss. For that, keratinocytes must migrate over the wound area and proliferate there. In the intact skin basal keratinocytes are connected via hemidesmosomes with the basal membrane, whereas in suprabasal epidermal layers cell-cell contacts of adjacent keratinocytes are formed by desmosomes. These cell contacts have to be decomposed during re-epithelialization to allow the migration of keratinocytes into the wound and their proliferation as well as their differentiation to reconstitute the epidermal layers [23, 24]. Besides keratinocytes, other cell types like fibroblasts, immune cells, or macrophages are active during this re-epithelialization phase. Each cell type releases a distinct set of signaling molecules including growth factors, integrins, chemokines, or metalloproteinases. These factors mediate the strictly directed epidermal remodeling at the wound site. Fibroblasts play an important role because they release high concentrations of TGF-β, which trigger the expression of metalloproteinases, collagen, proteoglycanes, and fibronectin. Additionally, protease inhibitors are stimulated and simultaneously the release of proteases is reduced [25, 26]. Further details regarding the biologic mechanisms of wound healing mediated by keratinocytes can be found in the review of Pastar et al. [24]. The authors also depict structural and chemical changes of keratinocytes in chronic wounds.

### 7.2.3 Remodeling

During the last phase of wound healing skin layers are remodeled including cellular connective tissue and blood vessels. Macrophages produce IL-10 that inhibits the chemotactic invasion of granulocytes as well as the release of IL-1β, monocyte chemoattractant protein 1 (MCP-1), macrophage inflammatory protein 1 alpha (MIP-1α), IL-6, and TNF-α [27]. Additional growth factors are released from fibroblasts, macrophages, keratinocytes, endothelial cells, and thrombocytes (epidermal growth factor (EGF), TGF-α, vascular endothelial growth factor (VEGF), bFGF, TGF-β). Together, these processes lead to remodeling of connective tissue, neoangiogenesis, and renewal of the skin layers. Surrounding cofactors like a reduced pH value and partial oxygen pressure as well as increased lactate levels play important roles in the remodeling and the recruitment of blood vessels [17, 28, 29].

In any stage the healing process of a wound can be disturbed and may lead to a chronic wound condition.

## 7.3 Modern Wound Therapy

The therapy of chronic venous ulceration includes the symptomatic therapy of the wound in addition to the causal therapy. The local wound treatment depends on the stage of wound healing. It is also based on the extent of the wound exudation, the extent of the bacterial colonization, and the location, size, and depth of the wound.

The most common and promising standard therapy of ulcerations includes repetitive debridements of the wound, i.e. removing necrotic and dead tissue. This can be done in different ways. The golden standard is the surgical removal with a sharp scalpel [30]. Other debridement techniques e.g. use ultrasonic waves for cleaning. The pulse-lavage system is a mechanical wound rinse where saline solution is being sprayed directly into the wound and onto tissue parts. Enzymatic ointments are also used for debridements [30]. After successful removal of dead and necrotic tissue the wound is washed out with physiological saline solution and modern wound dressings are applied to keep the wound moist. In venous ulcers, which are caused by hypertension of the veins, a continuous compression treatment with compression stockings is usually used [31]. The greatest challenge in chronically infected wounds is to control the multipathogenic overload. Here, active dressings such as antibiotic or antiseptic containing dressings (e.g. Fucidine® or Betaisodona® gaze) can be used to prevent a wound infection. In case of excessive use, however, resistance or allergies may develop. Further active dressings e.g. include silver ions (i.e. Silvercel®, Urgosorb® Silver, Aquacel® Ag), which have antimicrobial activity or growth factors (e.g. Regranex®) which are intended to stimulate the proliferation of skin cells. Furthermore, operations or skin transplantations may be necessary.

Plasma medicine is a very promising and innovative approach to treat chronic wounds.

In physical terms plasma is defined as partially or completely ionized gas, which is why it is also considered as the fourth state of matter. In partially ionized gas, free charged carriers such as ions and electrons as well as neutral molecules are present. As a result of the directed movement of the charged carriers, plasma contains electric current. Furthermore, different types of radiations are generated in the plasma by spontaneous emission of excited atoms, ions or molecules, such as VUV and optical radiation (UV, VIS, IR), which leads to the characteristic glow of the plasma. It can be generated at different temperatures and pressures so that a variety of different plasma sources are available [32–34].

Because of the bactericidal effect, the use of hot plasma has proved to be an effective method for sterilizing e.g. of medical devices and implants, but also for the cauterization and cutting of tissue [35–38]. The sterilization or disinfecting effect is based on the interaction of the individual plasma components [39]. Furthermore, plasmas has been used for a long time for coagulation purposes [36, 40].

### 7.3.1 Cold Atmospheric Plasma Devices for Medical Use

So-called biocompatible, cold plasma sources, operating with temperatures of less than 40 °C, allowed the direct application of biological tissues [38, 41, 42]. Many research groups started to investigate this promising technology. These groups needed an interdisciplinary approach, which have brought together researchers from plasma physics, chemistry, technology, microbiology, biochemistry, biophysics, medicine, and hygiene. Many of these groups focused on interactions between plasma and biological materials [38, 42, 43].

Current research mainly investigate the application of cold plasma under atmospheric pressure. Numerous *in-vitro* and *in-vivo* studies already demonstrated the antimicrobial potential of plasma not only against individual pathogens, but also against resistant microorganisms as well as biofilms [44–50]. Daeschlein et al. [51] showed the efficacy of plasma against most pathogens of wound infections *in-vitro*. Cultured bacterial mixtures taken from the human skin were inactivated within a few seconds by dielectric barrier discharge (DBD) treatment [52]. The bactericidal effect of plasma was also shown *in-vivo*; the skin of mice was sterilized by the application of plasma without harming the animals [38]. The treatment of artificially contaminated pig eyes led to a significant reduction in bacterial load without any histological damages detectable [53]. Antiseptic treatments are extremely important for infected wounds, because in such wounds the healing process is impaired and therefore cannot proceed correctly. It is well known, that microbial colonization of wounds delays or prevents the wound healing process [54], resulting in the development of a chronic condition. Plasmas can act as very good superficial antibiotic/antiseptic due to its previously described properties and, thus, it is not surprising that these properties are already used for treatments of superficial disease, especially like e.g. chronic wounds that are negatively affected by bacteria.

So far, the standard therapy of infected ulcerations is based on topical or systemic antibiotic therapy. Besides the allergic potential which can be developed by patients against the antibiotics, an additional major drawback is the development of resistance. Here, plasma therapy combines two advantages: (1) the effective elimination of multi-resistant germs and (2) it is extremely unlikely that microorganisms will develop resistance against plasma due to its physical-chemical properties. Further advantages of plasma treatments are the non-invasive and painless application, as well as its gaseous state, which allows the penetration into smallest areas, e.g. the marginal area of fistulated ulcers. Recently it was shown that plasma even promotes proliferation of endothelial cells by stimulating angiogenesis through the release of growth factors [55]. Furthermore, there is evidence that the use of plasma influences the pH value [56, 57], which also may be of advantage in wound therapy. It is well known, that the body naturally responses with acidification of wounds upon skin injury [58]. Moreover, the pH value in the environment of chronic wounds influences numerous factors of wound healing. This is e.g. utilized in the therapeutically induced acidosis within the wound bed.

Cold atmospheric pressure plasma has an antibacterial effect, can promote tissue generation, and enhance blood flow.

Arndt et al. [59] showed that atmospheric low-temperature plasma (produced with the device MicroPlaSter β) positively influences the expression of several factors relevant for wound healing. *In-vitro*, pro-inflammatory cytokines and growth factors were stimulated or activated, such as IL-6, IL-8, MCP-1, TGF-β1, and TGF-β2. Furthermore, migration rates of fibroblasts were increased by plasma whereas the proliferation rate of fibroblasts were unaffected in the study. Pro-apoptotic and anti-apoptotic markers remained unchanged. However, expression rates of type I collagen and alpha-smooth muscle actin (alpha-SMA) were increased. Similar observations were made in *in-vitro* and *in-vivo* experiments on keratinocytes [60]. Increased expression rates of IL-8, TGF-β1, and TGF-β2 were induced by plasma (with the MicroPlaSter β). Here, the proliferation and migration of keratinocytes were unaffected.

So far, no side effects were reported for plasma applications. Experiments with mice, *ex-vivo* studies on pig skin and human skin biopsies, as well as *in-vitro* experiments on living human cells showed no cell damage (necrosis) after plasma treatments [38, 49, 61–63].

Up today, no side effects could be detected after cold atmospheric pressure plasma applications.

## 7.4 Clinical Trials on Chronic Wounds and Ulcers

In two randomized controlled clinical phase II trials, patients with chronic infected wounds of different etiology received plasma treatments, in addition to the daily modern wound treatment (Fig. 7.5) [64, 65]. The patients acted as their own control.

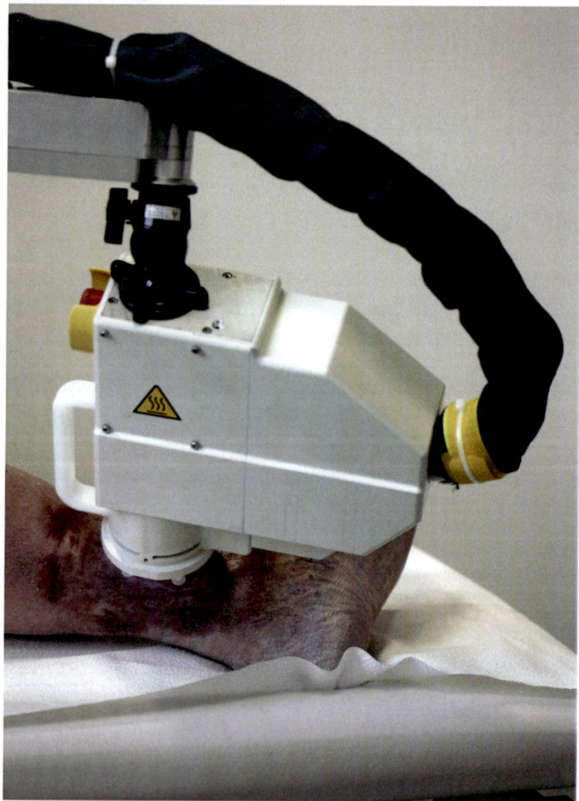

**Fig. 7.5** Treatment of a leg ulcer with the MicroPlaSter β. (after Isbary et al. [65] with reprint permission)

Plasma was applied using one of two different indirect plasma devices (MicroPlaSter α and MicroPlaSter β) over 2 or 5 min. Irrespective of the device used and the treatment duration, significantly higher reduction rates of bacteria were achieved in plasma-treated wounds (Fig. 7.6) without any side effects for the patients in both studies.

A retrospective randomized controlled trial demonstrated the beneficial effect of indirect plasma treatment (with the MicroPlaSter α) in a patient group with chronically infected ulcers of different etiology [66]. The patients were divided into three groups and treated with plasma between 3 and 7 min. In the most heterogeneous group (different ulcers and different treatment times), no significant differences in wound width or length were measured. However, in the more homogenous two groups (chronic venous ulcers treated with for different application times and chronic venous ulcers treated for 5 min) significant reductions in wound width were detected.

Despite the limitations of this retrospective study, these results suggest for the first time that plasma can accelerate wound healing in patients with chronic ulcers.

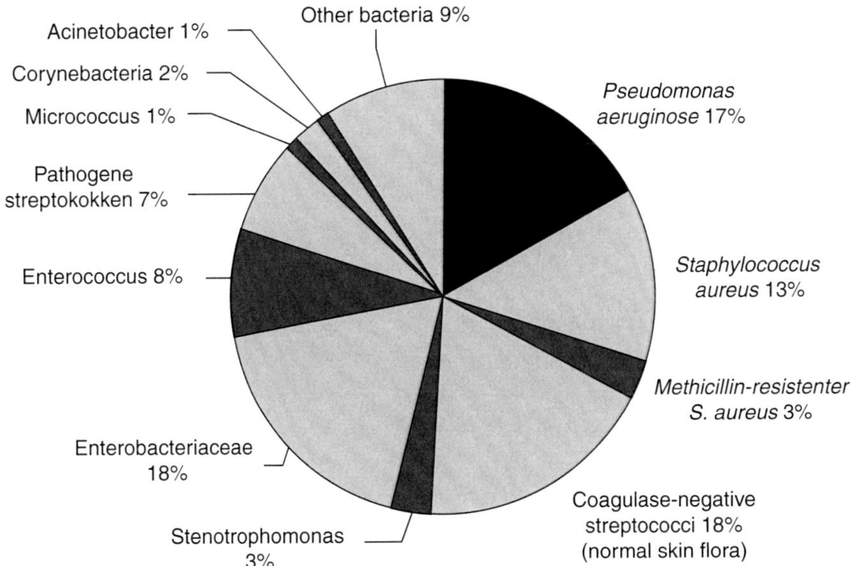


**Fig. 7.6** Bacterial strains that were detected *in-vivo* on chronic colonized wounds (Isbary et al. [64] with reprint permission)

These results were supported by a prospective randomized placebo controlled clinical trial on acute wounds [67]. Forty patients with skin graft donor sites on the upper leg were randomized and either treated with plasma (MicroPlaSter β) or placebo (argon gas) for 2 min. Positive effects were observed in terms of improved re-epithelialization, fewer fibrin layers, and blood crusts, whereas wound surroundings were always normal, independent of the type of treatment. In general, the treatment was very well tolerated and no side effects occurred. This trial on acute wounds demonstrated that cold, biocompatible plasma has beneficial effects even in the absence of pathogens and is therefore not limited to infected or chronic wounds.

In the meantime, some devices that generate cold atmospheric pressure plasma are approved for the treatment of chronic wounds as a medical device and gained a CE certification; i.e. the kINPen® MED device (INP Greifswald/neoplas tools GmbH, Greifswald) (Fig. 7.7) and the PlasmaDerm® device from CINOGY GmbH in Duderstadt (Fig. 7.8). Clinical trials were also conducted with these devices, demonstrating positive effects related to wound healing [68, 69].

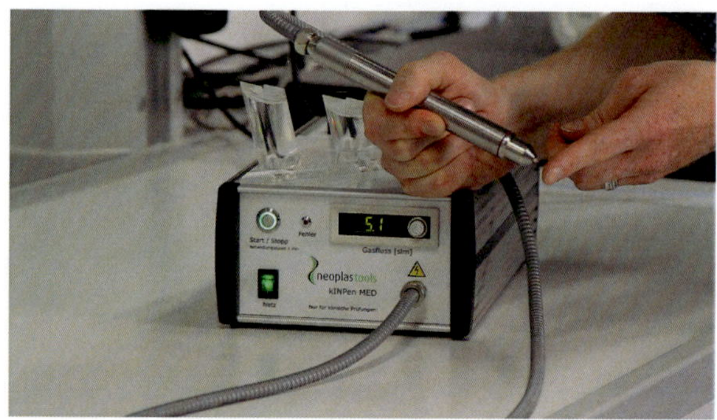


**Fig. 7.7** kINPen® MED (neoplas tools GmbH, Greifswald)

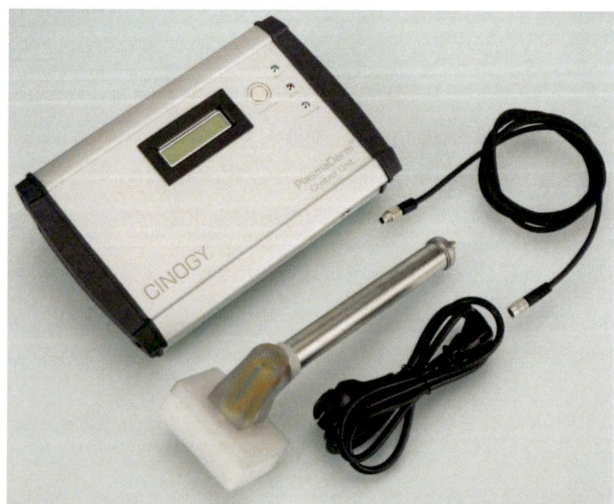


**Fig. 7.8** PlasmaDerm® (CINOGY GmbH, Duderstadt)

The aim of the study by Brehmer et al. [68] was to demonstrate the safety and efficacy of plasma application in chronic venous ulceration in the clinic as an add-on therapy to the standard wound therapy.

In the monocentric, two-arm, randomized, and controlled pilot study seven patients with venous leg ulcers were treated over a period of eight weeks, three times a week, for 45 s/cm$^2$ wound area with the PlasmaDerm® device and in addition to the standard care. Seven other patients only received the standard wound therapy. The standard therapy included repeated debridements of the wound, wound washing with physiological saline solution, and application of a modern wound dressing (Mepitel® or Mepilex®) to keep the wound moist, as well as a continuous compression treatment with compression stockings (Ulcer X®) to prevent hypertension of the veins [31].

Regarding the efficacy of the plasma application, there was a significant reduction in bacterial load in the wound immediately after plasma application.

Beside the significantly higher reduction of bacterial load immediately after plasma application there was no difference detectable in the relative wound sizes between the two compared patients' groups. However, the mean initial wound size was larger in the plasma group and plasma treated wounds showed a greater absolute decrease until the end of the treatment period (Fig. 7.9a). In three patients the ulcer reduced of about 50%.

The only patient with a complete cure of the ulcer was in the plasma group (Fig. 7.9b).

It is important to mention that patients of the plasma group reported less pain during the therapy and the plasma therapy received a positive assessment by doctors, too. Despite the low number of patients, it can be stated that the plasma treatment with the PlasmaDerm® device was safe and feasible.

Another clinical pilot study used a plasma jet device (kINPen® MED) on patients with multiple chronic venous ulcers [69]. Results demonstrated that the wound healing was not negatively influenced by the plasma jet, but the device was only partially suitable for large ulcers. Due to the thin plasma effluent streaming out of the device the application is very spot-like with a small exposure area. Therefore, small-size wounds were chosen for plasma treatments, which, however, makes the interpretation of the results more difficult. Upcoming clinical studies are intended to re-evaluate the effect with a device adapted for larger wound surfaces.

Further prospective clinical trials with large patient groups and sufficient statistical power are necessary to confirm the demonstrated first positive clinical effects of the plasma on accelerated wound healing.

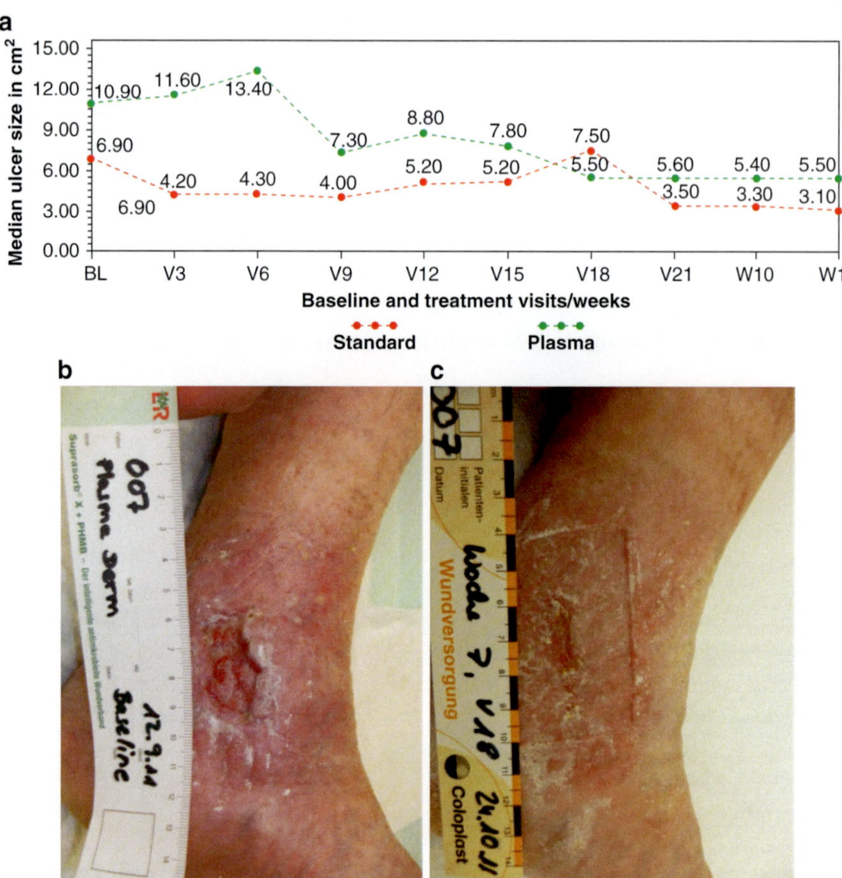


**Fig. 7.9** Assessment of ulcer size in cm² by Visitrak®. (**a**) The median ulcer sizes in the plasma and standard group in cm²; BL: baseline; V: Visit (3 visits per week); W: week after baseline. (**b**) Ulcer at baseline and (**c**) just before closure at week 7 (plasma treatment in addition to modern wound care; after Brehmer et al. [68] with reprint permisssion)

## 7.5 Safety and Efficacy Aspects for Comparison and Standardization of Medical Plasma Devices

The huge potential of cold atmospheric pressure plasma for the treatment of wounds has been widely demonstrated in clinical *in-vivo* and *in-vitro* studies as outlined above [52, 64, 65, 68, 70–72]. Along those studies fast track developments of medical plasma devices occur. This leads to a fast rising availability of different plasma devices that are already licensed as medical product or strive towards gaining one. Not all of these already commercially available plasma devices carry the CE label necessary in Europe for a medical device to be applied on humans. As mentioned above, the devices kINPen® MED and PlasmaDerm® already obtained the CE certification of the category IIa in 2013. In conformity with the EU guidelines 93/42/EWG and 90/385/EWG this guarantees the safety in use of the devices and confirms that they are medically and therapeutically efficient. Potential side effects during application are not excluded by these guidelines.

As plasma is composed of different biologically active components, already existing guidelines and threshold values, e.g. for UV radiation, electrical current, or reactive gas species like ozone, are utilized for safety evaluations. Some studies and publications already addressed the issue of risk assessment of medical plasma devices [33, 72–74] and additionally suggested some plasma-specific parameters as well as biomedical efficacy criteria that should be assessed to allow for a comprehensive evaluation of safety and efficacy of new plasma devices.

World-wide there is only one pre-norm available in accordance with the German standardization guidelines (DIN institute) that presents plasma-specific parameters for a safe and effective medical use of plasma devices: DIN-Specification 91315 "General requirements for plasma sources in medicine" [75]. This document can serve as a starting point for the development of an international plasma-specific guideline including other, already existing physical, chemical, biological, and medical guidelines. The DIN-SPEC 91315 includes physical and biological test systems for simple measurements of basic performance parameters to allow a first characterization of medical plasma sources and a comparison with other devices.

Based on the basic characterization the best possible therapeutic use of a plasma device can be determined. In Table 7.2 the plasma-specific test systems after the DIN-SPEC 91315 are listed and briefly described.

However, the DIN-SPEC does not include tests for the assessment of genotoxic and mutagenic potentials of plasma. Several studies already showed that the DNA indeed is damaged by plasma due to reactive gas species and UV radiation, but especially due to reactive oxygen species (ROS). ROS-mediated direct oxidative DNA damage can be expected upon plasma treatment [76–79]. However, in all studies isolated DNA dissolved in aqueous solutions were exposed to the plasma. This allowed a direct impact of ROS and UV on DNA and resulted in strand breaks, exchange of base pairs, or complete fragmentation of DNA. A recent review by Arjunan et al. [80] describes in detail potential DNA damages due to ROS and reactive nitrogen species (RNS) as well as the impact of plasma on isolated and cellular DNA. This potential genotoxic property of plasma regarding long-term therapeutic side effects is of quite importance. If too much DNA damages accumulate in the cell it will initiate apoptosis (programed cell death). If, however, DNA lesions manifest as DNA mutations the cell may likely undergo tumorigenic transformation. Therefore, in addition to the suggested test systems in the DIN-SPEC 91315 assays and tests have to be developed and composed regarding the mutagenic potential of medical plasma devices. The work of Tiede [81] presents a compilation of test

**Table 7.2** Test criteria according to DIN-specification 91315

| |
|---|
| • *Physical and technical criteria* |
| – Temperature: Should be below 40 °C to prevent thermal damage of biological materials. Temperature measurements over the entire plasma area can be performed with a fiber optic temperature detector |
| – Thermal power: To sustain a constant power of the device during the treatment time, the time-dependent heating of a substrate (e.g. copper plate) should be measured. The thermal power can be calculated according to<br>$P = m \times c_w \times \frac{\Delta T}{\Delta T}$<br>(P = thermal power; m = mass of the substrate; cw = heating of the substrate [J/(kg × K)]; ΔT/Δt = time dependent heating of the substrate) |
| – Artificial optical radiation: Using optical emission spectrometry the emission within 200–900 nm should be measured. Radiation within the ultraviolet range (200–400 nm) is especially important as it leads to DNA damage |
| – Gas emission: The quantification of potentially toxic gases produced by plasma should be measured according to DIN EN ISO 12100, e.g. $O_3$ or $H_2O_2$ which can damage mucosal skin and especially the respiratory tracts |
| – Electrical current: According to DIN EN 60601-1 and DIN EN 60601-2-57 different electric currents should be measured to avoid electrical harm |
| • *Biological criteria* |
| – Inactivation efficacy against microorganisms: Especially for wound treatments with plasma the antimicrobial activity is of importance and should be measured using the inhibition zone test as well as the germ reduction test by treatment of cell suspensions with five different microorganisms (*Staphylococcus aureus*, *Staphylococcus epidermidis*, *Escherichia coli*, *Pseudomonas aeruginosa,* and *Candida albicans*) |
| – Cytotoxicity: Exclusion of skin cell damage is mandatory for plasma application. Thus, a plasma dose-dependent cytotoxicity against the human fibroblast cell line GM00637 should be assessed applying MTS or MTT test systems |
| – Plasma-induced ROS and RNS production in liquids: The biologic efficacy of a plasma source strongly depends on the type and amount of reactive gas species generated. The plasma-induced concentrations of nitrite and nitrate should be assessed according to DIN EN 26777 and DIN 38405-9 in water or phosphate-buffered saline as well as the concentration of $H_2O_2$ according to DIN 38409-15. Additionally the change of the pH-value (acidification) of the fluid should be assessed |

systems that allow for a detailed genotoxic and mutagenic evaluation of plasma sources using human skin fibroblasts.

Results on isolated DNA revealed a plasma dose-dependent genotoxicity and a plasma specific mutagenicity (different in comparison with UVC radiation). Plasma treatments of cellular DNA within the fibroblasts during treatments induced mutation frequencies similar to the spontaneous one.

However, further investigations are necessary for verification as the mutagenic potential of both tested plasma sources (i.e. kINPen® MED and μs-pulsed DBD) could not be excluded [81]. Nonetheless, since 2013 plasma is used by an increasing number of doctors to treat chronic wounds and no single long-term side effect including carcinogenicity was reported so far. This adds to the notion of the *in-vitro* tests systems that there is no carcinogenic risk of plasma used in the current settings.

In summary, future developments of medical plasma devices should be carried out following standardized processes along with plasma-specific criteria and guidelines. Moreover, it is crucial to clinically and experimentally monitor potential long-term side effects of plasma applications. Specific international guidelines for medical plasma devices seem, therefore, mandatory.

## References


1. German Society for Pediatric Surgery. Leitlinie zu Wunden und Wundbehandlung AWMF-Leitlinienregister Nr 006/129. 2014.
2. German Society for Wound Healing and Wound Treatment e.V. Lokaltherapie chronischer Wunden bei Patienten mit den Risiken periphere arterielle Verschlusskrankheit, Diabetes mellitus, chronische venöse Insuffizienz. AWMF-Leitlinienregister Nr. 091/001. 2012.
3. Jung E. Duale Reihe Dermatologie. 7th ed. Stuttgart: Thieme; 2010. Moll I.
4. German Society for Phlebology. Leitlinien zur Diagnostik und Therapie des Ulcus cruris venosum AWMF-Leitlinien-Register Nr 037/009. 2008.
5. Valencia IC, Falabella A, Kirsner RS, Eaglstein WH. Chronic venous insufficiency and venous leg ulceration. J Am Acad Dermatol. 2001;44:401–24.
6. Etufugh CN, Phillips TJ. Venous ulcers. Clin Dermatol. 2007;25:121–30.
7. Nord D. Kosteneffektivität in der Wundbehandlung. Zentralbl Chir. 2006;131:185–8. https://doi.org/10.1055/s-2006-921433.
8. De Araujo T, Valencia I, Federman DG, Kirsner RS. Managing the patient with venous ulcers. Ann Intern Med. 2003;138:326–34.
9. Heit JA. Venous thromboembolism epidemiology: implications for prevention and management. Semin Thromb Hemost. 2002;28:3–13.
10. Kurz X, Kahn SR, Abenhaim L, et al. Chronic venous disorders of the leg: epidemiology, outcomes, diagnosis and management. Summary of an evidence-based report of the VEINES task force. Venous insufficiency epidemiologic and economic studies. Int Angiol. 1999;18:83–102.
11. German Society for Angiology and Society for Vascular Medicine e.V. Leitlinien zur Diagnostik und Therapie der peripheren arteriellen Verschlusskrankheit (PAVK). AWMF-Leitlinienregister Nr. 065/003. 2009.
12. Programm für Nationale Versorgungs-Leitlinien. Nationale Versorgungs-Leitlinie Typ-2-Diabetes: Präventions- und Behandlungsstrategien für Fußkomplikationen. AWMF-Leitlinienregister Nr nvl/001c Version 2.8. 2010.
13. Nordrheinische Gemeinsame Einrichtung Disease Management Programme. Qualitätssicherungsbericht 2009. Disease-Management-Programme in Nordrhein-Westfalen, Düsseldorf. 2010.
14. Purwins S, Herberger K, Debus ES, Rustenbach SJ, Pelzer P, Rabe E, Schäfer E, Stadler R, Augustin M. Cost-of-illness of chronic leg ulcers in Germany. Int Wound J. 2010;7:97–102.
15. Bosanquet N, Franks P. Venous disease: the new international challenge. Phlebology. 1996;11:6–9.

16. Robson MC. Wound infection: a failure of wound healing caused by an imbalance of bacteria. Surg Clin North Am. 1997;77:637–50.
17. Diegelmann RF, Evans MC. Wound healing: an overview of acute, fibrotic and delayed healing. Front Biosci. 2004;9:283–9.
18. Hart CA, Scott LJ, Bagley S, Bryden AA, Clarke NW, Lang SH. Role of proteolytic enzymes in human prostate bone metastasis formation: in vivo and in vitro studies. Br J Cancer. 2002;86:1136–42.
19. Sylvia CJ. The role of neutrophil apoptosis in influencing tissue repair. J Wound Care. 2003;12:13–6.
20. Broughton IG, Janis JE, Attinger CE. The basic science of wound healing. Plast Reconstr Surg. 2006;117:12–34.
21. Artuc M, Hermes B, Steckelings UM, Grützkau A, Henz BM. Mast cells and their mediators in cutaneous wound healing—active participants or innocent bystanders? Exp Dermatol. 1999;8:1–16.
22. Diegelmann RFPD, Cohen IKMD, Kaplan AMPD. The role of macrophages in wound repair: a review. Plast Reconstr Surg. 1981;68:107–13.
23. Heng MCY. Wound healing in adult skin: aiming for perfect regeneration. Int J Dermatol. 2011;50:1058–66.
24. Pastar I, Stojadinovic O, Yin NC, Ramirez H, Nusbaum AG, Sawaya A, Patel SB, Khalid L, Isseroff RR, Tomic-Canic M. Epithelialization in wound healing: a comprehensive review. Adv Wound Care. 2014;3:445–64.
25. Roberts AB, McCune BK, Sporn MB. TGF-**β**: Regulation of extracellular matrix. Kidney Int. 1992;41:557–9.
26. Hall MC, Young DA, Waters JG, Rowan AD, Chantry A, Edwards DR, Clark IM. The comparative role of activator protein 1 and Smad factors in the regulation of Timp-1 and MMP-1 gene expression by transforming growth factor-beta1. J Biol Chem. 2003;278:10304–13.
27. Peranteau WH, Zhang L, Muvarak N, Badillo AT, Radu A, Zoltick PW, Liechty KW. IL-10 Overexpression decreases inflammatory mediators and promotes regenerative healing in an adult model of scar formation. J Invest Dermatol. 2008;128:1852–60.
28. Knighton D, Hunt T, Scheuenstuhl H, Halliday B, Werb Z, Banda M. Oxygen tension regulates the expression of angiogenesis factor by macrophages. Science. 1983;221:1283–5.
29. LaVan FB, Hunt TK. Oxygen and wound healing. Clin Plast Surg. 1990;17:463–72.
30. Steed DL, Attinger C, Brem H, et al. Guidelines for the prevention of diabetic ulcers. Wound Repair Regen. 2008;16:169–74.
31. Dissemond J. Moderne Wundauflagen für die Therapie chronischer Wunden. Hautarzt. 2006;57:881–7.
32. Isbary G, Shimizu T, Li Y-F, Stolz W, Thomas HM, Morfill GE, Zimmermann JL. Cold atmospheric plasma devices for medical issues. Expert Rev Med Devices. 2013;10:367–77.
33. Tiede R, Hirschberg J, Daeschlein G, von Woedtke T, Vioel W, Emmert S. Plasma applications: a dermatological view. Contrib Plasma Phys. 2014;54:118–30.
34. Tiede R, Mann M, Viöl W, Welz C, Daeschlein G, Wolff HA, Von Woedtke T, Lademann J, Emmert S. New therapeutic options: plasma medicine in dermatology|Neue therapiemöglichkeiten: plasmamedizin in der dermatologie. HAUT. 2014;6:283–9.
35. Baxter HC, Campbell GA, Richardson PR, Jones AC, Whittle IR, Casey M, Whittaker AG, Baxter RL. Surgical instrument decontamination: efficacy of introducing an Argon: oxygen RF gas-plasma cleaning step as part of the cleaning cycle for stainless steel instruments. IEEE Trans Plasma Sci. 2006;34:1337–44.
36. Raiser J, Zenker M. Argon plasma coagulation for open surgical and endoscopic applications: state of the art. J Phys D Appl Phys. 2006;39:3520–3.
37. Koban I, Holtfreter B, Hübner NO, Matthes R, Sietmann R, Kindel E, Weltmann KD, Welk A, Kramer A, Kocher T. Antimicrobial efficacy of non-thermal plasma in comparison to chlorhexidine against dental biofilms on titanium discs in vitro—proof of principle experiment. J Clin Periodontol. 2011;38:956–65.

38. Fridman G, Friedman G, Gutsol A, Shekhter AB, Vasilets VN, Fridman A. Applied plasma medicine. Plasma Process Polym. 2008;5:503–33.
39. Shimizu T, Steffes B, Pompl R, et al. Characterization of microwave plasma torch for decontamination. Plasma Process Polym. 2008;5:577–82.
40. Farin G, Grund KE. Technology of argon plasma coagulation with particular regard to endoscopic applications. Endosc Surg Allied Technol. 1994;2:71–7.
41. Stoffels E, Flikweert AJ, Stoffels WW, Kroesen GMW. Plasma needle: a non-destructive atmospheric plasma source for fine surface treatment of (bio)materials. Plasma Sources Sci Technol. 2002;11:383–8.
42. Moreau M, Orange N, Feuilloley MGJ. Non-thermal plasma technologies: new tools for biodecontamination. Biotechnol Adv. 2008;26:610–7.
43. Dobrynin D, Fridman G, Friedman G, Fridman A. Physical and biological mechanisms of direct plasma interaction with living tissue. New J Phys. 2009;11:115020. (26pp)
44. Joaquin JC, Kwan C, Abramzon N, Vandervoort K, Brelles-Marino G. Is gas-discharge plasma a new solution to the old problem of biofilm inactivation? Microbiology. 2009;155:724–32.
45. Ehlbeck J, Schnabel U, Polak M, Winter J, von Woedtke T, Brandenburg R, von dem Hagen T, Weltmann K-D. Low temperature atmospheric pressure plasma sources for microbial decontamination. J Phys D Appl Phys. 2011;44:013002. (18pp).
46. Daeschlein G, Scholz S, von Woedtke T, Niggemeier M, Kindel E, Brandenburg R, Weltmann K, Junger M. In vitro killing of clinical fungal strains by low-temperature atmospheric-pressure plasma jet. IEEE Trans Plasma Sci. 2011;39:815–21.
47. Zimmermann JL, Dumler K, Shimizu T, Morfill GE, Wolf A, Boxhammer V, Schlegel J, Gansbacher B, Anton M. Effects of cold atmospheric plasmas on adenoviruses in solution. J Phys D Appl Phys. 2011;44:505201. (9pp).
48. Klämpfl TG, Isbary G, Shimizu T, Li YF, Zimmermann JL, Stolz W, Schlegel J, Morfill GE, Schmidt HU. Cold atmospheric air plasma sterilization against spores and other microorganisms of clinical interest. Appl Environ Microbiol. 2012;78:5077–82.
49. Maisch T, Shimizu T, Li YF, Heinlin J, Karrer S, Morfill G, Zimmermann JL. Decolonisation of MRSA, S. aureus and E. coli by cold-atmospheric plasma using a porcine skin model in vitro. PLoS One. 2012;7:1–9.
50. Daeschlein G, Napp M, von Podewils S, et al. In vitro susceptibility of multidrug resistant skin and wound pathogens against low temperature atmospheric pressure plasma jet (APPJ) and dielectric barrier discharge plasma (DBD). Plasma Process Polym. 2014;11:175–83.
51. Daeschlein G, von Woedtke T, Kindel E, Brandenburg R, Weltmann K-D, Jünger M. Antibacterial activity of an atmospheric pressure plasma jet against relevant wound Pathogens in vitro on a simulated wound environment. Plasma Process Polym. 2010;7:224–30.
52. Fridman G, Peddinghaus M, Ayan H, Fridman A, Balasubramanian M, Gutsol A, Brooks A, Friedman G. Blood coagulation and living tissue sterilization by floating-electrode dielectric barrier discharge in air. Plasma Chem Plasma Process. 2006;26:425–42.
53. Hammann A, Huebner NO, Bender C, et al. Antiseptic efficacy and tolerance of tissue-tolerable plasma compared with two wound antiseptics on artificially bacterially contaminated eyes from commercially slaughtered pigs. Skin Pharmacol Physiol. 2010;23:328–32.
54. Edwards R, Harding KG. Bacteria and wound healing. Curr Opin Infect Dis. 2004;17:91–6.
55. Kalghatgi S, Friedman G, Fridman A, Clyne AM. Endothelial cell proliferation is enhanced by low dose non-thermal plasma through fibroblast growth factor-2 release. Ann Biomed Eng. 2010;38:748–57.
56. Fridman G, Shereshevsky A, Jost MM, Brooks AD, Fridman A, Gutsol A, Vasilets V, Friedman G. Floating electrode dielectric barrier discharge plasma in air promoting apoptotic behavior in Melanoma skin cancer cell lines. Plasma Chem Plasma Process. 2007;27:163–76.
57. Helmke A, Hoffmeister D, Mertens N, Emmert S, Schuette J, Vioel W. The acidification of lipid film surfaces by non-thermal DBD at atmospheric pressure in air. New J Phys. 2009;11:115025. (10pp)

58. Schneider LA, Korber A, Grabbe S, Dissemond J. Influence of pH on wound-healing: a new perspective for wound-therapy? Arch Dermatol Res. 2007;298:413–20.
59. Arndt S, Unger P, Wacker E, et al. Cold atmospheric plasma (CAP) changes gene expression of key molecules of the wound healing machinery and improves wound healing in vitro and in vivo. PLoS One. 2013;8:e79325. (9pp).
60. Arndt S, Landthaler M, Zimmermann JL, Unger P, Wacker E, Shimizu T, Li YF, Morfill GE, Bosserhoff AK, Karrer S. Effects of cold atmospheric plasma (CAP) on ß-defensins, inflammatory cytokines, and apoptosis-related molecules in keratinocytes in vitro and in vivo. PLoS One. 2015;10:1–16.
61. Sosnin EA, Stoffels E, Erofeev MV, Kieft IE, Kunts SE. The effects of UV irradiation and gas plasma treatment on living mammalian cells and bacteria: a comparative approach. IEEE Trans Plasma Sci. 2004;32:1544–50.
62. Awakowicz P, Bibinov N, Born M, et al. Biological stimulation of the human skin applying healthpromoting light and plasma sources. Contrib Plasma Phys. 2009;49:641–7.
63. Wende K, Landsberg K, Lindequist U, Weltmann K-D, von Woedtke T. Distinctive activity of a nonthermal atmospheric-pressure plasma jet on eukaryotic and prokaryotic cells in a cocultivation approach of keratinocytes and microorganisms. IEEE Trans Plasma Sci. 2010;38:2479–85.
64. Isbary G, Morfill G, Schmidt HU, et al. A first prospective randomized controlled trial to decrease bacterial load using cold atmospheric argon plasma on chronic wounds in patients. Br J Dermatol. 2010;163:78–82.
65. Isbary G, Heinlin J, Shimizu T, et al. Successful and safe use of 2 min cold atmospheric argon plasma in chronic wounds: results of a randomized controlled trial. Br J Dermatol. 2012;167:404–10.
66. Isbary G, Stolz W, Shimizu T, et al. Cold atmospheric argon plasma treatment may accelerate wound healing in chronic wounds: results of an open retrospective randomized controlled study in vivo. Clin Plasma Med. 2013;1:25–30.
67. Heinlin J, Isbary G, Stolz W, Zeman F, Landthaler M, Morfill G, Shimizu T, Zimmermann JL, Karrer S. A randomized two-sided placebo-controlled study on the efficacy and safety of atmospheric non-thermal argon plasma for pruritus. J Eur Acad Dermatol Venereol. 2013;27:324–31.
68. Brehmer F, Haenssle HA, Daeschlein G, Ahmed R, Pfeiffer S, Görlitz A, Simon D, Schön MP, Wandke D, Emmert S. Alleviation of chronic venous leg ulcers with a hand-held dielectric barrier discharge plasma generator (PlasmaDerm® VU-2010): results of a monocentric, two-armed, open, prospective, randomized and controlled trial (NCT01415622). J Eur Acad Dermatol Venereol. 2015;29:148–55.
69. Ulrich C, Kluschke F, Patzelt A, et al. Clinical use of cold atmospheric pressure argon plasma in chronic leg ulcers: a pilot study. J Wound Care. 2015;24:196–203.
70. Daeschlein G, Scholz S, Arnold A, von Woedtke T, Kindel E, Niggemeier M, Weltmann K, Junger M. In vitro activity of atmospheric pressure plasma jet (APPJ) plasma against clinical isolates of demodex folliculorum. IEEE Trans Plasma Sci. 2010;38:2969.
71. Ermolaeva SA, Varfolomeev AF, Chernukha MY, et al. Bactericidal effects of non-thermal argon plasma in vitro, in biofilms and in the animal model of infected wounds. J Med Microbiol. 2011;60:75–83.
72. Heinlin J, Morfill G, Landthaler M, Stolz W, Isbary G, Zimmermann JL, Shimizu T, Karrer S. Plasma medicine: possible applications in dermatology. J Dtsch Dermatol Ges. 2010;8:968–76.
73. Lademann J, Richter H, Alborova A, et al. Risk assessment of the application of a plasma jet in dermatology. J Biomed Opt. 2009;14:054025. (6pp).
74. von Woedtke T, Reuter S, Masur K, Weltmann K-D. Plasmas for medicine. Phys Rep. 2013;530:291–320.
75. DIN SPEC 91315: General requirements for plasma sources in medicine. Berlin: Beuth-Verlag; 2014.

76. Yan X, Zou F, Lu XP, et al. Effect of the atmospheric pressure nonequilibrium plasmas on the conformational changes of plasmid DNA. Appl Phys Lett. 2009;95:083702. (3pp).
77. Leduc M, Guay D, Leask RL, Coulombe S. Cell permeabilization using a non-thermal plasma. New J Phys. 2009;11:115021. (12pp).
78. Bahnev B, Bowden MD, Stypczyńska A, Ptasińska S, Mason NJ, Braithwaite NSJ. A novel method for the detection of plasma jet boundaries by exploring DNA damage. Eur Phys J D. 2014;68:140. (5pp).
79. Alkawareek MY, Gorman SP, Graham WG, Gilmore BF. Potential cellular targets and antibacterial efficacy of atmospheric pressure non-thermal plasma. Int J Antimicrob Agents. 2014;43:154–60.
80. Arjunan K, Sharma V, Ptasinska S. Effects of atmospheric pressure plasmas on isolated and cellular DNA—a review. Int J Mol Sci. 2015;16:2971–3016.
81. Tiede R. Evaluation strategies for risk assessment and usability of medical plasma sources in dermatology. Georg-Göttingen: August University Göttingen; 2017.

# Cold Atmospheric Plasma in Context of Surgical Site Infection

# 8

Rico Rutkowski, Matthias Schuster, Julia Unger, Isabella Metelmann, and Tran Thi Trung Chien

## 8.1 Introduction

Thermal atmospheric plasma has been established for several decades in medical technology (including surface conditioning, technical sterilization and disinfection) and direct application to biological tissue (including electro-surgery) [1, 2]. Based on technological progress various concepts for generation of cold atmospheric plasma (CAP) have been developed in recent years [3–5]. Within a biomedical application horizon that is constantly growing in theory as well as in practice, wound therapy similarly as the handling of infectious skin diseases are one of the best investigated treatment indications. Despite the fact that the subcellular, immunological and molecular biological signaling cascades, mechanisms and interactions between plasma and tissue are not completely understood yet, a wide antimicrobial and wound healing promoting potential is demonstrated in several in vitro and in vivo studies [6–11]. The combination of antimicrobial efficacy and high biocompatibility within the scope of wound healing disorders and by infections endangered skin and mucous membrane

R. Rutkowski, M.D., D.D.S. (✉) • M. Schuster, M.D., D.D.S.
Department of Oral and Maxillofacial Surgery/Plastic Surgery,
University Medicine Greifswald, Greifswald, Germany
e-mail: rutkowskir@uni-greifswald.de; schusterm@uni-greifswald.de

J. Unger, M.D.
Department of Obstetrics and Gynecology,
University Medicine Greifswald, Greifswald, Germany
e-mail: jk114735@uni-greifswald.de

I. Metelmann, M.D., M.A. Pol.Sc.
Department of Visceral, Vascular, Transplant and Thoracic Surgery,
University Medicine Leipzig, Leipzig, Germany
e-mail: isabella.metelmann@medizin.uni-leipzig.de

T. T. T. Chien, M.D., Ph.D.
Vietnam Association of HIV/AIDS Prevention, Hanoi, Vietnam



H.-R. Metelmann et al. (eds.), *Comprehensive Clinical Plasma Medicine*,
https://doi.org/10.1007/978-3-319-67627-2_8

allows to consider, that the innovative technique of plasma medicine should not only be used to reduce an existing pathology but also as part of prevention measures.

## 8.2 Role of Surgical Site Infection (SSI)

Despite an enormous improvement in surgical techniques, sterilization methods, pharmacological prophylaxis and an increasing pathophysiological understanding of wound healing in the last decades, surgical site infections are among the most common healthcare-associated nosocomial infections [12, 13]. Notwithstanding differences regarding incidence and prevalence, SSIs occur not only in low-income developing countries but as well represent an important epidemiological burden in high-income countries that affect millions of people worldwide [14–16]. SSIs are infections that occur in or next to the surgical incision during the first 30 days after surgery (if an implant is inserted up to 1 year), and can inter alia be classified clinically based on their anatomical depth (incisional (superficial or deep) or organ/space) [17].

Surgical site infections are directly associated with increased morbidity and mortality in all surgical disciplines [12, 18, 19]. For affected patients these circumstances are frequently connected with an extension of pain and functional limitations, prolonged hospital stay, recurrent surgeries or death as a result of progressive, systemically spreading infection in the worst case. Demographic change and closely associated conditions like a rising number of surgical interventions (especially in the ambulant sector), multimorbidity and polypharmacy as well as the growing challenge of global microbial resistance problems are directly linked to an increased expenditure for diagnostic and treatment [20–23]. Many studies have shown a wide range of variables like surgical procedures, variances in inclusion of certain cost items as well as differences in methods and design of performed studies. Concerning the impact of health economics these studies and variables are hardly to compare. While there exists an undeniably estimated number of unknown SSI cases on the one hand and although there is no widely accepted method to evaluate healthcare costs due to complications on the other hand, it is highly evident that SSIs are responsible for a substantial increase in healthcare-related costs [24–26].

## 8.3 Risk Factors

Pathogens that are directly related to SSI can be of endogenous or exogenous origin. The most pronounced risk lies in the time between surgical cutting and wound closure [27, 28]. A major exogenous factor is the pathogen spectrum. Especially the resident flora of the patient is of particular importance [29, 30]. With regard to the most common pathogens, a clear dependence on the type of surgical intervention performed is shown. In consideration of the distribution shown in Table. 8.1, it becomes clear that the body's physiological flora, which is also referred as standard flora, carries a significant proportion of causative pathogens. Overall, the percentage of multi resistant organisms in context of wound infection has been increasing

**Table. 8.1** Most common SSI-causing pathogens in Germany depending on the surgical area (Data from KISS-Surveillance-System (Modul OP KISS), 01/2012–12/2016) [60]

| | Abdominal surgery | | Traumatology | | Gynecology | | Overall | |
|---|---|---|---|---|---|---|---|---|
| Frequency # | Pathogen | Ratio (%) | Pathogen | Ratio (%) | Pathogen | Ratio (%) | Pathogen | Ratio (%) |
| 1 | E. coli | 31.39 | S. aureus<br>- MRSA ratio | 29.95<br>11.96 | S. aureus<br>- MRSA ratio | 19.96<br>11.05 | S. aureus<br>- MRSA ratio | 18.92<br>14.19 |
| 2 | Enterococcus spp. | 30.02 | Koagulase neg. Staph. | 21.25 | E. coli | 12.90 | Enterococcus spp. | 17.82 |
| 3 | P. aeroguinosa | 6.22 | Enterococcus spp. | 11.41 | Enterococcus spp. | 10.36 | E. coli | 15.61 |
| 4 | Klebsiella spp. | 6.20 | E. coli | 5.17 | Koagulase neg. Staph. | 8.38 | Koagulase neg. Staph. | 14.64 |
| 5 | Bacteroides spp. | 5.13 | Enterobacter spp. | 2.94 | Proteus spp. | 5.29 | P. aeroguinosa | 4.51 |

**Table. 8.2** Selection of various risk factors that affect SSI occurrence

| Preoperative | Perioperative | Postoperative |
|---|---|---|
| General<br>• Low/high age<br>• Malnutrition<br>• Obesity<br>• Nicotine/alkohol<br>• Local and systemic infections<br>• ASA-Score >2<br>• Cortisone therapy<br>Comorbidities<br>• Diabetes mellitus<br>• Renal insufficiency (requiring dialysis)<br>• Disease of blood forming system<br>• Liver disease<br>• Cytotoxic therapy | General<br>• Insufficient disinfection of hands and operations area<br>• Deficient sterilization of instruments and implants<br>• Hypothermia<br>• Hypoxia<br>• Mismatching perioperative antibiotic therapy<br>Operation specific<br>• High NNIS-Score<br>• Delayed or extended operation time<br>• Type of operation (e.g. emergency, recurrence, contaminated, infected)<br>• Surgical technique<br>• Expertise of the surgeon | General<br>• Inadequate wound care<br>• Drains<br>• Improperly prolonged parenteral nutrition<br>• Not indicated prolongation of systemic antibiotic therapy<br>• Stress ulcer<br>• Incorrect adjusted blood glucose<br>• Pain<br>• Hypothermia<br>• Hypoxia<br>• Numerous preoperative risk factors |

*ASA* Classification of the American Society of Anesthesiologists, *NNIS* National Nosocomial Infections Surveillance Score

for decades [31, 32]. Quantitatively it could be shown that a microbial colonization of $>10^5$ microorganisms per gram of tissue significantly enhances the risk of developing surgical site infections [33]. In addition to the large microbiological risk component there are various other predisposing factors that can also impact the risk of SSI [34–40]. Knowledge about certain dependent and independent risk factors allows the implementation of an adequate risk assessment as well as conception and use of targeted prevention and therapeutic measures. Table. 8.2 shows an overview of selected risk factors.

## 8.4 Preventive and Therapeutic Strategies

Based on the enormous personal and economic consequences, the need for appropriate preventive and therapeutic strategies is rising. It has been estimated that approximately half of SSIs are preventable by the use of evidence-based strategies [13]. Considering individual and general risk factors, this requires a combination of different interdisciplinary preoperative, intraoperative and postoperative approaches including risk reduction of bacterial colonization as a key challenge. It was shown that such approaches can cause a significant reduction in SSI rates in numerous surgical disciplines and patient-specific subpopulations. Beside basic hygienic measures like hand disinfection, also professional treatment of medical devices, weight reduction, smoking cessation, risk-adjusted screening and remediation measures, nutritional supplementation, pharmacological adjustments as well as various measures to prepare the patient and the surgical site for the upcoming surgery are important in preoperative setting [41–45]. Furthermore, there was shown an increased significance for intraoperative factors such as skin antiseptic, antimicrobial prophylaxis, surgical techniques, measures for the reduction of dead space, and monitoring acid-base and electrolyte balance as well as blood and glycemic control under anesthesia [46–50]. By definition the risk of SSI can persist for up to 30 days after a surgical operation (1 year if the patient has received an implant) and a significant proportion (12–84%, depending on study) of SSIs are first detected after the patient has been discharged from hospital [51]. Accordingly, there are various evidence-based strategies in the postoperative period which essentially comprise type and duration of antimicrobial prophylaxis as well as wound management [52–56]. Current recommendations come from worldwide leading institutions such as World Health Organization (WHO) and Center for Disease Control and Prevention (CDC) [12, 13]. The latest version of CDC Guideline for Prevention of Surgical Site Infection (2017) provides updated and new recommendations for prevention of surgical site infection. Table. 8.3 gives an overview about actual recommended strategies. Focusing on a few selected areas this updated version is intended to be used by surgeons, physician assistants, perioperative nurses and other allied perioperative assistive personnel as well as persons who are responsible for developing, implementing, delivering, and evaluating infection prevention.

**Table. 8.3** In 2014 by HICPAC reviewed and suggested strong recommendations (mod.) of CDC (1999), that should be accepted as practice for preventing surgical site infections [61]

| | |
|---|---|
| Preparation of the patient | • Identify and treat all infections remote to the surgical site before elective operations and postpone elective operations on patients with remote site infections until the infection has resolved<br>• Do not remove hair preoperatively unless the hair at or around the incision site will interfere with the operation. If hair removal is necessary, remove immediately before the operation, with clippers<br>• Tobacco cessation for a minimum of at least 30 days before elective operations<br>• Skin around the incision site should be free of gross contamination before performing antiseptic skin preparation |
| Hand/forearm antisepsis for surgical team | • Perform preoperative surgical hand/forearm antisepsis according to manufacturer's recommendations for the product being used |
| Operating room ventilation | • Maintain positive pressure ventilation in the operating room and adjoining spaces<br>• Maintain the number of air exchanges, airflow patterns, temperature, humidity, location of vents, and use of filters |
| Cleaning and disinfection of environmental surfaces | • Do not perform special cleaning or closing of operating rooms after contaminated or dirty operations |
| Reprocessing of surgical instruments | • Sterilize all surgical instruments according to published guidelines and manufacturer's recommendations<br>• Immediate-use steam sterilization should never be used for reasons of convenience, as an alternative to purchasing additional instrument sets, or to save time (exception: patient care items that will be used immediately in emergency situations when no other options are available) |

(continued)

**Table. 8.3** (continued)

| | |
|---|---|
| Surgical attire and drapes | • Wear a surgical mask that fully covers the mouth and nose when entering the operating room if an operation is about to begin or already under way, or if sterile instruments are exposed (throughout the operation)<br>• Wear a new, disposable, or hospital laundered head covering for each case, when entering the operating room and ensure it fully covers all hair on the head and all facial hair not covered by the surgical mask<br>• Wear sterile gloves if serving as a member of the scrubbed surgical team and put on sterile gloves after donning a sterile gown<br>• Use surgical gowns and drapes that are effective barriers when wet (i.e., materials that resist liquid penetration)<br>• Change scrub suits that are visibly soiled, contaminated, and/or penetrated by blood or other potentially infectious materials |
| Sterile and surgical technique | • Adhere to principles of sterile technique when performing all invasive surgical procedures<br>• If drainage is necessary, use a closed suction drain<br>• Place a drain through a separate incision distant from the operative incision and remove the drain as soon as possible |
| Post-op incision care | • Protect primarily closed incisions with a sterile dressing for 24–48 h postoperatively |

## 8.5 CAP as Part of Anti SSI Strategy

Summarizing all scientifically and clinically evidence based findings, there is a considerable common intersection between preventative and therapeutic anti SSI approaches and the indications and potentials of clinical use of cold atmospheric plasma. Particularly against the background of best possible reduction of bacterial load as a key challenge, different approaches result for plasma medicine.

### 8.5.1 Current Clinical Applications

In head and neck surgery a fundamental perioperative risk for occurrence of surgical site infection is closely related to the typically high proportion of facultative pathogens, particularly in the area of the oral cavity, oropharynx and hypopharynx.

Besides the essential tumor resection the removal of cervical lymph nodes is another important part of surgical first-line therapy of head and neck tumors. During surgery a temporary connection between oral cavity, tumor mass and neck wound is not uncommon. Due to the high risk for spreading of microbiological colonization (intra- and postoperatively) with a subsequent increased hazard for SSI, we applied CAP with the intention of reducing the microbial load (Fig. 8.1, currently treatment of ten patients completed).

Furthermore, tracheostomies and their surgical closures are occasionally associated with postoperative wound infections. Consequently we started to support early wound healing by daily application of cold atmospheric plasma (Fig. 8.2, currently treatment of five patients completed).

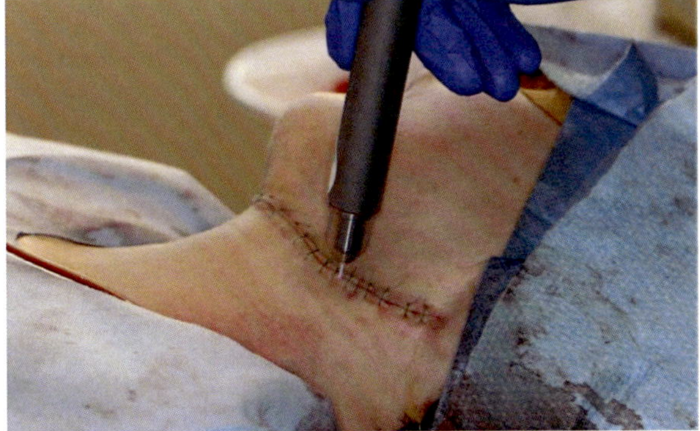

**Fig. 8.1** Reducing microbial load and supporting wound healing in early wound healing period after neck dissection by CAP (intraoperative setting immediately after wound closure)

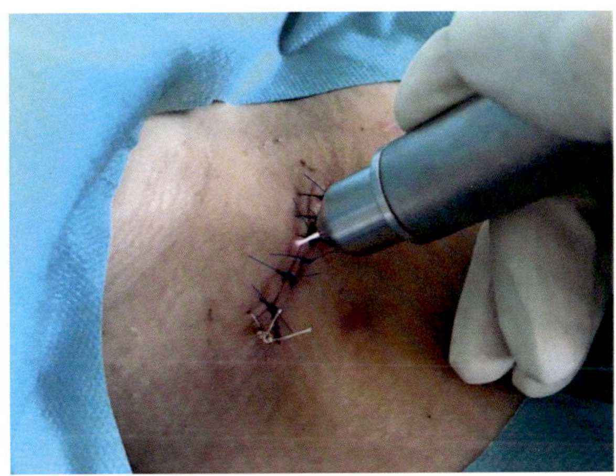

**Fig. 8.2** Application of cold atmospheric plasma after surgical tracheostomy closure

Donor site wound healing disorders after raising of radial forearm flap for reconstructive surgery in context of tumor surgery represents another indication for plasma treatment (Fig. 8.3, currently treatment of four patients completed). Ideally suited for reconstruction of orofacial defects with good functional and cosmetic results, this fasciocutaneous flap is often criticized for donor site complications and morbidity [57].

Moreover, we increasingly use CAP for patients who underwent abdominoplasty. Following significant weight loss, patients show residual problems due to the redundant skin and functional restriction. Several studies identified independent risk factors for development of SSI and consequential prolonged hospital stay [58, 59]. In addition to general risk factors resulting from different comorbidities (i. a. diabetes mellitus, immunosuppression, smoking), abdominoplasty-specific variables increase the overall risk. These include hygienic difficulties, insufficient microcirculation in fat tissue and chronically recurring skin infections. We started to support early wound healing from the first postoperative day after abdominoplasty (Fig. 8.4).

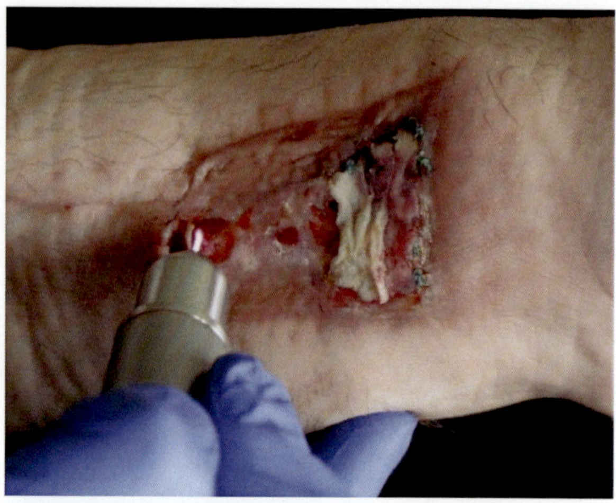

**Fig. 8.3** CAP treatment for donor site wound healing disorder after raising of microvascular radial forearm flap

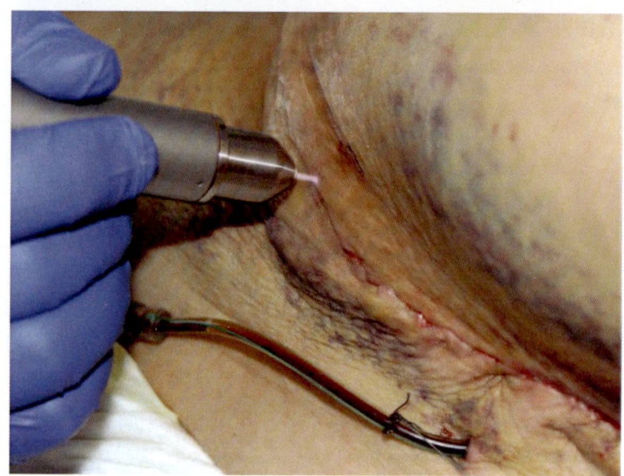

**Fig. 8.4** Application of cold atmospheric plasma in the area of the right abdomen after abdominoplasty

In all cases plasma-specific combination of chemical and physical active components was used for reduction of microbial load, stimulation of cell proliferation and optimizing wound healing. Plasma therapy was performed with kINPen© MED (neoplas tools GmbH, Greifswald, Germany). Application was carried out preoperatively in addition to the normal skin antiseptic (four slow sinusoidal pathways in the area of the planned incision) and was continued postoperatively for 7 days (2 times a day, 10 s/cm$^2$). Evaluation of wound healing including CAP impact on local quantitative microbial load and the aesthetic-reconstructive result, both from patient's as well as observer's view, were collected. Additionally hyperspectral imaging (HSI) was used to monitor and objectify the impact of CAP on microcirculation in and around plasma treated area. Within the preoperative approach, analysis of microbial contamination was performed by quantitative microbiological tests in the incision area at different times (before skin antiseptics, after skin antiseptics, after surgical closure and at the time of first dressing change). The collected data were evaluated against comparative data without plasma therapy. Concerning a still ongoing data collection, the evaluation could not be completed yet. However, an interim evaluation already indicates various clinical advantages in the patient group treated with cold atmospheric plasma. These benefits include the following facts:

- Higher reduction of bacterial load in preoperative setting (added to normal skin antiseptic, publication under review)
- Efficient reduction of bacterial load in postoperative setting (quantitative comparison to the standard wound treatment still pending, publication under review)
- Reduction of postoperative pain level
- Shortening the period of wound healing
- Significant increased oxygen saturation superficially and deeply immediately after CAP treatment, lasting for a longer time (Plasma-associated impact on microcirculation exceeds the field of actual plasma application, publication under review)
- Decrease of functional rehabilitation time of the hand after CAP treatment on donor site of radial forearm flap
- Functional-aesthetic improvement of scars (analyzed by POSAS score)
- Sure indication for reduction of hospitalization (for example oncology patients could be treated more quickly with adjuvant therapy)

Both the preoperative as well as the postoperative CAP application could be performed without the occurrence of acute therapy-associated complications or side effects. A large amount of patients felt comfortable during the application of CAP. Current long time follow ups (between 6 and 60 months after last CAP treatment) are without any sign of negative long-term side effects.

## 8.6 Summary and Future Prospects

Surgical site infections are one of the most common nosocomial infections worldwide and impact the increase of morbidity and mortality as well as healthcare-related costs significantly. Exceeding the limit of actual health care system, there is the urgent need for additional and new evidence-based anti SSI strategies. Especially due to the central task of best possible reduction of bacterial load within anti SSI concept, cold atmospheric plasma could be the missing key for this complicated challenge. Plasma could be a solution for the lack of complete removal of the resident flora in deeper skin layers known for normal skin antiseptic. Own research results as well as numerous external studies illustrate the enormous potential of plasma medicine in context of anti SSI strategy. According to our clinical experience CAP can easily be integrated into the preoperative and postoperative setting. Especially in postoperative care there is the possibility of delegation, stationary as well as ambulant. Cross-sectional areas such as the interaction of plasma with liquids, for example to increase the antiseptic effects, will expand current scientific and clinical questions. However, there is still a need for further evidence-based prospective research to further on improve the clinical use of cold atmospheric plasma, extend existing indications and fulfill the integration into daily clinical practice.

## References


1. Moisan M, Barbeau J, Crevier M-C, Pelletier J, Philip N, Saoudi B. Plasma sterilization. Methods and mechanisms. Pure Appl Chem. 2002;74(3):349–58.
2. Von Woedtke T, Kramer A, Weltmann KD. Plasma sterilization: what are the conditions to meet this claim? Plasma Process Polym. 2008;5(6):534–9.
3. Bárdos L, Baránková H. Cold atmospheric plasma: sources, processes, and applications. Thin Solid Films. 2010;518(23):6705–13.
4. Bekeschus S, Schmidt A, Weltmann K-D, von Woedtke T. The plasma jet kINPen—a powerful tool for wound healing. Clin Plasma Med. 2016;4(1):19–28.
5. Conrads H, Schmidt M. Plasma generation and plasma sources. Plasma Sources Sci Technol. 2000;9(4):441.
6. Daeschlein G, Scholz S, Ahmed R, Von Woedtke T, Haase H, Niggemeier M, et al. Skin decontamination by low-temperature atmospheric pressure plasma jet and dielectric barrier discharge plasma. J Hosp Infect. 2012;81(3):177–83.
7. Daeschlein G, Scholz S, Arnold A, von Podewils S, Haase H, Emmert S, et al. In vitro susceptibility of important skin and wound pathogens against low temperature atmospheric pressure plasma jet (APPJ) and dielectric barrier discharge plasma (DBD). Plasma Process Polym. 2012;9(4):380–9.
8. Daeschlein G, von Woedtke T, Kindel E, Brandenburg R, Weltmann KD, Jünger M. Antibacterial activity of an atmospheric pressure plasma jet against relevant wound pathogens in vitro on a simulated wound environment. Plasma Process Polym. 2010;7(3–4):224–30.
9. Isbary G, Morfill G, Schmidt H, Georgi M, Ramrath K, Heinlin J, et al. A first prospective randomized controlled trial to decrease bacterial load using cold atmospheric argon plasma on chronic wounds in patients. Br J Dermatol. 2010;163(1):78–82.
10. Isbary G, Stolz W, Shimizu T, Monetti R, Bunk W, Schmidt H-U, et al. Cold atmospheric argon plasma treatment may accelerate wound healing in chronic wounds: results of an open retrospective randomized controlled study in vivo. Clin Plasma Med. 2013;1(2):25–30.
11. Tipa RS, Kroesen GM. Plasma-stimulated wound healing. IEEE Trans Plasma Sci. 2011;39(11):2978–9.
12. Allegranzi B, Zayed B, Bischoff P, Kubilay NZ, de Jonge S, de Vries F, et al. New WHO recommendations on intraoperative and postoperative measures for surgical site infection prevention: an evidence-based global perspective. Lancet Infect Dis. 2016;16(12):e288–303.
13. Berríos-Torres SI, Umscheid CA, Bratzler DW, Leas B, Stone EC, Kelz RR, et al. Centers for disease control and prevention guideline for the prevention of surgical site infection. JAMA Surg. 2017;152(8):784–91.
14. Allegranzi B, Nejad SB, Combescure C, Graafmans W, Attar H, Donaldson L, et al. Burden of endemic health-care-associated infection in developing countries: systematic review and meta-analysis. Lancet. 2011;377(9761):228–41.
15. Magill SS, Edwards JR, Bamberg W, Beldavs ZG, Dumyati G, Kainer MA, et al. Multistate point-prevalence survey of health care–associated infections. N Engl J Med. 2014;370(13):1198–208.
16. Suetens C, Hopkins S, Kolman J, Högberg LD. Point prevalence survey of healthcare-associated infections and antimicrobial use in European acute care hospitals: 2011–2012. Publications Office of the European Union; 2013.
17. Horan TC, Andrus M, Dudeck MA. CDC/NHSN surveillance definition of health care–associated infection and criteria for specific types of infections in the acute care setting. Am J Infect Control. 2008;36(5):309–32.
18. Jarvis WR. Selected aspects of the socioeconomic impact of nosocomial infections: morbidity, mortality, cost, and prevention. Infect Control Hosp Epidemiol. 1996;17(8):552–7.
19. Kirkland KB, Briggs JP, Trivette SL, Wilkinson WE, Sexton DJ. The impact of surgical-site infections in the 1990s: attributable mortality, excess length of hospitalization, and extra costs. Infect Control Hosp Epidemiol. 1999;20(11):725–30.
20. Barnett K, Mercer SW, Norbury M, Watt G, Wyke S, Guthrie B. Epidemiology of multimorbidity and implications for health care, research, and medical education: a cross-sectional study. Lancet. 2012;380(9836):37–43.

21. Laxminarayan R, Duse A, Wattal C, Zaidi AK, Wertheim HF, Sumpradit N, et al. Antibiotic resistance—the need for global solutions. Lancet Infect Dis. 2013;13(12):1057–98.
22. Maher RL, Hanlon J, Hajjar ER. Clinical consequences of polypharmacy in elderly. Expert Opin Drug Saf. 2014;13(1):57–65.
23. Organization WH. Antimicrobial resistance: global report on surveillance. Geneva: World Health Organization; 2014.
24. Magill SS, Hellinger W, Cohen J, Kay R, Bailey C, Boland B, et al. Prevalence of healthcare-associated infections in acute care hospitals in Jacksonville, Florida. Infect Control Hosp Epidemiol. 2012;33(3):283–91.
25. Broex E, Van Asselt A, Bruggeman C, Van Tiel F. Surgical site infections: how high are the costs? J Hosp Infect. 2009;72(3):193–201.
26. Umscheid CA, Mitchell MD, Doshi JA, Agarwal R, Williams K, Brennan PJ. Estimating the proportion of healthcare-associated infections that are reasonably preventable and the related mortality and costs. Infect Control Hosp Epidemiol. 2011;32(2):101–14.
27. Bowler P, Duerden B, Armstrong DG. Wound microbiology and associated approaches to wound management. Clin Microbiol Rev. 2001;14(2):244–69.
28. Singh R, Singla P, Chaudhary U. Surgical site infections: classification, risk factors, pathogenesis and preventive management. Int J Pharma Res Health Sci. 2014;2(3):203–14.
29. Geffers C, Baerwolff S, Schwab F, Gastmeier P. Incidence of healthcare-associated infections in high-risk neonates: results from the German surveillance system for very-low-birthweight infants. J Hosp Infect. 2008;68(3):214–21.
30. Towfigh S, Cheadle WG, Lowry SF, Malangoni MA, Wilson SE. Significant reduction in incidence of wound contamination by skin flora through use of microbial sealant. Arch Surg. 2008;143(9):885–91.
31. Gjødsbøl K, Christensen JJ, Karlsmark T, Jørgensen B, Klein BM, Krogfelt KA. Multiple bacterial species reside in chronic wounds: a longitudinal study. Int Wound J. 2006;3(3):225–31.
32. Neu HC. The crisis in antibiotic resistance. Science. 1992;257(5073):1064–74.
33. Krizek TJ, Robson MC. Evolution of quantitative bacteriology in wound management. Am J Surg. 1975;130(5):579–84.
34. Chen S, Anderson MV, Cheng WK, Wongworawat MD. Diabetes associated with increased surgical site infections in spinal arthrodesis. Clin Orthop Relat Res. 2009;467(7):1670–3.
35. Gaynes RP, Culver DH, Horan TC, Edwards JR, Richards C, Tolson JS, et al. Surgical site infection (SSI) rates in the United States, 1992–1998: the National Nosocomial Infections Surveillance System basic SSI risk index. Clin Infect Dis. 2001;33(Supplement_2):S69–77.
36. Harrington G, Russo P, Spelman D, Borrell S, Watson K, Barr W, et al. Surgical-site infection rates and risk factor analysis in coronary artery bypass graft surgery. Infect Control Hosp Epidemiol. 2004;25(6):472–6.
37. Leong G, Wilson J, Charlett A. Duration of operation as a risk factor for surgical site infection: comparison of English and US data. J Hosp Infect. 2006;63(3):255–62.
38. Malone DL, Genuit T, Tracy JK, Gannon C, Napolitano LM. Surgical site infections: reanalysis of risk factors. J Surg Res. 2002;103(1):89–95.
39. ter Gunne AFP, Cohen DB. Incidence, prevalence, and analysis of risk factors for surgical site infection following adult spinal surgery. Spine. 2009;34(13):1422–8.
40. Vilar-Compte D, de Iturbe IÁ, Martín-Onraet A, Pérez-Amador M, Sánchez-Hernández C, Volkow P. Hyperglycemia as a risk factor for surgical site infections in patients undergoing mastectomy. Am J Infect Control. 2008;36(3):192–8.
41. Melling AC, Ali B, Scott EM, Leaper DJ. Effects of preoperative warming on the incidence of wound infection after clean surgery: a randomised controlled trial. Lancet. 2001;358(9285):876–80.
42. Hetem DJ, Bootsma MC, Bonten MJ. Prevention of surgical site infections: decontamination with mupirocin based on preoperative screening for Staphylococcus Aureus carriers or universal decontamination? Clin Infect Dis. 2015;62(5):631–6.
43. Darouiche RO, Wall MJ Jr, Itani KM, Otterson MF, Webb AL, Carrick MM, et al. Chlorhexidine–alcohol versus povidone–iodine for surgical-site antisepsis. N Engl J Med. 2010;362(1):18–26.

44. Tanner J, Norrie P, Melen K. Preoperative hair removal to reduce surgical site infection. London: The Cochrane Library; 2011.
45. Parienti JJ, Thibon P, Heller R, Le Roux Y, von Theobald P, Bensadoun H, et al. Hand-rubbing with an aqueous alcoholic solution vs traditional surgical hand-scrubbing and 30-day surgical site infection rates: a randomized equivalence study. JAMA. 2002;288(6):722–7.
46. Obermeier A, Schneider J, Wehner S, Matl FD, Schieker M, von Eisenhart-Rothe R, et al. Novel high efficient coatings for anti-microbial surgical sutures using chlorhexidine in fatty acid slow-release carrier systems. PLoS One. 2014;9(7):e101426.
47. Kurz A, Sessler DI, Lenhardt R. Perioperative normothermia to reduce the incidence of surgical-wound infection and shorten hospitalization. N Engl J Med. 1996;334(19):1209–16.
48. Buchleitner AM, Martínez-Alonso M, Hernández M, Solà I, Mauricio D. Perioperative glycaemic control for diabetic patients undergoing surgery. London: The Cochrane Library; 2012.
49. Meyhoff CS, Wetterslev J, Jorgensen LN, Henneberg SW, Høgdall C, Lundvall L, et al. Effect of high perioperative oxygen fraction on surgical site infection and pulmonary complications after abdominal surgery: the PROXI randomized clinical trial. JAMA. 2009;302(14):1543–50.
50. Beldi G, Bisch-Knaden S, Banz V, Mühlemann K, Candinas D. Impact of intraoperative behavior on surgical site infections. Am J Surg. 2009;198(2):157–62.
51. Mangram AJ, Horan TC, Pearson ML, Silver LC, Jarvis WR, Committee HICPA. Guideline for prevention of surgical site infection, 1999. Am J Infect Control. 1999;27(2):97–134.
52. Silva JM, de Oliveira AMR, Nogueira FAM, Vianna PMM, Pereira Filho MC, Dias LF, et al. The effect of excess fluid balance on the mortality rate of surgical patients: a multicenter prospective study. Crit Care. 2013;17(6):R288.
53. Masden D, Goldstein J, Endara M, Xu K, Steinberg J, Attinger C. Negative pressure wound therapy for at-risk surgical closures in patients with multiple comorbidities: a prospective randomized controlled study. Ann Surg. 2012;255(6):1043–7.
54. Dumville JC, Gray TA, Walter CJ, Sharp CA, Page T, Macefield R, et al. Dressings for the prevention of surgical site infection. London: The Cochrane Library; 2016.
55. Ata A, Lee J, Bestle SL, Desemone J, Stain SC. Postoperative hyperglycemia and surgical site infection in general surgery patients. Arch Surg. 2010;145(9):858–64.
56. Gyssens IC. Preventing postoperative infections: current treatment recommendations. Drugs. 1999;57(2):175–85.
57. Richardson D, Fisher SE, Vaughan DE, Brown JS. Radial forearm flap donor-site complications and morbidity: a prospective study. Plast Reconstr Surg. 1997;99(1):109–15.
58. Vu MM, Gutowski KA, Blough JT, Simmons CJ, Kim JY. Development of an individualized surgical risk calculator for abdominoplasty procedures. Plast Reconstr Surg. 2015;136(4S):95–6.
59. Massenburg BB, Sanati-Mehrizy P, Jablonka EM, Taub PJ. Risk factors for prolonged length of stay in Abdominoplasty. Plast Reconstr Surg. 2015;136(4S):164–5.
60. Infektionen NRfrSvn. Modul OP-KISS, Referenzdaten Berechnungszeitraum: Januar 2012 bis Dezember 2016. 2017.
61. U.S. Department of Health and Human Services CfDCaP. Meeting Minutes: Healthcare Infection Control Practices Advisory Committee (HICPAC). 2014.

# Cold Atmospheric Plasma (CAP) Combined with Chemo-Radiation and Cytoreductive Surgery: The First Clinical Experience for Stage IV Metastatic Colon Cancer

9

Jerome Canady, Steven Gordon, Taisen Zhuang, Shruti Wigh, Warren Rowe, Alexey Shashurin, Dereck Chiu, Sterlyn Jones, Kimberly Wiley, Emil Cohen, Tammy Naab, Barry Trink, Victor Priego, Anu Gupta, Giacomo Basadonna, Robert Dewitty, and Michael Keidar

J. Canady, M.D. (✉)
Jerome Canady Research Institute for Advanced Biological and Technological Sciences, Translational and Molecular Center, Takoma Park, MD, USA

Plasma Medicine Life Sciences, Takoma Park, MD, USA

Department of Mechanical and Aerospace Engineering, School of Engineering and Applied Science, The George Washington University, Washington, DC, USA
e-mail: drjcanady@canadysurgicalgroup.com

S. Gordon, M.D.
Department of Surgery, Baton Rouge General Hospital (Bluebonnet), Baton Rouge, LA, USA

T. Zhuang, Ph.D. • S. Wigh • D. Chiu
Plasma Medicine Life Sciences, Takoma Park, MD, USA

W. Rowe, Ph.D. • S. Jones • K. Wiley, M.D.

Jerome Canady Research Institute for Advanced Biological and Technological Sciences, Translational and Molecular Center, Takoma Park, MD, USA

A. Shashurin, Ph.D. • M. Keidar, Ph.D.
Jerome Canady Research Institute for Advanced Biological and Technological Sciences, Translational and Molecular Center, Takoma Park, MD, USA

George Washington University, Washington, DC, USA

E. Cohen, M.D.
Department of Radiology, Washington Hospital Center, Washington, DC, USA

T. Naab, M.D.
Department of Pathology and Surgery, Howard University Hospital, Washington, DC, USA

B. Trink, Ph.D.
Department of Otolaryngology, Rambam Medical Center, Haifa, Israel


H.-R. Metelmann et al. (eds.), *Comprehensive Clinical Plasma Medicine*,
https://doi.org/10.1007/978-3-319-67627-2_9

V. Priego, M.D.
Medical Oncology Section, Cancer for Center and Blood Disorder,
Bethesda, MD, USA

A. Gupta, M.D.
Cancer Center @ Gaithersburg, Radiation Oncology, Gaithersburg, MD, USA

G. Basadonna, M.D., Ph.D.
Jerome Canady Research Institute for Advanced Biological and Technological Sciences,
Translational and Molecular Center, Takoma Park, MD, USA

Department of Surgery, University of Massachusetts School of Medicine,
Worcester, MA, USA

R. Dewitty, M.D.
Jerome Canady Research Institute for Advanced Biological and Technological Sciences,
Translational and Molecular Center, Takoma Park, MD, USA

Department of Pathology and Surgery, Howard University Hospital,
Washington, DC, USA

## 9.1 Introduction

Colorectal cancer (CRC) is the third most common cancer in the world and the second leading cause of cancer death in the United States. In 2012 an estimated 103,170 new cases of colon cancer and approximately 40,290 rectal cases were newly diagnosed with 51,690 related deaths from these combined cancers [1]. There is evidence of peritoneal carcinomatosis (PC) in 8–10% of these patients at the time of diagnosis and 25% during the progression of their disease [2–5].

PC is associated with a poor prognosis. Patients are considered to have a terminal condition with a 6–10 month median survival time [2–7]. The standard treatment for advanced stage CRC and PC is systemic chemotherapy which is considered palliative with minimal improvement in patient survival. Advanced chemotherapeutic regimens such as FOLFOX have been reported to improve survival to a median of 15.7 months [8, 9].

Cytoreductive surgery (CRS) combined with hyperthermic intraoperative peritoneal chemotherapy (HIPEC) has evolved over the past 20 years as a new approach for the treatment of PC. CRS is described as removal of gross tumor follow by HIPEC treatment. Despite limited evidence to support CRS and HIPEC, there are some reports that this new approach has reported beneficial results [10]. Although there are promising results, CRS and HIPEC is associated with a significant morbidity, mortality, increase operating time, prolonged ICU care which results in an increase cost in patient care. This new multimodality approach is limited to several factors; age, extra abdominal disease (liver or lung metastasis), and peritoneal cancer index (PCI) which is the most common prognostic indicator and relies on the spread of the disease based on a scoring systems and the capability of complete removal of the gross tumor. PCI score calculates the spread of tumor in 13 areas of the abdomen in combination with tumor size. It ranges from 0 to 39 points.

An elevated score indicates significant increase tumor load [11]. Elias et al. [12] reported a 4 year survival rate of 44% if the PCI score is <6, score between 7 and 12 (22%) and >19 (7%) respectively. CRS and HIPEC is not recommended if the PCI score is >20. Controversy still exists whether CRS and HIPEC is considered "experimental".

Plasma medicine has qualified as a new scientific field after intense research effort in low-temperature or cold atmospheric plasma applications [13–15]. It is known that cold atmospheric plasmas (CAP) produce various chemically reactive species including reactive oxygen species (ROS) and reactive nitrogen species (RNS). CAP is a cocktail containing ROS and RNS in combination with transient electric fields, UV and charged species.

CAP has already been proven to be effective in wound healing, skin diseases, hospital hygiene, sterilization, antifungal treatments, dental care, and cosmetics targeted cell/tissue removal [16–18]. One of the most recent applications of CAP is in cancer therapy [19–21]. Multiple studies have convincingly demonstrated that the CAP treatment leads to selective eradication of cancer cells *in vitro* and reduction of tumor size *in vivo*. While most studies were done in vitro, some work was done in vivo [1–3, 7–9]. Recently, clinical cases of CAP application in cancer therapy were presented at the 2nd International Workshop on Plasma for Cancer Therapy in Nagoya (Japan) [22, 23] and one of these studies involving 12 patients afflicted with advanced squamous cell carcinoma of the head and neck has been documented in a recent paper [24].

The authors report a novel treatment approach for peritoneal carcinomatosis secondary to colon cancer using Cold Atmospheric Plasma combined with chemotherapy, radiation and cytoreductive surgery.

## 9.2 Clinical Patients Descriptions

A 56 year-old female previously underwent a laparoscopic right hemi-colectomy on April 18th 2011 at a local hospital in Lanham, MD. Pathology revealed adenocarcinoma, moderately differentiated with focal mucinous areas arising in villous adenoma at cecum proximal ascending colon and positive for one out of seven regional lymph nodes ($T_3N_1M_0$). She was originally treated with adjuvant chemotherapy FOLFOX after primary resection but developed an allergic reaction to oxaliplatin toward the end of treatment. She received two courses of FOLFIRI. In December 2012, CT scan revealed a solitary liver lesion and extensive tumors throughout the abdomen consistent with peritoneal carcinomatosis. She has a mutated K-ras (codon 12). Her CEA was 3014.5, CA19-9 2682 on 11.27.13.

Patient was referred for consultation on November 2013. Her CT scan showed widespread peritoneal carcinomatosis Stage $IV_b$ ($T_3N_1M_{1b}$). PET scan performed on November 2013 showed hepatic metastasis, numerous omental and abdominal wall masses, hyper-metabolic masses in the right lower quadrant next to the colon, mass at the ileocolonic anastomotic site intraluminal respectively, and increase activity in the pelvis posterior to uterus, cul de sac consistent with metastatic disease. A multi-disciplinary approach was started to cytoreduce the gastrointestinal tumors.

Patient received 14 cycles of FOLFIRI with the last dose on 9.22.14. Patient was subsequently treated using IMRT to all sites of disease based on 3D Conformal Computerized Contours combined with Xeloda. Nine gantry angles were used for the abdominal areas and eight gantry angles were used for the pelvic gutters. Summary of radiation treatment entailed abdominal regions dose 4500 cGY, 25 fractions from March 6th 2014 to April 24th 2014, Pelvic Gutters 4500 cGY 25 fractions from March 6th 2014 to April 23rd 2014. CT scan of chest, abdomen and pelvis on June 2014 showed good response to chemotherapy with a decrease in size of peritoneal metastatic implants with the exception of lesions on the surface of the spleen and nodule in the pelvis.

### 9.2.1 Methods

The Institutional Review Boards at Baton Rouge General Hospital (Bluebonnet campus), Baton Rouge reviewed and approved the study protocol. Approval was obtained from the Food and Drug Administration (FDA) for Compassionate and Emergency Use prior to surgical treatment as well as informed surgical consent. Human tissue was handled according to the tenets of the Declaration of Helsinki. SS-601 Electrosurgical generator integrated with Canady Plasma™ Coagulator and Canady Hybrid Plasma™ Scalpel (US Medical Innovations, LLC (USMI) Takoma Park, MD) was used for gross dissection of tumor and afterwards the Canady Helios™ Cold Plasma Ablator (USMI Takoma Park, MD) was used to treat the margins at the tumor site. March 2015 the patient underwent exploratory laparotomy, liver segmentectomy, cholecystectomy, right partial diaphragm resection with reconstruction using alloderm patch, en bloc resection of distal small bowel, transverse, left colon, sigmoid colon, distal pancreas with spleen and omentum, small bowel resection, resection of tumors from the mesentery and abdominal wall and supracervical total abdominal hysterectomy with bilateral salpingoophorectomy. A R0 resection was completed. Time of procedure and estimated blood loss were 7.5 h and 800cc respectively. Specimens sent to pathology were positive for metastatic adenocarcinoma from the liver, peritoneal implants, small bowel tumor with implants in the mesentery, bilateral tumor involvement adjacent to the ovaries, en bloc resection of the transverse, left and sigmoid colon, prior anastomosis to the small bowel, spleen with the tail of the pancreas, multiple tumor deposits of the mesentery, mesocolon, peripancreatic, perisplenic, adipose tissue and the small bowel prior anastomostic staple line. The patient's peritoneal cancer index (PCI) was >23 intra-operatively.

### 9.2.2 Hospital Course

After surgery the patient was transferred to the ICU and subsequently transferred to the floor. Patient was taken back to the operating room on 3.22.15 for anastomotic leak at the ileoproctostomy site. Take down of the rectal anastomosis and Brook ileostomy was performed. Patient returned to the OR on 3.24.15 and 3.27.14 for abdominal washing of abdomen and closure of the fascia. Postoperatively the patient developed an enterocutaneous fistula which was managed by TPN and abdominal wound vac. Patient was discharged to home on 5.15.15. On June 25th, 2015 postoperative CT scan of the abdomen and pelvis revealed no evidence of tumor in the abdomen. Patient and family decided hospice care August 2015.

## 9.3 Treatment of the Resected Surgical Margins Using Cold Atmospheric Plasma (CAP)

In the course of surgery, CAP treatment of the surgical margins (diaphragm, abdominal wall, mesentery, left colic gutter, mesenteric area, area of the splenic bed) was performed using the Canady Helios Cold Plasma™, Images of treatment of surgical margins by CAP are shown in Fig. 9.1c, d. Figure 9.1c show partial resection of the diaphragm using the Canady Hybrid Plasma™ scalpel and cold plasma jet treatment of surgical margins after resection are shown (Fig. 9.1d).

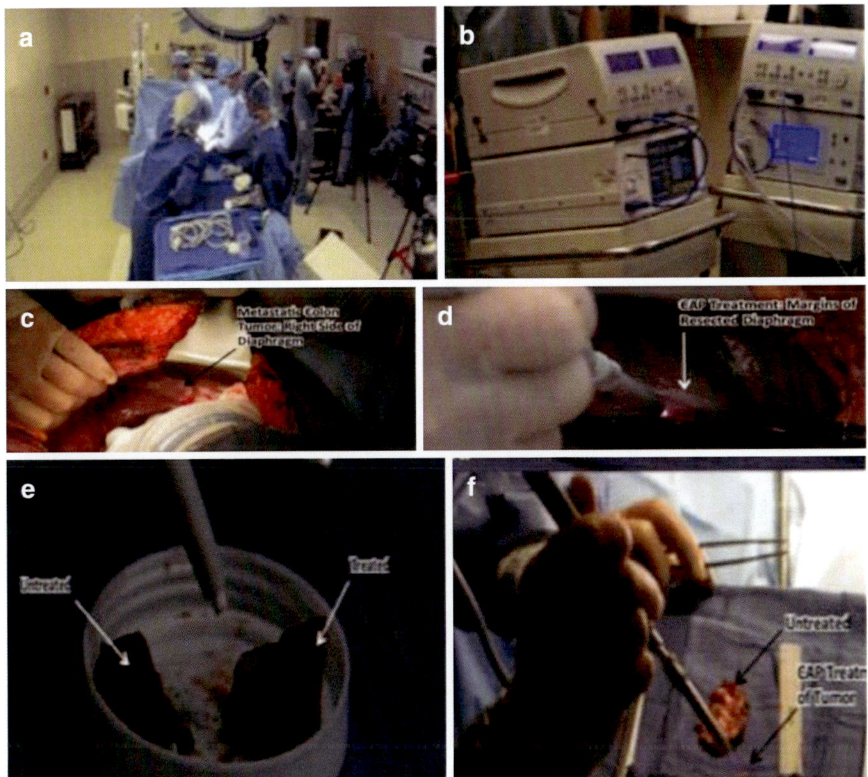


**Fig. 9.1** (**a**) OR set up. (**b**) Cold Plasma Generator (USMI). (**c, d**) Partial resection and Cold plasma treatment of surgical margins, ex vivo. (**e**) Treatment of liver. (**f**) Treatment of diaphragm

In addition to treatment of surgical margins we performed cold plasma treatment of the ex vivo sample of liver (shown in Fig. 9.1e) and diaphragm (shown in Fig. 9.1f). Treated and untreated samples were imaged and analyzed using various assays (see Sect. 9.5).

## 9.4 Body Temperature Measurements During Surgery

In this section we present body temperature measurements during surgery using USMI Helios cold plasma device. Schematics of experimental set up is shown in Fig. 9.2.

### 9.4.1 Experiment Setup and Procedure

A thermal camera (FLIR A35) with a 19 mm lens and a 60 Hz frame-rate was used to collect the plasma object and patient body's thermal data. The FLIR A35 camera was mounted approximately 3 ft above the patient to observe the treatment area. To get a better viewing angle and to ensure that the camera is less intrusive to the surgeon's procedure, a less than 20° view angle was applied to the camera. The FLIR A35 thermal camera's area of view at approximately 3 ft is 2.7 ft by 2 ft area, which is larger

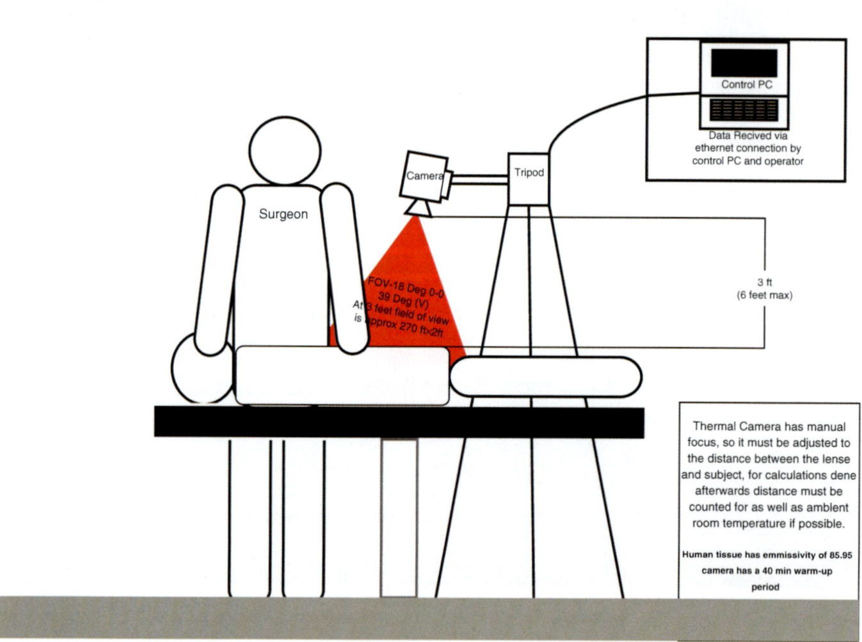


**Fig. 9.2** Setup of the thermal camera during the intraoperative cold plasma treatments

than the 1 foot by 1 foot of the patient's procedure area. In total, 5 h of thermal video was captured by the camera and stored onto the hard drive of the control PC. During the procedure, the patient was treated with the Canady Hybrid Plasma™ and the Canady Helios Cold Plasma™ scalpels. The treatments consisted of "spraying" the margins of the cancerous area with the cold plasma jet created at the distal end of the Helios Cold Plasma Scalpel. The settings for the Canady Helios Cold Plasma™ Ablator's settings were 1.6 W and helium flow rate 5 L/min for a duration of 2 min per treatment area.

The data captured by the FLIR camera was later processed using **FLIR tools+** [25]. To compare the cold plasma intraoperative thermal performance and patient's tissue reaction to the cold plasma scalpel, the patient's pre-treatment area tissue temperature and post-treatment tissue area temperature were measured. Tissue area temperature was calculated by taking the average of the temperature data in the treatment area by using the built in functions of FLIR tools+, Fig. 9.3 demonstrate a side by side comparison of tissue temperature pre-treatment and post-treatment.

Along with intraoperative cold plasma treatments, the thermal camera recorded several cold plasma ex vivo treatments as shown in Fig. 9.1. The tumor cells and a small amount of normal cells were removed from the patient for a comparison study; tumor and control samples were treated with the cold plasma scalpel with the same settings as the intraoperative treatments. The pre-treatment and post-treatment thermal images for ex vivo were processed identically to the intraoperative treatments as shown in Fig. 9.4.

During the data processing, **FLIR tools+** built in functions were selected to measure the treatment area's minimum, maximum, and average temperatures. Based on the background reference material [25], a thermal emissivity of 0.95 was selected, so as to best represent the actual temperature of live body tissues for the spectral range of the camera (7.5–13 μm). During the procedure, the patients End Tidal $CO_2$ and $O_2$ level were recorded via the ventilator and the pulse oximeter respectively.

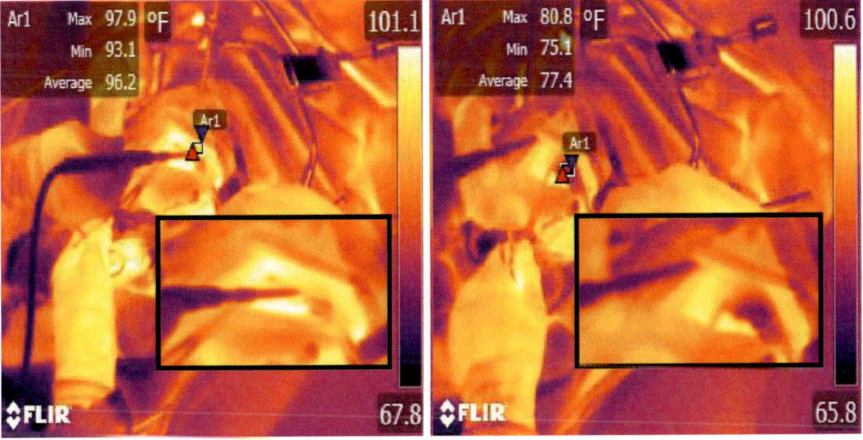


**Fig. 9.3** Thermal stills of the cold plasma intraoperative treatment. The left figure is the pre-treatment tissue temperature; the right figure is post-treatment tissue temperature

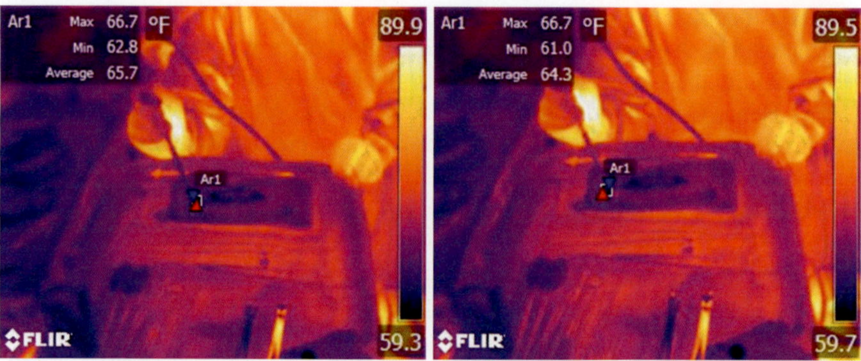


**Fig. 9.4** Thermal stills of the cold plasma ex vivo treatment. The left figure is the pre-treatment tissue temperature; the right figure is post-treatment tissue temperature

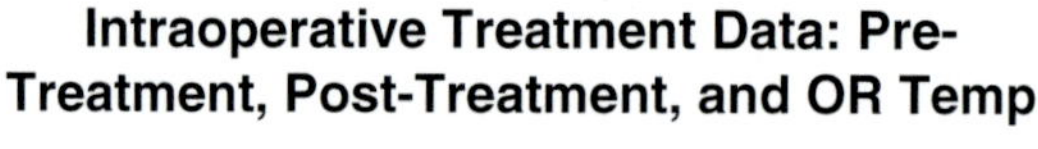


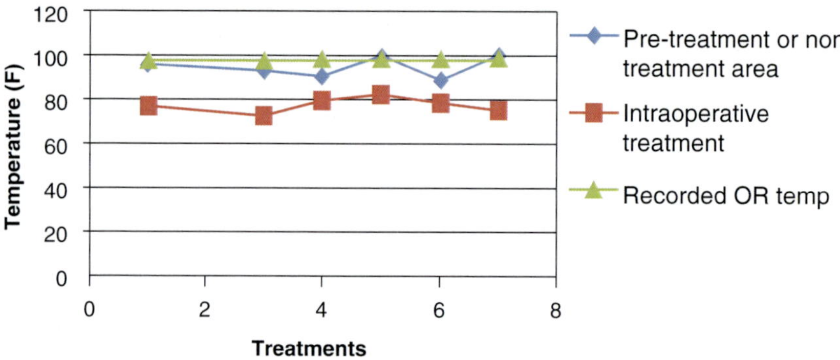


**Fig. 9.5** Graph of intraoperative temperature, showing the temperature before and after treatment as well as the temperature measured by the OR equipment

### 9.4.2 Experiment Results

Thermal measurements from the in vivo treatments are shown in Fig. 9.5. Significant temperature change occurs in the area of treatment for each case. A temperature drop of 10–20° across the surface of the tissue occurs in all six treatments. Temperature measurements of the surrounding tissue and tissues pre-treatment are displayed as well and are consistent with the core temperature measured with the hospitals equipment.

## 9.5 Expansion In Vitro, Characterization and Immunohistological Analysis of Human Primary Colon Cancer Epithelial Cells Isolated After Surgery

In this Section we describe characterization of the human primary colon cancer cells. Identification of colon stem cell markers CD44 and TRAIL receptor 1 were performed (Figs. 9.6 and 9.7)

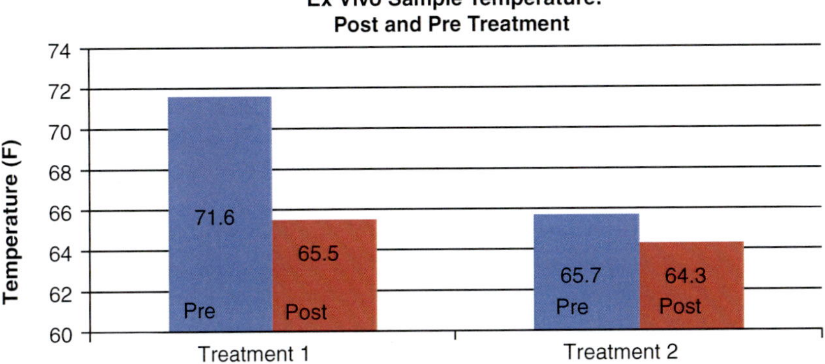


**Fig. 9.6** Ex vivo cold plasma treatment results, showing the temperature measured before and after the treatments. The thermal measurements for the ex vivo are shown in figure. There is a slight temperature decrease between pre-treatment and intraoperative treatment, but not as large as in the case of the patient

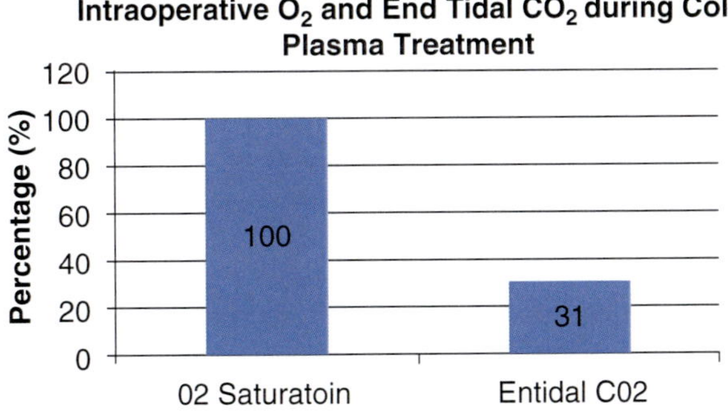


**Fig. 9.7** $O_2$ and End Tidal $CO_2$ results for the patient during the treatments. The patient intraoperative $O_2$ and End Tidal $CO_2$ measurements were unaffected by the treatment and were well within the normal range throughout the treatments as shown in figure

### 9.5.1 Materials and Methods

#### 9.5.1.1 Human Tissue Preparation and Sample Collection

Human tissue was handled according to the tenets of the Declaration of Helsinki. On the basis of our studies in vitro using primary LT-97-3 colon cancer stem cells (Generous gift of Dr. Brigitte Marian, Univ. of Vienna Medical Center, Austria; J Pathol. 2007 Oct;213(2):152–60), HCT-116 ATCC derived Colon cancer cells and normal colon epithelial cells (unpublished data) we chose to use the LT-97-3 medium for developing primary cultures. Medium used to culture the human LT-97 includes the following components, 4 parts Ham F12, 1 part L15, 2% FCS, insulin, 20 nm Triiodotyronin, Trasnferrin-20 μL for 500 mL, 1 μg/mL hydrocortisone- 20 μL, 30 ng/mL EGF- 15 μL, Penicillin 10,000 μg/mL (5 mL) / Streptomycin (5 mL)/gentamycin (2.5 mL) (Sigma Aldrich). The samples were collected in 20 mL sample collection vials containing the above medium at 4 °C and brought back to the lab within 10 h from the sample collection site and processed immediately.

Colon tumor explants was minced to 1 mm size and was processed to isolate epithelial cells using enzymatic digestion with 1 mg/mL collagenase type IV for 10 min at 37 °C and some of the 1 mm samples were expanded in vitro as explant cultures. The human colon epithelial cultures were expanded in a BSL2 classified laboratory (Jerome Canady Research Institute for Advanced Biological and Technological Sciences, Takoma Park, MD) for maintaining cell lines for biomedical, translational and regenerative biology applications. Five freshly isolated human colon cancer samples were procured within 10 h of patient's surgery in sterile 20 mL borosilicate sample collection vials containing the above mentioned medium composition. 3–5 $cm^2$ or larger size of the colon tumor and normal tissue samples excised from the patient were used in the current study: (1) liver tissue with colon cancer treated with CAP (2) liver tissue with colon cancer treated without CAP (3) Subphrenic Diaphragm with colon cancer treated with CAP (4) Subphrenic Diaphragm with colon cancer treated without CAP and (5) normal diaphragm with and without CAP. Tissues were treated with penicillin streptomycin in PBS and minced and processed as described previously [26]. Normal diaphragm tissues were processed for cryosectioning and H&E staining. These two methods of cell culture namely, explant cultures and isolated cells cultures were used in the current study to generate primary using the patient's biopsy samples. Only two explants developed into epithelial cultures from tissues isolated with enzymatic treatments. The cells were serially diluted (into six 35 mm well plates) with the hope that the stem cells would develop and proliferate into colonies. All cultures were terminated for the following tests for histology, confocal microscopy to detect various proteins/antigens. Images were acquired periodically to assess the morphology of the cells.

#### 9.5.1.2 Immunofluorescence Analysis for Identification of Colon Stem Cells and Colon Cancer Markers in Tissues Excised Using Cold Plasma Scalpel

Some of the tissues procured from the patient were immediately cryosectioned using Leica cryostat. 5–6 μm sections at −20 °C were stained with H&E and double immunofluorescence for localization of colon stem cell marker human CD44 FITC (Bio Legend), anti TRAIL receptor1 (Santa Cruz) and second antibody anti-alexaflour 594 or 488(molecular probes), respectively was used along with nuclear counterstaining with DAPI (Vectashield, Molecular Probes). Appropriate isotype controls (Life Technologies) were maintained. Zeiss confocal images were acquired to analyze the cold plasma excised tissue for remnant colon cancer markers.

#### 9.5.1.3 Confocal Imaging

Zeiss 1um tick Z-stack images were acquired and 3D–reconstruction of the images (Jerome Canady Research Institute for Advanced Biological and Technological Sciences, Takoma, Park, MD) were analyzed for surface expression of TRAIL-R1 and CD44 or Ki67 in the cryosections (n = 3) and in cultured colon cancer cells after 30 days in culture. The entire dish was assessed and images were captured for the remnant cells and the % of positive cells was calculated. 15 images per dish were acquired to record the % total number of cells remaining and % of cells positive for the above markers.

#### 9.5.1.4 Statistical Analysis

The following test was carried out for n = 3 samples.

Nonparametric Tests: Independent Samples. NP tests/independent Test-Mann Whitney Wald Wolfowitz Kruskal Wallis test compared pair wise; median(test value = sample = compare = pairwise) Hodges Lehmann/missing Scope = analysis usermissing = exclude/criteria with alpha = 0.05 Cilevel = 95.

### 9.5.2 Results

#### 9.5.2.1 Metastatic Liver With and Without CAP Treatments

Figure 9.8 shows cross sections images along the thickness of the sample excised from the patient. Note the intactness of the tissue sections in a and b showing no damage at the site of CAP treatments (arrow). Arrowhead indicates the metastatic colon cancer area in the liver. These tissues were used to isolate the colon cancer cells to be cultured and expanded in vitro for further analysis.

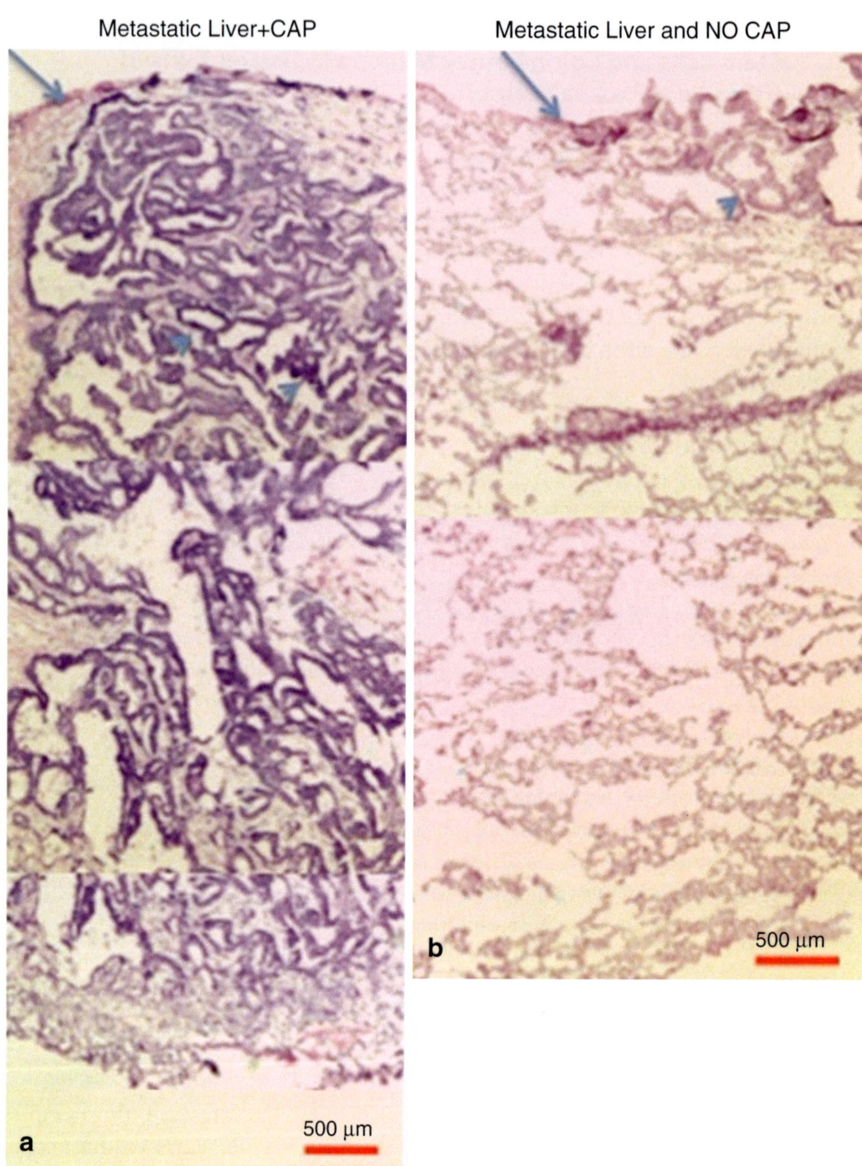


**Fig. 9.8** (**a**, **b**) H&E stained showing (**a**) Metastatic liver treated with cold plasma (**b**) without Cold Plasma

#### 9.5.2.2 Metastatic Tumor from Sub Phrenic Diaphragm With and Without CAP Treatments

Figure 9.9 shows images, which are cross sections along the entire thickness of the sample excised from the patient. Note the intactness of the tissue sections in a and b showing no damage at the site of CAP treatments (arrow). Arrowhead indicates the metastatic colon cancer area in the sub phrenic diaphragm. These tissues were used to isolate the colon cancer cells to be cultured and expanded in vitro for further analysis.

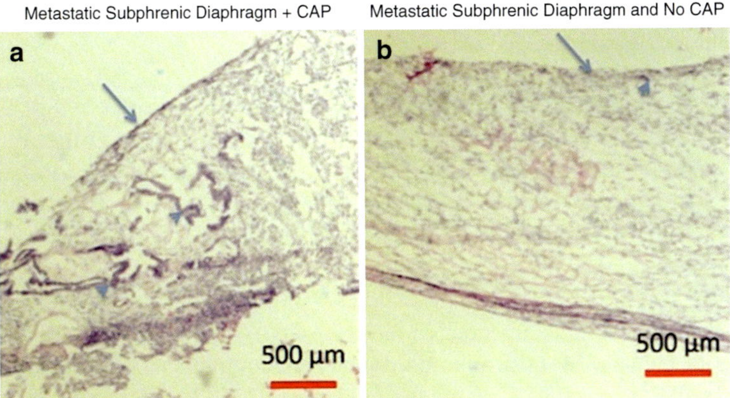


**Fig. 9.9** (**a, b**) H&E stained sections showing Metastatic Tumor Sub phrenic Diaphragm (**a**) treated with cold plasma (**b**) without Cold Plasma

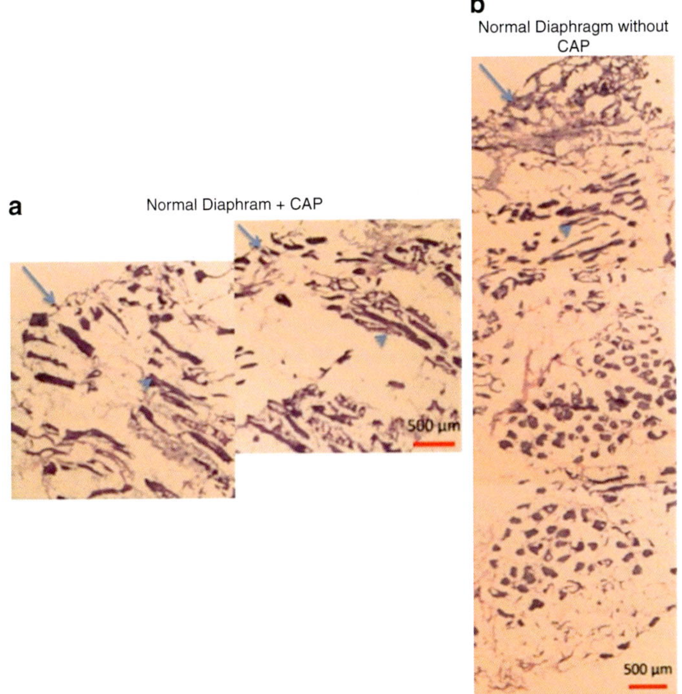


**Fig. 9.10** (**a**, **b**) H&E stained sections showing (**a**) Normal Diaphragm treated with CAP (**b**) without CAP

#### 9.5.2.3 Normal Diaphragm With and Without CAP Treatments, to Demonstrate That CAP Does Not Cause Injury to the Healthy Tissues

Images in Fig. 9.10 are cross sections along the thickness of the sample excised from the patient. Note the intactness of the tissue sections in a and b showing no damage at the site of CAP treatments (arrow). Arrowhead shows muscle fibers of the diaphragm separated by loose connective tissue.

#### 9.5.2.4 Confocal Double-Immunofluorescence Images of Human Liver Showing Localization of Colon Stem Cells (CD44 Positive Red) and TRAIL -Receptor 1 (Green)

Figures a, b are samples without CAP treatments and figures c, d are with CAP treatments. Note the bright TRAIL R-1 staining in (c and d) in presence of CAP and the absence of bright TRAIL-R1 in (a and b).

Freshly procured human tumor samples from liver treated with and without CAP were oriented and embedded in the cryostat. 6–7μm thick sections and fixed in ice-cold methanol for 15 min and double-immunostained for TRAIL-R1 and CD44. In the presence of CAP treatments, the TRAIL-R1 expression increases. Moreover, the double positive cells expressing CD44 and TRAIL-R1, typical of a stem cell was observed in all the tumor samples as shown in Fig. 9.11a–d. It was found that the localization and expression of TRAIL-R1 in the CAP treated CD44 positive cell was greater in both number and expression (c, d). These results suggest that CAP triggering of TRAIL-R1 in colon cancer stem cells may play a role in apoptosis. Therefore, we isolated and expanded the cells from these CAP treated and untreated tumor samples to further characterize the cellular profile.

#### 9.5.2.5 In Vitro Expansion of Human Colon Cancer Cells from Liver Samples Treated with CAP

In order to test for characterization of cellular profile generated from tissue explants with and without CAP, two different in vitro culture methods were employed (materials and methods). It was interesting to note that explant cultures of liver did not show any outgrowth of cells, while cells isolated using enzymatic treatments, yield a varied population of cells. Figure 9.12 demonstrate that the CAP treated tissue yielded a population of epithelial cells, which over a period of time showed morphology of mostly differentiated cells in the terminal phase of apoptosis. Most of the cells were floating in culture demonstrating an apoptotic phenotype.

#### 9.5.2.6 In Vitro Expansion of Human Colon Cancer Cells from Liver Samples Without CAP Treatment.

The explant cultures showed no outgrowth, while the cells isolated from liver samples showed small colonies and proliferating colonies as shown in Fig. 9.13 (arrowhead **a, b**). This colony was tracked and the colony size increased over time (**a, b**). After more than 3-weeks of culture these cells were still proliferating (arrowhead). These cultures were terminated to assess the molecular characteristics using various markers.

#### 9.5.2.7 In Vitro Expansion of Human Colon Cancer Cells from Subphrenic Diaphragm Samples Treated with CAP

The cellular profile and phenotype from CAP treated sub phrenic diaphragm (Fig. 9.14) showed epithelial cells going through apoptosis. However, the explant

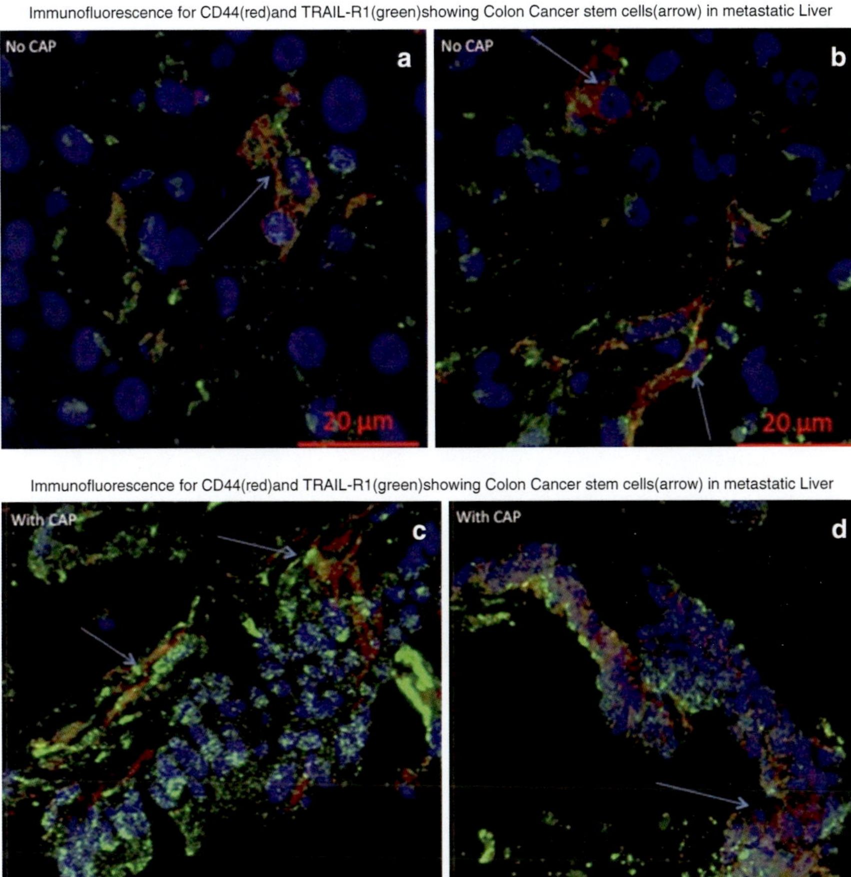


**Fig. 9.11** Confocal Immunofluorescence images of human Liver demonstrate localization of colon stem cells (CD44 positive red) and TRAIL-Receptor 1 (green) (arrow-**a** to **d**). DAPI was used for nuclear counterstaining

cultures showed fibroblast-like cells, which may not be of colon cancer origin and may be from the remnant diaphragm tissue. The isolated cell cultures showed floating dead cells at the end of 27th day.

#### 9.5.2.8 In Vitro Expansion of Human Colon Cancer Cells from Sub Phrenic Diaphragm Samples Without CAP Treatment

Sub phrenic diaphragm without CAP treatment (Fig. 9.15) showed colon epithelial stem cell phenotype. The small colony enlarged over a period of time showing colon stem cell phenotype (**b, d, f**). However, the explant cultures showed fibroblast-like cells, which may not be of colon cancer origin and may be from the remnant diaphragm tissue.

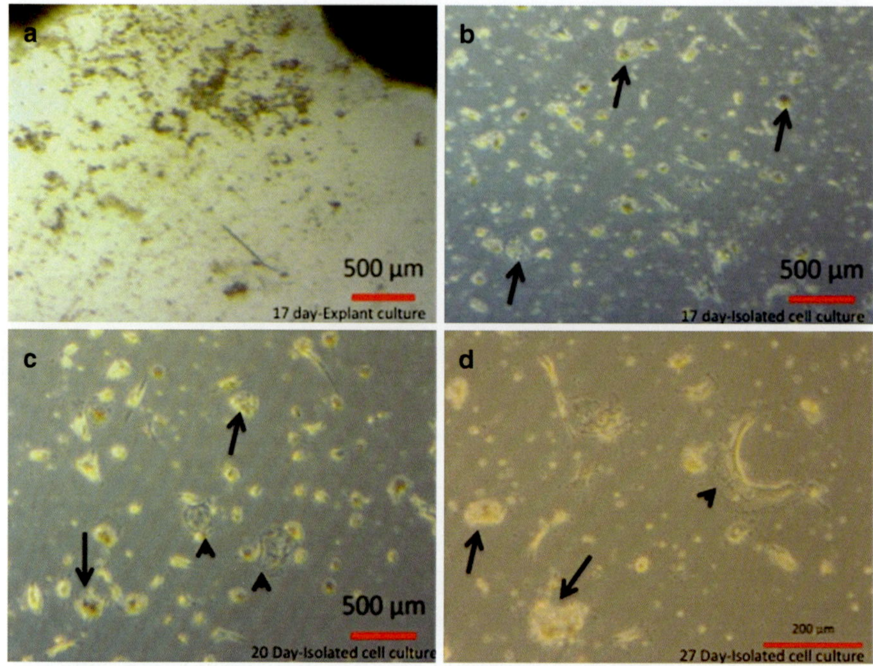


**Fig. 9.12** In vitro expansion of Human colon Cancer cells from liver samples treated with CAP. Representative images of explant (**a**) and isolated cell cultures (**b–d**) of colon cells from liver showing cell death and many floating dead cells (arrow) and differentiated cells (arrowhead) in the presence of CAP after 17–27 days in culture (**b–d**). Note the absence of outgrowth in the liver explant cultures

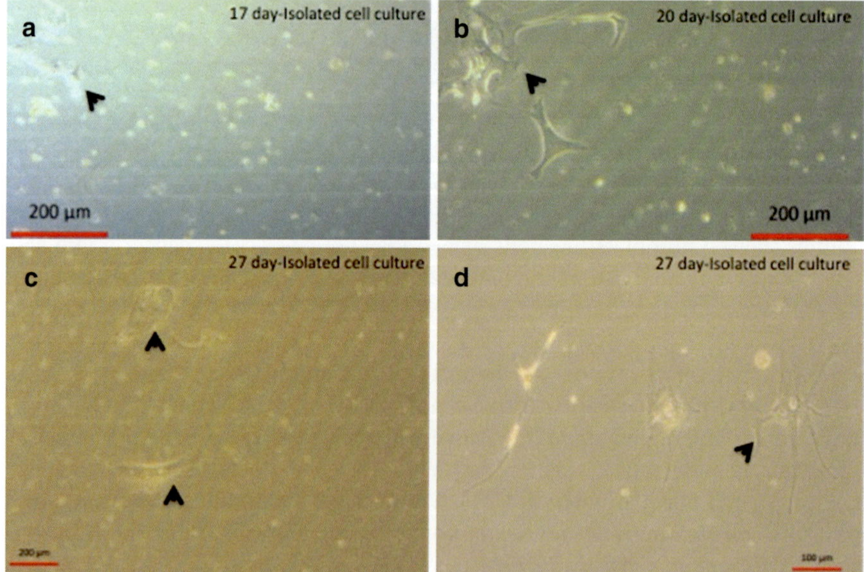


**Fig. 9.13** Representative images of isolated cell cultures of colon cells from liver showing healthy proliferating colony of cells (arrowhead) without CAP after 17 (**a**) to 24 days (**b–d**) in culture

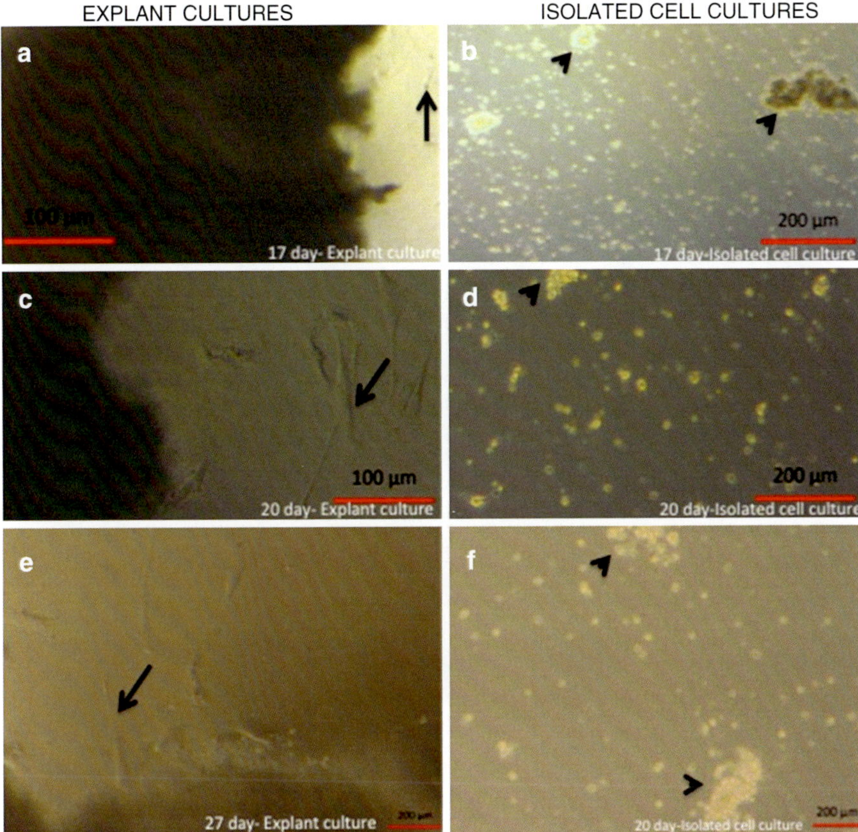


**Fig. 9.14** In vitro expansion of Human Colon Cancer cells from Sub phrenic Diaphragm samples treated with CAP. Explant (**a**, **c**, **e**) and isolated cell cultures (**b**, **d**, **f**) of colon cells from Sub phrenic Diaphragm showing cell death and many floating dead cells (arrowhead) in the presence of CAP after 17–27 days in culture. Arrow shows fibroblast-like cells from the tissue explants

#### 9.5.2.9 Characterization of Colon Cancer Cells Expanded In Vitro Isolated from Liver

Isolated cell cultures of colon cells from liver showing disintegrating nuclei of smaller size in (arrowhead in a, b) Note these cells are negative for Ki67 and TRAIL-r1, suggesting that these cells are in last phase of apoptosis. (b) Showing healthy proliferating colony of cells (arrow; green Ki67 positive and red-TRAIL-R1 positive) without CAP after 30 days in culture.

Most of the cells display disintegrated nuclei and a few differentiated large cells in the presence of CAP treatment as shown in Fig. 9.16. The smaller size of the nuclei and absence of any cytoplasmic material was suggestive of a dead cell phenotype after CAP treatment. Large number of proliferating Ki67 positive cells were observed in cultures without CAP treatment and such cells were more in number when compared to the CAP treated. These results suggested that the profile of cells after CAP treatment was significantly different from the healthy proliferating tumor cells, generated from samples without CAP treatment. Therefore in order to further

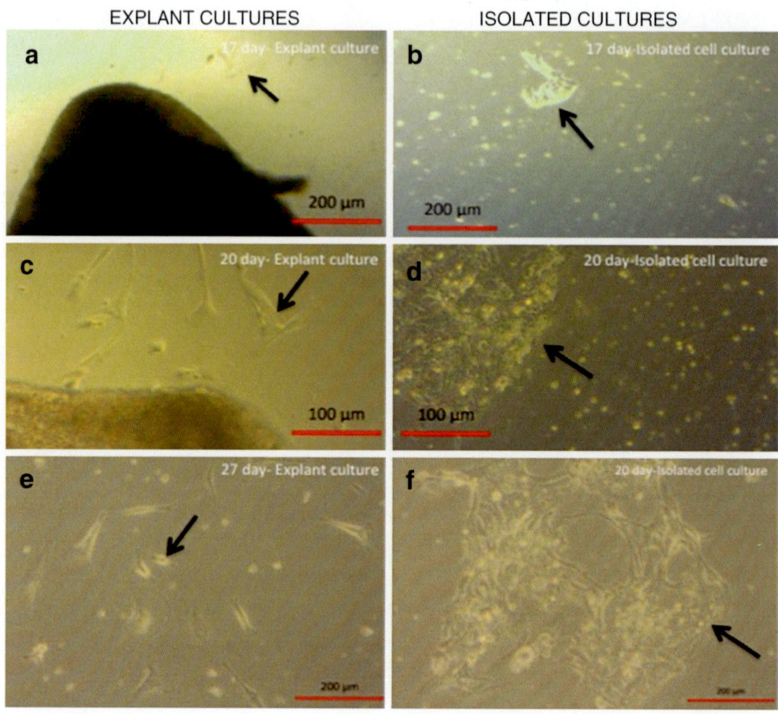


**Fig. 9.15** In vitro expansion of Human Colon Cancer cells from Sub phrenic Diaphragm samples without CAP treatment. Cellular profile of the sub phrenic diaphragm showing proliferating colony of cells (arrow) without CAP after 17–27 days in culture (**b**, **d**, **f**). Note the large colony, a property of a tumor stem cell. Explant cultures show fibroblast-like phenotype

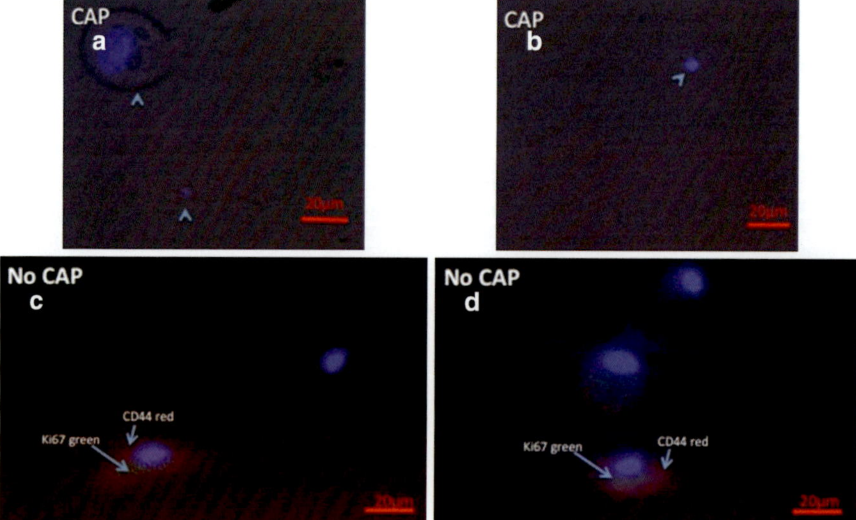


**Fig. 9.16** Characterization of colon cancer cells expanded in vitro isolated from liver nuclear counterstaining with DAPI (blue)

characterize these cells for their proliferation we measured Ki67 along with TRAIL-R1 and the % total of positive and double positive cells in CAP treated and untreated cells was calculated.

#### 9.5.2.10 Characterization of Cellular Profile of Human Colon Cancer Cells Expanded In Vitro

Our analysis suggests that all the cells went through cell death and apoptosis in the CAP treated case. Recall that this proliferative population of cells was absent in the CAP untreated samples. About 40% cells were proliferating (Ki67 positive) and 24% cells expressed TRAIL-R1 in CAP untreated, while CAP treatment lead to cell death and apoptosis as shown in Table 9.1. None of the CAP treated cells expressed TRAIL-R1 and were not proliferating, suggesting that these cells were no longer viable and their apoptotic mechanism was initiated by CAP treatment. These results suggest that CAP has an effect in inducing colon stem cell death by triggering TRAIL Receptor -1 expression.

## 9.6 Concluding Remarks

The authors report the first use of cold atmospheric plasma in a clinical setting for the treatment of metastatic stage IV colon cancer and demonstrate the safety and efficacy of cold atmospheric plasma.

The human colon cancer in the patient samples expressed colon stem cells in liver and was positive for CD44 and TRAIL-R1 expression. TRAIl-R1 expression increases in the CAP treated liver tissues, suggesting that the death receptor molecule may be involved in inducing apoptosis. Isolation of colon epithelial cells from these liver and subphrenic diaphragm explants after CAP treatment, induced cell death within 3 weeks of culture. CAP untreated tissues yields a population of cells that are healthy and colonies increase in size, typical of tumor stem cells. These colonies proliferated even after 4 weeks in culture. In addition explant cultures after treatments with CAP and without treatments yielded fibroblast-like cell phenotype only in the subphrenic diaphragm samples and not from liver explants. These results suggest that these may be normal healthy cells and not the colon cancer epithelial cells and may require further investigation. It has to be noted that none of the CAP treated cells after 3-weeks of culture expressed TRAIL-R1. Moreover, the nuclei of

**Table 9.1** Characterization of cellular profile of human colon cancer cells expanded in vitro

| | %Double positive cells | Ki67% positive cells | %Trail-r1 positive cells | %DAPI positive cells |
|---|---|---|---|---|
| Colon tumor cells without CAP* | 24 | 16 | 32 | 28 |
| Colon tumor cells with CAP | NIL | NIL | NIL | 24 disintegrating cells |

The entire culture dish was analyzed to calculate proportion of total number of cells. Significant (*$p \leq 0.05$) difference in the profile was cells with CAP treatment and without treatment was observed. Note the absence of TRAIL-R1 and Ki67 positivity in CAP treated samples remnant cells were all disintegrated and were significantly different from the population of CAP untreated proliferating Ki67 positive cells.

Overall the results suggest that CAP has an effect on colon epithelial cells and colon stem cells and induces tumor cell death and the use of CAP had no adverse event to the patient.

## References

1. Siegel R, Naishadham D, Jemal A. Cancer statistics, 2012. CA Cancer J Clin. 2012;62:10–29.
2. Chu DZ, Lang NP, Thompson C, Osteen PK, Westbrook KC. Peritoneal Carcinomatosis in non gynecologic malignancy. Cancer. 1989;63:364–7.
3. Sadeghi B, Arvieux C, Glehen O, et al. Peritoneal carcinomatosis from non-gynecologic Smalignancies. Results from the EVOCAPE 1 multicentric prospective study. Cancer. 2000;88:358–63.
4. Glehen O, Osinky D, Cotte E, Kwiatkowski F, Freyer G, Issac S, Trillet-lenoir V, Sayag-beaujard AC, Francois Y, Vignal J, et al. Intraperitoneal chemohyperthermia using a closed abdominal procedure and cytoreductive surgery for the treatment of peritoneal carcinomatosis: morbidity and mortality analysis of 216 concsecutive procedures. Ann Surg Oncol. 2003;10(8):863–9.
5. Glockzin G, Rochon J, Arnold D, Sa L, Klebl F, Zeman F, Koller M, Schlitt HJ, Piso P. A prospective multicenter phase II study evaluating multimodality treatment of patients with peritoneal carcinomatosis arising from appendiceal and colorectal cancer: the combatac trial. BMC Cancer. 2013;13:67. https://doi.org/10.1186/1471-2407-13-67.
6. Jayne DG, Fook S, Loi C, Seow-Choen F. Peritoneal carcinomatosis from colorectal cancer. Br J Surg. 2002;89:1545–50.
7. Piso P, Arnold D. Multimodal treatment approaches for peritoneal carcinosis in colorectal cancer. Dtsch Arztebl Int. 2011;108(47):802–8.
8. Kulu Y, Muller-stich B, Buchler MW, Ulrich A. Surgical treatment of peritoneal carcinomatosis: current treatment modalities. Langenbeck's Arch Surg. 2013;399(1):41–53.
9. Franko J, Shi Q, Goldman CD, et al. Treatment of Colorectal peritoneal carcinomatosis with systemic chemotherapy: a pooled analysis of north central cancer treatment group phase III trials n9741 and n9841. J Clin Oncol. 2012;30:263–7. https://doi.org/10.1016/ejso2013.06.001.
10. Verwaal VJ, van Ruth S, de Bree E, et al. Randomized trial of cytoreduction and hyperthermic intraperitoneal chemotherapy versus systemic chemotherapy and palliative surgery in patients with peritoneal carcinomatosis of colorectal cancer. J Clin Oncol. 2003;21:3737–43.
11. Riss S, Mohamed F, Dayal S, Cecil T, Stift A, Bachleitner-Hofmann T, Moran B. Peritoneal Metasases from colorectal cancer: patient selection for cytoreductive surgery and Hyperthermic Intraperitoneal chemotherapy. Eur J Surg Oncol. 2013;39(9):931–7.
12. Elias D, Gilly F, Quenet F, et al. Peritoneal colorectal carcinomatosis treated with surgery and Perioperative Intraperitoneal Chemotherapy: Retrospective analysis of 523 patients from a multicentric French study. J Clin Oncol. 2010;28:63–8.
13. Laroussi M, Kong M, Morfill G, Stolz W, editors. Plasma medicine. Cambridge; 2012.
14. Friedman A, Friedman G. Plasma medicine. Hoboken: Wiley; 2013.
15. Keidar M, Beilis II. Plasma Engineering: application in aerospace, nanotechnology and bionanotechnology. Oxford: Elsevier; 2013.
16. Morfill GE, Kong MG, Zimmermann JL. Focus on plasma medicine. Review. New J Phys. 2009;11:115011.
17. Keidar M. Plasma for cancer treatment. Plasma Source Sci Technol. 2015;24:033001.
18. Fridman G, Friedman G, Gutsol A, Shekhter AB, Vasilets VN, Fridman A. Applied plasma medicine. Plasma Process Polym. 2008;5:503.

19. Vandamme M, Robert E, Pesnel S, Barbosa E, Dozias S, Sobilo J, Lerondel S, Le Pape A, Pouvesle JM. Antitumor effect of plasma treatment on U87 Glioma Xenografts: preliminary results. Plasma Process Polym. 2010;7:264.
20. Keidar M, Walk R, Shashurin A, Srinivasan P, Sandler A, Dasgupta S, Ravi R, Guerrero-Preston R, Trink B. Cold plasma selectivity and the possibility of a paradigm shift in cancer therapy. Br J Cancer. 2011;105:1295.
21. Vandamme M, Robert E, Lerondel S, Sarron V, Ries D, Dozias S, Sobilo J, Gosset D, Kieda C, Legrain B, Pouvesle J-M, Le Pape A. ROS implication in a new antitumor strategy based on non-thermal plasma. Int J Cancer. 2011;130:2185.
22. Metelmann HR. What kind of impact is possible by plasma-jet in head and neck cancer?", The 2nd International Workshop on Plasma for Cancer Treatment, Nagoya, Japan, March, 2015.
23. Canady J. "Development and clinical application of hybrid and cold atmospheric plasma combined with systemic chemotherapy and selective 3D conformal radiation therapy: A novel approach to the treatment of peritoneal metastases from colorectal cancer." The 2nd International Workshop on Plasma for Cancer Treatment, Nagoya, Japan, March, 2015.
24. Metelmann HR, Nedrelow DS, Seebauer C, Schuster M, von Woedtke T, Weltmann K-D, Kindler S, Metelmann PH, Finkelstein SE, Von Hoff DD, Podmelle F. Head and neck cancer treatment and physical plasma. Clin Plasma Med. 2015;3:17–23.
25. Lahiri BB, Bagavathiappan S, Jayakumar T, Philip J. Medical applications of infrared thermography: a review. Infrared Phys Technol. 2012;55(4):221–35.
26. Ray S, et al. Establishment of human ultra-low passage colorectal cancer cell lines using spheroids from fresh surgical specimens suitable for in vitro and in vivo studies. J Cancer. 2012;3:196–206.

# 10 Palliative Treatment of Head and Neck Cancer

Christian Seebauer, Hans-Robert Metelmann, Katherina Witzke, and Jean-Michel Pouvesle

## 10.1 Introduction

Since the first report about the cell destructive effect of cold atmospheric plasma (CAP) on malignant melanoma in 2007, the potential spectrum of CAP application in cancer treatment has quickly expanded [1–10]. To date, the CAP treatment has demonstrated its significant anti-cancer capacity in several experimental settings in approximately 20 more types of malignant tumor cells including skin cancer [11–17], brain cancer [18–26], breast cancer [27–29], cervical cancer [30–36], lung cancer [8, 37–42], gastric cancer [43], pancreatic cancer [44, 45], colorectal cancer [18, 46–50], bladder cancer [8], prostatic cancer [51], leukemia [52–55], hepatic cancer [32, 56–58], thyroid cancer [59, 60], as well as head & neck cancer [61–65]. Among diverse plasma-originated species (RONS: reactive oxygen and nitrogen species), $H_2O_2$ has been proved to be the main anti-cancer reactive species causing the death of cancer cells in-vitro [10]. Nevertheless, the understanding of the precise anti-cancer mechanism is very limited. Case reports and scientific studies of in-vivo applications of CAP are rare and generally limited

C. Seebauer, M.D., D.D.S. (✉)
Department of Oral and Maxillofacial Surgery/Plastic Surgery,
University Medicine Greifswald, Greifswald, Germany

Leibniz Institute for Plasma Science and Technology, Greifswald, Germany

National Center of Plasma Medicine, Berlin, Germany
e-mail: seebauerc@uni-greifswald.de

H.-R. Metelmann • K. Witzke
Department of Oral and Maxillofacial Surgery/Plastic Surgery,
University Medicine Greifswald, Greifswald, Germany

National Center of Plasma Medicine, Berlin, Germany

J.-M. Pouvesle
GREMI, Orlcans, France


H.-R. Metelmann et al. (eds.), *Comprehensive Clinical Plasma Medicine*,
https://doi.org/10.1007/978-3-319-67627-2_10

to animal investigations. These animal studies have supported the previous in-vitro findings of tumor growth reduction by the CAP treatment [5] and show much promise of therapeutic value in treating humans.

## 10.2 Palliative Care: Current Status of Clinical Application

Treatment of advanced head and neck carcinoma is multifaceted, challenging and has to be performed on an individualized basis. Complexity and variability of different tumor entities require specific and individualized cancer therapy including the main pillars of evidence based medicine, namely surgery, chemotherapy and radiotherapy. When a patient enters a stage a curative approach to destroy the tumor and heal the disease is no longer in reach, palliative care becomes the focus of care. Treatment goals now are managing pain, taking care of nutrition and open airways, facilitating social contacts, in summary alleviate the symptoms and emotional issues of cancer. Head and neck cancer ulcerations present both exceedingly physical and emotional challenges to the patient, family, and even the most experienced nurse. Patients with advanced incurable tumors frequently suffer from superinfected chronic wounds caused by necrotic tissue due to progressive tumor growth, weak systemic and local immunological response and various accompanying illnesses. These wounds may be associated with pain, odor, exsudate, bleeding, and repulsive appearance. They may adversely affect self-esteem and body image, causing patients to isolate themselves at a time when social support is critically needed. Due to strong wound vulnerability, local antiseptic wound care of microbial contaminated tumor areas is frequently complicated by bleeding, pain and patient dissatisfaction. Plasma is clinically known for inactivating microbial pathogens, making it the key concept of palliative care of these patients to manage odor, bleeding, preventing infections, and optimizing the emotional well-being of the patient and family.

In 2015, the study group of Metelmann, Seebauer and co-workers introduced the first in-vivo application of CAP in the care of patients suffering from advanced head and neck cancers [66]. In a prospective descriptive clinical evaluation, 12 patients received plasma treatment as part of the palliative treatment concept for reduction of bacterial colonization of ulcerated cancer wounds. Effects of CAP treatment beyond successful palliation as characterized above have been described either as a flat area with vascular stimulation or as a contraction of tumor ulceration rims forming recesses covered with scabs that were surrounded by tumor tissue in visible progress [67].

In a recent study, clinical benefit and histological changes have been prospectively evaluated during the standardized CAP treatment intended for palliation of six patients with locally advanced head and neck cancer [68]. CAP treatment was implemented in conventional palliative therapy of contaminated exulcerative cancer wounds. The survival time of the patients, the plasma related effects on contamination, tumor growth, and need of pain medication, the side effects and quality of life under treatment, as well as changes of tumor size have been recorded.

Plasma was applied with a kINPen® MED plasma jet (neoplas tools GmbH, Greifswald, Germany), size dependent like 1 min/cm$^2$ of cancer wound with a distance of approximately 10 mm and in a meandering manner. Plasma treatment was continued to be performed every 2–3 days and was implemented in conjunction with conventional cancer wound care including antiseptic wound treatment and antiseptic dressing.

## 10.3 Clinical Cases

### 10.3.1 Case History 1 (Fig. 10.1)

In February 2015, a 51-year-old Caucasian male patient presented himself in the department of oral and maxillofacial surgery with an ulcerating lesion on the left cheek extending to the molar and retromolar region of the upper alveolar ridge. The patient's medical history was significant for long-term tobacco addiction of more than 25 years. The tumor measured approximately 4 × 5 cm in size (cT3) and revealed an irregular diffuse growth with irregular and indurated margins. After incisional biopsy from the area suspected to be tumor, the histopathological examination revealed well-differentiated squamous cell carcinoma. Pre-operative computed tomography scan indicated no tumor suspect cervical lymph nodes or distant metastases. In March, the patient had undergone the curatively intended tumor surgery removing the cancer tissue with safety distance and cervical lymph drainage ducts (Neck dissection) on both sides. According to the TNM system proposed by American Joint commitee on Cancer (AJCC) the tumor was found to be stage II (pT2 pN0 cM0 pL0 pV0 p R0 G1). Since June 2015, the patient noticed a rapidly progressive swelling on the left neck. Computed tomography scan indicated a large contrast enhancing mass, which superposed the external carotid suspected to be tumor recurrence. In July, operative findings revealed tumor tissue of Level 1–3 infiltrating the vascular wall of the external carotid, so that a resection in healthy tissue could not be performed. The tumor recurrence was classified as a large lymph node metastasis of the aforesaid well to moderately differentiated squamous cell carcinoma at the AJCC

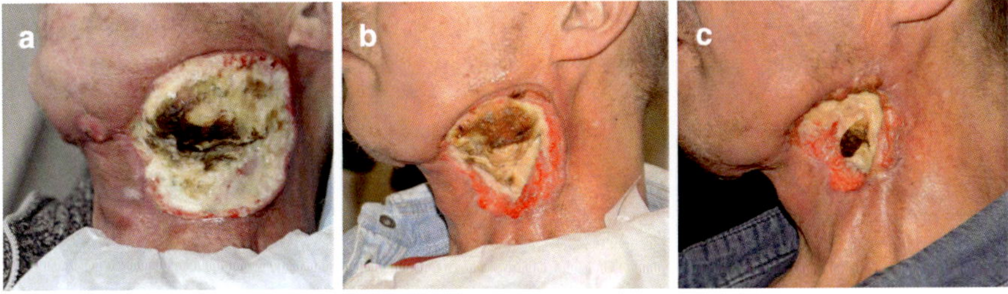

**Fig. 10.1** Clinical tumor development of a 51-year-old Caucasian male patient suffering from bacterially contaminated cancer wound on the left neck during CAP treatment in terms of supportive palliative cancer care. (**a**) April 2016, (**b**) June 2016, (**c**) August 2016

stage IVb (pT2 pN2c cM0 pL1 pV1 pR2 G2). Between July and August 2015 the patient had undergone a palliative radiotherapy with a daily dosage of 2 Gy up to a total radiation dosage of 66.0 Gy. Simultaneously, 2 cycles of a cisplatin chemotherapy have been administered. In October 2015 after this therapy, the tumor was characterised by extensive and progressive growth with exulceration. Due to the vulnerability of the extended bacterially contaminated wound and the underlying carotid artery, wound care of the exulcerated lymph node was difficult. Since October 2015, a supportive palliavtive cancer treatment using cold atmospheric plasma (CAP) has been started with the patients' written consent.

The exulcerative tumor growth region, located on the left neck, received treatment with the kINPen® MED (neoplas tools GmbH, Greifswald, Germany) for nearly 5–6 min with a distance of approximately 10 mm in a meandering manner, monitoring plasma related effects, side effects and responses to CAP. Plasma treatment was continued to be performed every 2–3 days. Wound care was implemented in conjunction with an antiseptic wound dressing.

### 10.3.2 Case History 2 (Fig. 10.2)

In March 2015, the 55-year-old male patient presented himself in the department of oral and maxillofacial surgery, with an alio loco histologically proven moderately-differentiated squamous cell carcinoma of the anterior floor of the mouth.

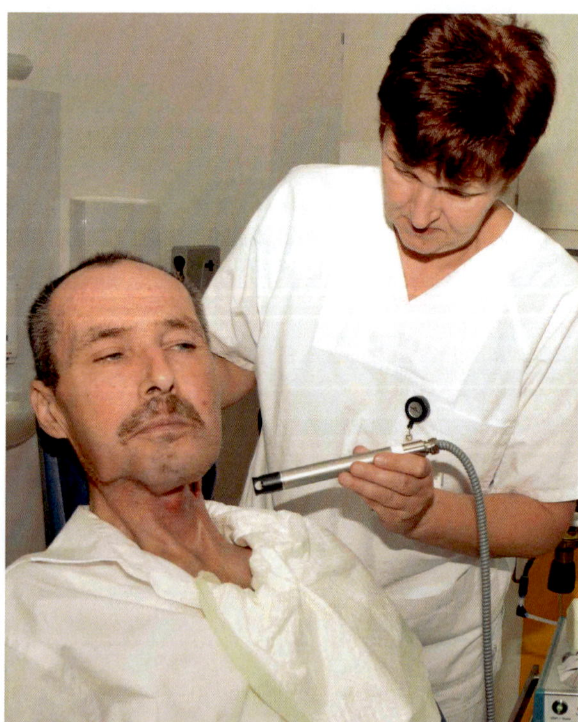

**Fig. 10.2** Plasma application by the kINPen® MED (neoplas tools GmbH, Greifswald, Germany) during the cancer wound treatment of the patient of Fig. 10.1 by a nurse

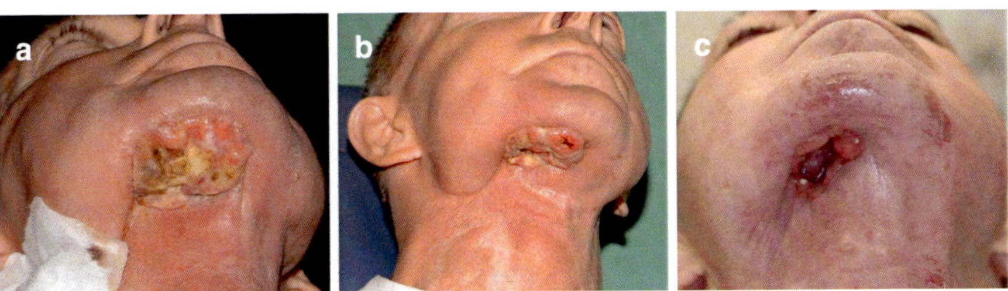


**Fig. 10.3** Clinical tumor development of a 55-year-old Caucasian male patient suffering from bacterially contaminated submental cancer wound during CAP treatment in terms of supportive palliative cancer care. (**a**) August 2016, (**b**) October 2016, (**c**) February 2017

The patient's medical history was significant for long term tobacco addiction of more than 20 years. Pre-operative computed tomography scan indicated no tumor suspect cervical lymph nodes or distant metastases. In March, the patient had undergone the curatively intended tumor surgery removing the cancer tissue with safety distance and cervical lymph drainage ducts (Neck dissection) on both sides. According to the TNM system proposed by American Joint commitee on Cancer (AJCC) the tumor was found to be stage II (pT2 pN0 cM0 pL0 pV0 pR0 G2). In October 2015, a local recurrence of the pretreated squamous cell carcinoma was noticed on the anterior floor of the mouth. Computed tomography scan indicated contrast enhancing on the floor of the mouth and submental, which was suspected to be a large tumor recurrence. In addition, between December 2015 and February 2016 the patient had undergone an adjuvant curative radiotherapy with a daily dosage of 2 Gy up to a total radiation dosage of 70.0 Gy. Simultaneously, 3 cycles of a cisplatin chemotherapy have been administered. After this combined radio-chemotherapy, the tumor was characterised by progressive growth with exulceration, pronounced inflammatory reactions and cancer wound vulnerability. Since March 2016, a supportive palliative cancer treatment using cold atmospheric plasma (CAP) has been started with the patients' written consent. The exulcerative tumor growth region, located submental, received treatment with the kINPen® MED (neoplas tools GmbH, Greifswald, Germany) for near 4–5 min every 2–3 days. Wound care was implemented in conjunction with an antiseptic wound dressing (Fig. 10.3).

## 10.4 Clinical Findings (Table 10.1)

Antimicrobial, anti-inflammatory, tissue stimulation, stimulation of microcirculation, and other therapeutic effects are achieved during CAP treatment and are most commonly described in literature [1–10]. Many dermatological trials have demonstrated that CAP is a useful tool for decontaminating severely infected wounds and ulcerations [69, 70].

By treating bacterially contaminated chronic cancer wounds of advanced head and neck cancers, local CAP application has been proven to reduce microbial colonization, especially pathogenic anaerobic germs, and inflammatory response gently and sufficiently in a non-contact manner. CAP treated superinfected necrotic tumor

**Table 10.1** Clinical and histological effects achieved with CAP during palliative cancer care

| Clinical effects | Histological effects |
|---|---|
| Reduction of bacterial colonization | Selective apoptosis of cancer cells |
| Reduction of inflammatory response and wound vulnerability | Desmoplastic reaction of conjunctive tissue |
| Reduction of pain and demand for pain medication | Reduction and change of inflammatory cells |
| Reduction of wound odour | Modulation of immune response |
| Increase of quality of life | |
| Reduction of cancer wound size, partial tumor remission | |

areas appear to be clean of cell detritus and bacteria and lead to a decrease of bacterial decomposition products. The wound bed is covered with a physiological fibrin coating. Due to the decrease of local and perifocal inflammation, vulnerability, wound algesia, and demand of pain medication can be reduced significantly. By reducing bacterial colonization, inflammatory response and the related symptoms, e.g. pain, bleeding, and wound odor, the emotional and physical burden of cancer can be reduced and quality of life improved.

In some cases, the ulcerated tumor areas could be reduced noticeably during CAP therapy. In the case series published by the study group of Metelmann and Seebauer, a reduction of tumor size could be achieved up to 80% [68]. This fact and the reduction of wound odor inspire hope and improve living conditions in the end stage of the patient's cancer disease. However, the described effect of tumor size reduction was only of an uncertain period. Therefore, it is still unclear how to establish a standstill regarding the persistence of the tumor and the cancer disease.

## 10.5 Histological Findings (Table 10.1)

TUNEL analyses of the tissue samples collected during CAP treatment demonstrated an increased amount of apoptotic tumor cells in-vivo whereas healthy cells remained nearly unaffected. This is well known and most commonly described in literature based upon in-vitro investigations. Furthermore, a desmoplastic reaction of the conjunctive tissue represented by an increased production rate of collagen and extracellular matrix in terms of scarring is depicted histologically within CAP treated cancer areas.

One further promising effect is that CAP treatment locally modulates immune response in-vivo to attack the tumor. Vandana Miller as a pioneer regarding plasma related immune response provided a comprehensive introduction about the promising cancer immunotherapy based on the CAP treatment in a recent review [71]. By optimizing the parameters of CAP to induce immunogenic cell death in tumors locally, it is possible to trigger specific, protective immune responses systematically. Metelmann and co-workers could verify an inactivation and reduction of myeloid cells such as tissue-resident macrophages, the increased presence is known to be correlated with poor prognosis in the progression of the cancer disease [68].

## 10.6 Side Effects

The gentle and non-contact CAP treatment does not guarantee a complete absence of side effects. But, all the side effects present and described were just slightly to moderate and did not influence patient's treatment willingness.

Due to the time consuming CAP treatment of large tumor areas, exhaustion is reported by some patients. But for an effective treatment a wound size dependent plasma application of 1 min/cm$^2$ of cancer wound is necessary. Longer and more frequent CAP applications may lead to a local inflammatory response accompanied by hypervascularization, redness, edema, bleeding and pain. Unpleasant sensations and pain may occur if the plasma jet is pausing for some time on the same place. In rare cases a stimulation of salivation was reported. A longer CAP application may lead to unpleasant ozone odor.

## 10.7 Impact and Outlook

The evidence to date suggests that CAP has a significant apoptotic effect on cancer cells as demonstrated in several tumor lines, tumor models in in-vitro and in-vivo studies. But, the local and superficial induction of apoptosis is of minor importance for treating palliatively intended cancer patients in the end stage of their cancer disease. Rather, the treatment of local complaints in consequence of the bacterial colonization and its accompanying symptoms, e.g. wound odour, inflammation and pain are of major priority for these patients. First clinical studies have shown the CAP's effectiveness and impact in palliative cancer wound care [66–68]. By reducing inflammation, wound vulnerability, pain and wound odor patients satisfaction and quality of life are improved.

The CAP-induced tumor mass reduction described in some cases is an unexpected, promising, but not yet entirely understood manifestation. The nutrient competition between cancer cells and the increased production rate of collagen and extracellular matrix in the term of desmoplastic reaction could be a reason as well as the changed immunologic response after CAP application. Furthermore, the reduction of inflammation in consequence of the reduction of bacterial colonization may also be understood as a loss of stimulant for tumor progression.

In contrast to common cancer treatment modalities such as chemotherapy and radiotherapy, the primary advantage of CAP is its selective anti-cancer capacity [1–65]. CAP tends to address the growth of cancer cells rather than the growth of healthy cells by triggering more apoptosis in cancer cells than normal cells. Due to stronger metabolism in cancer cells, the basal RONS level in cancer cells is thought to be higher and rather than that in normal cells.

In addition to addressing the growth of cancer cells, CAP is also able to restore the sensitivity of chemo-resistant cancer cells to specific drugs [24, 72].

The first in-vivo studies concerning CAP treatment of bacterially contaminated cancer wounds in palliative cancer care are promising and at the moment the only reports of clinical plasma medicine in human cancer care. Understanding of the impact of CAP and its verification of clinical evidence in controlled human clinical trials are still pending.

## References


1. Fridman G, Shereshevsky A, Jost MM, Brooks AD, Fridman A, Gutsol A, Vasilets V, Friedman G. Floating electrode dielectric barrier discharge plasma in air promoting apoptotic behavior in melanoma skin cancer cell lines. Plasma Chem Plasma Process. 2007;27(2):163–76.
2. vonWoedtke T, Metelmann HR, Weltmann KD. Clinical plasma medicine: state and perspectives of in vivo application of cold atmospheric plasma. Contrib Plasma Phys. 2014;54(2):104–17.
3. von Woedtke T, Reuter S, Masur K, Weltmanna KD. Plasmas for medicine. Phys Rep. 2013; 530:291–320.
4. Kim SJ, Chung TH. Cold atmospheric plasma jet-generated RONS and their selective effects on normal and carcinoma cells. Sci Rep. 2016;3(6):20332.
5. Yan D, Sherman JH, Keidar M. Cold atmospheric plasma, a novel promising anti-cancer treatment modality. Oncotarget. 2017;8(9):15977–95.
6. Gay-Mimbrera J, García MC, Isla-Tejera B, Rodero-Serrano A, García-Nieto AV, Ruano J. Clinical and biological principles of cold atmospheric plasma application in skin cancer. Adv Ther. 2016;33(6):894–909.
7. Volotskova O, Hawley TS, Stepp MA, Keidar M. Targeting the cancer cell cycle by cold atmospheric plasma. Sci Rep. 2012;2:636.
8. Keidar M, Walk R, Shashurin A, Srinivasan P, Sandler A, Dasgupta S, Ravi R, Guerrero-Preston R, Trink B. Cold plasma selectivity and the possibility of a paradigm shift in cancer therapy. Br J Cancer. 2011;105(9):1295–301.
9. Hirst AM, Frame FM, Arya M, Maitland NJ, O'Connell D. Low temperature plasmas as emerging cancer therapeutics: the state of play and thoughts for the future. Tumour Biol. 2016;37(6):7021–31.
10. Bauer G. The antitumor effect of singlet oxygen. Anitcancer Res. 2016;36:5649–64.
11. Lee HJ, Shon CH, Kim YS, Kim S, Kim GC, Kong MG. Degradation of adhesion molecules of G361 melanoma cells by a non-thermal atmospheric pressure microplasma. New J Phys. 2009;11(11):115026.
12. Kim GC, Kim GJ, Park SR, Jeon SM, Seo HJ, Iza F, Lee JK. Air plasma coupled with antibody-conjugated nanoparticles: a new weapon against cancer. J Phys D Appl Phys. 2009;42(3):032005.
13. Daeschlein G, Scholz S, Lutze S, Arnold A, et al. Comparison between cold plasma, electro chemotherapy and combined therapy in a melanoma mouse model. Exp Dermatol. 2013;22:582–6.
14. Yajima I, Iida M, Kumasaka MY, Omata Y, Ohgami N, Chang J, Ichihara S, Hori M, Kato M. Non-equilibrium atmospheric pressure plasmas modulate cell cycle-related gene expressions in melanocytic tumors of RET-transgenic mice. Exp Dermatol. 2014;23(6):424–5.
15. Iida M, Yajima I, Ohgami N, Tamura H, Takeda K, Ichihara S, Hori M, Kato M. The effects of non-thermal atmospheric pressure plasma irradiation on expression levels of matrix metalloproteinases in benign melanocytic tumors in RETtransgenic mice. Eur J Dermatol. 2014;24(3):392–4.
16. Sensenig R, Kalghatgi S, Cerchar E, Fridman G, Shereshevsky A, Torabi B, et al. Non-thermal plasma induces apoptosis in melanoma cells via production of intracellular reactive oxygen species. Ann Biomed Eng. 2011;39(2):674–87.
17. Zirnheld JL, Zucker SN, DiSanto TM, Berezney R, Etemadi K. Nonthermal plasma needle: development and targeting of melanoma cells. IEEE Trans Plasma Sci. 2010;38(4):948–52.
18. Vandamme M, Robert E, Lerondel S, Sarron V, Ries D, Dozias S, Sobilo J, Gosset D, Kieda C, Legrain B, Pouvesle JM, Pape AL. ROS implication in a new antitumor strategy based on non-thermal plasma. Int J Cancer. 2012;130(9):2185–94.
19. Tanaka H, Mizuno M, Ishikawa K, Nakamura K, Kajiyama H, Kano H, Kikkawa F, Hori M. Plasma-activated medium selectively kills glioblastoma brain tumor cells by down-regulating a survival signaling molecule, AKT kinase. Plasma Med. 2011;1(3–4).

20. Kaushik NK, Attri P, Kaushik N, Choi EH. A preliminary study of the effect of DBD plasma and osmolytes on T98G brain cancer and HEK non-malignant cells. Molecules. 2013;18(5):4917–28.
21. Tanaka H, Mizuno M, Ishikawa K, Nakamura K, Kajiyama H, Kano H, Kikkawa F, Hori M. Plasma-activated medium selectively kills Glioblastoma brain tumor cells by downregulating a survival Signaling molecule, AKT kinase. Plasma Med. 2011;1(3–4):265–77.
22. Tanaka H, Mizuno M, Ishikawa K, Nakamura K, Utsumi F, Kajiyama H, Kano H, Maruyama S, Kikkawa F, Hori M. Cell survival and proliferation signaling pathways are downregulated by plasma-activated medium in glioblastoma brain tumor cells. Plasma Med. 2012;2(4):207–20.
23. Vandamme M, Robert E, Pesnel S, Barbosa E, Dozias S, Sobilo J, Lerondel S, Le Pape A, Pouvesle JM. Antitumor effect of plasma treatment on U87 glioma xenografts: preliminary results. Plasma Process Polym. 2010;7(3–4):264–73.
24. Koritzer J, Boxhammer V, Schafer A, Shimizu T, Klampfl TG, Li YF, Welz C, Schwenk-Zieger S, Morfill GE, Zimmermann JL, Schlegel J. Restoration of sensitivity in chemo—resistant glioma cells by cold atmospheric plasma. PLoS One. 2013;8(5):e64498. https://doi.org/10.1371/journal.pone.0064498.
25. Kaushik NK, Uhm H, Choi EH. Micronucleus formation induced by dielectric barrier discharge plasma exposure in brain cancer cells. Appl Phys Lett. 2012;100(8):084102. https://doi.org/10.1063/1.3687172.
26. Kaushik NK, Kim YH, Han YG, Choi EH. Effect of jet plasma on T98G human brain cancer cells (vol 13, pg 176, 2012). Curr Appl Phys. 2013;13(3):614–8. https://doi.org/10.1016/j.cap.2012.10.009.
27. Kim SJ, Chung TH, Bae SH, Leem SH. Induction of apoptosis in human breast cancer cells by a pulsed atmospheric pressure plasma jet. Appl Phys Lett. 2010;97(2):023702.
28. Ninomiya K, Ishijima T, Imamura M, Yamahara T, Enomoto H, Takahashi K, Tanaka Y, Uesugi Y, Shimizu N. Evaluation of extra- and intracellular OH radical generation, cancer cell injury, and apoptosis induced by a non thermal atmospheric-pressure plasma jet. J Phys D Appl Phys. 2013;46(42):425401.
29. Wang M, Holmes B, Cheng X, Zhu W, Keidar M, Zhang LG. Cold atmospheric plasma for selectively ablating metastatic breast cancer cells. PLoS One. 2013;8(9):e73741.
30. Ahn HJ, Kim KI, Hoan NN, Kim CH, Moon E, Choi KS, Yang SS, Lee JS. Targeting cancer cells with reactive oxygen and nitrogen species generated by atmosphericpressure air plasma. PLoS One. 2014;9(1):e86173.
31. Kim K, Jun Ahn H, Lee J-H, Kim J-H, Sik Yang S, Lee J-S. Cellular membrane collapse by atmospheric-pressure plasma jet. Appl Phys Lett. 2014;104(1):013701.
32. Tan X, Zhao S, Lei Q, Lu X, He G, Ostrikov K. Single-cell-precision microplasma-induced cancer cell apoptosis. PLoS One. 2014;9(6):e101299.
33. Leduc M, Guay D, Leask RL, Coulombe S. Cell permeabilization using a non-thermal plasma. New J Phys. 2009;11:115021. https://doi.org/10.1088/1367-2630/11/11/115021.
34. Ahn HJ, Kim KI, Kim G, Moon E, Yang SS, Lee JS. Atmospheric-pressure plasma jet induces apoptosis involving mitochondria via generation of free radicals. PLoS One. 2011;6(11):e28154. https://doi.org/10.1371/journal.pone.0028154.
35. Sato T, Yokoyama M, Johkura K. A key inactivation factor of HeLa cell viability by a plasma flow. J Phys D Appl Phys. 2011;44(37):372001. https://doi.org/10.1088/0022-3727/44/37/372001.
36. Huang J, Chen W, Li H, Wang PY, Yang SZ. Inactivation of He la cancer cells by an atmospheric pressure cold plasma jet. Acta Phys Sin-Ch Ed. 2013;62(6):065201. https://doi.org/10.7498/Aps.62.065201.
37. Ja Kim S, Min Joh H, Chung TH. Production of intracellular reactive oxygen species and change of cellviability induced by atmospheric pressure plasma in normal and cancer cells. Appl Phys Lett. 2013;103(15):153705.
38. Kim JY, Ballato J, Foy P, Hawkins T, Wei Y, Li J, Kim SO. Apoptosis of lung carcinoma cells induced by a flexible optical fiber-based cold microplasma. Biosens Bioelectron. 2011;28(1):333–8.

39. Huang J, Chen W, Li H, Wang XQ, Lv GH, Khosa ML, Guo M, Feng KC, Wang PY, Yang SZ. Deactivation of A549 cancer cells in vitro by a dielectric barrier discharge plasma needle. J Appl Phys. 2011;109(5):053305. https://doi.org/10.1063/1.3553873.
40. Kim K, Choi JD, Hong YC, Kim G, Noh EJ, Lee JS, Yang SS. Atmospheric-pressure plasma-jet from micronozzle array and its biological effects on living cells for cancer therapy. Appl Phys Lett. 2011;98(7):073701. https://doi.org/10.1063/1.3555434.
41. Adachi T, Tanaka H, Nonomura S, Hara H, Kondo SI, Hori M. Plasma-activated medium induces A549 cell injury via a spiral apoptotic cascade involving the mitochondrial- nuclear network. Free Radic Biol Med. 2014;79C:28–44. https://doi.org/10.1016/j.freeradbiomed.2014.11.014.
42. Panngom K, Baik KY, Nam MK, Han JH, Rhim H, Choi EH. Preferential killing of human lung cancer cell lines with mitochondrial dysfunction by nonthermal dielectric barrier discharge plasma. Cell Death Dis. 2013;4:e642. https://doi.org/10.1038/cddis.2013.168.
43. Torii K, Yamada S, Nakamura K, Tanaka H, Kajiyama H, Tanahashi K, Iwata N, Kanda M, Kobayashi D, Tanaka C, Fujii T, Nakayama G, Koike M, Sugimoto H, Nomoto S, Natsume A, Fujiwara M, Mizuno M, Hori M, Saya H, Kodera Y. Effectiveness of plasma treatment on gastric cancer cells. Gastric Cancer. 2014;18(3):635–43. https://doi.org/10.1007/s10120-014-0395-6.
44. Brullé L, Vandamme M, Ries D, Martel E, Robert E, Lerondel S, Trichet V, Richard S, Pouvesle JM, Le Pape A. Effects of a non thermal plasma treatment alone or in combination with gemcitabine in a MIA PaCa2-luc orthotopic pancreatic carcinoma model. PLoS One. 2012;7(12):e52653. https://doi.org/10.1371/journal.pone.0052653.
45. Partecke LI, Evert K, Haugk J, Doering F, Normann L, Diedrich S, Weiss FU, Evert M, Huebner NO, Guenther C, Heidecke CD, Kramer A, Bussiahn R, Weltmann KD, Pati O, Bender C, von Bernstorff W. Tissue tolerable plasma (TTP) induces apoptosis in pancreatic cancer cells in vitro and in vivo. BMC Cancer. 2012;12:473. https://doi.org/10.1186/1471-2407-12-473.
46. Georgescu N, Lupu AR. Tumoral and normal cells treatment with high-voltage pulsed cold atmospheric plasma jets. IEEE T Plasma Sci. 2010;38(8):1949–55.
47. Ishaq M, Evans MDM, Ostrikov K. Atmospheric pressure gas plasma-induced colorectal cancer cell death is mediated by Nox2–ASK1 apoptosis pathways and oxidative stress is mitigated by Srx–Nrf2 anti-oxidant system. Biochim Biophys Acta. 2014;1843(12):2827–37.
48. Plewa J-M, Yousfi M, Frongia C, Eichwald O, Ducommun B, Merbahi N, Lobjois V. Low-temperature plasmainduced antiproliferative effects on multi-cellular tumor spheroids. New J Phys. 2014;16(4):043027.
49. Lupu AR, Georgescu N, Calugaru A, Cremer L, Szegli G, Kerek F. The effects of cold atmospheric plasma jets on B16 and COLO320 tumoral cells. Roum Arch Microbiol Immunol. 2009;68(3):136–44.
50. Kim CH, Kwon S, Bahn JH, Lee K, Jun SI, Rack PD, Baek SJ. Effects of atmospheric nonthermal plasma on invasion of colorectal cancer cells. Appl Phys Lett. 2010;96(24):243701. https://doi.org/10.1063/1.3449575.
51. Hirst AM, Frame FM, Maitland NJ, O'Connell D. Low temperature plasma: a novel focal therapy for localized prostate cancer? Biomed Res Int. 2014;2014:878319. https://doi.org/10.1155/2014/878319.
52. Barekzi N, Laroussi M. Dose-dependent killing of leukemia cells by low-temperature plasma. J Phys D Appl Phys. 2012;45(42):422002.
53. Thiyagarajan M, Waldbeser L, Whitmill A. THP-1 leukemia cancer treatment using a portable plasma device. Stud Health Technol Inform. 2011;173:515–7.
54. Thiyagarajan M, Anderson H, Gonzales XF. Induction of apoptosis in human myeloid leukemia cells by remote exposure of resistive barrier cold plasma. Biotechnol Bioeng. 2014;111(3):565–74.
55. Thiyagarajan M, Sarani A, Gonzales X. Characterization of portable resistive barrier plasma jet and its direct and indirect treatment for antibiotic resistant bacteria and THP-1 leukemia cancer cells. IEEE T Plasma Sci. 2012;40(12):3533–45.
56. Zhang X, Li M, Zhou R, Feng K, Yang S. Ablation of liver cancer cells in vitro by a plasma needle. Appl Phys Lett. 2008;93(2):021502.

57. Zhao S, Xiong Z, Mao X, Meng D, Lei Q, Li Y, Deng P, Chen M, Tu M, Lu X, Yang G, He G. Atmospheric pressure room temperature plasma jets facilitate oxidative and nitrative stress and lead to endoplasmic reticulum stress dependent apoptosis in HepG2 cells. PLoS One. 2013;8(8):e73665.
58. Gweon B, Kim M, Kim DB, Kim D, Kim H, Jung H, Shin JH, Choe W. Differential responses of human liver cancer and normal cells to atmospheric pressure plasma. Appl Phys Lett. 2011;99(6):063701. https://doi.org/10.1063/1.3622631.
59. Kaushik NK, Kaushik N, Park D, Choi EH. Altered antioxidant system stimulates dielectric barrier discharge plasma- induced cell death for solid tumor cell treatment. PLoS One. 2014;9(7):e103349. https://doi.org/10.1371/journal.pone.0103349.
60. Chang JW, Kang SU, Shin YS, Kim KI, Seo SJ, Yang SS, Lee JS, Moon E, Lee K, Kim CH. Non-thermal atmospheric pressure plasma inhibits thyroid papillary cancer cell invasion via cytoskeletal modulation, altered MMP-2/-9/ uPA activity. PLoS One. 2014;9(3):e92198. https://doi.org/10.1371/journal.pone.0092198.
61. Guerrero-Preston R, Ogawa T, Uemura M, Shumulinsky G, Valle BL, Pirini F, Ravi R, Sidransky D, Keidar M, Trink B. Cold atmospheric plasma treatment selectively targets head and neck squamous cell carcinoma cells. Int J Mol Med. 2014;34(4):941–6.
62. Kang SU, Cho JH, Chang JW, Shin YS, Kim KI, Park JK, Yang SS, Lee JS, Moon E, Lee K, Kim CH. Nonthermal plasma induces head and neck cancer cell death: the potential involvement of mitogen-activated protein kinasedependent mitochondrial reactive oxygen species. Cell Death Dis. 2014;5:e1056.
63. Hasse S, Tran TD, Hahn O, Weltmann KD, Metelmann HR, Masur K. Plasma application in human skin—molecular analyses in situ. Exp Dermatol. 2014;23:e51.
64. Han X, Klas M, Liu YY, Stack MS, Ptasinska S. DNA damage in oral cancer cells induced by nitrogen atmospheric pressure plasma jets. Appl Phys Lett. 2013;102(23):233703. https://doi.org/10.1063/1.4809830.
65. Chang JW, Kang SU, Shin YS, Kim KI, Seo SJ, Yang SS, Lee JS, Moon E, Baek SJ, Lee K, Kim CH. Non-thermal atmospheric pressure plasma induces apoptosis in oral cavity squamous cell carcinoma: Involvement of DNA-damage- triggering sub-G(1) arrest via the ATM/p53 pathway. Arch Biochem Biophys. 2014a;545:133–40.
66. Metelmann H-R, Nedrelow DS, Seebauer C, Schuster M, von Woedtke T, Weltmann K-D, Kindler S, Metelmann PH, Finkelstein SE, Von Hoff DD, Podmelle F. Head and neck cancer treatment and physical plasma. Clin Plasma Med. 2015;3(1):17–23.
67. Schuster M, Seebauer C, Rutkowski R, Hauschild A, Podmelle F, Metelmann C, Metelmann B, von Woedtke T, Hasse S, Weltmann KD, Metelmann HR. Visible tumor surface response to physical plasma and apoptotic cell kill in head and neck cancer. J Craniomaxillofac Surg. 2016;44(9):1445–52.
68. Metelmann HR, Seebauer C, Miller V, Friedman A, Bauer G, Graves DB, Pouvesle JM, Rutkowski R, Schuster M, Bekeschus S, Wende K, Masur K, Hasse S, Gerling T, Hori M, Tanaka H, Choi EH, Weltmann KD, Metelmann PH, Von Hoff DD, von Woedtke T. Clinical experience with cold plasma in the treatment of locally advanced head and neck cancer. Clin Plasma Med. 2017. https://doi.org/10.1016/j.cpme.2017.09.001.
69. Isbary G, Morfill G, Schmidt HU, Georgi M, Ramrath K, Heinlin J, et al. A first prospective randomized controlled trial to decrease bacterial load using cold atmospheric argon plasma on chronic wounds in patients. Br J Dermatol. 2010;163:78–82.
70. Isbary G, Zimmermann JL, Shimizu T, Li YF, Morfill GE, Thomas HM, et al. Non-thermal plasma – more than five years of clinical experience. J Clin Plasma Med. 2013;1:19–23.
71. Miller V, Lin A, Fridman A. Why target immune cells for plasma treatment of cancer. Plasma Chem Plasma Process. 2016;36(1):259–68.
72. Ishaq M, Han ZJ, Kumar S, Evans MD, Ostrikov KK. Atmospheric pressure plasma-and TRAIL-induced apoptosis in TRAIL-resistant colorectal cancer cells. Plasma Process Polym. 2015;12(6):574–82.

# 11 Treatment of Split Skin Draft Donor and Recipient Sites

Saskia Preissner, Jan-Dirk Raguse, and Stefan Hartwig

## 11.1 Background

Split-thickness skin graft (STSG) is a reliable workhorse in soft tissue reconstruction within reconstructive surgery [1, 2]. Wound healing disorders of the STSG donor sites (e.g. the thigh) are seldom and research in this matter deals with accelerated healing and reduced pain and itching [3, 4]. In contrast, wound healing disorders of the STSG recipient sites are more frequent due to challenging wound conditions (e.g. chronic wounds, infected or complex wounds) or sytemic impairment (elderly patients, diabetes) [5–8], see Fig. 11.1.

S. Preissner (✉)
Department of Operative and Preventive Dentistry, Charité—Universitätsmedizin Berlin, Berlin, Germany

Freie Universität Berlin, Humboldt-Universität zu, Berlin, Germany

Berlin Institute of Health, Berlin, Germany
e-mail: saskia.preissner@charite.de

J.-D. Raguse
Freie Universität Berlin, Humboldt-Universität zu, Berlin, Germany

Berlin Institute of Health, Berlin, Germany

Department of Oral and Maxillofacial Surgery, Charité—Universitätsmedizin Berlin, Berlin, Germany

S. Hartwig
Department for Oral and Maxillofacial and Facial Plastic Surgery, Johannes Wesling Hospital Minden, University Hospital of the Ruhr University Bochum (RUB), Minden, Germany



H.-R. Metelmann et al. (eds.), *Comprehensive Clinical Plasma Medicine*,
https://doi.org/10.1007/978-3-319-67627-2_11

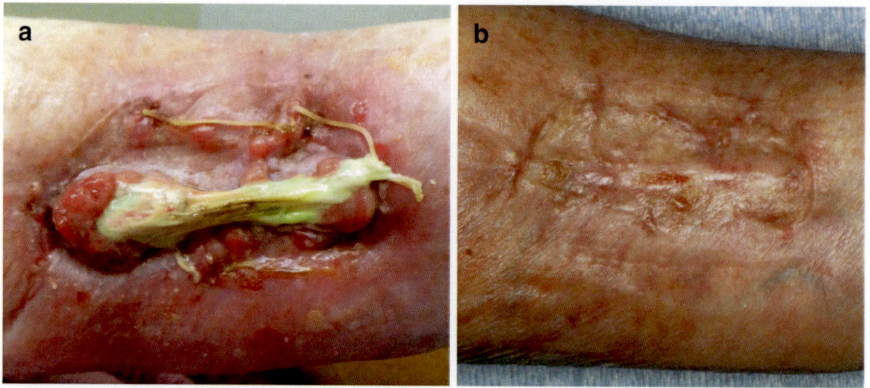


**Fig. 11.1** (**a**, **b**) Impaired wound healing at the radial forearm free flap donor site of a patient with partial split-thickness skin graft necrosis and exposed tendon and infection with methicillin resistant *Staphylococcus aureus* **a**, before and **b**, after 4.9 weeks of plasma treatment (Photographs from [9])

## 11.2 Current Treatment

### 11.2.1 Donor Site

As conventional dressing methods are established since decades, a 14-centre, six armed randomized clinical trial compared six wound dressing materials (alginate/semipermeable film/gauze dressing/hydrocolloid/hydrofibre/silicone) showed the speediest healing with hydrocolloid dressing in median 16 days while the highest rate of infections occured in the gauze dressing group [10]. Another prospective randomized controlled trial showed no difference between calcium alginate and polyurethane film dressing [11]. A new approach without clinical experience is diathermy [12]. Until to date, there exists one randomized placebo-controlled study of cold atmospheric plasma on skin graft donor sites. In the pilot-study of *Heinlin et al.*, 40 wounds were treated in a split-wound model with CAP and presented an improved reepithelialization and fewer fibrin layers and blood crusts [13].

### 11.2.2 Recipient Site

One of the main recipient sites for STSGs in reconstructive surgery are the donor sites of free flaps, e.g. the fibula and radialis free flaps. As current options for wound healing therapy solely or in combination of free flap donor sites include open wound healing [14], full-thickness skin graft [15, 16] or negative pressure dressing [17], the STSG remain a proven option [16, 18]. Common complications after STSG include wound breakdo wn and skin graft loss, resulting in delayed wound healing and/or infection. For the radialis free flap donor site the tendon exposure of the forearm is an additional possible complication [9, 19, 20].

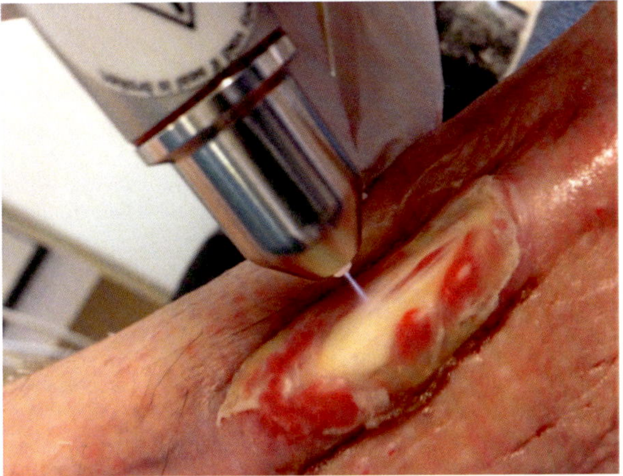

**Fig. 11.2** Cold atmospheric plasma (CAP) treatment of the radial forearm free flap wound with exposed tendon. Note that the spacer has been removed for better presentation of the plasma jet. (Photograph from [9])

CAP as a treatment option was shown singularly for wound healing disorders of the STSGs donor sites of forearm after radialis free flaps, see Fig. 11.2 [9] and fibula free flaps [9] and presented treatment periods between 4 and 38 weeks for succesful wound closure.

Regardless of the limitations of the studys, CAP presented promising results with wound closure of chronic, infected and unsuccessful treated wounds in the head and neck surgery related wounds.

## 11.3 Outlook

CAP and its multifactorial effects on wound healing may serve as a standard of care in the armamentarium of therapy of these particular type of wounds. Further studies should be initiated to evaluate the plasma approach in a larger group of patients and to compare the outcomes with a control group to reveal the supposed positive effect of CAP in regular postoperative wound care and in case of infection and/or wound healing disorder.

## References


1. Davis WJ, Wu C, Sieber D, Vandevender DK. A comparison of full and split thickness skin grafts in radial forearm donor sites. J Hand Microsurg. 2011;3(1):18–24.
2. Ho T, Couch M, Carson K, Schimberg A, Manley K, Byrne PJ. Radial forearm free flap donor site outcomes comparison by closure methods. Otolaryngol Head Neck Surg. 2006;134(2):309–15.
3. Bradow BP, Hallock GG, Wilcock SP. Immediate regrafting of the split thickness skin graft donor site assists healing. Plast Reconstr Surg Glob Open. 2017;5(5):e1339.
4. Prather JL, Tummel EK, Patel AB, Smith DJ, Gould LJ. Prospective randomized controlled trial comparing the effects of noncontact low-frequency ultrasound with standard care in healing split-thickness donor sites. J Am Coll Surg. 2015;221(2):309–18.

5. Knott PD, Seth R, Waters HH, Revenaugh PC, Alam D, Scharpf J, et al. Short-term donor site morbidity: a comparison of the anterolateral thigh and radial forearm fasciocutaneous free flaps. Head Neck. 2016;38(S1):E945–8.
6. Liang J, Yu T, Wang X, Zhao Y, Fang F, Zeng W, et al. Free tissue flaps in head and neck reconstruction: clinical application and analysis of 93 patients of a single institution. Braz J Otorhinolaryngol. 2017.
7. Loeffelbein DJ, Al-Benna S, Steinsträßer L, Satanovskij RM, Rohleder NH, Mücke T, et al. Reduction of donor site morbidity of free radial forearm flaps: what level of evidence is available? Eplasty. 2012;12:e9.
8. Yun TK, Yoon ES, Ahn DS, Park SH, Lee BI, Kim HS, et al. Stabilizing morbidity and predicting the aesthetic results of radial forearm free flap donor sites. Arch Plast Surg. 2015;42(6):769–75.
9. Hartwig S, Doll C, Voss JO, Hertel M, Preissner S, Raguse JD. Treatment of wound healing disorders of radial forearm free flap donor sites using cold atmospheric plasma: a proof of concept. J Oral Maxillofac Surg. 2017;75(2):429–35.
10. Brölmann FE, Eskes AM, Goslings JC, Niessen FB, de Bree R, Vahl AC, et al. Randomized clinical trial of donor-site wound dressings after split-skin grafting. Br J Surg. 2013;100(5):619–27.
11. Läuchli S, Hafner J, Ostheeren S, Mayer D, Barysch MJ, French LE. Management of split-thickness skin graft donor sites: a randomized controlled trial of calcium alginate versus polyurethane film dressing. Dermatology. 2013;227(4):361–6.
12. Holden AM, Beech AN, Farrier JN. Diathermy of split-thickness skin graft donor site: a new technique. Br J Oral Maxillofac Surg. 2017;55(7):734–5. https://doi.org/10.1016/j.bjoms.2017.05.011.
13. Heinlin J, Zimmermann JL, Zeman F, Bunk W, Isbary G, Landthaler M, et al. Randomized placebo-controlled human pilot study of cold atmospheric argon plasma on skin graft donor sites. Wound Repair Regen. 2013;21(6):800–7.
14. Fry AM, Patterson A, Orr RL, Colver GB. Open wound healing of the osseocutaneous fibula flap donor site. Br J Oral Maxillofac Surg. 2014;52(9):861–3.
15. Riecke B, Assaf AT, Heiland M, Al-Dam A, Gröbe A, Blessmann M, et al. Local full-thickness skin graft of the donor arm--a novel technique for the reduction of donor site morbidity in radial forearm free flap. Int J Oral Maxillofac Surg. 2015;44(8):937–41.
16. Zuidam JM, Coert JH, Hofer SOP. Closure of the donor site of the free radial forearm flap: a comparison of full-thickness graft and split-thickness skin graft. Ann Plast Surg. 2005;55(6):612–6.
17. Chio EG, Agrawal A. A randomized, prospective, controlled study of forearm donor site healing when using a vacuum dressing. Otolaryngol Head Neck Surg. 2010;142(2):174–8.
18. Shiba K, Iida Y, Numata T. Ipsilateral full-thickness forearm skin graft for covering the radial forearm flap donor site. Laryngoscope. 2003;113(6):1043–6.
19. Hekner DD, Abbink JH, van Es RJ, Rosenberg A, Koole R, Van Cann EM. Donor-site morbidity of the radial forearm free flap versus the ulnar forearm free flap. Plast Reconstr Surg. 2013;132(2):387–93.
20. Richardson D, Fisher SE, Vaughan ED, Brown JS. Radial forearm flap donor-site complications and morbidity: a prospective study. Plast Reconstr Surg. 1997;99(1):109–15.

# 12 The Use of Cold Atmospheric Pressure Plasma (CAP) in Cardiac Surgery

Lutz Hilker, Thomas von Woedtke, Rüdiger Titze, Klaus-Dieter Weltmann, Wolfgang Motz, and Hans-Georg Wollert

## 12.1 Wound Healing Disturbances in Cardiac Surgery

"During the 80s we saw an outbreak of nosocomial sternal wound infections caused by atypical mycobacteria. Five patients died, and the others all eventually were healed. The source of the infections was never really solved, but we now think that it was tap water. We were using topical ice slush for myocardial protection. … The bacteria may have been in the ice, that was used to produce the slush in glass bottles. If this had happened more recently, we would have used muscle flaps after debridement and the outcomes would have been much better. Their use has greatly reduced the mortality of and recovery time from sternal wound infections. The surgeons who described the use of muscle flaps should get the Nobel Prize and every cardiac surgeon should mention their names in evening prayer…".

These words from Francis Robicsek, one of the pioneers of open heart surgery, bear witness to the persisting importance that measures for successfully avoiding and treating mediastinal or sternal dehiscences have always had in heart surgery [1].

Sternal osteomyelitis continues to be one of the most severe complications after cardiac surgery. It occurs in 0.4–8% of the treated patients. With regard to the

L. Hilker (✉) • W. Motz • H.-G. Wollert
Clinic for Cardiovascular Surgery, Klinikum Karlsburg, Heart and Diabetes Center, Karlsburg, Germany
e-mail: hilker@drguth.de; motz@drguth.de; wollert@drguth.de

T. von Woedtke
Leibniz Institute for Plasma Science and Technology (INP Greifswald) and University Medicine Greifswald, Institute for Hygiene and Environmental Medicine, Greifswald, Germany
e-mail: woedtke@inp-greifswald.de

R. Titze • K.-D. Weltmann
Leibniz Institute for Plasma Science and Technology (INP), Greifswald, Germany
e-mail: titze@inp-greifswald.de; weltmann@inp-greifswald.de



H.-R. Metelmann et al. (eds.), *Comprehensive Clinical Plasma Medicine*,
https://doi.org/10.1007/978-3-319-67627-2_12

mortality rate, various sources describe rates between 14 and 50% [2, 3]. Further surgical treatment methods such as the latissimus dorsi flap, the rectus abdominus flap and the omentum majus flap [4, 5], as well as the application of postoperative thorax support systems and, in particular, the stabilizing vacuum therapy of the open thorax if seen to be infected, have led to an improvement of the results with a noticeably reduced mortality rate in recent years.

Wound-healing disturbances in the areas around the saphenous vein harvesting site following graft harvesting and, in particular, the groin for peripheral vascular interventions or minimally invasive aortic valve or aortic interventions, are generally not as serious, but just as time consuming and onerous for the patients affected. Due to the multimorbid and partly very obese and usually also diabetic pool of patients, it is not rare that a proportion of the previously mentioned patients have a mycotic groin area prior to operation.

Furthermore, critically ill patients on heart surgery intensive care wards regularly contract wounds due to long periods of non-movement. Sacral, gluteal, trochanteric, spinal and heel decubitis and inguinal or inframammary intertriginous mycoses often require long periods of treatment.

Particularly after valve surgery or in cases of incorporated foreign bodies (e.g. endoprostheses, pacemakers or defibrillator devices, heart support systems), there is danger of severe infectious conditions such as endoplastitis and endocarditis due to possible recurring bacteremia in local wounds and which frequently lead to fatal outcomes.

## 12.2 Clinical Experience with the Use of Atmospheric Pressure Plasma (CAP) at Klinikum Karlsburg

Working closely with the INP in Greifswald, our research group in the Clinic for Heart, Thorax and Vascular Surgery at Klinikum Karlsburg has been examining the possibilities of using atmospheric pressure plasma to support the wound-healing in selected therapy trials since 2014. For this, we have been using the kinpen Med from the neoplas tools GmbH Greifswald, which has been authorized for the treatment of chronic wounds according to the *Medizinprodukte-Gesetz* (Act on Medical Devices).

We were able to attain good treatment results for the preoperative treatment of intertriginous mycoses or fissures, for the cleansing and induction of granulation tissue of infected ulcers on diabetic foot with accompanying peripheral arterial occlusive disease, for incipient pressure ulcers caused by sustained pressure and for incipient infections of the exit site of foreign bodies (e.g. Driveline of HeartWare—left ventricular assist devices).

### 12.2.1 Patient 1: Ulcus Cruris with Peripheral Arterial Occlusive Disease

This was a 61-year-old male with generalized arteriosclerosis, who had contracted an ulcus cruris in his left medial malleolus in mid-2015. A surgical debridement with subsequent vacuum therapy was carried out on an increasingly moist necrosis. At the

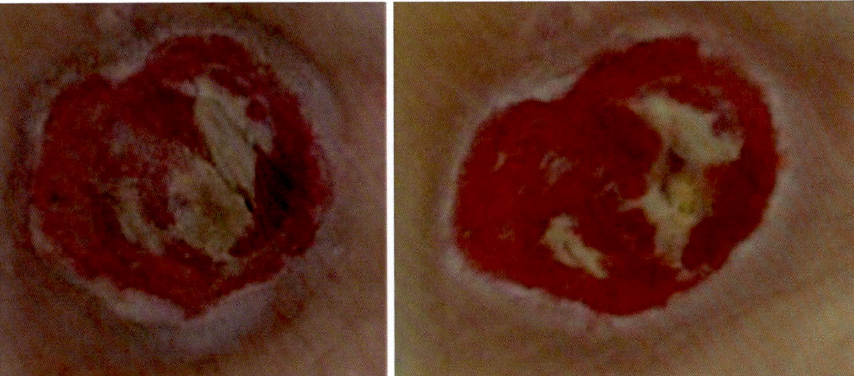

**Figs. 12.1 and 12.2** Ulcer on the left medial malleolus with PAOD, left three weeks after wound debridement and VAC therapy, right after a further 9 days VAC therapy and three CAP applications

same time a PTA of the left arteria femoralis superficialis took place to improve the circulation situation. Two days after this intervention, an acute coronary syndrome emerged, which led to the patient being admitted to our clinic for further cardiac diagnosis. The results presented a severe three vessel coronary disease also affecting the coronary artery. This indicated an operative myocardial revascularization was needed.

When the patient was admitted, the ulcer, after 20 days of VAC therapy, was moderately anergic with a low granulation tendency. We then started straight away with preoperative intermittent CAP application during the three-day interval between the changes of VAC dressing, each time after local disinfection with octenidine. Four treatments displayed an impressive induction of granulation tissue and an improved epithelialization starting at the edges of the wound (Figs. 12.1 and 12.2).

### 12.2.2 Patient 2: Intertriginous Mycoses Prior to Planned Transfemoral Aortic Valve Replacement

Patients who are obese and less mobile due to their age and who also have diabetes mellitus are more likely to have wound-healing disturbances. Particularly the hygienically critical groin areas, which is where access is gained for minimally invasive interventions (e.g. transfemoral aortic valve replacements), are predestined for such complications. Regularly, patients first display serous secretion with a reddening of the wound, this can lead to mechanical macerations or wound dehiscence and finally to a super infection with putrid drainage. Usually this results in lengthy healing periods with a risk of secondary complications. Our example shows the partially macerated groins and the abdominal crease of an 80-year-old, obese, female patient prior to a planned transfemoral aortic valve implantation with symptoms of an aortic stenosis.

Six days prior to the operation one application of CAP at 1 min/cm$^2$ was carried out after disinfection with octenidine. This was followed by a daily change of dry dressing with gauze. The results showed dry skin conditions and increasingly less irritation. The planned transfemoral aortic valve implantation was completed without complications (Figs. 12.3, 12.4, 12.5, 12.6, 12.7 and 12.8).

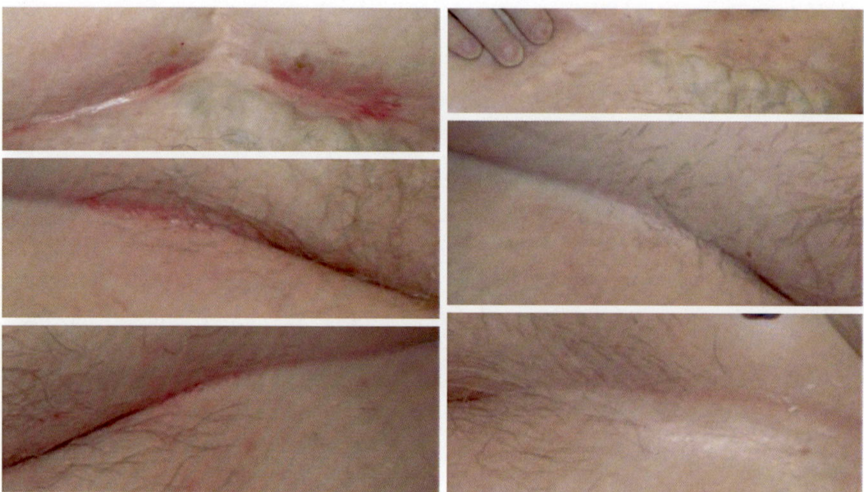

**Figs. 12.3, 12.4, 12.5, 12.6, 12.7 and 12.8** Macerated groin and abdominal crease prior to planned transfemoral aortic valve implantation. Wound development on the left before and right 6 days after CAP application

### 12.2.3 Patient 3: Incipient Infection of the Driveline Exit Site on a Patient with a Left Ventricular Assist Device

Patients with foreign bodies that have contact points on the skin are generally at risk of infection. In the worst-case scenario, it can come to increasing wound infection with subsequent bacteremia and the resulting septitides. The mortality rate in such cases is very high. Even for patients who have the most common heart assist systems at present from the company HeartWare, the energy supply of the pump has to come from an electric cable, which is coated with polyurethane and partially covered by Teflon, the so-called Driveline, which exits the body via the left or right central abdomen. This means that there is a serious infection potential and ascending Driveline infections and their effects regularly curtail the length of life. The author had access to investigations on an ex vivo powered pump system that showed no indication of negative impacts to the controller or pump function, nor to the protective insulation of the Driveline during CAP application. We then used CAP on patients with impending ascending Driveline infections on several occasions (Fig. 12.9).

Our example shows the course of an incipient infection of the Driveline exit site of a 68-year-old male patient, 2 years after implantation of a HeartWare-LVAD who had cardiogenic shock after a heart attack. The wound which started out reddened and secreting pus (pathogen: clostridum difficile), worsened during a suitably resistant course of antibiotics with clindyamycin and ended up in the formation of a distinct hypergranulation. A further smear after one week verified the development of a resistance to the applied antibiotics. The course of antibiotics was then terminated.

After one single application of silver nitrate, CAP was applied on the following 12 consecutive days for one minute respectively. The hypergranulation, secretion

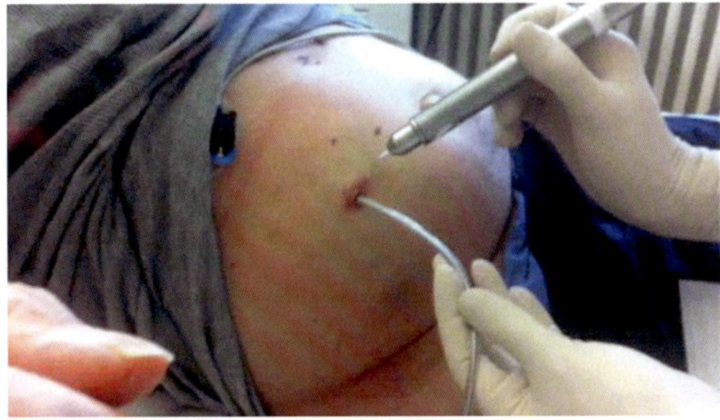

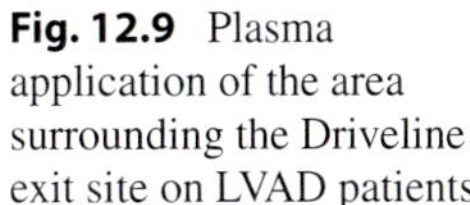

**Fig. 12.9** Plasma application of the area surrounding the Driveline exit site on LVAD patients

and reddening immediately decreased, meaning that the patient could be sent home. Following four other outpatient treatments once a week, the wound had healed completely (Figs. 12.10, 12.11, 12.12, 12.13 and 12.14).

After 6 further months, this patient once again contracted an incipient Driveline infection with hypergranulation, which was again treated successfully in the manner described above (Figs. 12.15, 12.16, 12.17, 12.18 and 12.19).

In order to be able to carry out perspective outpatient CAP treatments of this patient as part of the Karlsburger KARLA Home Visit Program for artificial heart patients at home, the INP Greifswald has just recently developed the kinpen Med mobile pocket. This device is equipped with a 2-L pressure gas cylinder, which can be re-filled thanks to a special adapter, allowing manual transport and causing no problems with fitting it into the boot of the outpatient unit's vehicle (Figs. 12.20 and 12.21).

### 12.2.4 Patient 4: Inframammary Mycoses on Critically Ill Intensive Patients

Serious complications in heart surgery often lead to lengthy periods of stay on intensive care wards. Particularly for patients who are critically ill, have recurring septic wounds or weak immune systems, this increases the risk of skin lesions due to non-movement and long-term care. In this case, a 75-year-old female patient who, after an emergency myocardial revascularization operation, was put on an external weaning station due to protracted pulmonary weaning caused by severe COPD, and then developed a late sternal wound healing disturbance and was consequently relocated back to our clinic to treat the open wound.

A prominent inframammary candidiasis was found on both sides with emerging fissures, which were not healed by the nursing measures which were implemented.

This was followed by the application of CAP to the patient's right-hand side on four consecutive days and after each application the wound was dressed with gauze. After twelve days, the patient's right side shew almost complete healing of the wound. The left-hand side was then treated three times with CAP application in the same manner and after 15 days, we documented the completion of wound-healing (Figs. 12.22, 12.23, 12.24, 12.25, 12.26 and 12.27).

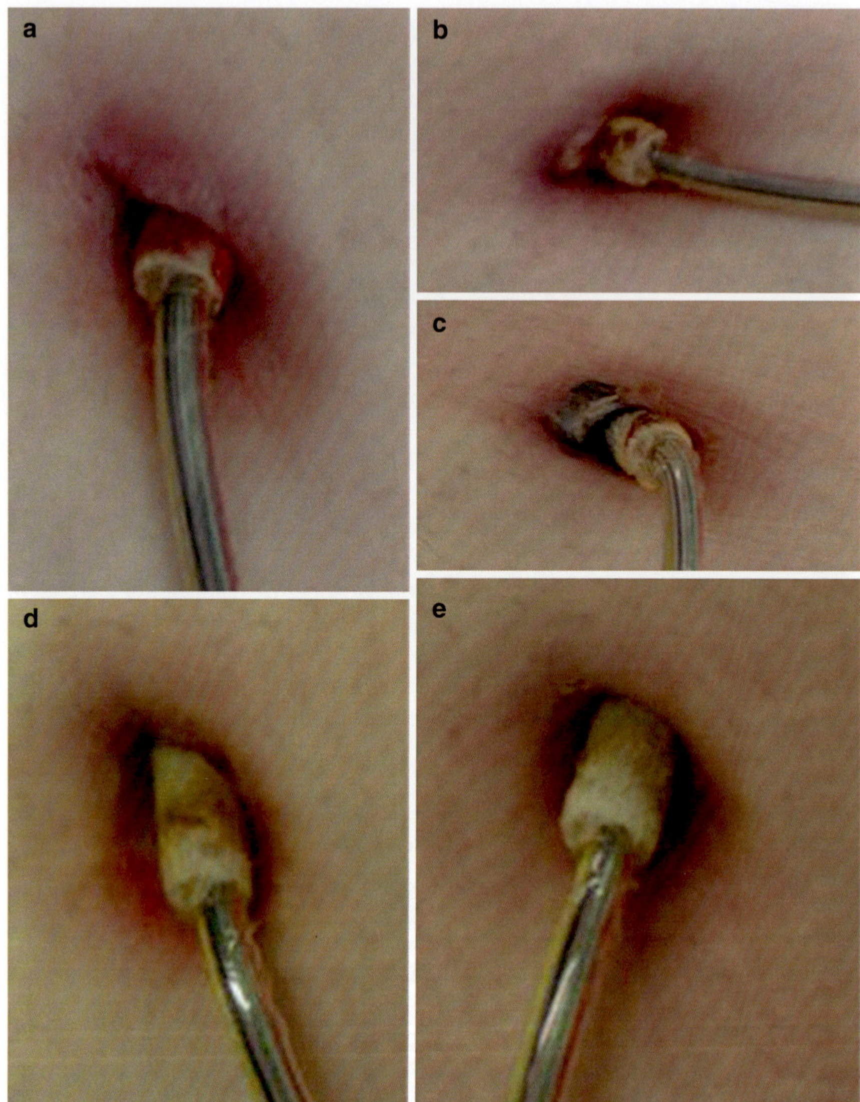


**Figs. 12.10, 12.11, 12.12, 12.13 and 12.14** Course of wound healing with an incipient Driveline infection: (**a**) Day 0: secreting exit site, (**b**) Day 7 hypergranulation at 9–11 o'clock after a week of conventional changes of dressing and course of antibiotics with Clindamycin, (**c**) Day 8 after one single application of silver nitrate, (**d**) Day 35 after 15 CAP applications, (**e**) Day 57 wound situation 1 month after completed therapy

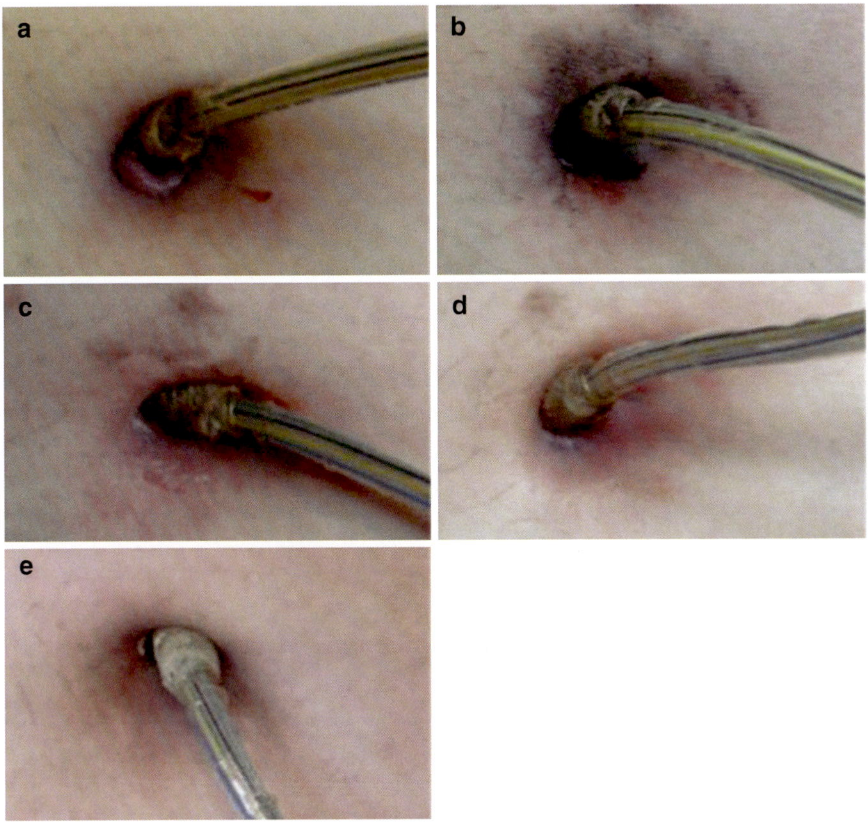

**Figs. 12.15, 12.16, 12.17, 12.18 and 12.19** (**a**) Day 0 reoccurrence of hypergranulation at 5–8 o'clock, (**b**) Day 7 after one single local application of silver nitrate, (**c**) Day 10 after 3 CAP applications, (**d**) Day 14 after 7 CAP applications, (**e**) Day 102 3 months after end of therapy

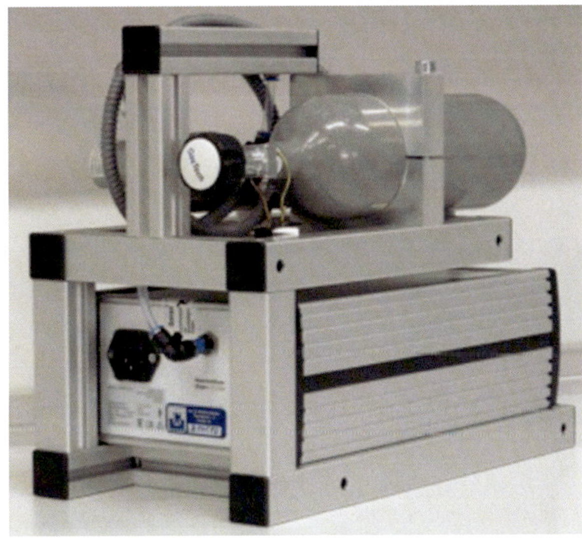

**Fig. 12.20** kinpen Med mobile pocket for outpatient CAP therapy of patients with implanted heart support systems

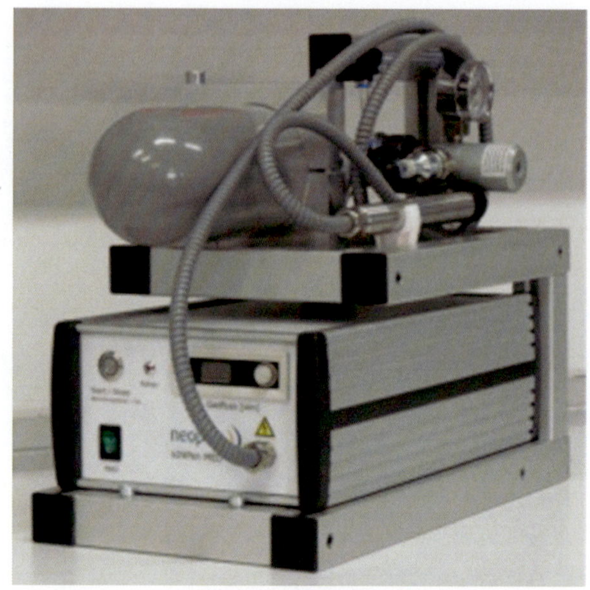

**Fig. 12.21** kinpen Med mobile pocket for outpatient CAP therapy of patients with implanted heart support systems

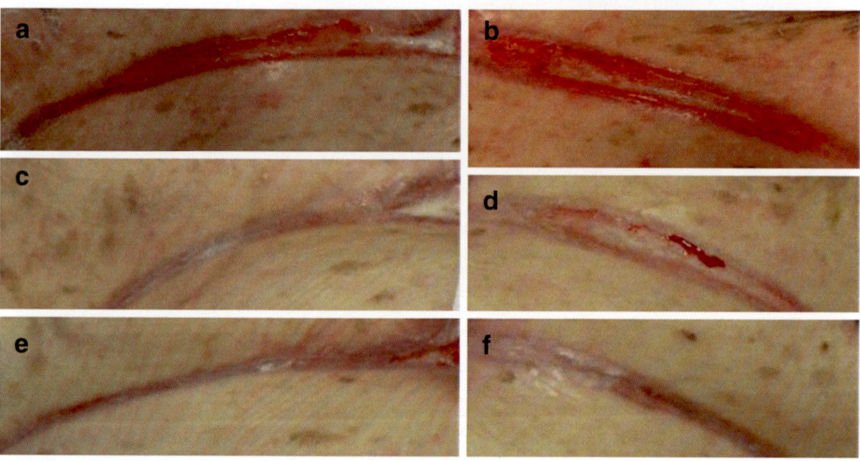

**Figs. 12.22, 12.23, 12.24, 12.25, 12.26 and 12.27** Inframammary fissures due to candidiasis on a critically ill patient after an emergency myocardial revascularization operation. (**a**) and (**b**) initial state, (**c**) after 4 CAP treatments on the right-hand side after 12 days, (**d**) left side at the same stage, (**e**) state after a further 15 days, (**f**) at the same stage after 3 CAP treatments to the left-hand side

## 12.3 Current Limitations and Risks of Plasma Therapy

In order to attain the initial goal of avoiding wound healing disturbances in the thorax region as best as possible, or the acceleration of their healing without unwanted effects for the patient or examiner, more detailed tests are needed. Firstly, plasma applicators that cover larger surfaces are needed to reduce the amount of time needed per application and to avoid local plasma overdoses. Secondly, a handpiece which can be sterilized is needed for possible intraoperative use. And last, but not least, it must be guaranteed that no unwanted effects are seen in either the patient, or the operator when used for long periods of time.

### 12.3.1 Ozone Concentrations During Permanent Plasma Application

When using plasma devices, ozone is released and can actually be faintly smelled. Ozone that occurs close to the earth's atmosphere is usually created by photochemical processes between nitrogen oxides and volatile organic compounds during intensive periods of sunshine. Ozone is classified as a secondary pollutant, because it can trigger respiratory problems due to inflammation. The MAK-Commission (Permanent Senate Commission for the Investigation of Health Hazards of Chemical Compounds in the Work Area) from the DFG (Deutsche Forschungsgemeinschaft) assessed ozone as a substance that "is suspected of causing cancer in humans". The reform of the *Gefahrstoffverordnung* (Hazardous Substances Ordinance—GefStoffV) meant that the maximum workplace concentration (MAK-Wert) was replaced by the *Arbeitsplatzgrenzwert* (workplace exposure limit—AGW). The MAK-Wert for ozone was 0.2 mg/m$^3$ or 0.1 mL/m$^3$. As no AGW has been set yet for ozone, the previous MAK-Wert or international exposure limits of 0.12 mg/m$^3$ (BG ETEM Information Sheet No. 526) serve as orientation for concentrations at the workplace, which after conversion, corresponds to 0.06 ppm.

A measurement of the ozone concentration during permanent plasma application, which took place in a 39.1 m$^3$ unventilated examination room at our clinic, using a APOA-360-Measuring device from the manufacturer HORIBA, revealed that using the kinpen Med from the manufacturer neoplas tools with a feeding gas flow (Argon) of 5 L/min was safe to use externally for operator and patient regarding its ozone pollution, as long as the distance between the patient's or operator's head to the source of pollution was greater than 40 cm (see Figs. 12.28 and 12.29).

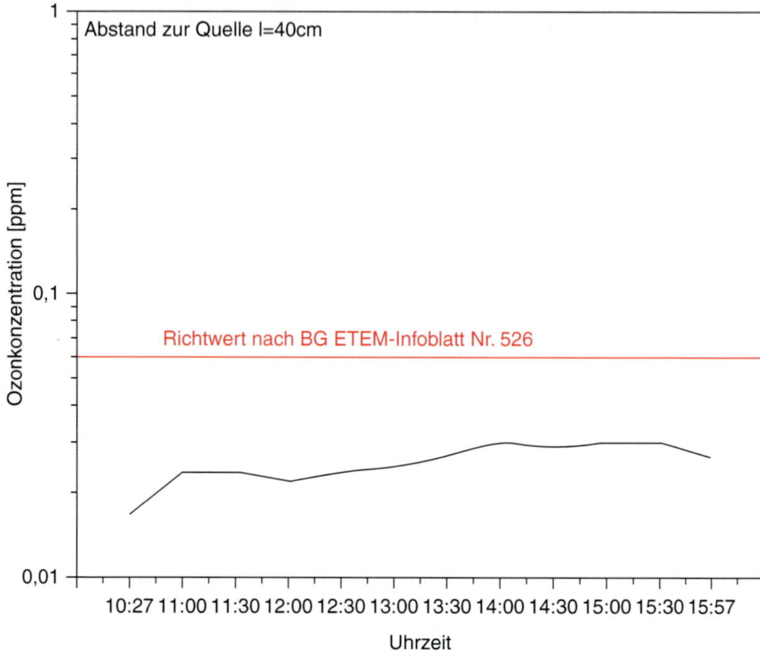


**Fig. 12.28** Ozone concentration [ppm] in an unventilated examination room, 40 cm from the kinpen Med handpiece during permanent therapy

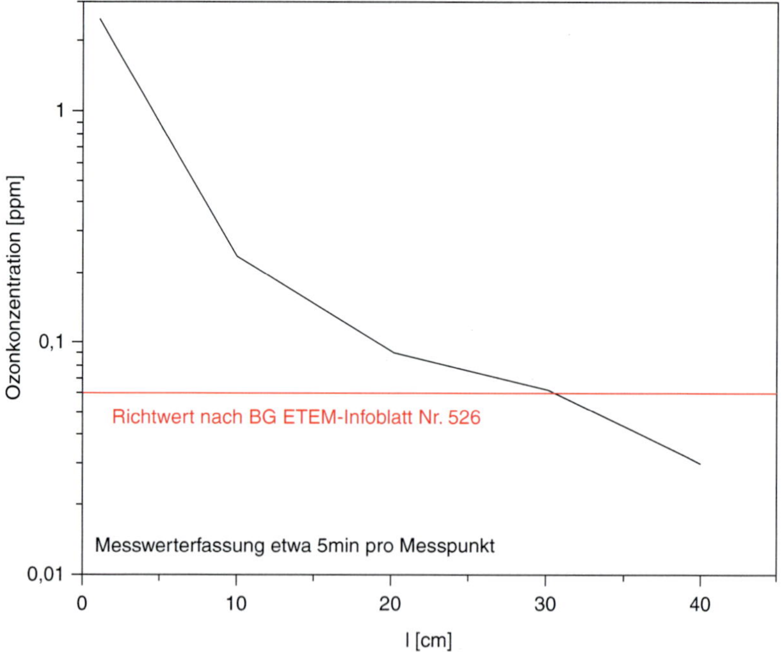


**Fig. 12.29** Ozone concentration [ppm] in an unventilated examination room, depending on the distance (l) of the handpiece to the measuring device

## 12.4 Outlook

We have not yet been able to fulfill our hope of preserving our heart surgery patients fully from the extensive complications of a profound wound healing disturbance and its effects. However, the experience we have made so far with the use of plasma has confirmed our expectations that the further development of plasma generators made to meet cardiac surgery demands in particular, can be expected to achieve a considerable advancement in surgical wound prophylaxis and therapy, as well as the reduction of resistances to antibiotics. It is not clear at this moment in time as to whether postoperative mediastinitis or sternum osteomyelitis will be avoidable in the future. It is, however, a fact that surface wound healing disturbances can be healed significantly faster when using plasma therapy.

In our opinion, this opens up the following areas of work at the interface between plasma medicine and cardiac surgery or surgery in general for the coming years:

- Plasma modifications for the optimal application on wounds with different etiologies in different areas of the body and with the presence of various pathogens
- Possibilities of plasma sterilization of surgical instruments during operative interventions
- Effects of plasma atmosphere during operations in body cavities
- Plasma wound disinfection of primary or secondary wound closures
- Plasma suture treatment in the early postoperative phase
- Plasma surface activation prior to introduction of implants
- Plasma surface modification to improve the biocompatibility of implants

## References


1. Stoney WS. Pioneers of cardiac surgery. 1st ed. Nashville: Vanderbilt University Press; 2008. p. 316–21. ISBN 978-0-8265-1594-0.
2. Loop FD, Lytle BW, Cosgrove DM, Mahfood S, McHenry MC, Goormastic M, Stewart RW, Golding LAR, Taylor PC. Sternal wound complications after isolated coronary artery bypass grafting: early and late mortality, morbidity and cost of care. Ann Thorac Surg. 1990;49:179–87.
3. Ahumada LA, de la Torre JI, Ray PD, Espinosa-de-los-Monteros A, Long JN, Grant JH, Gardner PM, Fix RJ, Vasconez LG. Comorbidity trends in patients requiring sternectomy and reconstruction. Ann Plast Surg. 2005;54(3):264–8.
4. Klesius AA, Simon A, Kleine P, Abdel-Rahman U, Herzog C, Wimmer-Greinecker G, Moritz A. Successful treatment of deep sternal wound infections following open heart surgery by bilateral pectoralis major flaps. Eur J Cardiothorac Surg. 2004;25(5):218–23.
5. Ghazi BH, Carlson GW, Losken A. Use of the greater omentum for reconstruction of infected sternotomy wounds: a prognostic indicator. Ann Plast Surg. 2008;60(2):169–73.

# Selected Settings of Clinical Plasma Treatment

# 13

T. Urayama and M. McGovern

## 13.1 Development of Plasma Device for Chronic Wound Treatment

### 13.1.1 Introduction

Plasma generated from atmospheric pressure to high pressure has been mainly used as a high temperature heat source for large scale facilities such as melting of metals and incineration of garbage. Additionally, low pressure plasma is widely used in semiconductor manufacturing processes and flat panel display manufacturing processes. It has recently been used for material processing applications including surface modification processing such as coating. On the other hand, application of atmospheric pressure plasma which does not require pressurization or decompression has also been studied for industrial applications. It has become possible to develop semiconductor and flat panel display manufacturing processing applications currently in widespread use [1–5]. Atmospheric pressure plasma had limited applications due to the high temperature of the plasma generated or it is generated at a low temperature but the effective use area is extremely limited. However, recent research and development has made it possible to diversify plasma sources such as low temperature regardless of the torch structure, atmospheric pressure plasma has started to expand to various fields including thin films such as semiconductors, flat panel displays, and solar cells. Additionally, application development in the field of biotechnology and medicine is also emerging, especially deployment for therapeutic applications using plasma technology for disinfection with wounds care

T. Urayama (✉)
ADTEC Europe Limited, Middlesex, UK
e mail: Takuyaurayama@adtec.eu.com

M. McGovern
Adtec Europe Ltd, Hounslow, UK
e-mail: mary@adtec.eu.com



H.-R. Metelmann et al. (eds.), *Comprehensive Clinical Plasma Medicine*,
https://doi.org/10.1007/978-3-319-67627-2_13

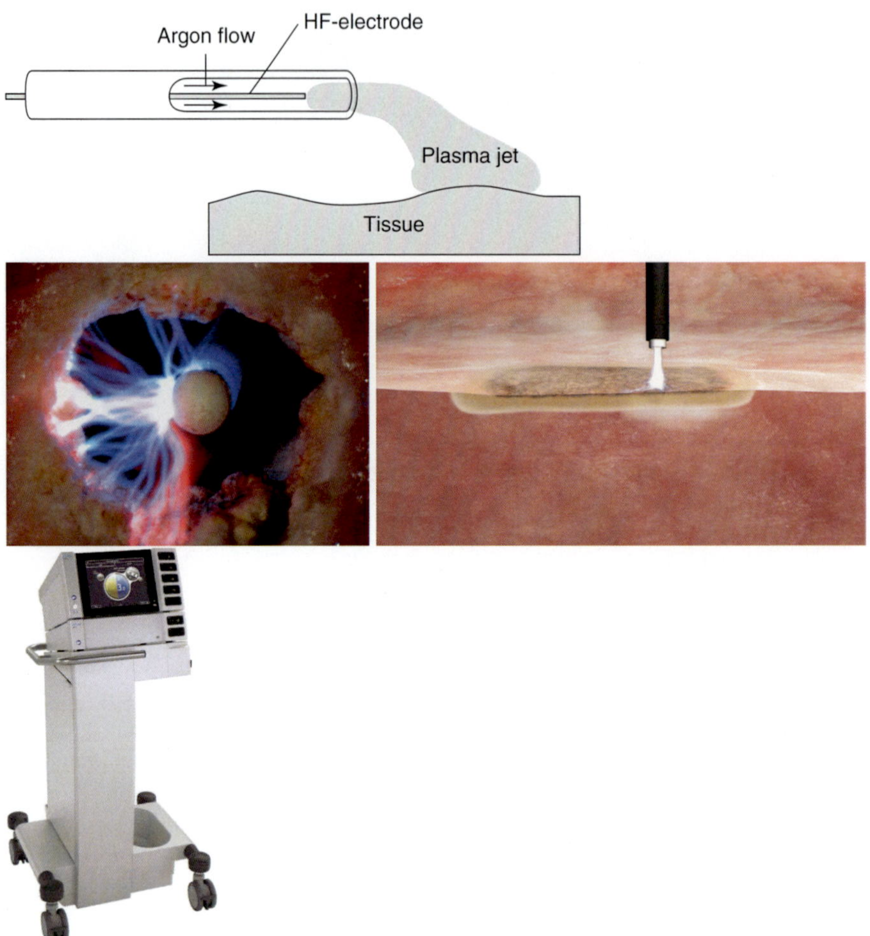


**Fig. 13.1** Plasma coagulation device APC 3(ERBE)

in addition to conventional plasma sterilization technology. In October 2007, the International Conference on Plasma Medicine (ICPM) was held in Texas, USA, and six meetings have been held so far. The seventh time will be held in Philadelphia, USA in June 2018. The conference has been growing and interest in plasma therapy has increased. ERBE (Erbe Elektromedizin GmbH [6]) Germany has developed and marketed a therapeutic plasma device—an argon plasma coagulation device APC 2 (Fig. 13.1). This device is mainly used in postoperative hemostasis, burn tissue locally by using Joule heat at discharge, and coagulate the blood. It can also be used with an endoscope so, it is used for hemostasis after incision surgery such as internal organs. Meanwhile, medical devices using atmospheric pressure low temperature plasmas, which have been actively researched and developed in recent years, are still in the process of commercialization. In 2017 ADTEC Steriplas gained the first commercial achievement for surgical site effect. The atmospheric pressure low temperature plasma generates a plasma that can be used at a temperature (40 °C or lower) and low enough to be touched. The characteristic of atmospheric pressure low temperature plasma is that it is possible to treat by plasma an object at low temperature and has potential applications in treating heat-sensitive materials which could not be treated with high temperature (several hundred degrees or more) plastic, films, paper also including biomaterials. The disinfection efficacy of plasma treatment for microorganisms such as E. coli [7] has been confirmed in a clinical study for wound care treatment concluded in 2014 with the MicroPlaster© developed by Max-Planck institute and ADTEC Plasma Technology. Clinical study results of more than 4000 plasma treatments on more than 350 patients confirmed the safety of plasma treatment in MicroPlaster©. Clinical trials are continuing post market supported by Adtec Europe ltd after 2014, and efficacy on Surgical site infections and biofilms have also been confirmed. In 2016 ADTEC EUROPE Ltd. launched business as ADTEC Health care with product "Adtec SteriPlas©". First sales achieved in early 2017.

## 13.2 Plasma Device at Atmospheric Pressure

The atmospheric pressure low temperature plasma device is shown in Fig. 13.2 This device was developed by Adtec PlasmaTechnology, Co. Ltd in Hiroshima JAPAN, in 2002. This device uses microwave power (2.45 GHz) as an energy source, the microwave power is fed through to the antenna in the torch via coaxial cable, and at the same time, gas is passed around the antenna to generate plasma. The generated plasma emerges from bottom of torch and the jet generated at low temperature can be touched. The length of the jet is from several cm to 10 cm, but the length depends on the gas flow rate and input power, and the colour of the jet depends on the gas materials. This device can generate atmospheric pressure plasma with argon gas mixed with nitrogen gas. The input power is from a few watt to several hundred watt, the gas flow rate can be from 0.5 slm to several tens slm, the plasma temperatures can be controlled from room temperature to several hundred by adjusting the input power, gas flow rate, and type of gas. Waveguides have been used for the propagation of high-power microwaves so far, however, coaxial cables are used to propagate in this device. Coaxial cables improve the flexibility regarding the operation of the plasma torch. This flexibility improvement makes it possible to develop various applications that could not be considered in conventional waveguide. In general, a magnetron type has been mainly used for the microwave power source because of cost and technical problems which the usable output range of the magnetron type microwave power source is 100 W or more. This is not suitable for use at several watts to several tens watt like our plasma torch. Therefore, solid state type microwave power supply and coaxial type automatic tuning device has been developed with ADTEC Plasma Technology Co., Ltd. and Nagano Japan Radio Co., Ltd. The maximum power is 150 W and

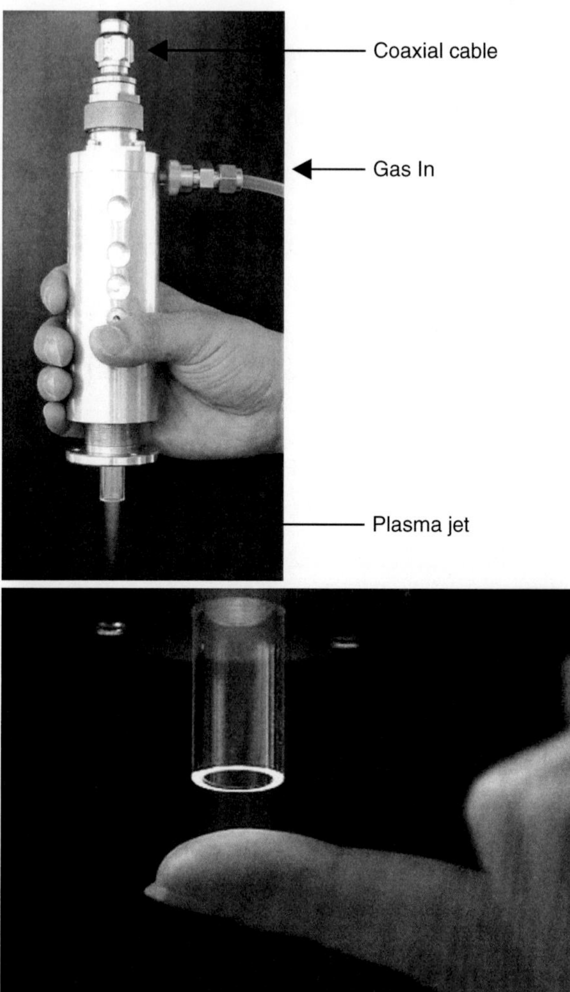


**Fig. 13.2** Microwave atmospheric pressure gas plasma torch (Adtec Plasma Technology Co., Ltd)

utilizes the characteristics of the solid state, it can control the output power from 1 W with coaxial output. The automatic tuning device withstands through power up to 500 W. With this microwave power supply and automatic tuning device put into practical use, it is possible to connect all microwave components by coaxial cable. As a result, the system as a whole has more flexibility, and it is possible to design a scalable smaller microwave system. An example is shown in Fig. 13.3. This device is an all-in-one atmospheric pressure plasma system built in the solid-state microwave power supply, automatic tuning, gas control and control PC. Basically, a simple automatic control that can generate plasma with one start switch has been realized. It is able to control microwave output, gas flow rate by

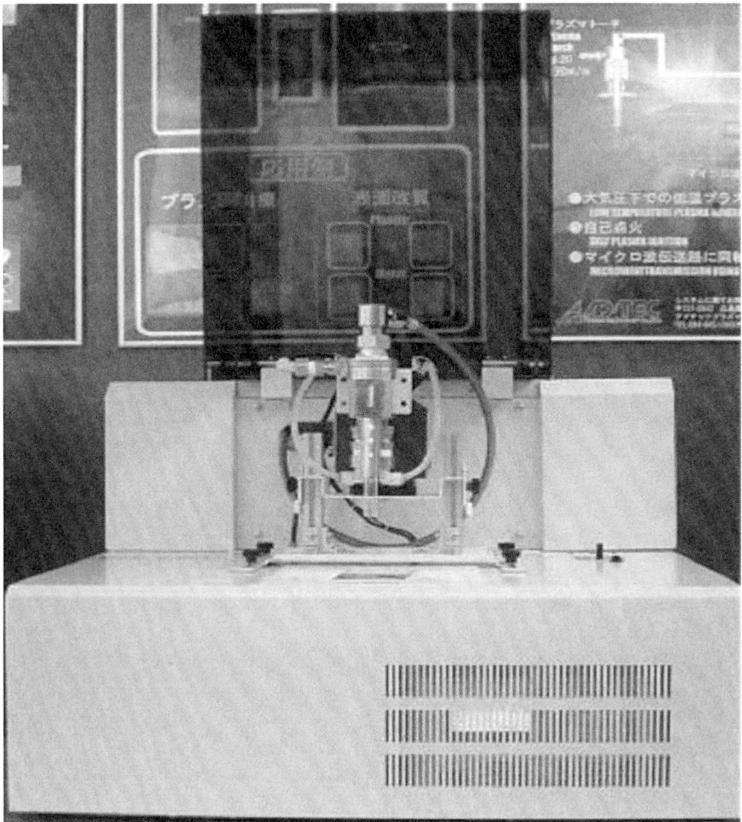

**Fig. 13.3** Microwave Atmospheric pressure plasma device APTN-150 (Adtec Plasma Technology Co., Ltd)

connected PC if it is necessary. In additionally, rack mounted model and low power model with less than 1 W generated plasma has also been developed (Adtec Plasma Technology Co., Ltd). Figure 13.4 shows the results of plasma treatment for metal plate, plastic plate and polyimide film by these plasma devices. Although it has been able to improve the hydrophilicity of the surface by generating plasma with argon gas as the main and mixing a small amount of oxygen, nitrogen etc., there is no melting or damaging on the surface at that time. From these result, it can be said that the plasma is able to treat at low temperature. From this result, plasma treatment to biomaterial was attempted. It was confirmed that plasma was able to reduce activity of E. coli which is treated by argon gas plasma at 40 W microwave power with 40 °C as a gas temperature. In general, plasma sterilization devices were considered toxic to human body using hydrogen peroxide at higher temperature. Results shows this device is able to inactivate microorganisms with

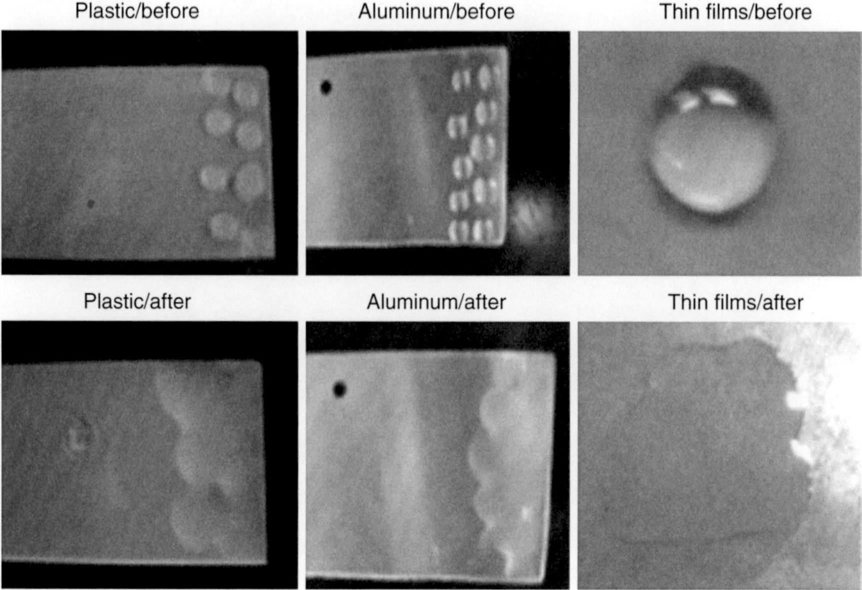


**Fig. 13.4** Surface treatment result of microwave

argon gas which is an extremely stable fundamentally harmless gas at low temperature and is said to be harmless to the human body.

## 13.3 Disinfection by Plasma

From these result, it was found that there is a possibility of inactivation of bacteria such as disinfection/sterilization by microwave.

atmospheric pressure low temperature plasma (disinfection). Please also refer to disinfection result with plasma treatment for Bacillus subtilis in a spore state with a plasma jet of 80 °C [8–10]. It has been the theory that high temperature disinfection is treated at 120 °C or higher, however, in this experiment disinfection of spores with argon plasma at about 80 °C was confirmed. The result of plasma treatment for active bacteria. Figure 13.5 shows treatment result by microwave atmospheric pressure argon plasma for E. coli on agar plate with 2 min and culturing for 16 h. The plasma gas temperature at that time is 40 °C or less. It is shown that there is a region which is sterilized around centre. It shows that it is able to be disinfection by microwave atmospheric pressure plasma generated by argon gas only not by a thermal factor. Regarding the mechanism of this disinfection has not been established yet and is under discussion with researchers. However, here are some possibilities that can be considered from the result so far.

Figure 13.6 shows the gas temperature distribution in the axial direction of the plasma gas. Z = 0 mm is the outlet of the torch, plasma gas temperature has dropped

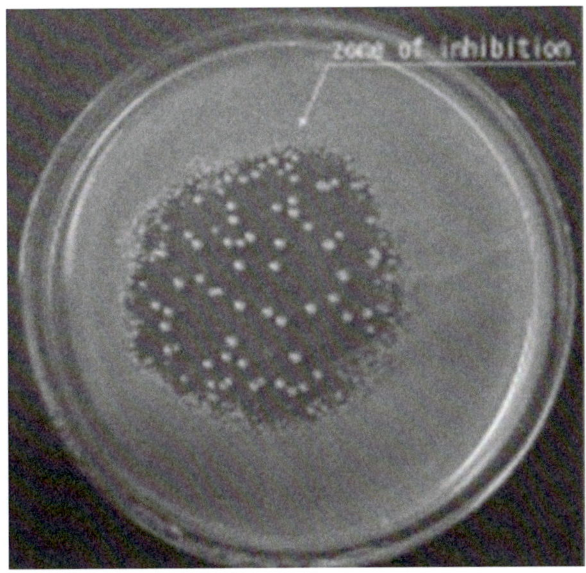


**Fig. 13.5** Plasma treatment for E. coli

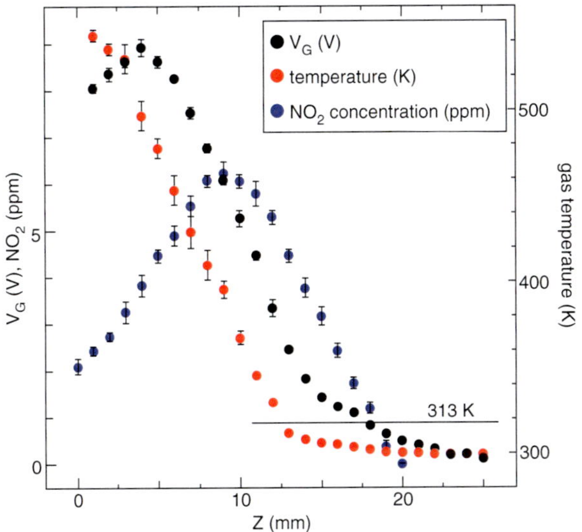


**Fig. 13.6** Gas temperature distribution in the axial direction

to 40 °C or less at Z = 20 mm. Otherwise, there is higher plasma gas temperature within Z = 20 mm which can be imagined that there are many active species (Fig. 13.7). The various active species arc produced by higher energy active species mixing with air around the torch outlet and they include $NO_2$ or ozone which seems

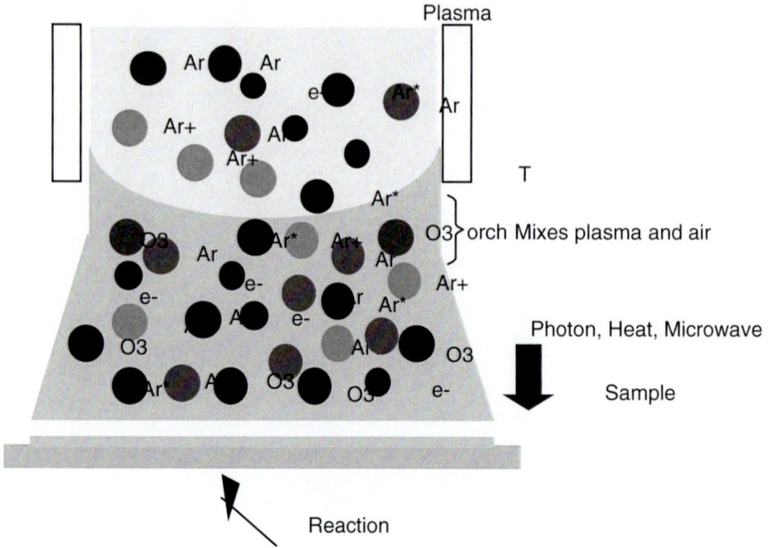


**Fig. 13.7** Plasma reaction

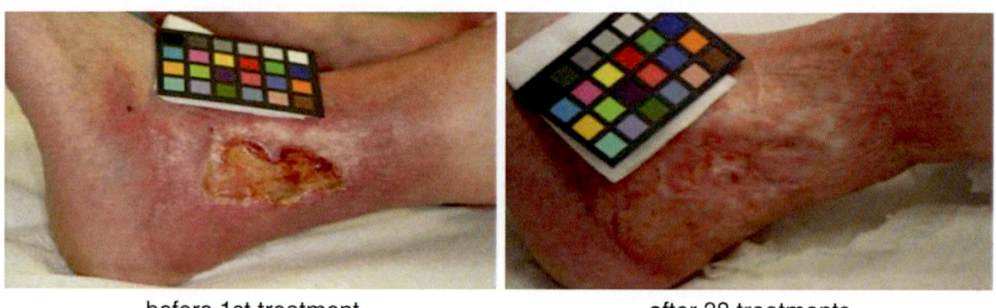


**Fig. 13.8** Example of wounds

to be active in disinfection. It is considered that these secondary produced species are the main active agents on disinfection. In additionally, collision by argon ion or UV from plasma are also considered to have a role in disinfection. The important point is that non-toxic gas plasma generated at almost human body temperature is able to deactivate bacteria. This means that it is able to disinfect bacteria on human body by plasma directly, for example, bacteria on the skin.

## 13.4 Clinical Study for Clinical Wounds

Figure 13.8 shows one example of clinical wounds. Plasma treatment was tested on clinical wounds. From the result so far, it has been confirmed that atmospheric pressure argon gas plasma is able to disinfect bacteria in 40 °C or less. Therefore, it is treated by plasma directly for clinical wounds for disinfection. It is a clinical study to stop progress of disease condition by disinfection and to promote treatment by encouraging skin regeneration ability. Clinical trials were conducted on patients at multiple hospitals. Clinical study was conducted Phase I and Phase II and no side effects or adverse events were reported. Here is short explanation about clinical trials, although a lot of countries take their own approval, generally similar methods are taken and roughly exist from Phase I to Phase VI. Phase I is generally a basic experiment including animal experiments, and the possibility of effects and side effects is examined. In addition, clinical study on the human body are conducted by Phase II, and tests are carried out on the effects and side effects. As an advantage of this atmospheric pressure low temperature gas plasma treatment method, there is no concern about allergic symptoms caused by drugs and the greatest advantage is that it does not cause pain to the patient. In particular, patients suffering such wounds complain of pain even if a little movement. In addition, Fig. 13.9 shows skin condition at 3 and 7 min after atmospheric pressure argon plasma treatment. As shown in this figure, the skin is composed of overlapping of various layers, but the epidermis close to the surface layer is generally newly regenerated from about 4 weeks to 6 weeks, and the dermis under the epidermis, its It consists of the underlying subcutaneous tissue [11–13]. Epidermis is newly born with the basal layer at the lowermost layer of the epidermis and nutrients for epidermal neogenesis are sent from the dermis but when these tissues seem to die it will be late or stop. Therefore, it is also important in clinical study to investigate how far the effect of plasma effectives. Table 13.1 shows the main items to be carried out in clinical study. In clinical study Phase I, we conducted experiments on human body including animal experiments. In additional, Phase II has been tested for a considerable number of patients (Table 13.2). In addition to this item, we verified the placebo effect, conducted more cases and clinical trials on patients. It shows the marketing research result how many patients having such symptoms are in the world. Figure 13.10 is the top five treatment costs in particular for skin diseases in the United States. Among them, the proportion of medical expenses for wounds accounts for a considerable number, and it is reported that there are more than 800,000 patients. There are various types of

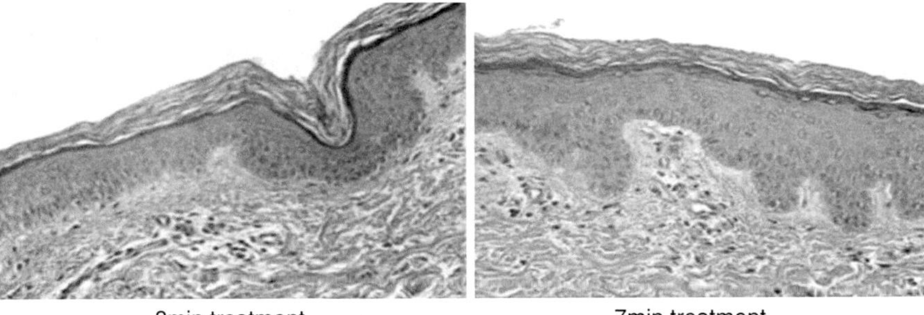


**Fig. 13.9** Skin section after plasma treatment

**Table 13.1** Characteristics of the patient group and wounds

| Characteristics | Group A | Group B | Group C |
|---|---|---|---|
| Number of patients | 70 | 27 | 18 |
| Female | 32 | 17 | 12 |
| Average age (years) | 69.7 | 74.9 | 75.2 |
| Age > 80 years (%) | 27.1 | 48.1 | 50.0 |
| Anteil systemischer Antibiotika (%) | 80.0 | 88.9 | 83.3 |
| Patients with heart disease (%) | 58.6 | 55.6 | 72.2 |
| Patients with diabetes (%) | 24.3 | 14.8 | 11.1 |
| Patients with lung disease (%) | 15.8 | 7.4 | 5.6 |
| Anteil chronisches Lymphödem (%) | 14.3 | 18.5 | 16.7 |
| Immobile patients (%) | 10.0 | 14.8 | 13.8 |
| Overweight patients (%) | 30.0 | 29.6 | 27.8 |
| Smokers (%) | 12.9 | 7.4 | 0 |
| Patients who regularly consume alcohol (%) | 7.2 | 11.1 | 11.1 |
| Patients suffering from allergies (Type I or IV) (%) | 35.7 | 55.2 | 55.5 |
| Patients with more than one wound (%) | 67 (81.4) | 21 (77.8) | 16 (88.9) |
| Number of plasma treatments (Timespan) | 8.39 (4–39) | 8.22 (4–39) | 7.1 (4–19) |
| Initial average length of wound (plasma) (cm) | 4.5 | 4.1 | 3.2 |
| Initial average length of wound (control) (cm) | 4.4 | 4.3 | 4.8 |
| Initial average width of wound (plasma) (cm) | 3.8 | 3.6 | 3.2 |
| Initial average width of wound (control) (cm) | 3.8 | 3.9 | 3.6 |
| Average change in wound length (plasma) (%) | 8.2 | 4.4 | 2.7 |
| Average change in wound length (control) (%) | 5.1 | 8.7 | 8.4 |
| Average change in wound width (plasma) (%) | 10.4 | 11.4 | 14.6 |
| Average change in wound width (control) (%) | 4.2 | 0 | 0 |
| Presence of wound (<3 months) (%) | 17.1 | 7.4 | 5.6 |
| Presence of wound (3–12 months) (%) | 44.3 | 48.4 | 50.0 |
| Presence of wound (>12 months) (%) | 38.6 | 44.4 | 44.4 |

skin diseases, some example is shown in Fig. 13.11. It is necessary to contact with the affected area such as applying medicine for disinfection. However, as able to be seen from Fig. 13.11, it is not hard to imagine that contact may be painful with treatment. On the other hand, the painless treatment by atmospheric pressure gas plasma treatment may have a big impact with advantage for treatment and quality of life for the patient.

## 13.5 Development of Atmospheric Pressure Plasma Treatment Device

From these points of view, there was considered that there is sufficient superiority in developing a treatment device using atmospheric pressure plasma which can disinfect without pain. ADTEC Plasma Technology. (Japan) and Max Planck Institute (Germany) has developed "MicroPlaSter©" for atmospheric pressure plasma

**Table 13.2** Characteristics of the patient group of the placebo-controlled clinical study with Herpes Zoster

| | Treatment (plasma 5 min) | Control (Argon gas 5 min) |
|---|---|---|
| Patients | 19 | 18 |
| Average age (span) in years | 64.3 (19–94) | 61.8 (27–91) |
| Ratio of females | 8/19 (42.1%) | 7/18 (38.9%) |
| Trigeminal region affected | 8/19 (42.1%) | 10/18 (55.6%) |
| History of cancer | 2/19 (10.5%) | 2/18 (11.1%) |
| Cardiovascular disease | 6/19 (31.6%) | 9/18 (50%) |
| Number of treatments (average per patient) | 89 (4.68) | 81 (4.5) |
| Initial pain, VAS span (median) | 0–10 (3) | 0–8 (2.5) |
| Pain during follow-up 2, VAS span (median) | 0–3.5 (0) | 0–3.2 (0.5) |
| Improvement of pain—patient numbers | 54/89 (60.7%) | 33/81 (40.7%) |
| Deterioration of pain—patient numbers | 0% | 10/81 (12.3%) |
| No change in pain—patient numbers | 35/89 (39.3%) | 38/81 (46.9%) |
| Average pain reduction, VAS Span (median) | 0–4.5 (0.6) | 0–3.5 (0.3) |
| Participant follow-up 1 (2 weeks) | 10/19 (52.6%) | 11/18 (61.1%) |
| Pain during follow-up 1 | 4/10 (40%) | 5/11 (45.5%) |
| Participant follow-up 2 (4 weeks) | 9/19 (47.4%) | 10/18 (55.6%) |
| Pain during follow-up 2 | 2/9 (22.2%) | 4/10 (40%) |
| DLQI during first visit 1, span (median) | 0–18 (6) | 1–20 (8) |
| DLQI after last treatment, span (median) | 0–23 (8) | 0–17 (5) |
| DLQI follow-up 1, span (median) | 1–18 (4) | 0–19 (7) |
| DLQI follow-up 2, span (median) | 0–16 (3.5) | 0–7 (1) |
| Number of patients with improved of DLQUI after discharge | 8 | 9 |
| Number of patients with no change in DLQUI after discharge | 2 | 0 |
| Number of patients with deteriorated DLQUI after discharge | 7 | 7 |

treatment device using microwaves. Figure 13.12 shows MicroPlaSter© be-ta model. This device has 150 W solid state type microwave generator and auto tuning unit and also, this device has mass flow controller that is controlled automatically by computer. It is designed to be simple to use and able to control everything by touch panel screen in front panel for operator who is doctors or nurses. On the other hand, there is another operation panel inside of device which is for various conditions to use, so it is designed to operate anywhere there is electric power supply plug. Figure 13.13 shows the plasma torch for MicroPlaSter©. From Fig. 13.11 shows, affected area varies, our plasma torch has six electrode which is for generated plasma that is covered for 40 mm diameter treatment area. This plasma torch is attached to the tip of the arm in this device and this arm is freely moved to the affected area of the patient for plasma treatment. The device had a function for placebo effect which is mechanism for warmed argon gas heated by an electric heater from the torch instead of plasma. It is able to create a state where it is unknown for

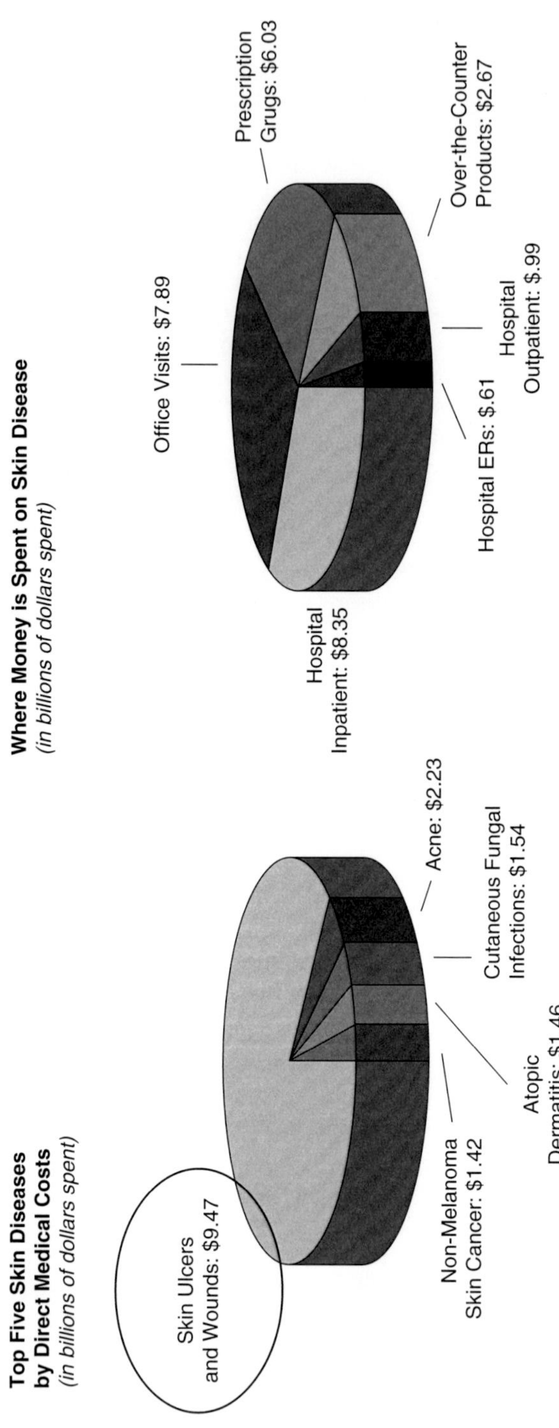


**Fig. 13.10** Top five treatment costs for skin diseases in USA [14]

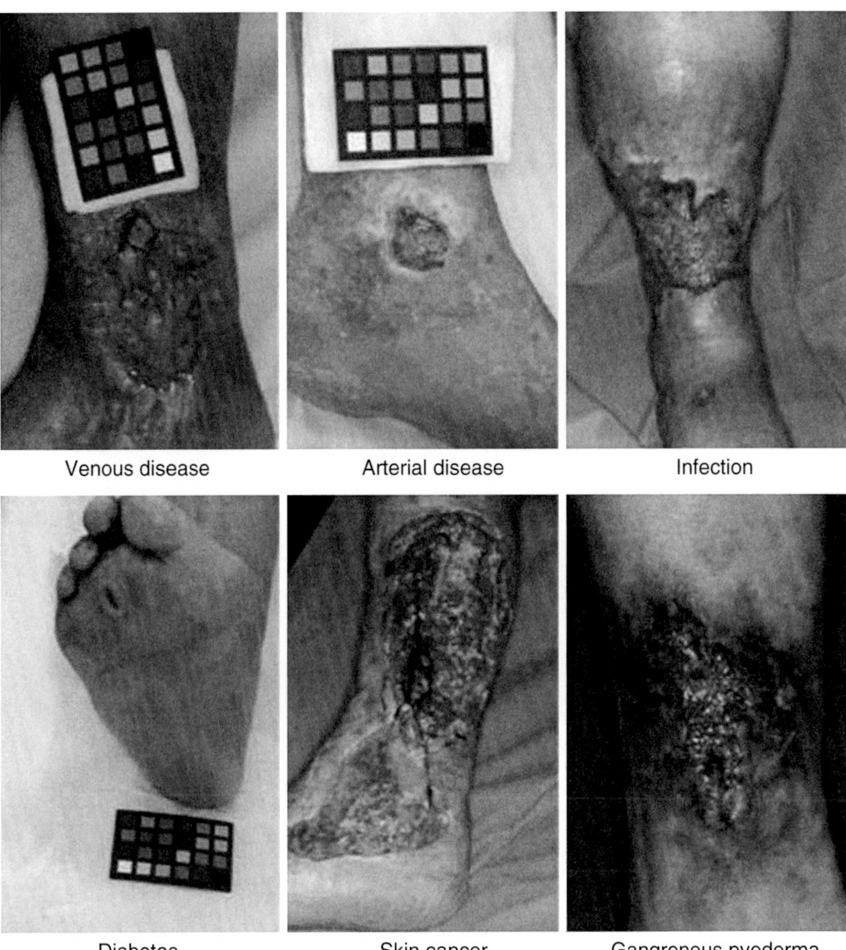


**Fig. 13.11** Chronic skin ulcer

patients whether it is treated by plasma or warm argon gas. Further, Fig. 13.14 shows main screen of this device. The device has two screens for displaying current status and information input. The operator selected a plasma generation mode which is plasma treatment or placebo and pressed the start button only. Treatment timer is selected time and the treatment is started. This device has been developed with the knowledge that expert knowledge and experience is unnecessary for operation, so it is even possible to operate from that day on which it is delivered. We had developed an atmospheric pressure plasma treatment device with such a function and this device was released in multiple units for clinical study conducted at hospitals in Germany and Russia.

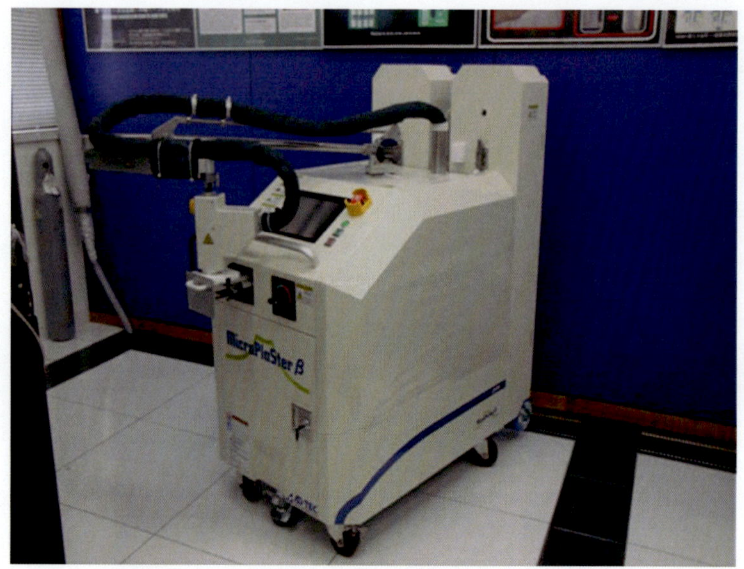


Fig. 13.12 MicroPlaSter©

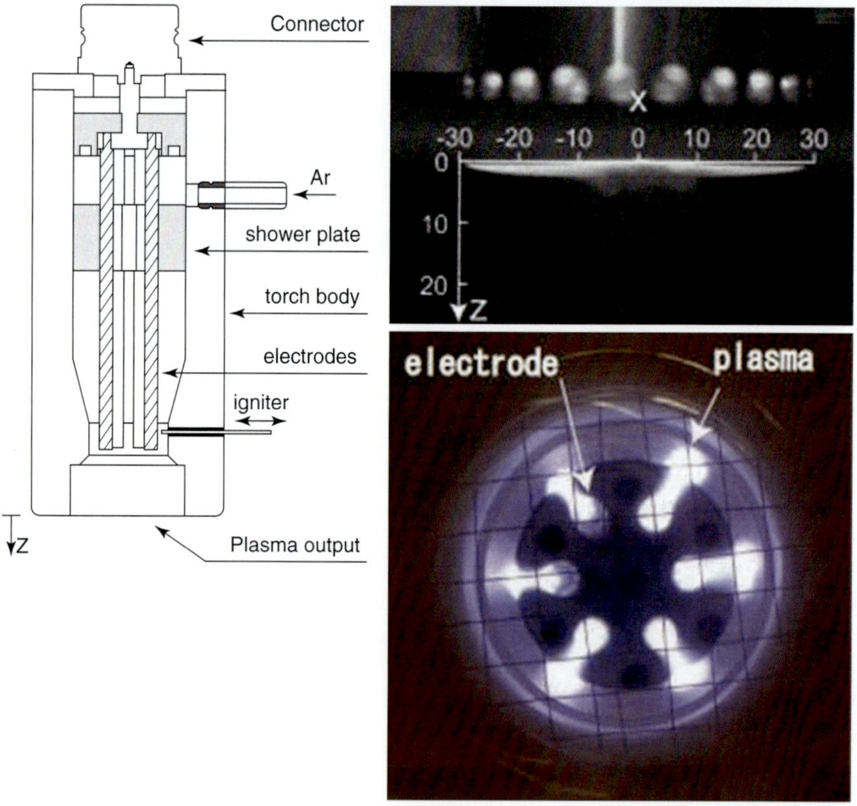

Fig. 13.13 Atmospheric plasma torch for MicroPlaSter©

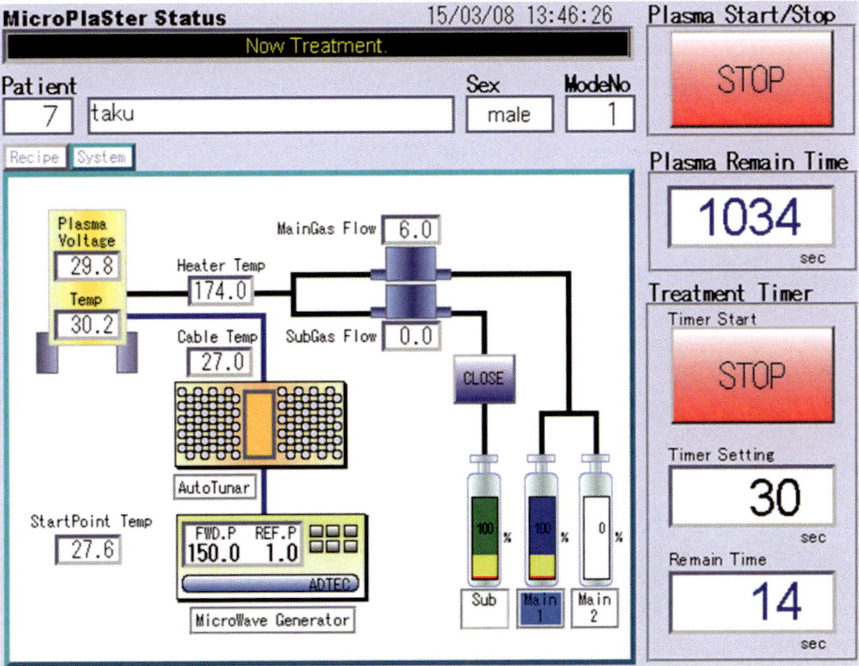


**Fig. 13.14** One of example for operation display

## 13.6 Commercialization

In this way, it was found that atmospheric pressure plasma can be generated at low temperature that is able to use for a new application which has never existed before. We have developed the atmospheric pressure gas plasma device which treated plasma directly to the human body for disinfection which is first time in the world. The results of clinical study in this device led to propose new possibilities to conventional medical devices, which leads to gentle treatment to reduce the burden on patients. After completing the clinical study in 2014, we confirmed clinical efficacy with no side effect or adverse events reported. It is a proven safe device, it is difficult to create resistant bacteria and it is a painless treatment. From these result, we have commercialized this device. ADTEC Europe ltd is a subsidiary of ADTEC Plasma technology in Japan which has offices in London, U.K. ADTEC EUROPE Ltd. acquired ISO 13485 in 2015 and obtained approval as a medical device manufacturer. We commercialized MicroPlaSter© as a evaluation model and commercialized Adtec SteriPlas© as an atmospheric pressure plasma medical device in Adtec Healthcare Brand in 2016 (Fig. 13.15). Adtec SteriPlas© further developed the MicroPlaSter© technology, succeeded in miniaturization with half the weight and more simple operations. After commercialization, positive evaluation and sales activities have been carried out, clinical trials have been conducted on wound treatment of diabetic patients, Surgical site infections, actinic keratoses, etc. in addition to usual wound treatment, and good results have been obtained.

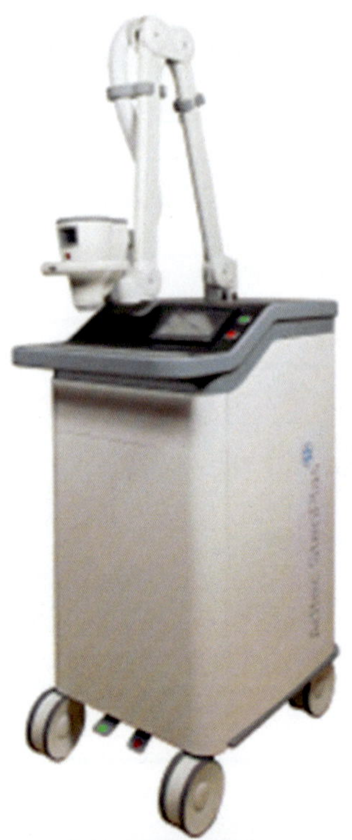

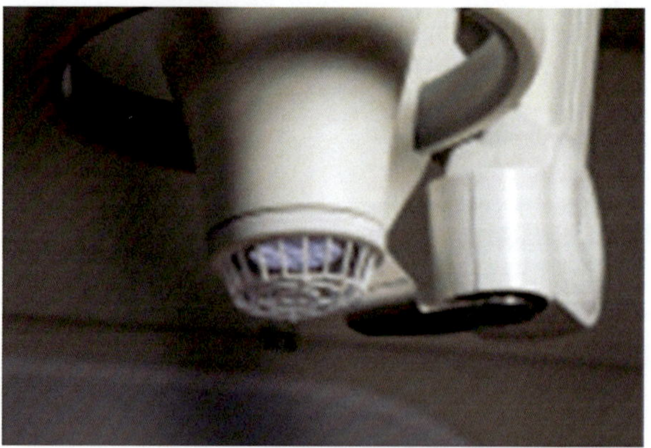

**Fig. 13.15** Adtec SteriPlas©

## 13.7 Clinical Evidence of ADTEC MicroPlaSter/SteriPlas

### 13.7.1 Introduction

This document concerns the overall clinical evaluation of ADTEC Healthcare non-thermal gas plasma generating devices (NTGP). The following devices fall within this group:

- MicroPlaSter—ARPP-MS-02
- SteriPlas—ARPP-SP-01

The ARPP-SP-01 is a new product in the MicroPlaSter family. The ARPP-SP-01 (SteriPlas) is the next generation of the ARPP-MS-02. (MicroPlaSter). The Plasma generating device used in the treatment head is exactly the same in the MicroPlaSter and SteriPlas.

The clinical efficacy and results are therefore the same in the MicroPlaSter and SteriPlas and we use the data from the MicroPlaSter Clinical report to justify the clinical evidence of the SteriPlas.

## 13.8 Applicable Regulations, Standards and Guidelines

The present evaluation was performed according to the requirements and guidance of

- MDD 93/42/EC Annex II.
- EN ISO 14155 Clinical investigation of medical devices for human subjects—Good Clinical Practice.
- EN ISO 14971 "Medical devices—Application of risk management to medical devices".
- MEDDEV 2.7.1 Evaluation of clinical data: A guide for the manufacturers and notified body.
- BS EN 60601-1 Medical electrical equipment—Part 1: General requirements for basic safety and essential performance.
- IEC 60601-1-2 Medical electrical equipment—Part 1–2: General requirements for basic safety and essential performance—Collateral standard: Electromagnetic compatibility—Requirements and tests.
- BS EN 62304 Medical device software. Software life-cycle processes.
- BS EN 62366-1 Medical devices. Application of usability engineering to medical devices.

## 13.9 Safety Precautions/Contraindications

Full Risk assessment of the device has been carried out following EN ISO 14971.

The toxicity and mutagenicity of argon plasma has been investigated [15].

## 13.10 Claims and Studies

Gas Plasma has been shown to have a greater microbial load reduction than antibiotics on wounds in Randomized Controlled Clinical Trials [16] and has efficacy against biofilms [17–19]. It has proven efficacy in management of infection in surgical site infections [20, 21]. Gas Plasma is also a broad spectrum antimicrobial (including multi-resistant strains) and with a physical mode of action, resistance is unlikely [22].

### 13.10.1 Chronic Wounds

This research project initiated the first study using such a low temperature argon plasma machine in an "Add-on" capacity on patients with chronically infected wounds, due to those already mentioned problems in the treatment of chronic ulcers and rising resistance among bacteria [23]. The patients received 1× daily plasma treatment lasting 5 min with the MicroPlaSter Alpha machine, on a random wound (in case of multiple ulcers) or a randomly chosen half of a wound (in case of a larger wound). The patient served as a self check. This made it possible that the antibacterial effect could clearly be attributed to the plasma treatment—both wounds and wound halves received the identical wound treatment. Also any systematically provided antibiotics always affected the treated wound as well as the control area.

During this stage a blind/double blind test was not possible, because the first machine (MicroPlaSter alpha) did not contain a placebo mode and the patient as well as the operator could see and smell the plasma.

After testing with 36 patients who suffered from 38 infected ulcers of differing aetiology (Fig. 13.16), it could be shown that as a result of the Plasma treatment (a total of 291 treatments, meaning the average treatment interval per patient was 7.86) significantly more bacteria could be reduced, regardless of the type of infection or the resistance pattern (microbial spectrum, see Fig. 13.17).

The additional benefit for the area treated with plasma was around 34% ($p < 0.01$) (Fig. 13.18).

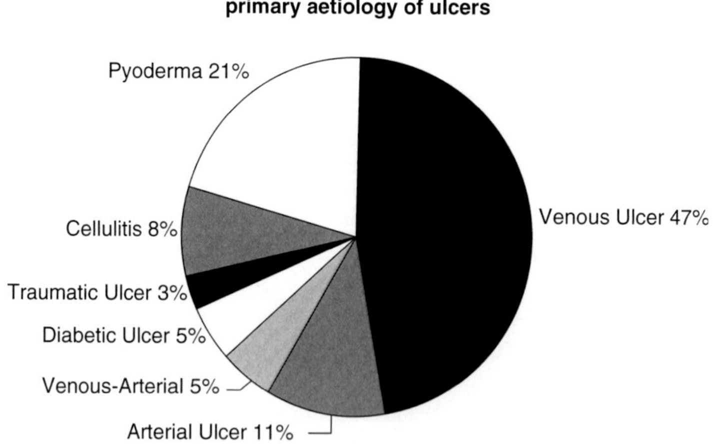


**Fig. 13.16** Aetiology of the chronic ulcers

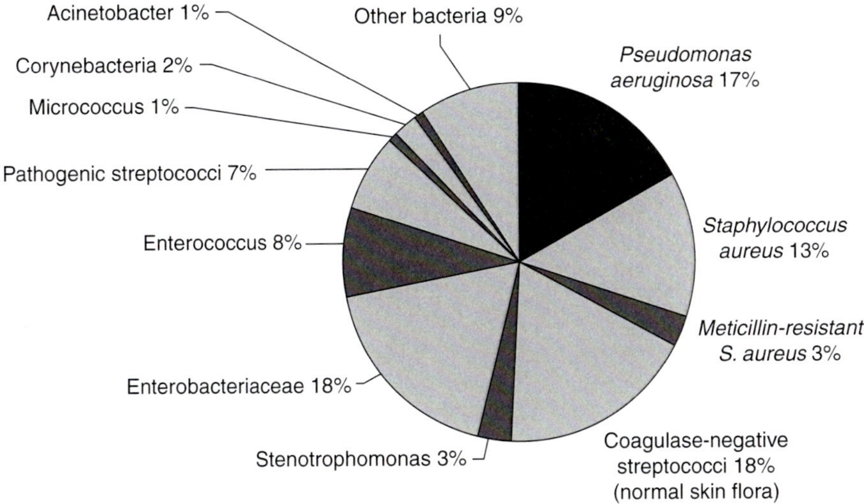


**Fig. 13.17** Microbial spectrum of the chronically infected ulcers

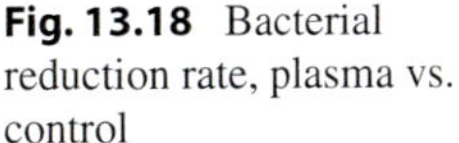

**Fig. 13.18** Bacterial reduction rate, plasma vs. control

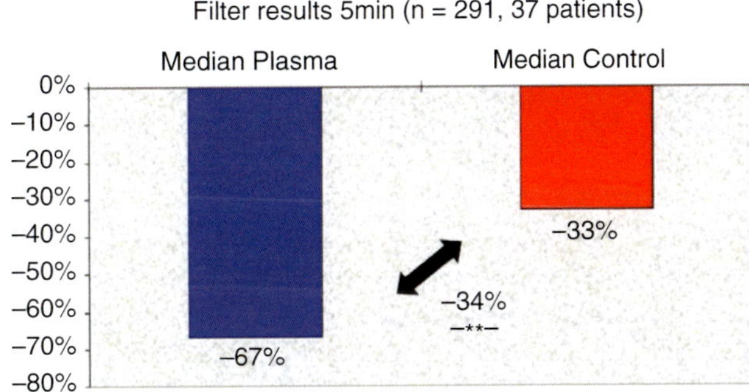


The relatively high rate of reduction of around 33% in the control area can happen due to various factors.

Firstly, the filter method represents a light debridement. Additionally the 5 min treatment time in the treated area means a certain drying effect could not be avoided. Also, 14 patients with a large ulcer were recruited. Here, despite the >0.5 cm safety distance, it is possible that plasma components made their way into the control area, or that the wound fluids themselves were altered by the plasma, and so the control area was inadvertently treated as well to some extent.

Another important finding of the study was that the plasma treatment was completely painless and did not cause side effects. The patients merely experienced a "warm breath of air", which depending on environmental temperature could vary from 20 to 33 °C and which patients experienced as pleasant.

After tests that found that the UV dosage produced by the plasma treatment were already negligible according to international standards, [24] the efficacy of a reduced

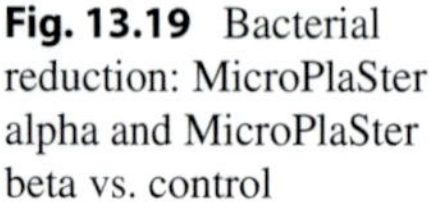

**Fig. 13.19** Bacterial reduction: MicroPlaSter alpha and MicroPlaSter beta vs. control

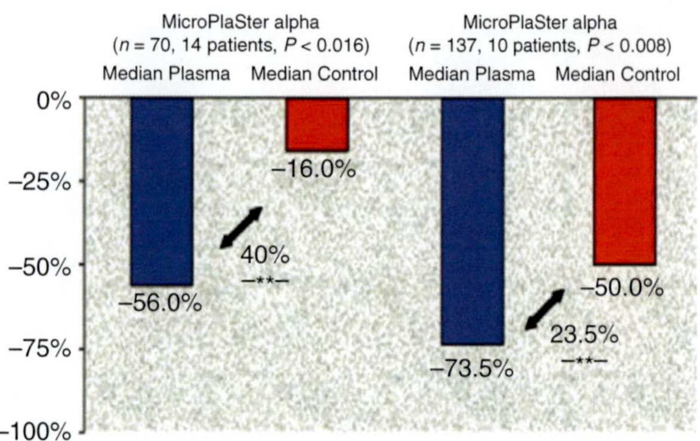


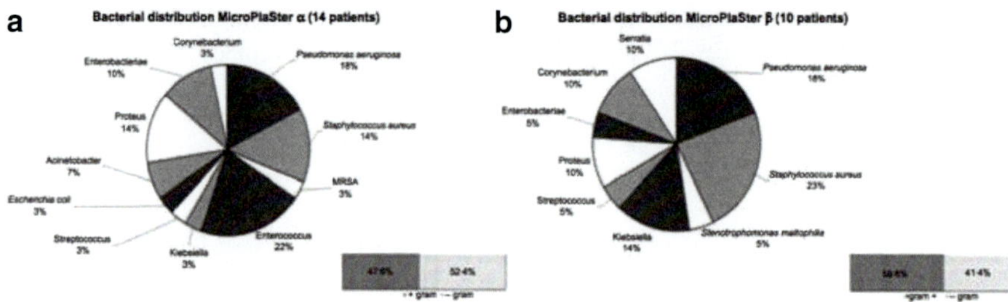


**Fig. 13.20** Microbial spectrum of both treatment groups. (**a**) MicroPlaSter alpha. (**b**) MicroPlaSter beta

treatment time of 2 min was to be tested. Furthermore the plasma machine was improved. The machine (MicroPlaSter beta) became visibly more compact, benefitted from a much better arm and allowed for mixing in further gases, as well as a placebo treatment mode with pure Argon gas. The latter was not yet employed at this point—other gas mixtures were not used during the entire duration of the study.

Within a different group of patients, now the efficacy of a 2 min plasma treatment with reduced UV-load and clear timesaving was to be tested, subject to approval of the amendment by the ethics committee. At the same time, the efficiency of both generations of machine (MicroPlaSter alpha and beta) was to be compared.

24 patients with chronically infected wounds were treated according to the same schedule as during the study previous—however employing a plasma therapy lasting 2 min (Isbary et al. 2012, publication 4). 14 patients (aged 49–85, average 72.4 years old) received the treatment with the MicroPlaSter alpha machine—a total of 70 treatments. 10 Patients (aged 41–88, average 76.0 years old) were treated 137 times in total with the newer MicroPlaSter beta. The result was significant reductions with a benefit of around 40% ($p < 0.016$) with plasma treatment using the alpha machine and highly significant reductions of 23.5% ($p < 0.008$) using the beta machine (Fig. 13.19).

The reduction once again was achieved regardless of type of infection (microbial spectrum of both treatment groups, see Fig. 13.20).

Once again no side effects were observed and the plasma treatment as painless.

Until now, the pain-free and so far side effect free plasma treatments on wound patients could only demonstrate that the treatment brings with it an additional antibacterial effect. *In vitro* and *in vivo* results from the study of Arndt et al. [23, 25] however showed, that with the help of low temperature plasma (MicroPlaSter beta) important genes for the wound healing mechanism could be induced and therefore sped up wound healing in tests with mice.

*In vitro* it could be demonstrated that the 2 min plasma treatment—analogous to the *in vivo* treatment time on a patient—stimulates/induces pro-inflammatory Zytokine and growth factors, meaning respectively IL-6, IL-8, MCP-1, TGF-ß1 and TGF-ß2. Furthermore, the treatment did not lead to a change of proapoptotic factors or anti-apoptopic markers Migration rates of Fibroblasts had increased after the 2 min treatment—an important factor in the context of wound healing. At the same time no increased proliferation rate could be detected—this is also important in the avoidance of hypertrophic scars or keloids. Also, collagen type 1 and alpha-SMA were activated by the plasma treatment *in vitro*—this is important for the end phase of wound healing.

*In vivo*, the artificially created wounds at the back of mice healed better in the area treated by plasma, than they did in the control area with the placebo treatment (pure argon treatment). On the third and fifth treatment day, the wounds were significantly smaller. Looking at histology, the wounds treated with plasma showed heightened Macrophage counts. Also, plasma increased the chemical attractor for neutrophil granulocytes GRO alpha and serpine E, which are important in the remodelling phase and also attracts leukocytes. These facts, as well as the results from the previous *in vitro* studies demonstrate that plasma can especially support the healing during the initial stage of infection. On the 15th treatment day it was observed that plasma treated wounds showed a more homogenous and thicker epidermis layer than control wounds. The collagen fibres in the treatment area were taut and well ordered. In contrast, the connective tissue in the control area was very loosely structured.

### 13.10.2 Acute Wounds

Another part of this research project was the study of using plasma to possibly speed up wound healing in patients with acute wounds [26]. For this, patients with split skin crafts after excisions of skin tumours were recruited.

In a randomised placebo controlled study, 40 patients (aged 26–92 years old, average age 64.7 years) received a daily 2 min plasma treatment (MicroPlaSter beta) on the skin graft donor site. The skin graft donor sites on different patients were very homogenous acute wounds in terms of wound depth and location, due to the technique used to remove the skin grafts. The control treatment consisted of pure argon gas treatment on the opposing wound half. The size of the graft donor site varied between 9.0 and 78.8 $cm^2$ (average size 30.9 $cm^2$). The success was judged by two independent researchers according to a double blind procedure,

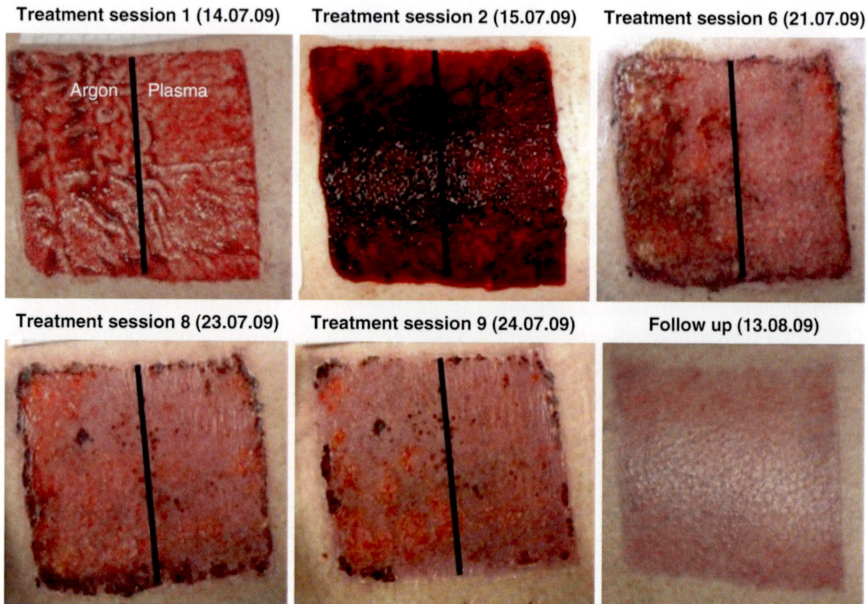


**Fig. 13.21** Skin graft donor sites treated with placebo (Argon) and plasma

considering reepithelialisation, number of blood crusts, fibrin layers and wound surroundings. The results showed that from the second treatment day, those wounds treated with plasma showed significant improvements in wound healing when compared with control wounds (Fig. 13.21). Positive effects were seen in the reepithelialisation, reduction of fibrin layers and blood crusts. The wound surroundings did not change significantly in both treatment areas. In no case did any wound infection take place during the study. This study supports the assumption, that plasma also supports wound healing in non infected wounds. Once again the pain-free treatment was well tolerated.

Evaluated by two independent researchers according to double blind procedure. The benefit for the side treated with plasma becomes clear after the second, respectively third plasma treatment.

### 13.10.3 Chronic Wounds

Based on the results of the study on acute wounds, another open, retrospective randomly controlled study was begun to research the effect of the MicroPlaSter alpha on wound healing (as a secondary endpoint) (Fig. 13.22) [27].

It remains to be noted that wound healing in this study is only the secondary end point and that the study design was conceptualised for proving a reduction in microbial load and not to judge wound healing. The maximum wound lengths and breadths in the treatment and control areas were compared to the same markers during the

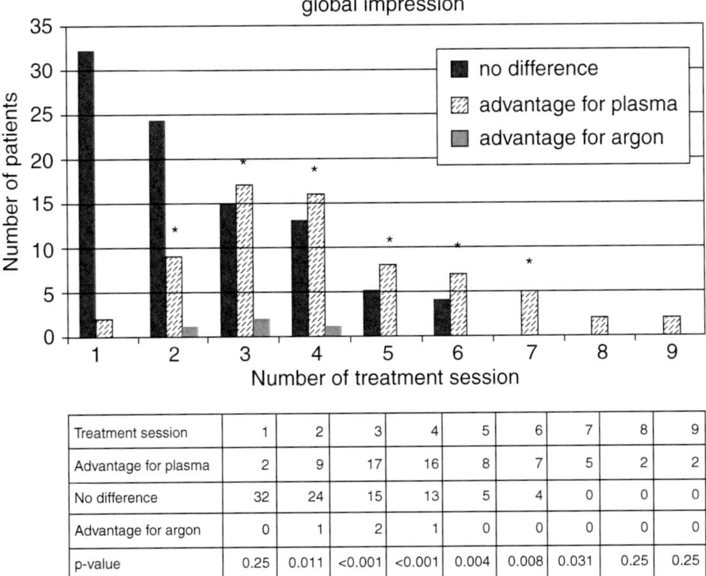


| Treatment session | 1 | 2 | 3 | 4 | 5 | 6 | 7 | 8 | 9 |
|---|---|---|---|---|---|---|---|---|---|
| Advantage for plasma | 2 | 9 | 17 | 16 | 8 | 7 | 5 | 2 | 2 |
| No difference | 32 | 24 | 15 | 13 | 5 | 4 | 0 | 0 | 0 |
| Advantage for argon | 0 | 1 | 2 | 1 | 0 | 0 | 0 | 0 | 0 |
| p-value | 0.25 | 0.011 | <0.001 | <0.001 | 0.004 | 0.008 | 0.031 | 0.25 | 0.25 |

**Fig. 13.22** Results of the study

previous treatment. Neither the wound depth and wound area calculation were recorded. This was for the following reasons: when the wound area is calculated (length × breadth), the total area will constantly be estimated as bigger than what it actually is. Adding wound depth as a third dimension would have worsened the above mentioned calculation error. It was not possible to use a computer to measure the wound size by using digital images, because of the number of larger wounds in various locations on the body with different angles and distances towards the digital camera, meaning wounds would not always fit into one digital figure. For this reason the very simple method of recording the wound lengths and breadths was used.

Patients in this study were divided into three groups.

(a) Group A contained 70 patients with chronic infected wounds of different aetiology (Fig. 13.23) who were treated between 3 and 7 min with plasma in an add-on procedure. In this group significantly larger reductions in wound length and breadth compared to control wounds were observed.
(b) Group B was a sub group of Group A, contained 27 patients with chronic venous ulcers, who were also treated between 3 and 7 min with plasma. Within this group, the plasma treated wounds significantly improved in terms of breadth when compared to the control. However there was no significant change in the wound length.
(c) In the sub group C, a very homogenous group, there were only patients with chronic venous wounds who received a 5 min plasma treatment. In this group the plasma again led to a significant improvement in wound breadth, but not in wound length.

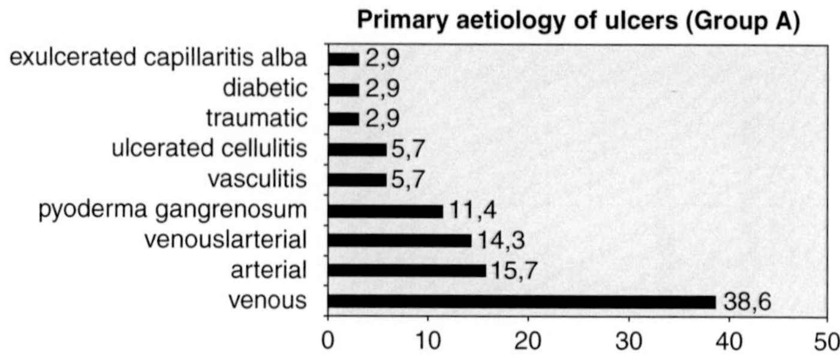


**Fig. 13.23** The different aetiologies of the wounds included in Group A

The fact that the wound lengths in group B and C did not improve significantly, can be caused by the location of most of the wounds, on the calf. The wound breadth would experience less mechanical stress, since it opposes the natural direction in which the body experiences tension. Furthermore the possibility exists that the wounds in order to achieve healing in the wound length, the wound must first become broader in order to make a length reduction under a lot of stress possible. A further point that needs to be noted is the randomisation process. The randomisation took place according to distal, or proximal localisation. The wound length in these solitary wounds however is calculated by adding the length of the control and treatment half. This means that a potentially positive effect in the treatment area is less obvious than when plasma is applied on the entire length of the wound.

When interpreting the results, further points need to be noted. The collective of patients contained some negative predictive values in terms of wound healing. Table 13.1 shows the various patient and wound characteristics. In this study included chronic wounds regardless of aetiogenesis, localisation, wound size, duration, and age of the patient (except for inclusion criteria which state that all patients must be of legal age). All these factors can influence wound healing.

A further limitation is the short inclusion period caused by deciding microbial load as the primary end point. The patients received on average around eight plasma treatments, which means a very short treatment time of about 2 weeks. However, chronic wounds require a relatively long healing time, and the best timeframe to decide the success of the healing tendency has been set at 4 weeks. Possibly there was not enough time to show significant changes.

Despite these limitations, the results firstly show that wound healing has sped up in patients with chronic wounds, especially chronic venous ulcers. Side effects were not recorded in the context of this study.

With the help of these results it could be shown that the plasma treatment using the MicroPlaSter alpha and beta can be classified as safe, with over 8 years of clinical experience, and on the other hand that it is effective in the treatment of bacteria in wounds—regardless of type and resistance pattern. Furthermore it seems like plasma has a positive influence on wound healing.

### 13.10.4 Case Studies

The use of low temperature plasma is not just limited to patients with ulcers. Case studies can demonstrate that also other pathogen associated diseases can be treated successfully with plasma.

### 13.10.5 Hailey-Hailey Disease

The first case report [28] showed success of an additional plasma treatment on a patient with therapy resistant Hailey-Hailey disease (specifically Pemphigus chronicus benignus familiaris). With Haily-Haily disease an autosomal dominant genetic defect in the ATP2C1-gene causes acantholysis and the formation of blisters in areas which are mechanically stressed and prone to maceration. The patient with therapy resistant lesions of the right axilla and the right armpit and right groin received a daily 5 min plasma treatment (MicroPlaSter beta), in addition to the already initiated topical fusidic acid and betamethasone therapy. The groin was treated according to a randomised approach only with the localised treatment mentioned above. Both lesions were secondarily impetiginized with *Proteus mirabilis* and *Candida albicans*.

Within just four plasma treatments there was a clear improvement of the condition of the skin in the right armpit and also the reduction of the stabbing pain in this area, whereas the untreated, right groin, did not experience change. Furthermore both areas received four more plasma treatments, which caused a clear improvement in the groin, before the patient left for a vacation. There the skin condition clearly deteriorated in both areas while receiving topical external treatment which was sterile and contained steroids. Only after their return, there was an almost complete healing of the erosively moist lesions in the right armpit and right groin after 11 further plasma treatments, so that the patient then became symptom free (Fig. 13.24). The workings of the plasma could in this patient be explained on the one hand by the secondary impetiginization, and on the other hand possibly by the effect of the reactive species created by the plasma, which could have positively influenced the pathophysiologically disturbed redox-behaviour in Hailey-Hailey patients.

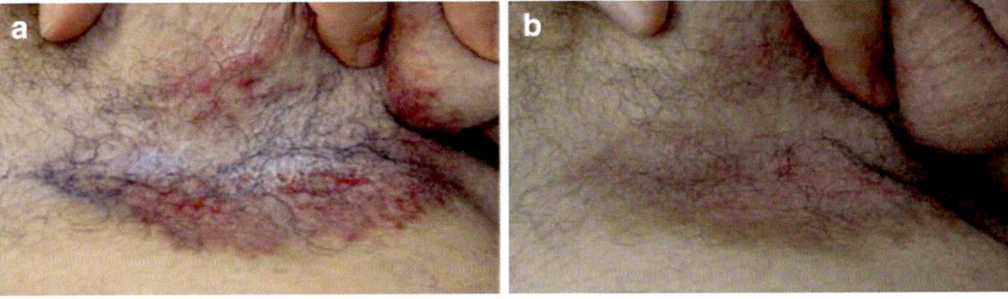


**Fig. 13.24** (**a**) Untreated right groin after the condition worsened during holiday (the blue and whitish film is created by the topical prior treatment) (**b**) After 11 further plasma treatments resulted in a clear improvement of the skin condition with some remaining mild remaining erythema [28]

### 13.10.6 Infection of External Ear Canal

A further publication outlined that plasmas can also be successfully used in other scenarios [29]. One patient suffered for 3 years from bacterial infections of the ear canal, as well as the nasopharynx following an operation due to a cholesteatoma in the left tympanic cavity, which subsequently caused him distinct pain. The antibiotic treatment of this very painful infection was made difficult by the presence of ESBL+ *Escherichia coli,* which only showed a sensitivity for Cotromoxazole. Before the plasma treatment the regular antibiotic treatment (over the past 6 months a continual systematic dose was given) with Cotrimoxazole, including a topical antiseptic treatment (consisting of Octenidin and 0.3% Hydroperoxide rinses), did not lead to any decontamination of germs.

Low temperature Argon plasma was applied daily for 5 min (MicroPlaSter beta, distance to the opening of the external ear canal 2 cm, see Fig. 13.25).

The therapy followed in 3 cycles at 8, 16 and 19 applications, which combine to a total of 43 treatments in 105 days. The treatment of the nasopharynx was not done because there is not enough study into the possible interactions of plasma with the respiratory tract in case inhalation takes place.

Directly connected to the exposure to plasma a highly significant pain reduction of 1.1 steps according to the visual analogue scale of 1–10 that measures pain intensity, as well as a highly significant improvement of pain during the longer term treatment (Fig. 13.26). Throughout the study period the patient did not have to systematically take pain medication. Also the systematic dosage of Cotrimoxazole could be stopped.

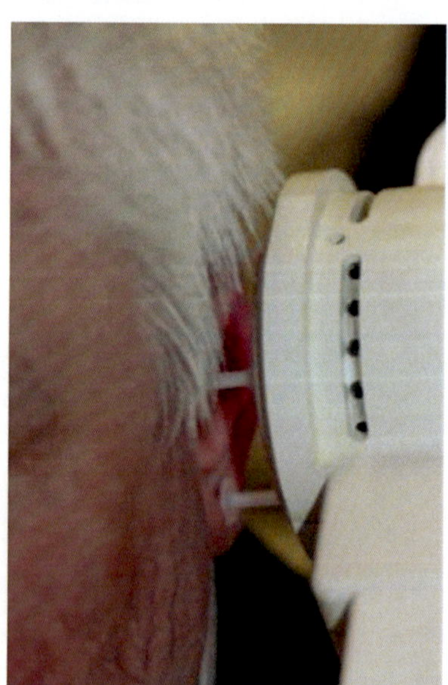

**Fig. 13.25** Plasma treatment of the infected ear canal

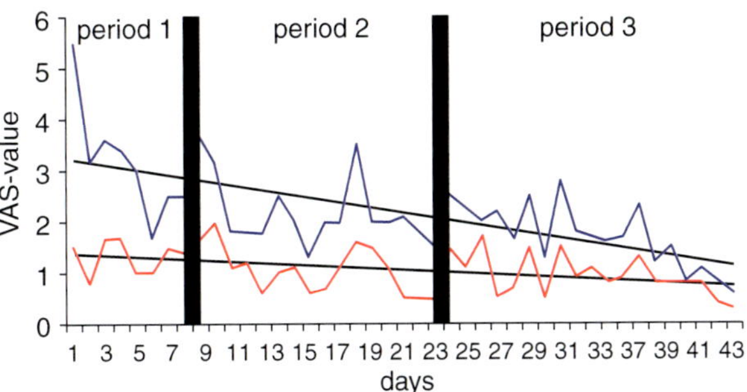


**Fig. 13.26** Development of pain during the long term treatment (blue: before plasma treatment, red: immediately after plasma treatment)

During and until 3 weeks after the last treatment with plasma there was no recurring infection in the treatment area, but after 3 weeks, ESBL+ *Escherichia coli* bacteria were detected in the untreated nasopharynx.

As noted during previous studies, no side effects were found and the plasma treatment was completely painless.

Despite the limitation, that the plasma machine was not conceptualised for treating the ear canal, and that the penetration of the plasma would have been clearly limited by diffusion, the patient could be treated successfully.

## 13.10.7 Herpes Zoster

In order to reduce the effect of subjective experiences, in the last large patient group of this research project, treatments were randomised by patient and not by localisation. The effect of low temperature argon plasma was investigated on the zoster rash and the acute pain [30]. In this randomised, placebo controlled prospective clinical study, patients received a daily 5 min plasma treatment per treatment area. The control group was treated with argon gas as a placebo for 5 min. Each patient received the standard therapy recorded in the study protocol (antiviral, analgetic and antiseptic treatment). In total at most four rashes were treated, because otherwise the treatment time would have totalled more than 20 min. The increase of the treatment time from 2 to 5 min was explained because Herpes Zoster is an intracellular viral disease. In order to achieve the desired effect, it was assumed that a longer treatment time with plasma would be necessary.

It should be noted that treatment of zoster rashes near the eyes was avoided, because there has been no detailed investigation into possible interactions of plasma with the eye.

In total 41 patients were included in the study (see Table 13.2). There were four drop-outs. Two patients were topically treated with Vioform lotion instead of the Polyhexanide mentioned in the study protocol and therefore the digital clinical figures could not be evaluated. In two further patients the PCR examination revealed that they did not suffer from an infection caused by the Varicella Zoster virus, but a Herpes simplex virus.

**Table 13.3** Characteristics of the pain treatment in the patient group

| | Treatment (plasma 5 min) | Control (argon gas 5 min) |
|---|---|---|
| Aciclovir 5 mg/kg i.v., initial dose | 8/19 (42.1%) | 7/18 (38.9%) |
| Aciclovir 7.5 mg/kg i.v., initial dose | 9/19 (47.4%) | 9/18 (50%) |
| Aciclovir 10 mg/kg i.v., initial dose | 2/19 (10.5%) | 2/18 (11.1%) |
| Aciclovir increased during study | 2/19 (10.5%) | 0 |
| Initial paracetamol use | 13/19 (68.4%) | 10/18 (55.6%) |
| Paracetamol increase during study | 1/19 (5.3%) | 3/18 (16.7%) |
| Paracetamol reduction during study | 3/19 (15.8%) | 1/18 (5.6%) |
| Initial tramadol use | 5/19 (26.3%) | 2/18 (11.1%) |
| Tramadol increase during study | 3/19 (15.8%) | 2/18 (11.1%) |
| Tramadol reduction during study | 1/19 (5.3%) | 0 |
| Initial Pregabalin use | 17/19 (89.5%) | 14/18 (77.8%) |
| Pregabalin increase during study | 0 | 1/18 (5.6%) |

The minimum treatment duration was 3 day, up to a maximum of 8 or 9 days, depending on treatment group.

It could be shown that one additional plasma treatment (19 patients, average age 64.3 years, 42.1% female, see Table 13.3), the acute zoster pain was reduced significantly more often ($p < 0.01$) and also significantly more strongly (median of 0.6 vs. 0.3, $p < 0.05$), when compared with patients of the control group (18 patients, average age 61.8 years, 38.9% female). Furthermore no patient in the plasma group showed a deterioration in pain after the treatment, vs. 12.3% in the argon group who complained of worsened pain. The initial pain (median) was higher in the plasma group, the pain at discharge (median) was higher in the control group.

The proportion of patients which were initially treated with Paracetamol or Tramadol, was higher in the plasma group (Table 13.3). However, in the control group the pain medication had to be increased more often, whereas they were reduced more often in the plasma group (Table 13.3).

This study only allowed for limited observations with regard to the possible influence of plasma on long term pain (so-called postherpes zoster). In order to remedy that a longer observation time would be checked. The voluntary follow-up examinations 2, respectively 4 weeks after the last treatment were at the 4 week period only performed on 47.3% of the patients in the plasma group and 55.6% of cases in the control group. Still, in the plasma group only 22.2% and in the control group however 40% of patients of pain. Three independent zoster specialists (two dermatologies and one internist) judged the evolution of the zoster lesions in the first days paying special attention to the development of blisters and erythema, and decided that the plasma treated areas were significantly better than the control areas (see Fig. 13.27). Also, the overall aspect looks better, but without a significant trend (Fig. 13.28).

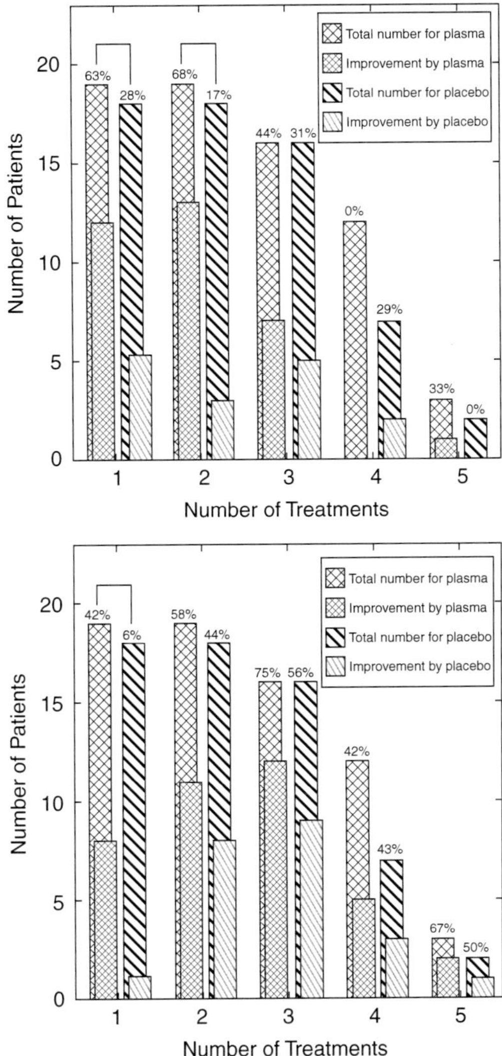


**Fig. 13.27** Comparison of plasma vs placebo treatment. Left: The healing process of the zoster blisters were evaluated by three independent Herpes Zoster specialists according to a double blind procedure. The Plasma treated rashes were judged as better than the control areas. Significant changes were noted on the first and second day of evaluation. Right: The healing process of the erythemas was also judged as better in the plasma treated rashes than the control areas. Significant changes were noted on the first day of evaluation (Fig. 13.28)

The clinical overall aspect of the Zoster rashes were evaluated by three independent Herpes Zoster specialists in a double blind procedure. The plasma treated rashes were judged as better than the control areas. Significant changes were not noted between the two treatment groups.

Again no side effects were recorded and the treatment was absolutely painfree.

In summary, this study of Herpes Zoster patients shows that plasma can significantly reduce acute pain in Zoster lesions and at the same time significantly improve the healing process.

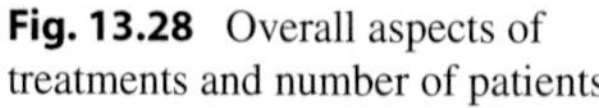

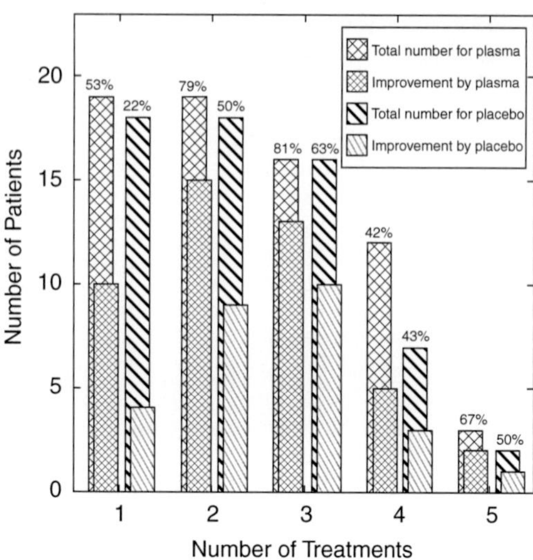


**Fig. 13.28** Overall aspects of treatments and number of patients

## 13.11 Post Market Case Studies

### 13.11.1 Adtec SteriPlas Use on Chronic Burn Wound

Non-thermal atmospheric gas plasma has already been shown to decrease the bacterial load in chronic wound dermatological applications. In this study, standard care is compared with standard care plus cold atmospheric argon plasma treatment for the treatment of a non-healing burn wound with exposed tibial bone on the left shin with the aim of increasing the rate of healing of the wound and reducing bacterial colonisation.

### 13.11.2 Study Outline

The patient had two sites on this left shin wound (separated by a bridge of granulation tissue,) which were selected for the study. The smaller proximal wound (4.37 cm$^2$) was used as the control, while the larger wound (15.32 cm$^2$) wound was selected to receive cold plasma treatment.

Both wound sites received the same standard care which included silver dressings. The distal wound received cold atmospheric argon plasma treatment for 2 min every 3–4 days for 16 days and wound swabs were taken from both sites before every treatment. The timing of the treatments was to occur at the same day of the routine dressing changes. Three dimensional pictures of the wounds were taken before each treatment session with a stereo 3-D camera (Eykona, Fuel 3D, UK) (Fig. 13.29).

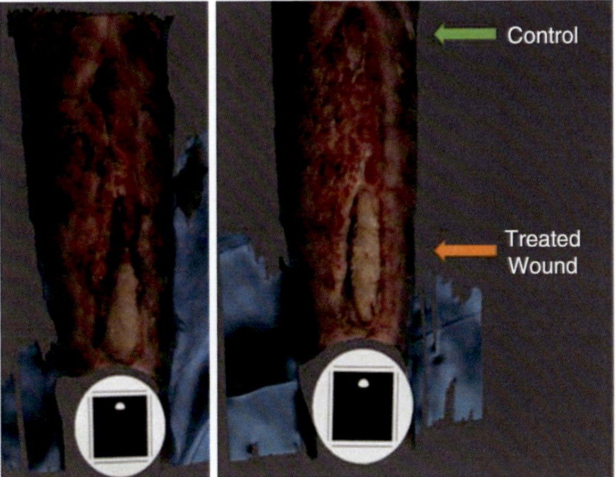


**Fig. 13.29** Comparison of wound day 1 (left) and day 15 (right)

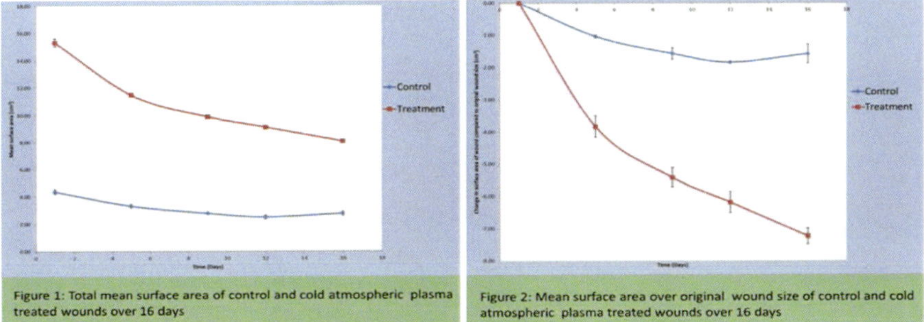


**Fig. 13.30** Comparison of surface area and absolute wound size for day 1 and 16

## 13.12 Results

The distal wound received a total of 5 treatments. Both the control and treatment wounds showed a significant decrease in surface area at day 16 (2.77 $cm^2$ for control, 8.07 $cm^2$ for treated wound, $p < 0.01$). However, the cold atmospheric argon plasma treated wound showed a greater reduction in absolute wound size (−7.24 $cm^2$ vs. −1.59 $cm^2$, $p < 0.01$) and percentage of original wound (−47.3% vs. −36.5%, $p = 0.005$) [31]. Full Study Details can be obtained (Fig. 13.30).

### 13.12.1 Adtec SteriPlas Treatment of Hard to Heal Wounds

Non-thermal atmospheric gas plasma has already been shown to decrease the bacterial load in chronic wound dermatological applications. In this study, a 68-year old patient at Regensburg Hospital with very chronic ulcers on the lower right leg since 2011 was selected for plasma treatment. The patient had known microangiopathy and chronic thrombosis of the right vena femoralis superficialis (postthrombotic syndrome). He also has polycythemia vera and had been treated with hydroxyurea, but the ulcers had not healed.

### 13.12.2 Study Outline

Plasma-treatment started on the 15th of July 2015, twice weekly until January 2016.

## 13.13 Results

During plasma treatment, the ulcers continuously improved and are now almost healed (he received a total of 51 plasma treatments between 15.07.2015 until 07.01.2016.) Professor Sigrid Karrer of Regensburg Hospital reported that 'the patent had a very long history of non-healing, very painful ulcers with a history of wound infections requiring antibiotics. Thus, we are very satisfied by this result' (Fig. 13.31).

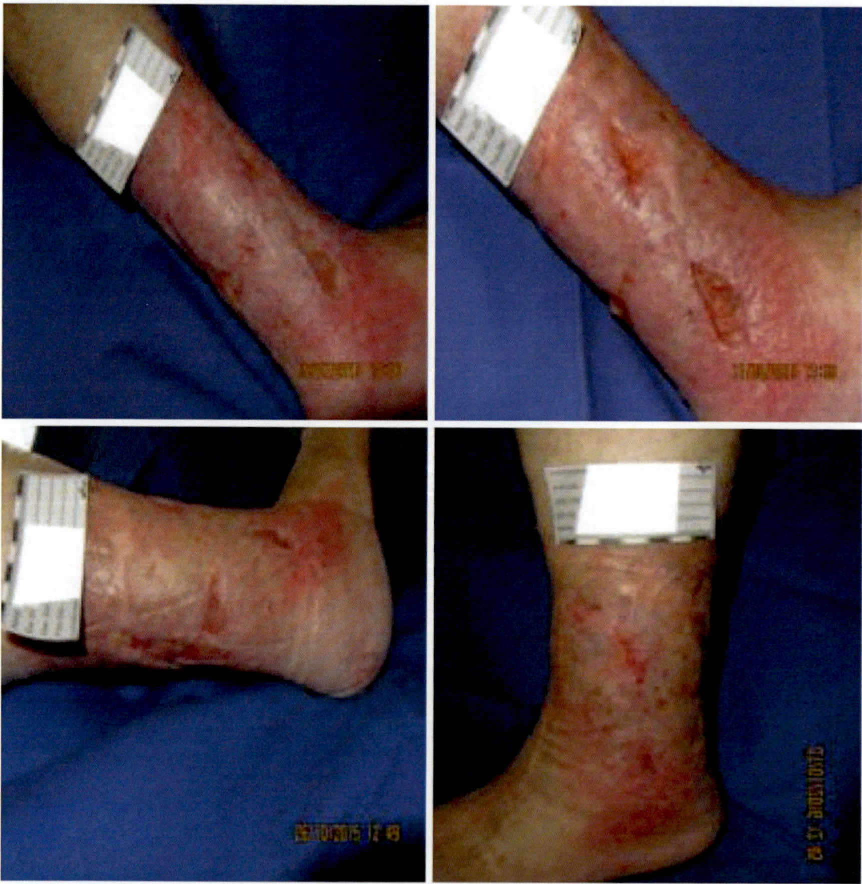

**Fig. 13.31** Comparison of plasma treatment results over 6 months

## 13.14 Adtec SteriPlas Treatment of Surgical Site Infections

Non-thermal atmospheric gas plasma has already been shown to decrease the bacterial load in chronic wound dermatological applications. Recent results on treatment of surgical site infections show promising results [24].

Patient 1—a male patient, 66 years, developed nearly 1 year after implantation of a LVAD an infection of the pump pocket with Enterobacter cloacae complex and was then selected for plasma treatment.

Patient 2—male 71 years with Coronary artery disease following CABG-operation BMI >40, Diabetes. The patient developed secondary a seroma after sternal refixation. The swabs taken from the seroma showed Staph epidermidis.

## 13.15 Study Outline

Patient 1—Plasma treatment started in January 2016 and the patient was treated with 3 min plasma three times a week for 3 weeks. First wound closure: In combination with NPWT, Secondary with ActiMaris.

Patient 2—Plasma treatment started in January 2016 and the patient was treated for 5 min three times a week. Treatment time 2 weeks in combination with NPWT in the small access area.

## 13.16 Results

Patient 1—Swabs were negative on plasma treatment and the wound showed good healing with complete closure of the wound after 3 weeks treatment (Figs. 13.32, 13.33 and 13.34).

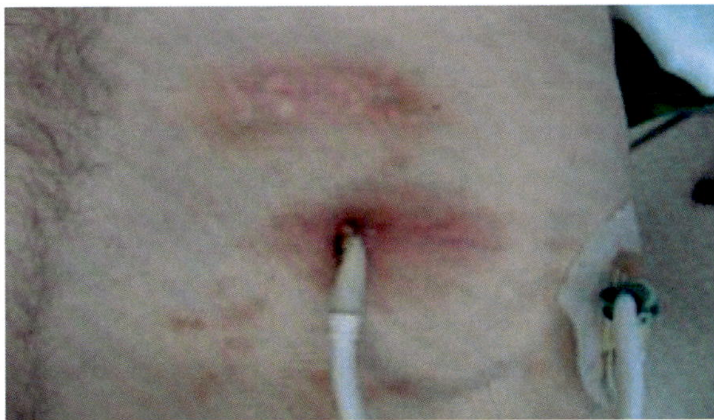

**Fig. 13.32** Driveline entry

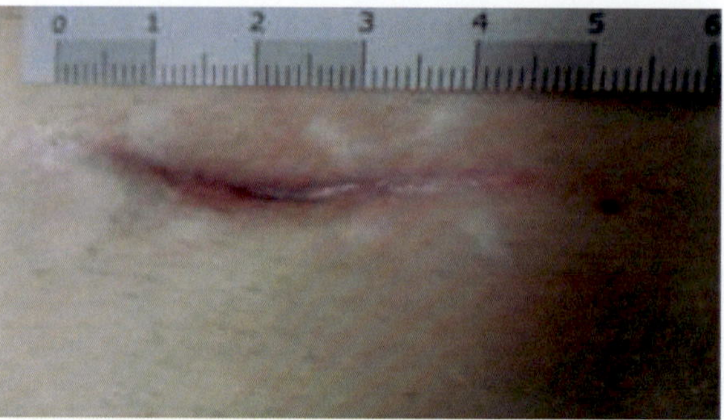


**Fig. 13.33** Closed wound. Patient 2—Patient showed good healing after treatment. Swabs were negative and wound closure was performed only with three sutures without opening the complete wound

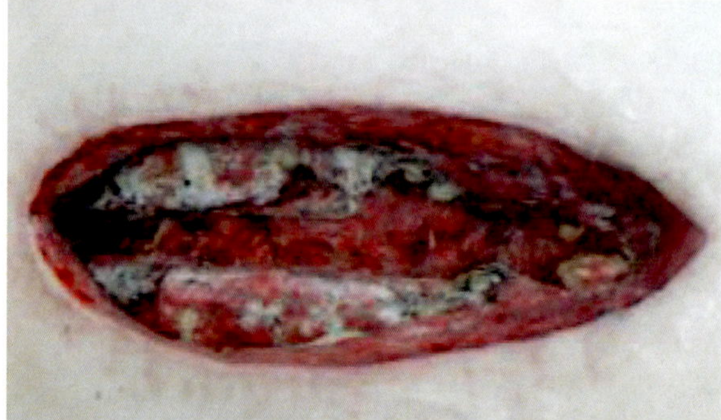

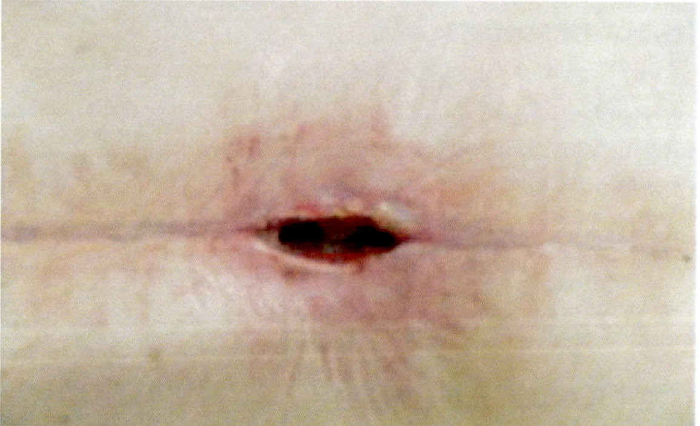

**Fig. 13.34** Comparison of wound before and after closure. These tests were carried out by Dr. Heinrich Rotering at the Universitätsklinik Münster, Germany and further research is planned on the use of plasma on surgical site infections

## 13.17 Adtec SteriPlas Treatment of Infected Drivelines

Gas plasma has already been shown to decrease the bacterial load in chronic wound dermatological applications. Recent results [21] on treatment of infected LVAD drivelines show promising results. Gas Plasma can migrate too hard to reach areas to treat infections.

## 13.18 Study Outline

Six patients were treated with Adtec SteriPlas as part of their post-surgery standard treatment.

## 13.19 Results (Fig. 13.35)

**Cold atmospheric plasma**

**CAP-Treatment of infected LVAD-systems**

| *Patient* | *Sex* | *Age* | *Localisation* | *Species* | *Treatment time* | *Result* |
|---|---|---|---|---|---|---|
| *H.P.G.* | *M* | *66* | *Pump pocket* | *Enterobacter cloacae complex* | *3 weeks* | *Complete healing* |
| *R.K.* | *M* | *28* | *Drivellne* | *Pseodomonas oeroginosa (4MRGN)* | *9 weeks* | *On going treatment* |
| *F.P.* | *M* | *42* | *Drivellne* | *Staph, aureus, Klebsiella penumonla* | *7 weeks* | *Healing nearly completed* |
| *U.R* | *M* | *61* | *Drivellne* | *Chronic fistula, Negativ swabs* | *2 weeks* | *Complete healing* |
| *U.T* | *F* | *49* | *Drivellne* | *Enterobacter cloacae complex, Staph, aureus* | *2 weeks* | *Complete healing* |
| *H.W.* | *M* | *64* | *Drivellne* | *Enterobacter cloacae complex* | *8 weeks* | *Wound size reduction* |

UKM

New treatment options for infected chronic implants with cold atmosheric plasma
H.Robering WUWHS Florence 2016

**Fig. 13.35** Summary of patients and results. These tests were carried out by Dr. Heinrich Rotering at the Universitätsklinik Münster, Germany and further research is planned on the use of plasma on surgical site infections

## 13.20 Plasma Treatment of Actinic Keratosis

Adtec Healthcare in collaboration with University Hospital Essen treated a small group of Actinic Keratosis patients with Adtec SteriPlas gas plasma.

In the case series, all treated lesions responded to plasma treatment with some showing complete clinical clearance after seven treatments. No side effects including inflammation or pain were recorded. Therefore, plasma might represent a novel, safe treatment method for AK that is worth being further investigated in prospective trials concerning application schemes and its exact biological effects.

The case series provided encouraging results leading to collaboration to do a clinical trial investigating the potential benefits and efficacy of plasma on Actinic Keratosis (start in August 2017).The case study results are published in the Journal of the European Academy of Dermatology and Venereology [32].

## 13.21 Efficacy of Plasma Treatment on Biofilm

Biofilms in wounds are considered to be one of the major challenges in infection management.

'Bacteria protected within biofilms are up to 1000 times more resistant to antibiotics…which severely complicates treatment options' [33].

Currently, either the physical method of debridement is used which is often time consuming, stressful for the patient and does not remove all of the microorganisms; wound dressings, which are changed on average twice a week '…but may take a considerable amount of time to achieve a granulating wound bed,' [34] or low doses of short term antibiotics that are given with little effect, 'Therefore there is great potential in this market for an alternative method of biofilm management that 'suppresses the biofilm without destroying the host cells' [35]. We believe Adtec SteriPlas technology has the potential to not only enable the healing of chronic wounds that are stalled by sub-clinical wound infection (biofilm) but accelerate healing time following intervention with our non-thermal gas plasma .

Earlier in vitro studies carried out by an independent microbiology testing laboratory (Perfectus Biomed) concluded that, 'Gas Plasma treatment may be an effective method of disrupting Staphylococcus aureus biofilms and has the potential to remove the challenge of persistent infection within a chronic wound thus allowing the wound to heal appropriately' [18, 19]. No organisms were detected after a 5 min treatment with Adtec SteriPlas (Fig. 13.36).

We are conducting a randomised controlled clinical trial in collaboration with Salford Royal NHS Foundation Trust UK (started February 2017). The primary objective of this project is to evaluate the efficacy of Adtec SteriPlas on sub-clinical wound infection (biofilm) in patients with diabetic foot ulcers (DFU) compared to those treated with standard care dressings. The secondary objective is to correlate

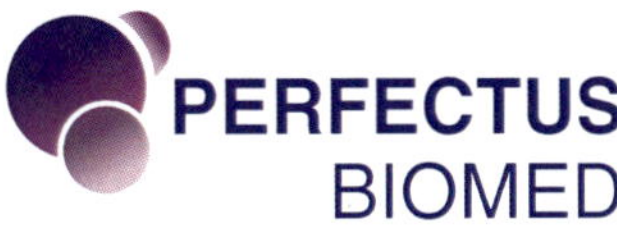


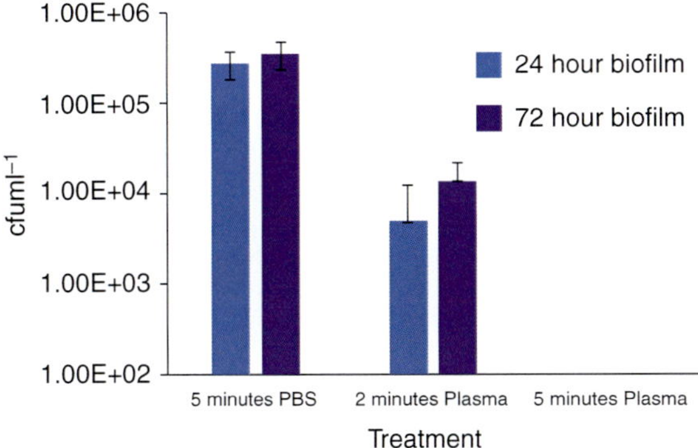


**Fig. 13.36** In-vitro results for biofilm

the clinical presentation of long standing DFUs with wound microbiology, biochemistry and histology.

**Acknowledgments** In writing this special issue, I would like to thank the Max—Planck Institute for Extraterrestrial Physics, Prof. G. Morfill, Dr. T. Shimizu, who collaborated on the research, and everyone else in the team.

## References

1. Shindo H, et al. High density plasma applied process technology: Realize Co. Ltd; 1993.
2. Jimbo Y, Kitamura Y, Kusaba K, Kikuchi M, Shindo H. Mode transition enhancement by permittivity of window materials in low frequency plasmas. Appl Phys Exp. 2009;2:016001.
3. Ishihara D, Noma T, Sai M, Stauss S, Tomai T, Terashima K. Development of a dielectric barrier discharge (DBD) cryo-microplasma: generation and diagnostics. Plasma Source Sci Technol. 2008;17:035008.
4. Ichiki T, Koidesawa T, Horiike Y. An atmospheric-pressure microplasma jet source for the optical emission spectroscopic analysis of liquid sample. Plasma Source Sci Technol. 2003;12:S16.
5. Akitsu T, et al. Micro/nano plasma technology and its applications. Frankfurt: CMC; 2006.
6. http:/www.erbe-med.de/.
7. Shimizu T, Steffes B, Pompl R, Jamitzky F, Bunk W, Morfill GE, Ramrath K, Georgi M, Stolz W, Schmidt H-U, Urayama T, Fujii S. Characterization of microwave plasma torch for decontamination. Plasma Process Polym. 2008;5:577–82. https://doi.org/10.1002/ppap.200800021.
8. Sato T, Miyahara T, Doi A, Ochiai S, Urayama T, Nakatani T. Sterilization mechanism for Escherichia Coli by plasma flow at atmospheric pressure. Appl Phys Lett. 2006;89: 73902.

9. Sato T, Fujioka K, Ramasamy R, Urayama T, Fujii S. Sterilization efficacy of a coaxial microwave plasma flow at atmospheric pressure. IEEE Trans Ind Appl. 2006;42:399–404.
10. Sato T, Doi A, Urayama T, Nakatani T, Miyahara T. Inactivation of Escherichia Coli by a coaxial microwave plasma flow. IEEE Trans Ind Appl. 2007;43:1159–63.
11. http://bken.net/hifu.htm/.
12. http://moltolice.livedoor.biz/archives/50202715.html.
13. http://www.wound-treatment.jp/title_kiso.htm.
14. Top five treatment costs of skin diseases. American Academy of Dermatology Report 2005. Prepared by the Lewin Group.
15. Maisch T, Bosserhoff AK, Unger P, Heider J, Shimizu T, Zimmermann JL, Morfill GE, Landthaler M, Karrer S. Investigation of toxicity and mutagenicity of cold atmospheric argon plasma. Environ Mol Mutagen. 2017;58(3):172–7.
16. Isbary G, Heinlin J, Shimizu T, Zimmermann JL, Morfill G, Schmidt H-U, Monetti R, Steffes B, Bunk W, Li Y, Klaempfl T, Karrer S, Landthaler M, Stolz W. Successful and safe use of 2 min cold atmospheric argon plasma in chronic wounds: results of a randomized controlled trial. Br J Dermatol. 2012;167(2):404–10.
17. Ermolaeva SA, Varfolomeev AF, Yu M, Chernukha DS, Yurov MM, Vasiliev AA, Kaminskaya MMM, Romanova JM, Murashev AN, Selezneva II, Shimizu T, Sysolyatina EV, Shaginyan IA, Petrov OF, Mayevsky EI, Fortov VE, Morfill GE, Naroditsky BS, Gintsburg AL. Bactericidal effects of non-thermal argon plasma in vitro, in biofilms and in the animal model of infected wounds. J Med Microbiol. 2011;60:75–83.
18. Booth R. Wounds UK 2015. Antibiofilm activity demonstrated following treatment with a novel plasma device (Poster presentation).
19. Westgate S. EWMA 2016. Antibiofilm activity demonstrated following treatment with a novel plasma device. Bremen (Poster presentation).
20. Rotering H. EWMA 2016. Cold atmospheric plasma- new options for infection control in wound management. Bremen (Oral presentation).
21. Rotering H. WUWHS 2016 cold atmospheric plasma- new treatment options for infected chronic implants. Florence (Oral presentation).
22. Isbary G, Morfill GE, Schmidt H-U, Georgi M, Ramrath K, Heinlin J, Karrer S, Landthaler M, Shimizu T, Steffes B, Bunk W, Monetti R, Zimmermann JL, Pompl R, Stolz W. A first prospective randomized controlled trial to decrease bacterial load using cold atmospheric argon plasma on chronic wounds in patients. Br J Dermatol. 2010;163(1):78–82.
23. Arndt S, Unger P, Wacker E, Shimizu T, Heinlin J, Li Y-F, Hubertus T, Morfill GE, Zimmermann JL, Bosserhoff A-K, Karrer S. Cold Atmospheric plasma (CAP) Changes gene expression of key molecules of the wound healing machinery and improves wound healing in vitro and in vivo. PLoS One. 2013;8(11):e79325.
24. Shimizu T, Nosenko T, Morfill GE, Sato T, Schmidt H-U, Urayama T. Characterization of low-temperature microwave plasma treatment with and without UV light for disinfection. Plasma Process Polym. 2010;7:288–93.
25. Arndt S, Landthaler M, Zimmemann JL, Unger P, Wacker E, Shimizu T, Li YF, Morfill GE, Bosserhoff AK, Karrer S. Effects of cold atmospheric plasma (CAP) on ß-defensins, inflammatory cytokines, and apoptosis-related molecules in keratinocytes in vitro and in vivo. PLoS One. 2015;10(3):e0120041.
26. Heinlin J, Zimmermann JL, Zeman F, Bunk W, Isbary G, Landthaler M, Maisch T, Monetti R, Morfill GE, Shimizu T, Steinbauer J, Stolz W, Karrer S. Randomized placebo-controlled human pilot study of cold atmospheric argon plasma on skin graft donor sites. Wound Repair Reg. 2013;21(6):800–7.
27. Isbary G, Stolz W, Shimizu T, Monetti R, Bunk W, Schmidt H-U, Morfill GE, Klaempfl TG, Steffes B, Thomas HM, Heinlin J, Karrer S, Landthaler M, Zimmermann JL. Cold atmospheric argon plasma treatment may accelerate wound healing in chronic wounds: results of a retrospective in vivo randomized controlled study. Clin Plasma Med. 2013;1(2):25–30.
28. Isbary G, Morfill G, Zimmermann J, Shimizu T, Stolz W. Cold atmospheric plasma: a successful treatment of lesions in Hailey-Hailey disease. Arch Dermatol. 2011;147(4):388–90.

29. Isbary G, Shimizu T, Zimmermann J, Hubertus T, Morfill G, Stolz W. Cold atmospheric plasma for local infection control and subsequent pain reduction in a patient with chronic post operative ear infection. New Microbes New Infect. 2013;1(3):41–3.
30. Isbary G, Shimizu T, Zimmermann JL, Heinlin J, Al-Zaabi S, Rechfeld M, Morfill GE, Karrer S, Stolz W. Randomized placebo-controlled clinical trial showed cold atmospheric argon plasma relieved acute pain and accelerated healing in herpes zoster. Clin Plasma Med. 2014;2(2):50–5.
31. Kwang CL. Wounds UK 2015. Use of cold atmospheric plasma treatment in a chronic burn wound (Poster presentation).
32. Wirtz M, Stoffels I, Dissemond J, Schadendorf D, Roesch A. Actinic keratoses treated with cold atmospheric plasma. J Eur Acad Dermatol Venereol. 2018;32(1):e37–9. https://doi.org/10.1111/jdv.14465.
33. Potera C. Antibiotic Resistance: biofilm dispersing agent rejuvenates older antibiotics. Environ Health Perspect. 2010;118(7):A288.
34. Ousey K, Fumarola S, Cook L, Bianchi J. The Missing Link: the key to improved wound assessment. Case Study. Br J Nurs. London. 2012. http://eprints.hud.ac.uk/15484/.
35. Heyman H, Van De Looverbosch DE, Meijer EP, Schols JM. Benefits of an oral nutritional supplement on pressure ulcer healing in long-term care residents. J Wound Care. 2008;17:476–8.

# Plasma Application for Hygienic Purposes in Medicine, Industry, and Biotechnology: Update 2017

14

Axel Kramer, Frieder Schauer, Roald Papke, and Sander Bekeschus

## 14.1 Introduction

This publication is an update of several fields of hygiene covered in a review and book chapter [1, 2]. It comprises the most prominent advances made in the past 2 years. To avoid redundancy, the literature cited in sources 1 and 2 have not been cited in the present paper.

## 14.2 Reasons for Application in Medicine, Industry and Biotechnology

**The use of cold atmospheric plasma (CAP) is successful or promising for hygienic indications when antimicrobial, antiviral, and/or antibiofilm activity is required. This is especially relevant for materials that are thermolabile or sensitive against chemical microbicidal active agents and/or when microbicidal chemical agents cannot or only insufficiently reach the site of action.**

A. Kramer (✉) • R. Papke
Institute of Hygiene and Environmental Medicine, University Medicine Greifswald, Greifswald, Germany
e-mail: kramer@uni-greifswald.de; roald.papke@uni-greifswald.de

F. Schauer
Department of Applied Microbiology, Ernst-Moritz-Arndt University of Greifswald, Greifswald, Germany
e-mail: schauer@uni-greifswald.de

S. Bekeschus
Leibniz-Institute for Plasma Science and Technology (INP Greifswald), Greifswald, Germany
e-mail: sander.bekeschus@inp-greifswald.de



H.-R. Metelmann et al. (eds.), *Comprehensive Clinical Plasma Medicine*,
https://doi.org/10.1007/978-3-319-67627-2_14

Because of the highly active antimicrobial components of CAP, the spectrum of its activity includes all vegetative bacteria species, including multidrug resistant organisms as well as viruses. An intrinsic resistance against CAP is not possible, given its mode of action. This has been confirmed by results with all organisms tested to date [3–13]. Bacterial inactivation via discharge plasma is highest with air plasma, followed by $N_2$ plasma, while $O_2$ plasma was the least effective [14]. Bacterial spores [15–21] and fungi [22–26] were also killed.

CAP partially or completely eliminates mono- or multispecies biofilms, depending on exposure time and source of plasma; quorum-sensing related virulence factors are also affected by the treatment [9, 27–36]. Although the adherence and viability of *Candida albicans* in biofilm was reduced, after short treatment times, CAP left some C. *albicans* in superficial infections of the skin or mucosa, for example [37]. The inactivation of biofilms in cereal-based media and beef extract is relevant for use in the food industry [38]. Vitamin C destabilizes bacterial biofilms and renders them more susceptible to CAP killing, which could also be relevant for pre-treatment of biofilms on living tissues [39].

Viruses [40, 41] and prions [42], pathogens known for their extraordinary resistances, are inactivated by CAP. Depending on the plasma source and exposure time, virucidal disinfection or sterilization is attainable. This was demonstrated for noroviruses, hepatitis A, B and C virus, Newcastle disease virus, avian influenza virus, adenoviruses, herpes simplex, influenza and paramyxo virus as well as bacteriophages [43–48]. Without destroying antigenic determinants, viruses can be inactivated to produce an inactivated vaccine [49].

The charged species of CAP interact chemically with biological material. Depending on the plasma force, this may be complemented by physical means, such as shear stress, ion bombardment damage, thermal effects, radiation, and/or electrical fields [46, 50, 51]. Many species produced by CAP act antimicrobially. This includes singlet oxygen ($^1O_2$), superoxide ($O_2^-$), ozone ($O_3$), hydroxyl radicals (OH•), nitrogen radicals (N•), nitric oxide (•NO), nitrogen dioxide ($NO_2^•$), peroxynitrite ($ONOO^-$), hydrogen peroxide ($H_2O_2$), organic radicals, electrons, energetic ions, and charged particles (RO•, $RO_2$•) [52–60]. Under specific operating conditions, plasma-derived UV photons can be a dominant microbicidal component [61, 62]. The targets in viruses are capsid proteins and nucleic acids as well as lipids in enveloped viruses [46]. Electrical fields and charged particles could play a significant role in inactivation [51], especially for He-$O_2$ cold atmospheric pressure plasmas [63].

In contrast to microbiostatic agents, no resistance development is to be expected for CAP. This may be due to the high flux of reactive species derived by CAP, a principle that has been employed for millions of years by phagocytes to kill microorganisms [64]. Defects in the reactive species-derived killing in chronic granulomatous disease exemplify the importance of this mechanism [65]. Combined with the action of UV radiation and electrical fields, CAP releases a large number of different reactive species that may complement each other's microbicidal activity. Additional advantages of CAP over traditional antimicrobial agents are the absence of toxic residues, reduced water consumption, low energy requirements, low costs, and a relative inertness on materials sensitive to the chemical reactivity of some agents. Moreover, some materials cannot withstand the chemical reactivity.

**By supporting somatic cell growth but not bacterial proliferation, surface treatment of implants with CAP promotes implant integration in the body.**

Analogous to the antiseptic agent polihexanide [66], CAP improves the bioactivity of surfaces and thus increases the tissue compatibility of implant materials or inhibits the attachment of pathogens. This results in various application possibilities for improving the function of alloplastic implant surfaces, as well as other surfaces upon which the attachment of somatic cells is to be supported and that of microorganisms inhibited.

**CAP changes the metabolic profiles of microorganisms.**

CAP can also induce metabolic modification in microorganisms, which may be useful to improve biodegradation or to increase the production of specific metabolites. This enables the use of CAP in food production, wastewater treatment, and a possible alteration of microorganisms to change their resistances, for example, by intracellular destruction of R-plasmids.

**CAP eliminates odors or noxae by oxidation.**

This property is used for air purification combined with inactivation of microorganisms.

## 14.3 Antimicrobial Applications in Medicine

### 14.3.1 Requirements on Antimicrobial and Antiviral Efficacy

Since the following requirements for antimicrobial efficacy must be fulfilled for a method or substance to qualify as a chemical disinfectant or antiseptic, they are also mandatory if CAP is used in this field.

#### 14.3.1.1 Sterilization

**A sterility assurance level (SAL) of $10^{-6}$ is generally accepted for sterilization.**

By extrapolating the reduction rates following extreme artificial initial contamination, a theoretical overall CAP performance of at least 12 $\log_{10}$ increments (overkill conditions) is demanded to assure an SAL of $10^{-6}$. Practical proof of the required sterility assurance level of $10^{-6}$ is not possible due to infeasible sample sizes. Moreover, the attainability of this SAL is fundamentally questionable, at least in non-thermal procedures. Thus, the question to discuss is whether undifferentiated adherence to the concept of sterility assurance on the basis of a single SAL of $10^{-6}$ is justifiable in terms of patient- or user-safety requirements, costs and energy efficiency. Therefore, in terms of practical considerations, a concept of tiered SALs is recommended, analogous to the comparable and well-established categorization into "High-level disinfection", "Intermediate-level disinfection" and "Low-level disinfection". In the case of aseptic preparation, filling and production procedures, a mean contamination probability of $10^{-3}$ is assumed. In automated processes, lower contamination rates can be realized. In the case of the production of re-usable medical devices, a reduction of at least 2 $\log_{10}$ increments can be achieved through prior cleaning in validated cleaning and disinfecting devices. With chemical disinfection, a further reduction of $\geq$5 $\log_{10}$ increments is achieved. Finally, the amount of pathogens necessary to cause an infection must be considered. Logically considering all aspects, it seems possible to partially reduce sterility assurance levels without any loss of safety.

Hence, we suggest the following tiered SAL values, tailored to the respective sterilization task [67]:

- SAL $10^{-6}$ for heat-resistant pharmaceutical preparations (parenterals), suggested term: "Pharmaceutical sterilization",
- SAL $10^{-4}$ for heat-resistant medical devices, suggested term: "High-level sterilization",
- SAL $10^{-3}$ for heat-sensitive re-usable medical devices, under the precondition of a validated cleaning efficacy of >4 lg increments, suggested term: "Low-level sterilization".

#### 14.3.1.2 Disinfection

**The quantitative suspension test requires a reduction of 5 $\log_{10}$ for bactericidal efficacy, and 4 $\log_{10}$ for fungicidal, tuberculocidal and virucidal activity** [68, 69].

Bactericidal efficacy for surface disinfection must be 5 $\log_{10}$, but for *Pseudomonas aeruginosa* and fungi with 4 h of exposure 4 $\log_{10}$. For instrument disinfection against bacteria, 5 $\log_{10}$ is also required, and against mycobacteria and *Aspergillus brasiliensis* 4 $\log_{10}$ is necessary [70].

The spectrum of activity of hand disinfection must encompass vegetative bacteria, yeasts and enveloped viruses (these agents possess "limited virucidal activity") [70]. The category "limited virucidal activity Plus" encompasses the activity of hand disinfection against noro-, rota- and adenoviruses, and "virucidal activity" also includes polio- and polyomaviruses [69, 71–73]. The range of activity for skin antiseptics encompasses vegetative bacteria and yeasts. For surface disinfection, the range of activity must encompass vegetative bacteria and yeasts. Depending on certain conditions, other pathogens such as *Mycobacterium tuberculosis*, dermatophytes and molds, spores of *Clostridium difficile*, noro-, rota-, adeno- or papilloma viruses need to be inactivated. Instrument disinfectants are required to be bactericidal, levurocidal, possess limited virucidal activity, and be effective against mycobacteria. If no sterilization step follows, they also need to be fungicidal (test organism *Aspergillus brasiliensis*) and virucidal.

Practical test methods for hygienic and surgical hand disinfection or skin antisepsis are required to at least reach the efficacy of the reference method (60%v/v propan-2-ol, 60%v/v propan-1-ol or 70%v/v propan-2-ol).

#### 14.3.1.3 Antisepsis

**Given a typical organic load of a wound, the efficacy of wound antiseptics must be a reduction of the tested organisms $\geq 3 \log_{10}$ in the declared exposure time in both the suspension test and on germ carriers** [74, 75].

### 14.3.2 Current Applications

Currently, CAP is only used for sterilization processes. Several methods of producing plasma for sterilization have been developed, including direct current discharge, radio-frequency discharge, dielectric barrier discharge (DBD) and pulsed corona discharge [76].

#### 14.3.2.1 Plasma-Supported Hydrogen Peroxide Gas Sterilization

**The use of CAP results in a SAL $\leq 10^{-6}$ within validated limits (as documented in the manual) of specified lumen diameters.**

As an innovation for the sterilization of polymeric and heat-sensitive medical devices (MDs), the first sterilization device (Sterrad) was commercialized in 1993 and thereafter successfully introduced in health care services as well as industrial sterilization. The process involves the application of hydrogen peroxide (HPO) gas at a chamber wall temperature of 45°C and a corresponding chamber pressure of 6–10 Torr. After exposing the material to the gas, plasma generated by a high-frequency electromagnetic field is used to remove any HPO gas residue [77]. In addition to bacterial inactivation, HPO gas also shows virucidal activity and partially inactivates prions if combined with alkaline cleaning agents. The low relative humidity (5%) required during the sterilization process facilitates the use of this technology for reprocessing moisture-sensitive MDs. For specimens with smooth surfaces, a sure sterilization procedure was verified for *Bacillus pumilus, B. athrophaeus,*

*Geobacillus stearothermophilus, Mycobacterium terrae*, and *Aspergillus brasiliensis,* the most resilient test organisms according to DIN EN ISO 14937 [78]. The packaging, Tyvek foil tube, cellophane or vial used in Cycle-shure bioindicators do not seem to be obstacles to sterilization. The necessary prerequisites for a successful sterilization procedure are clean, dry materials in hydrophobic packaging. Furthermore, the surface needs to be readily accessible, because complex and porous surfaces do not allow uniform penetration of the active components. Contamination with blood or salt strongly reduces the efficacy, and additional cleaning is needed prior to performing the procedure. Finally, the efficacy is greatly limited by the presence of metals in or on the MDs. Liquids or powders, cloth, fibrous cellulosic material such as swabs, long hollow bodies with blind ends, and sterilization material in metal containers cannot be sterilized in this way. The plasma-supported sterilization process follows these steps [77]: Vacuum phase to dry the goods, second vacuum phase to decrease the temperature to below the vaporization temperature of the sterilizing agent, single vaporization of the HPO-gas/water from a vial into the chamber (HPO 59%), diffusion phase with distribution of the HPO steam into the chamber, onto the surfaces and into the cavities of the to-be-sterilized material, third evacuation and creation of a high-frequency magnetic field between the chamber walls, the anode. The steps beginning with the second vacuum phase then repeat for a second cycle. New technologies allow an accumulation of the sterilizing agent in the most recent devices in order to improve penetration and efficiency.

Devices employed in industry for sterilization use comparable conditions. Now such devices use methods analogous to low-temperature steam-formaldehyde sterilization, where not only the concentration gradients but also mechanical pressure pulses enable the agent to enter cavities.

The performance qualification for the application situation is undertaken with a Process Challenge Device (PCD) with the Validation Kit in a half cycle. The PCD is configured to provide a greater challenge to the sterilization process than the validated lumen sizes [77]. For endoscopes of all types, sterilization (SAL of $10^{-6}$) was achieved in all test situations for all the Sterrad models tested, but the efficacy of Sterrad 200 and 100S sterilizers is greater than that of Sterrad 50 and 100 sterilizers [79].

#### 14.3.2.2 Peracetic Acid Plasma-Based Sterilization

Peracetic acid is the central component in this sterilization process, while the plasma just seems to decompose any chemical remnants of the gas that would otherwise remain on the sterilized item. The peracetic acid plasma-based sterilizer (Plazlyte) was found to be only partially satisfactory [1].

#### 14.3.2.3 Further Development in Plasma Sterilization

**$N_2$ or Ar-$N_2$ plasma.** Recent efforts to increase the plasma activity by using the afterglow of $N_2$ or Ar-$N_2$ plasma resulted in the required 6 $\log_{10}$ reduction of initial inoculum only after extremely long exposure times. Although the efficacy of the HPO gas alone could not be further enhanced, recent studies point to synergistic effects of plasma ions with nitrogen [1, 2]. This underlines the innovation potential of plasma in sterilization technology.

**Large-volume microwave-excited surface-wave and volume-wave plasma.** Successful inactivation of Tyvek-wrapped spore-forming bacteria at temperatures below 70°C and within 70–80 min was experimentally confirmed [80].

**Steam plasma flow autoclave.** When air was mixed with the steam flow at a rate of 1 or 4 L/min, sterilization was achieved within 30 min, because total OH radical generation increased with time. CAP was generated by a wire electrode toward the ground electrode, and the concentration of $H_2O_2$ increased after streamer propagation [81].

### 14.3.3 Prospective Applications

#### 14.3.3.1 Disinfection of Medical Devices and Surfaces

Traditional manual cleaning and disinfection practices in hospitals are often suboptimal. CAP technologies show potential for use in hospitals and can-together with different UV light systems-lead to newer "no-touch" (automated) decontamination technologies [82–84]. The degree of bacterial damage due to the inactivation processes is highly dependent on both treatment parameters and treated bacteria [85, 86]. On surfaces tested under real-life conditions, CAP-mediated disinfection can be reached within 30s–90s [1, 2, 87–89]. On cell phones, *Staphylococcus aureus* was eliminated within 10 min [90]. The potential of CAP for the decontamination of equipment used in outer space seems to be quite a promising alternative to the standard "dry heat" and $H_2O_2$ methods [91]. Ingress of CAP into cavities allows the disinfection of poorly accessible areas, such as the lumina of endoscopes [1, 2]. However, detailed technical solutions for CAP disinfection of MD and surfaces are still being developed. Of special interest is the development of mobile CAP devices. These could treat non-sterile goods, instruments, or other MDs right at the point of care, for example during surgery, to enable their reuse quickly. It might also be possible to use CAP with a specially configured plasma source to disinfect soft contact lenses, instead of the common, often insufficient treatment in disinfection solution overnight [1, 2]. Plasma jets show promise in decontaminating the surface of implants before wound closure, eliminating bacteria that adhered during surgery and improving the surface conditions [1, 92].

An alternative to direct plasma treatment is the large-scale generation of plasma-treated liquids. This approach is simple, inexpensive, and provides surface disinfection and sterilization [93].

#### 14.3.3.2 Disinfection of Hands

Alcohol-based hand disinfectants enable disinfecting the surface of both hands within 15 s and within 60 s for gels [94–97]. The absorption of the residual alcohol on the surface is considered harmless [71, 98]. Disinfectant dispensers must be available at every workplace [71, 100]. To date, no data exists which shows that CAP can match this efficacy [101] and tolerability, which are indispensible, since up to 162 daily hand disinfections are performed [99]. At present, the costs are also not comparable. A hospital with 1000 beds requires about thrice the amount of disinfectant dispensers as number of beds. Thus, the application of CAP would only be feasible if either its price was less than that of acquiring and maintaining this number of dispensers, or its performance and/or side effects on skin outperformed current antiseptics.

#### 14.3.3.3 Antisepsis

**Preoperative skin antisepsis**. This is one of the key components in the prevention of Surgical Site Infections (SSI), since antisepsis on the skin is intended to inhibit transfer of resident skin bacteria into the surgical wound [99, 102]. The bacterial flora mostly resides in the stratum corneum and distal areas of hair follicles and sebaceous glands. About a fifth of the flora is found at depths >0.3 mm [103]. Alcohols used in skin antiseptics do not completely deeply penetrate skin [104], but CAP efficiently spreads it into narrow channels [1, 2]. Especially surgery with high SSI risk due to the resident bacterial flora, such as shoulder and hip surgery, justify the use of CAP after initial antiseptic by alcohol-based products.

**Therapeutic skin antisepsis**. The combined treatment of silver nanoparticles with cold atmospheric-pressure air plasma was effective in healing and suppressing disease symptoms caused by clinical isolates of dermatophytes, such as species of *Epidermophyton*, *Trichophyton* and *Microsporum* [105]. *Trichophyton rubrum* growth was significantly inhibited by 62–91%, and CAP strongly suppressed fungal ergosterol biosynthesis by 27–54% [106]. Additionally, CAP strongly suppressed the growth of *Candida albicans* by 31–82%, its ergosterol biosynthesis by 40–91%, and its biofilm formation by 43–57%. Thus, CAP seems useful to treat *Candida*-related superficial and cutaneous infections in practice [107]. CAP treatment is also effective in onychomycosis and fungal nail infection [108].

**Oral cavity.** Since bacteria on teeth can penetrate up to 500–1000 μm into dentin, chemical disinfection is not very effective. After application of a micro jet to disinfect the root canal, a complete elimination of $10^6$ *Enterococcus faecalis* was achieved [109]. Up to a depth of 1 mm, complete destruction of endodontic biofilm in the root canal was documented [1, 2, 110]. CAP seems to be useful for treating *Streptococcus mitis* infected dentin and root surfaces [111, 112], as well as pathogenic oral biofilms of *Staphylococcus* and *Candida* spp. [28]. CAP was also used for treatment of Denture Stomatitis (DS). The successful inactivation of *Candida albicans* biofilms and the significant enhancement of its drug susceptibilities induced by the CAP present a promising strategy for the treatment of DS caused by drug-resistant *Candida* biofilms [113]. CAP can therefore help (also in combination with antiseptics) to reduce denture-associated candidiasis [31]. CAP also possesses bactericidal efficacy on *Streptococcus mitis* biofilms on microrough titanium dental implants [114]. CAP immobilizes antimicrobial peptides on dental implants [1, 2].

**Decolonization of MRSA**. Since only in vitro results are available on the elimination of MRSA by CAP [115], no predictions can currently be made on the decolonization success in colonized or infected MRSA patients. If the wound is solely colonized by MRSA, elimination by CAP can be achieved; otherwise, decontamination can only be successful if all reservoirs of MRSA are fought simultaneously (nasal vestibulum, oral cavity, antiseptic full-body wash). If the eyes are colonized, they have to be included into the process as well [116]. In contrast to alcohol, CAP does not possess remanent properties. This means that if decolonization is incomplete, recolonization will occur quickly.

**Wounds**. CAP seems to be effective for antisepsis of cutaneous wounds [3].

## 14.4 Applications in Environmental Technologies, Food Production, and Biotechnology

### 14.4.1 Decontamination of Food and Packaging

**CAP is highly effective against germs causing rot or food-related illness. Application in the food sector has the great advantage that no chemical residue remains and products suffer no reduction in quality**.

Since physical methods such as gamma and beta radiation, ultrasound, UV irradiation, high hydrostatic pressure, and pulsed electrical fields, as well as chemical methods such as ozonation or ethylene oxide have certain limitations, CAP was introduced into the food sector in 2006 [1, 2, 97, 117–120]. Successful application has been documented for the decontamination of raw foodstuffs, e.g., fish, meat, poultry, vegetables, fruit, seeds, spices, tea, eggs, milk, dried nuts, dry milk, and for surface decontamination inside the packaging, including bottles [121–152]. *Salmonella* spp., *Escherichia coli*, and *Listeria monocytogenes* were eliminated on tomatoes within reasonably short treatment times. On strawberries, however, even very long treatment times were insufficient for complete elimination, due to the more complex surface of these fruits [150]. *Escherichia* coli and *Salmonella* spp. were significantly reduced on lettuce and radicchio [137, 153–157]. Combined treatment with clove oil, thyme oil and lemongrass oil enhanced the antibacterial effect of CAP on eggs and pork loin, respectively [158–160]. *Erwinia* spp. were eliminated on potatoes by CAP application for a few seconds without damaging the vegetable. The reduction of 5 $\log_{10}$ levels that is required by the US Food and Drug Administration can be attained by CAP in a time between several seconds and 30 min, depending on the species of pathogen. Spores in spices were inactivated within 5 min [1, 2]. Dielectric Barrier Discharge (DBD) plasma sterilization allows reduction of *Pseudomonas aeruginosa* by 5.4 $\log_{10}$ in 60 s; after 300 s application time, no more bacteria were detectable. Using DBD, alkaline phosphatase (ALP), an enzyme naturally present in milk, was inactivated within a few seconds [161]. This highly efficient plasma source has various applications in the food industry [1, 2].

For decontamination and detoxification of foods at risk of fungal spoilage, plasma techniques are being increasingly used. Examples are walnuts, hazelnuts, pistachios, maize, palm fruits, mandarin oranges, onion powder, dried fish, or beef jerky contaminated with *Aspergillus flavus*, *A. parasiticus*, *A. brasiliensis*, *A. niger*, *Penicillium citrinum*, *P. italicum*, or *Cladosporium cladosporioides* [26, 162–170]. CAP reduced mycotoxins without affecting quality [165, 171–175].

Microbial biofilms and bacteria internalized in produce tissue or in vacuum package may reduce the effectiveness of decontamination methods. Consequently, advanced technologies including CAP techniques for biofilm control are constantly emerging [176]. The influence of CAP on different packaged foods or of different gas mixtures has thus been increasingly studied [36, 170, 177–182]. Changes in properties of edible films for food coating by CAP treatment were considered toxicologically irrelevant, as examined in a rat model [179]. Food-intrinsic factors and processing parameters can influence the efficacy of CAP treatment [142, 143, 183].

Treatment of seed soybeans with CAP not only reduced the microbial contamination, but also increased the speed of germination, water absorption, availability of seed nutrients, and increased the growth rate of the seedling. Moisture content, appearance of the foods, and nutrition levels were not altered [1, 2].

Allergens released during production onto the surface of the foodstuffs can be removed and any enzyme activity that influences the sensory and nutritional value of the foods can be deactivated [1, 2].

### 14.4.2 Improving the Properties of Food and Raw Materials

**CAP inhibits or reduces unwanted enzyme reactions. It can also be used to influence the content of desired and undesired ingredients** [184, 185].

During post-harvest processing of both freshly cut and dried fruits and vegetables, polyphenoloxidases and peroxidases need to be inactivated or inhibited to avoid undesirable browning reactions and thus loss of quality. CAP offers a promising "gentle" alternative to traditional chemical methods [186]. The content and residual activity of polyphenol oxidase was decreased in treated apple slices after treatment with gliding arc plasma. In parallel, an increase of total polysaccharide content in apple and sugarcane specimens was observed, which were induced by cell wall disintegration [187]. In addition, oxidases and peroxidases from potatoes and tomatoes were inactivated by CAP [186, 188]. CAP technology is considered a suitable non-conventional technique for the preparation of modified starch. The alterations are mainly due to depolymerization of amylose and amylopectin side chains. After CAP treatment, there is a decrease in molecular weight, viscosity, and gelatinization temperatures [189]. Changes in functional and rheological properties of corn and rice starch were evaluated [190–192]. CAP manipulates surface properties, increases the water absorption of parboiled rice, and reduces the cooking time by up to 8 min [193]. CAP also modifies the functionality of wheat flour or whey protein isolates [194, 195] and improves the adsorption properties of bentonite clay [196]. A hydrophobization of wood surfaces was achieved by combining liquid flame spray (LFS) and CAP treatment [197].

Corn steep liquor (CSL) is used for instance in the production of penicillin, animal food, and ethanol. By reverse vortex gliding arc and forward vortex gliding arc with droplet atomizer, a notable reduction of bacteria and $SO_2$ (60 resp. 20%) is achievable [198]. CAP increases not only the production yield of plants [199–201], but also improves their antioxidative properties [191]. The growth enhancement effect was not passed onto the next generation, and there was no change in gene expression in the second generation, allowing the conclusion that the growth enhancement of plants is brought about epigenetically [202]. Treatment of running water with CAP on *Arabidopsis thaliana* showed that the plants could tolerate longer periods of dehydration and required less water, in addition to exhibiting certain molecular changes [203, 204]. By applying CAP, the biomass and content of triterpene ergosterol and B-l-3-D-glucan of mycelial cultures of *Ganoderma lucidum* were increased. The changes observed seemed to depend on total energy input by the plasma sources and the kind of mycelial treatment (solid piece or suspension; direct treatment or application of plasma-treated medium). Thus, CAP might be a useful tool for optimizing biotechnological processes in medicinal mushrooms [205]. The endproducts are oxygen, water, and $CO_2$.

### 14.4.3 Control of Molds

**CAP is active against molds and may thus be an alternative to toxic fungicides.**

Since CAP proved to be effective against both the cause of blue stain, *Aureobasidium pullulans* and molds, the application onto wood or interior spaces in order to fight fungus might be an effective alternative to the use of biocides [206]. If chemical decontamination for fungal infestation is problematic due to remnants, the use of properly configured plasma sources is promising, since it also allows treating poorly accessible cavities, especially discharges where the afterglow is used enable directed gas flow into the cavities.

In agriculture, the surface microflora of seedlings can be altered by CAP in a manner that hinders saprophytic molds, which are phytopathogens and destroy seedlings. The efficacy of CAP treatment of wheat seedlings artificially contaminated with filamentous fungi decreased in the following order: *Fusarium nivale* > *F. culmorum* > *Trichothecium roseum* > *Aspergillus flavus* > *Aspergillus clavatus* [207]. Exposure of winter wheat grain to CAP resulted in the reduction of colonies of fungi forming on grain in 10 s [208]. In addition, strains of *Penicillium chrysogenum*, *Cladosporium cladosporioides*, and *Aspergillus fumigatus* were inactivated on artificial surfaces [209]. CAP treatment can also improve germination of canola (an oilseed) seedlings and protect them from damage caused by drought stress [210].

CAP can be also used for fungal decontamination of the washwater used for certain fruit (strawberries, cherries, red grapes) in the food and food-preservation sector, because the fungal counts in the washwater of moldy fruits are much higher than those recovered from healthy fruits. Treatment of the washwater with double atmospheric pressure cold plasma (DAPCP) for 7.5 min significantly reduced fungal cells, chiefly *Aspergillus* and *Penicillium* spp. [137]. During CAP treatment of fruit and vegetable processing wastewater (blackberries, date palm, tomato, beetroot), the bacterial count was also reduced and the endotoxins in the wastewater were reduced by up to 90.2% [211].

### 14.4.4 Decontamination and Degradation of Water, Wastewater and Soil

CAP can microbially decontaminate and chemically degrade water and soil [131, 212–217]. For water purification (organic pollution, contamination), dielectric barrier discharge, contact glow discharge electrolysis, and pulsed corona discharge may be utilized [218]. In the recirculation system of hydroponics for tomato seedlings, the plasma reactor consisted of a wire electrode placed in an insulating circular cylinder and a grounded electrode on a cylinder. The numbers of the plant pathogen *Ralstonia solanacearum* decreased (5 $\log_{10}$), while tomato plant seedlings with discharge plasma treatment were relatively healthy [219]. Using high-voltage pulsed plasma can decontaminate water involved in the food industry, for example, that used for poultry cleansing [220]. This reduces the load of wastewater containing chlorides or secondary reaction products, such as trihalogen methane. Similarly, the reduction of the microbial load in wastewater from animal feeding facilities, especially multi-resistant bacteria such as LA-MRSA, is of importance. The effect is mostly caused by oxidative reactive oxygen and nitrogen compounds in combination with acidification of the environment [1, 2]. An integrated microwave plasma source (partially) decontaminated or detoxified wastewater loaded with surfactants, pesticides, herbicides, toxins, dyes, and persistent organic compounds. Water loaded with cyanide, for example, from fertilizer or pesticides, can be removed almost completely by CAP. Oxidizing radicals react with dissolved pollutants and inactivate them. Plasma-derived UV radiation positively influences the deactivation of contaminants due to its oxidizing effect. Remnants of medications can also be removed effectively by short electrical impulses [1, 2, 212, 221–223]. CAP treatment can also improve the bioremediation and fertility of soils [1, 2].

### 14.4.5 Air Purification and Air Decontamination

**In air cleansing, CAP eliminates odors, noxae, and airborne microorganisms.**

CAP is used for air purification in combination with inactivation of microorganisms [1, 2, 224, 225]. The inactivation of bacteria or fungi is based primarily on ozonization. The decontamination of air polluted by volatile organic compounds, chlorofluorocarbons, and nitrogen oxides can be supported by CAP [226–229]. To degrade ethylene efficiently, a reactor of corona discharge coupled with $TiO_2$-activated carbon fiber is suitable [230]. CAP can also be used for the treatment of exhaust gas from engines, the removal of sulfur and nitrogen oxides of flue gases, the destruction of aromatics such as toluene, benzene and chlorobenzene, or the decomposition of trifluormethane or methylbutanal [231–237]. In some cases, the combination of biofiltration with CAP systems is useful [238]. The PlasmaNorm® procedure primarily filters particles and dust; afterwards, microorganisms and odor molecules are disintegrated by CAP. Non-disintegrated compounds are caught an activated carbon filter, which is continually regenerated by the plasma stream, and ozone is reduced to molecular oxygen [239].

### 14.4.6 Application in Biotechnological Processes

**The application of CAP can modify microorganisms to produce higher growth rates and biomass, modify enzymes, change metabolism or produce special metabolites.**

CAP can modify and inactivate proteins and enzymes, altering their secondary and tertiary structures and oxidizing the most sensitive amino acid residues of the proteins [83, 195, 240, 241]. A modification of functionality by CAP treatment was demonstrated i.e. for serum albumin, lysozyme, lactate dehydrogenase, phospholipase and alkaline phosphatase [161, 242–245]. During immobilization of enzymes, CAP treatment can change enzymes or sorbents to improve the absorption or entrapment process [246]. In general, CAP can enhance catalyst activity and stability in chemical or biotechnological processes [247, 248]. Amino acids in aqueous solutions can be influenced by CAP in different ways, namely by hydroxylation, nitration, dehydrogenation and dimerization. Derivatization of amino acids resulting from CAP treatment can be categorized in descending order as follows: amino acids containing sulfur > aromatic amino acids > five-carbon aromatic amino acids > basic carbon-chain amino acids [216].

CAP improves the production of metabolites such as alcohol, triterpenes, ergosterol, polysaccharides and hydrogen. CAP may induce mutations in microorganisms for more effective decomposition of wastewater or in solid waste treatment [1, 2]. CAP can modify and intensify the secondary metabolism in microorganisms and crop plants. This was shown for the flavonol glycoside profile of *Pisum sativum* [249]. Additionally, CAP seems to influence the demethylation level of energy metabolism-related genes in soybean sprouts and seed germination [250]. In addition, membrane transporters were influenced by CAP, which produced enhanced levels of $H_2O_2$ and influenced the function of aquaporins considered as potential inhibitors for glioblastoma cells [251].

The penetration of biomolecules promoted by CAP might open new applications in the field of biotechnology [1, 2].

## 14.5 Plasma-Based Modification and Functionalization of Surfaces

**Since CAP increases hydrophobicity of surfaces, induces oxidation processes and allows attachment of target molecules, it allows for various hygienic oriented applications.**

For the hardening and processing of surfaces and materials, plasmas are indispensable in the technical sector. CAP can be used to create polymer surface modifications with promising industrial and biomedical applications [252]. CAP treatment was used for the improvement of physicochemical and biodegradable properties of polylactic acid (PLA) films for food packaging [144], to create functionalized PLA with multifunctional properties [253], and prepare biorepellent or bioabsorptive surfaces [254]. In other cases, PLA surfaces were coated using CAP with a chitosan layer to provide antifungal and antibacterial activities [255]. A significant increase in hydrophilicity, surface roughness and structural compactness of chitosan films was observed after DBD plasma treatment [256]. CAP was also applied to modify surfaces of cellulosic substrates, cellulose textiles (functionalized with ZnO nanoparticles as antibacterial treatment), impregnated cotton and viscose fabrics or nanocoated polyester-cotton-blend curtains [257–260]. A surface modification of polyethylene films led to higher antimicrobial activity [261]. Furthermore, changes of denture-base acrylic resin surface properties can significantly reduce *Candida albicans* adherence [262, 263]. Additionally, CAP-assisted coating of surfaces with inorganic antimicrobials, e.g., copper, contributes to reduced adherence and growth of microorganisms [264].

In the functionalization of surfaces, for example changes to hydrophobicity, MDs can be changed so that impurities and pathogens do not attach as easily, and detachment of those substances for processing needs is facilitated [265]. The osseointegration of implants may be supported [92, 266]. Polymethyl methacrylate surface modification by DBD plasma improves the biocompatibility of this material and has antibacterial and antifungal effects [113, 267].

By attaching positively charged polymer layers on a nanoscale, adhesion and growth of bone cells onto implants are supported by plasma techniques. The production of allylamine-plasma-polymer films fixates silver nanoparticles onto the surface; similarly, titan-copper layers can be applied. These technologies can be used for many material types and enables new production methods of antimicrobially effective implants or other products, such as antiseptic wound dressings, surgical suture material or fabrics [1, 2].

By treating titanium with cold oxygen plasma, a surface with antimicrobial properties was maintained for 16 days; a microbicidal titanium oxide film is under discussion as the source. This might inhibit the formation of biofilms after the insertion of titanium implants. The treatment of implant surfaces with CAP also supports the integrative and angioprotective effects, which might be a crucial benefit for the integration of implants [1, 2].

## 14.6 Applications for Synthesis Processes

**As an alternative to classical synthesis methods, CAP allows the production of active substances or products.**

Aqueous plasma pharmacy describes the generation and distribution of reactive plasma-generated species in an aqueous solution, followed by use in disinfection, antisepsis, agriculture, cell stimulation, and cancer treatment. The future of this field is also being discussed, regarding necessary research efforts that will enable commercialization for clinical deployment [268]. Surfactant-free silver (Ag) nanoparticles (NPs) stable for months can be obtained by treatment of $AgNO_3$ solution with $He/H_2$ bipolar pulsed discharge [269].

Present agricultural technology uses reactive nitrogen inefficiently. Animal, human, and food waste all contain significant quantities of organic nitrogen that are transformed into ammonia ($NH_3$) by bacterial degradation of organic waste, which is lost into the environment and causes environmental problems. Nonequilibrium air plasma technology creates reactive nitrogen that can be readily converted to dilute aqueous nitric acid solutions. If mixed with decaying organic waste, the $NH_3$ loss is greatly reduced via the formation of involatile ammonium nitrate, a nitrogen fertilizer. This technology could play a significant role in improving nitrogen use efficiency and reducing environmental and other threats associated with the current systems [270].

**CAP applications in hygiene are conceivable in the fields of medicine, environmental technology, and industry (Fig.** 14.1).

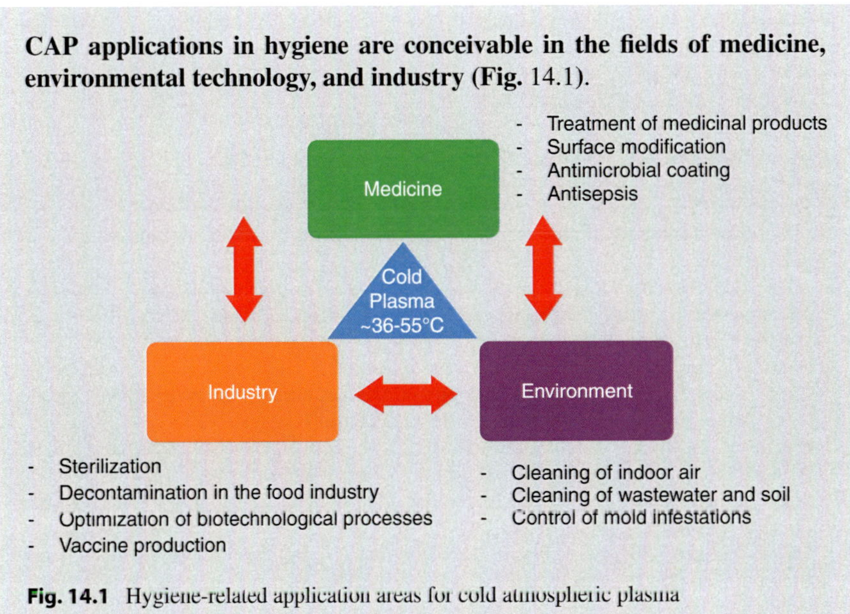


**Fig. 14.1** Hygiene-related application areas for cold atmospheric plasma

**Conclusion**

The applications of plasma for the sterilization or decontamination of inanimate materials is well established in the areas of medicine, the food industry, and air purification. A high potential exists in the sectors of water and wastewater management as well as soil treatment, especially regarding the removal of pharmaceutical remnants. Due to CAP-mediated biofunctionalization of surfaces and implant materials, other applications are likely to emerge. The development of easy-to-use, mobile devices for the creation of CAP will pave the way for innovations in many medical and industrial fields. It is therefore expected that the properties of CAP will be used for many more applications in the hygiene sector in the future.

## References

1. Kramer A, Bekeschus S, Matthes R, Bender C, Stope MB, Napp M, Lademann O, Lademann J, Weltmann KD, Schauer F. Cold physical plasmas in the field of hygiene—relevance, significance, and future applications. Plasma Process Polym. 2015;12:1410–22.
2. Kramer A, Matthes R, Bekeschus S, Bender C, Napp M, Lademann O, Weltmann KD. Aktueller und perspektivischer Einsatz kalter Plasmen aus hygienischer Sicht. In: Metelmann HR, von Woedtke T, Weltmann KD, editors. Plasmamedizin—Kaltplasma in der medizinischen Anwendung. Berlin: Springer; 2016. p. 137–55.
3. Daeschlein G, Napp M, Lutze S, Arnold A, von Podewils S, Gümbel D, Jünger M. Skin and wound decontamination of multidrug-resistant bacteria by cold atmospheric plasma coagulation. J Dtsch Dermatol Ges. 2015;13:143–50.
4. Daeschlein G, Napp M, Majumdar A, Richter E, Rüsch-Gerdes S, Aly F, von Podewils S, Sicher C, Haase H, Niggemeier M, Weltmann KD, Jünger M. In vitro killing of mycobacteria by low temperature atmospheric pressure plasma and dielectric barrier discharge plasma for treatment of tuberculosis. Clin Plasma Med. 2017;5-6:1–7.
5. Daeschlein G, Scholz S, Arnold A, von Podewils S, Haase H, Emmert S, von Woedtke T, Weltmann KD, Jünger M. In vitro susceptibility of multidrug resistant skin and wound pathogens against low temperature atmospheric pressure plasma jet (APPJ) and dielectric barrier discharge plasma (DBD). Plasma Proc Polym. 2014;11:175–83.
6. Daeschlein G, von Woedtke T, Kindel E, Brandenburg R, Weltmann KD, Jünger M. Antibacterial activity of an atmospheric pressure plasma jet against relevant wound pathogens in-vitro on a simulated wound environment. Plasma Process Polym. 2010;7(3–4):224–30.
7. Kulaga EM, Jacofsky DJ, McDonnell C, Jacofsky MC. The use of an atmospheric pressure plasma jet to inhibit common wound-related pathogenic strains of bacteria. Plasma Med. 2016;6(1):1–12.
8. Lührmann A, Matthes R, Kramer A. Impact of cold atmospheric pressure argon plasma on antibiotic sensitivity of methicillin-resistant Staphylococcus aureus strains in vitro. GMS Hyg Inf Contr. 2016;11:Doc17.
9. Maisch T, Shimizu T, Isbary G, Heinlin J, Karrer S, Klämpfl TG, Li YF, Morfill G, Zimmermann JL. Contact-free inactivation of Candida albicans biofilms by cold atmospheric air plasma. Appl Environ Microbiol. 2012;78(12):4242–7.
10. Matthes R, Lührman A, Holtfreter S, Kolata J, Radke D, Hübner NO, Assadian O, Kramer A. Antibacterial activity of cold atmospheric pressure argon plasma against 78 genetically different (mecA, luk-P, agr or capsular polysaccharide type) Staphylococcus aureus strains. Skin Pharmacol Physiol. 2016;29(2):83–91.
11. Misra NN, Tiwari BK, Raghavarao KSMS, Cullen PJ. Nonthermal plasma inactivation of food-borne pathogens. Food Eng Rev. 2011;3(3–4):159–70.

12. Napp M, Daeschlein G, von Podewils S, Hinz P, Emmert S, Haase H, Spitzmueller R, Gümbel D, Kasch R, Jünger M. In vitro susceptibility of methicillin-resistant and methicillin-susceptible strains of Staphylococcus aureus to two different cold atmospheric plasma sources. Infection. 2016;44(4):531–7.
13. Vukušić T, Stulić V, Jambrak AR, Milošević S, Stanzer D, Herceg Z. Effect of treatment by non-thermal plasma jet on the growth of various food spoilage bacteria in superfluous. Croat J Food Sci Technol. 2016;8(1):20–9.
14. Ke Z, Thopan P, Fridman G, Miller V, Yu L, Fridman A, Huang Q. Effect of $N_2/O_2$ composition on inactivation efficiency of Escherichia coli by discharge plasma at the gas-solution interface. Clin Plasma Med. 2017;7-8:1–8.
15. Claro T, Cahill OJ, O'Connor N, Daniels S, Humphreys H. Cold-air atmospheric plasma against Clostridium difficile spores: a potential alternative for the decontamination of hospital inanimate surfaces. Infect Control Hosp Epidemiol. 2015;36:742–4.
16. Connor M, Flynn PB, Fairley DJ, Marks N, Manesiotis P, Graham WG, Gilmore BF, McGrath JW. Evolutionary clade affects resistance of Clostridium difficile spores to cold atmospheric plasma. Sci Rep. 2017;7:41814.
17. Doona CJ, Feeherry FE, Kustin K, Olinger GG, Setlow P, Malkin AJ, Leighton T. Fighting Ebola with novel spore decontaminating technologies for the military. Front Microbiol. 2015;6:663.
18. Hertwig C, Steins V, Reineke K, Rademacher A, Klocke M, Rauh C, Schlueter O. Impact of surface structure and feed gas composition on Bacillus subtilis endospore inactivation during direct plasma treatment. Front Microbiol. 2015;6:774.
19. Raguse M, Fiebrandt M, Stapelmann K, Madela K, Laue M, Lackmann JW, Thwaite JE, Setlow P, Awakowicz P, Moeller R. Improvement of biological indicators by uniformly distributing Bacillus subtilis spores in monolayers to evaluate enhanced spore decontamination technologies. Appl Environ Microbiol. 2016;8:2031–8.
20. Wang SW, Doona CJ, Setlow P, Li YQ. Use of Raman spectroscopy and phase-contrast microscopy to characterize cold atmospheric plasma inactivation of individual bacterial spores. Appl Environ Microbiol. 2016;82:5775–84.
21. Klämpfl TG, Isbary G, Shimizu T, Li YF, Zimmermann JL, Stolz W, Schlegel J, Morfill GE, Schmidt HU. Cold atmospheric air plasma sterilization against spores and other microorganisms of clinical interest. Appl Environ Microbiol. 2012;78(15):5077–82.
22. Daeschlein G, Scholz S, von Woedtke T, Niggemeier M, Kindel E, Brandenburg R, Weltmann KD, Jünger M. In-vitro killing of clinical fungal strains by low temperature atmospheric pressure plasma (APPJ). IEEE Trans Plasma Sci. 2011;39(11):815–21.
23. Heinlin J, Maisch T, Zimmermann JL, Shimizu T, Holzmann T, Simon M, Heider J, Landthaler M, Morfill G, Karrer S. Contact-free inactivation of Trichophyton rubrum and Microsporum canis by cold atmospheric plasma treatment. Fut Microbiol. 2013;8(9):1097–106.
24. Itooka K, Takahashi K, Izawa S. Fluorescence microscopic analysis of antifungal effects of cold atmospheric pressure plasma in Saccharomyces cerevisiae. Appl Microbiol Biotechnol. 2016;100:9295–304.
25. Jambrak AR, Vukusic T, Stulic V, Mrvcic J, Milosevic S, Simunek M, Herceg Z. The effect of high power ultrasound and cold gas-phase plasma treatments on selected yeast in pure culture. Food Bioproc Technol. 2015;8:791–800.
26. Park SY, Ha SD. Application of cold oxygen plasma for the reduction of Cladosporium cladosporioides and Penicillium citrinum on the surface of dried filefish (Stephanolepis cirrhifer) fillets. Int J Food Sci Technol. 2015;50:966–73.
27. Brelles-Mariño G. Challenges in biofilm inactivation: the use of cold plasma as a new approach. J Bioproc Biotech. 2012;2:e107.
28. Delben JA, Zago CE, Tyhovych N, Duarte S, Vergani CE. Effect of atmospheric-pressure cold plasma on pathogenic oral biofilms and in vitro reconstituted oral epithelium. PLoS One. 2016;11:e0155427.
29. Ermolaeva SA, Varfolomeev AF, Chernukha MY, Yurov DS, Vasiliev MM, Kaminskaya AA, Moisenovich MM, Romanova JM, Murashev AN, Selezneva II, Shimizu T, Sysolyatina EV,

Shaginyan IA, Petrov OF, Mayevsky EI, Fortov VE, Morfill GE, Naroditsky BS, Gintsburg AL. Bactericidal effects of non-thermal argon plasma in vitro, in biofilms and in the animal model of infected wounds. J Med Microbiol. 2011;60(Pt 1):75–83.
30. Flynn PB, Busetti A, Wielogorska E, Chevallier OP, Elliott CT, Laverty G, Gorman SP, Graham WG, Gilmore BF. Non-thermal plasma exposure rapidly attenuates bacterial AHL-dependent quorum sensing and virulence. Sci Rep. 2016;6:26320.
31. Matthes R, Jablonowski L, Koban I, Quade A, Huebner NO, Schlueter R, Weltmann KD, von Woedtke T, Kramer A, Kocher T. In vitro treatment of Candida albicans biofilms on denture base material with volume dielectric barrier discharge plasma (VDBD) compared with common chemical antiseptics. Clin Oral Investig. 2015;19:2319–26.
32. Matthes R, Koban I, Bender C, Masur K, Kindel E, Weltmann KD, Kocher T, Kramer A, Hübner NO. Antimicrobial efficacy of an atmospheric pressure plasma jet against biofilms of pseudomonas aeruginosa and staphylococcus epidermidis. Plasma Process Polym. 2012;10(2):161–6.
33. Modic M, McLeod NP, Sutton JM, Walsh JL. Cold atmospheric pressure plasma elimination of clinically important single- and mixed-species biofilms. Int J Antimicrob Agents. 2017;49(3):375–8.
34. Rupf S, Idlibi AN, Umanskaya N, Hannig M, Nothdurft F, Lehmann A, Schindler A, von Müller L, Spitzer W. Disinfection and removal of biofilms on microstructured titanium by cold atmospheric plasma. J Dent Implant. 2012;28(2):126–37.
35. Ziuzina D, Boehm D, Patil S, Cullen PJ, Bourke P. Cold plasma inactivation of bacterial biofilms and reduction of quorum sensing regulated virulence factors. PLoS One. 2015;10(9):e0138209.
36. Ziuzina D, Han L, Cullen PJ, Bourke P. Cold plasma inactivation of internalised bacteria and biofilms for Salmonella enterica serovar typhimurium, Listeria monocytogenes and Escherichia coli. Int J Food Microbiol. 2015;210:53–61.
37. Borges AC, Nishime TMC, Kostov KG, Lima GMG, Gontijo AVL, Carvalho de JNMM, Honda RY, Koga-Ito CY. Cold atmospheric pressure plasma jet modulates Candida albicans virulence traits. Clin Plasma Med. 2017;7-8:9–15.
38. Patange A, Boehm D, Bueno-Ferrer C, Cullen PJ, Bourke P. Controlling Brochothrix thermosphacta as a spoilage risk using in-package atmospheric cold plasma. Food Microbiol. 2017;66:48–54.
39. Pandit S, Mokkapati VRSS, Helgadóttir SH, Westerlundan F, Mijakovic I. Combination of cold atmospheric plasma and vitamin C effectively disrupts bacterial biofilms. Clin Microbiol. 2017;6(283).
40. Pradeep P, Chulkyoon M. Non-thermal plasmas (NTPs) for inactivation of viruses in abiotic environment. Res J Biotechnol. 2016;11:91–6.
41. Weiss M, Daeschlein G, Kramer A, Burchardt M, Brucker S, Wallwiener D, Stope MB. Virucide properties of cold atmospheric plasma for future clinical applications. J Med Virol. 2017;89:952–9.
42. Bayliss DL, Walsh JL, Shama G, Iza F, Kong MG. Reduction and degradation of amyloid aggregates by a pulsed radio-frequency cold atmospheric plasma jet. New J Phys. 2009;11:115024.
43. Aboubakr HA, Gangal U, Youssef MM, Goyal SM, Bruggeman PJ. Inactivation of virus in solution by cold atmospheric pressure plasma: identification of chemical inactivation pathways. J Phys D Appl Phys. 2016;49:204001.
44. Aboubakr HA, Williams P, Gangal U, Youssef MM, El-Sohaimy SAA, Bruggeman PJ, Goyal SM. Virucidal effect of cold atmospheric gaseous plasma on feline calcivirus, a surrogate for human norovirus. Appl Environ Microbiol. 2015;81:3612–22.
45. Elaragi G. Inactivation of hepatitis C virus cells using gliding arc discharge. Plasma Med. 2015;5(1):49–55.
46. Puligundla P, Mok C. Non-thermal plasmas (NTPs) for inactivation of viruses in abiotic environment. Res J Biotechnol. 2016;11(6):91–6.
47. Wu Y, Liang YD, Wei K, Li W, Yao MS, Zhang J, Grinshpun SA. MS2 virus inactivation by atmospheric-pressure cold plasma using different gas carriers and power levels. Appl Environ Microbiol. 2015;81:996–1002.

48. Yasuda H, Miura T, Kurita H, Takashima K, Mizuno A. Biological evaluation of DANN damage in bacteriophages inactivated by atmospheric pressure cold plasma. Plasma Process Polym. 2010;7:301–8.
49. Wang GM, Zhu RH, Yang LC, Wang KL, Zhang Q, Su X, Yang B, Zhang J, Fang J. Non-thermal plasma for inactivated vaccine preparation. Vaccine. 2016;34:1126–32.
50. Guo J, Huang K, Wang J. Bactericidal effect of various non-thermal plasma agents and the influence of experimental conditions in microbial inactivation: a review. Food Control. 2015;50:482–90.
51. Mendis DA, Rosenberg M, Azam F. A note on the possible electrostatic disruption of bacteria. IEEE Trans Plasma Sci. 2000;28:1304–6.
52. Bekeschus S, Iséni S, Reuter S, Masur K, Weltmann KD. Nitrogen shielding of a plasma jet and its effects on human immune cells. IEEE Trans Plasma Sci. 2015;43(3):776–81.
53. Bekeschus S, Kolata J, Winterbourn C, Kramer A, Turner R, Weltmann KD, Bröker B, Masur K. Hydrogen peroxide: A central player in physical plasma-induced oxidative stress in human blood cells. Free Rad Res. 2014;48:542–9.
54. Fridman A. Plasma chemistry. New York: Cambridge University Press; 2008.
55. Kalghatgi S, Kelly CM, Cerchar E, Torabi B, Alekseev O, Fridman A, Friedman G, Azizkhan-Clifford J. Effects of non-thermal plasma on mammalian cells. PLoS One. 2011;6(1):e16270.
56. Laroussi M. Nonthermal decontamination of biological media by atmospheric pressure plasmas: review, analysis, and prospects. IEEE Trans Plasma Sci. 2002;30:1409–15.
57. Laroussi M. Low temperature plasma-based sterilization: overview and state of the art. Plasma Process Polym. 2005;2:391–400.
58. Reuter S, Winter J, Iseni S, Peters S, Schmidt-Bleker A, Dünnbier M, Schäfer J, Foest R, Weltmann KD. Detection of ozone in a MHz argon plasma bullet jet. Plasma Sources Sci Technol. 2012;21(3):034015.
59. Sakudo A, Misawa T, Shimizu N, Imanishi Y. $N_2$ gas plasma inactivates influenza virus mediated by oxidative stress. Front Biosci. 2014;6:69–79.
60. Weltmann KD, von Woedtke T. Plasma medicine—current state of research and medical application. Plasma Phys Control Fusion. 2016;59(1):014031.
61. Boudam MK, Moisan M, Saoudi B, Popovici C, Gherardi N, Massines F. Bacterial spore inactivation by atmospheric-pressure plasmas in the presence or absence of UV photons as obtained with the same gas mixture. J Phys D Appl Phys. 2006;39:3494–507.
62. Morent R, De Geyter N. Inactivation of bacteria by non-thermal plasmas. In: Fazel-Rezai R, editor. Biomedical engineering—frontiers and challenges. InTech; 2011. p. 25–54.
63. Dezest M, Bulteau AL, Quinton D, Chavatte L, Le Bechec M, Cambus JP, Arbault S, Nègre-Salvayre A, Clément F, Cousty S. Oxidative modification and electrochemical inactivation of Escherichia coli upon cold atmospheric pressure plasma exposure. PLoS One. 2017;12(3):e0173618.
64. Winterbourn CC, Hampton MB, Livesey JH, Kettle ASJ. Modeling the reactions of superoxide and myeloperoxidase in the neutrophil phagosome. Implications for microbial killing. J Biol Chem. 2006;281:39860–9.
65. Heyworth PG, Cross AR, Curnutte JT. Chronic granulomatous disease. Curr Opin Immunol. 2003;15(5):578–84.
66. Müller G, Benkhai H, Matthes R, Finke B, Friedrichs W, Geist N, Langel W, Kramer A. Poly(hexamethylene biguanide) adsorption on hydrogen peroxide treated Ti-Al-V alloys and effects on wettability, antimicrobial efficacy, and cytotoxicity. Biomaterials. 2014;35(20):5261–77.
67. von Woedtke T, Kramer A. The limits of sterility assurance. GMS Krankenhaushyg Interdiszip. 2008;3(3):Doc19.
68. Gebel J, Werner HP, Kirsch-Altena A, Bansemir K. Standardmethoden der DGHM zur Prüfung chemischer Desinfektionsverfahren. Wiesbaden: Mhp; 2001.
69. Schwebke I, Blümel J, Eggers M, Glebe D, Rapp I, von Rheinbaben F, Sauerbrei A, Steinmann E, Steinmann J, Willkommen H, Wutzler P, Rabenau HF. Mitteilung der Deutschen Vereinigung zur Bekämpfung der Viruskrankheiten e. V. (DVV) und des Robert Koch-Instituts (RKI) zur Veröffentlichung der aktualisierten Fassung der Leitlinie zur Prüfung von chemischen

Desinfektionsmitteln auf Wirksamkeit gegen Viren in der Humanmedizin (Suspensionstest)—Fassung 1. 12. 2014. Bgbl Gesundheitsforsch Gesundheitssch. 2015; 58(4):491–2.
70. Desinfektionsmittelkommission im VAH. Anforderungen und Methoden zur VAH-Zertifizierung chemischer Desinfektionscverfahren. Wiesbaden: Mhp; 2015.
71. Kramer A, Briesch H, Christiansen B, Löffler H, Perlitz C, Reichardt C. Empfehlungen zur Händehygiene. Mitteilung der Kommission für Krankenhaushygiene und Infektionsprävention am Robert Koch-Institut. BGBL. 2016;59:1189–220.
72. Robert Koch-Institut, Deutsche Vereinigung zur Bekämpfung der Viruskrankheiten e. V. Deutsche Gesellschaft für Hygiene und Mikrobiologie. Prüfung und Deklaration der Wirksamkeit von Desinfektionsmitteln gegen Viren—Stellungnahme des Arbeitskreises Viruzidie beim Robert Koch-Institut (RKI) sowie des Fachausschusses "Virusdesinfektion" der Deutschen Vereinigung zur Bekämpfung der Viruskrankheiten (DVV) und der Desinfektionsmittelkommission der Deutschen Gesellschaft für Hygiene und Mikrobiologie (DGHM). BGBL. 2004;47(1):62–6.
73. Schwebke I, Arvand M, Eggers M, Gebel J, Geisel B, Rapp I, Steinmann J, Rabenau HF. Empfehlung zur Auswahl viruzider Desinfektionsmittel—eine neue Stellungnahme des Arbeitskreises Viruzidie beim RKI. http://www.krankenhaushygiene.de/referate/d13b4982da4e67a8f40f1d8c674171ed.pdf.
74. Pitten FA, Werner HP, Kramer A. A standardized test to assess the impact of different organic challenges on the antimicrobial activity of antiseptics. J Hosp Infect. 2003;55:108–15.
75. Schedler K, Assadian O, Brautferger U, Müller G, Koburger T, Classen S, Kramer A. Proposed phase 2/ step 2 in-vitro test on basis of EN 14561 for standardised testing of the wound antiseptics PVP-iodine, chlorhexidine digluconate, polihexanide and octenidine dihydrochloride. BMC Infect Dis. 2017;17(1):143.
76. Moisan M, Barbeau J, Moreau S, Pelletier J, Tabrizian M, Yahia LH. Low-temperature sterilization using gas plasmas: a review of the experiments and an analysis of the inactivation mechanisms. Int J Pharm. 2001;226:1–21.
77. Kohnen W, Fleischhack R, Kaiser U, Kühne T, Salzbrunn R, Getreuer H, Wegner WD, Jatzwauk L. Grundlagen der Sterilisation. In: Kramer A, Assadian O, Exner M, Hübner N-O, Simon A, editors. Krankenhaus- und Praxishygiene—Hygienemanagement und Infektionsprävention in medizinischen und sozialen Einrichtungen. München. 3. Aufl.: Urban Fischer; 2016. p. 64–95.
78. DIN EN 14885. Chemical disinfectants and antiseptics - application of European standards for chemical disinfectants and antiseptics. Hamburg: Beuth; 2015–11.
79. Okpara-Hofmann J, Knoll M, Dürr M, Schmitt B, Borneff-Lipp M. Comparison of low-temperature hydrogen peroxide gas plasma sterilization for endoscopes using various Sterrad™ models. J Hosp Infect. 2005;59(4):280–5.
80. Singh MK, Nagatsu M. Large-volume plasma device with internally mounted face-type planar microwave launchers for low-temperature sterilization. Plasma Med. 2015;5(2–4):159–75.
81. Sato T, Furui T. Generation process and sterilization effect of oh radical in a steam plasma flow at atmospheric pressure for a plasma autoclave. Plasma Med. 2015;5(2–4):299–314.
82. Boyce JM. Modern technologies for improving cleaning and disinfection of environmental surfaces in hospitals. Antimicrob Resist Infect Control. 2016;5:10.
83. Mirmoghtadaie L, Aliabadi SS, Hosseini SM. Recent approaches in physical modification of protein functionality. Food Chem. 2016;199:619–27.
84. Scholtz V, Pazlarova J, Souskova H, Khun J, Julak J. Nonthermal plasma—a tool for decontamination and disinfection. Biotechnol Adv. 2015;33:1108–19.
85. Claro T, Fay R, Murphy C, O'Connor N, Daniels S, Humphreys H. Cold plasma technology and reducing surface bacterial counts: a pilot study. Infect Control Hosp Epidemiol. 2017;38:494–6.
86. Froehling A, Schlueter O. Flow cytometric evaluation of physico-chemical impact on gram-positive and gram-negative bacteria. Front Microbiol. 2015;6:939.
87. Cahill OJ, Claro T, O'Connor N, Cafolla AA, Steven NT, Daniels S, Humphreys H. Cold air plasma to decontaminate inanimate surfaces of the hospital environment. Appl Environ Microbiol. 2014;80(6):2004–10.

88. Golkowski M, Leszczynski J, Plimpton SR, McCollister B, Golkowski C. In vitro and in vivo analysis of hydrogen peroxide-enhanced plasma-induced effluent for infection and contamination mitigation at research and medical facilities. Plasma Med. 2015;5(2–4):109–23.
89. Li YF, Shimizu T, Zimmermann JL, Morfill GE. Cold atmospheric plasma for surface disinfection. Shimizu Plasma Proc Polym. 2012;9(6):585–9.
90. Morrison KA, Asanbe O, Dong X, Weinstein AL, Toyoda Y, Guevara D, Kirkels E, Landford W, Golkowski C, Golkowski M, Spector JA. Rapid sterilization of cell phones using a novel portable non-thermal plasma device. Plasma Med. 2015;5(1):57–70.
91. Müller M, Semenov I, Binder S, Zimmermann JL, Shimizu T, Morfill GE, Rettberg P, Thoma MH, Thomas HM. Cold atmospheric plasma technology for decontamination of space equipment. 6th Int Conf Plasma Medicine (ICPM-6), 2016, Bratislava, Slovakia. http://elib.dlr.de/106092/1/ME-SBA-2016-Mueller-Rettberg-icpm6.pdf.
92. Duske K, Jablonowski L, Koban I, Matthes R, Holtfreter B, Sckell A, Nebe JB, von Woedtke T, Weltmann KD, Kocher T. Cold atmospheric plasma in combination with mechanical treatment improves osteoblast growth on biofilm covered titanium discs. Biomaterials. 2015;52:327–34.
93. Krcma F, Klimova E, Mazankova V, Dostal L, Obradovic B, Nikiforov A, Vanraes P. Novel plasma source based on pin-hole discharge configuration. Plasma Med. 2016;6(1):21–31.
94. Kramer A, Pittet D, Klasinc R, Krebs S, Koburger T, Fusch C, Assadian O. Shortening the application time of alcohol-based hand rubs to 15 s may improve frequency of hand antisepsis. ICHE. In rev.
95. Kramer A, Rudolph P, Kampf G, Pittet D. Limited efficacy of alcohol-based hand gels. Lancet. 2002;359(9316):1489–90.
96. Paula H, Krebs U, Becker R, Assadian O, Heidecke CD, Kramer A. Wettability of hands during 15s and 30s contact intervals: a prospective, randomized cross-over study. J Hosp Inf. In rev.
97. Pires D, Soule H, Bellissimo-Rodrigues F, Pittet D. Hand hygiene with alcohol-based hand rub: how long is long enough? Infect Control Hosp Epidemiol. 2017;6:65.
98. Gessner S, Below E, Diedrich S, Wegner C, Gessner W, Kohlmann T, Heidecke CD, Bockholdt B, Kramer A, Assadian O, Below H. Ethanol and ethyl glucuronide urine concentrations after ethanol-based hand antisepsis with and without permitted alcohol consumption. Am J Infect Control. 2016;44(9):999–1003.
99. Kramer A, Harnoss JC, Walger P, Heidecke CD, Schreiber A, Maier S, Pochhammer J. Hygiene in der Allgemein- und Viszeralchirurgie—Fachspezifische Maßnahmen zur Prävention von Surgical Site Infections (SSI). Zbl Chir. 2016;141(06):591–6.
100. Kampf G, Kramer A. Epidemiologic background of hand hygiene and evaluation of the most important agents for scrubs and rubs. Clin Microbiol Rev. 2004;17(4):863–93.
101. Osman I, Ponukumati A, Vargas M, Bhakta D, Ozoglu B, Bailey C. Plasma-activated vapor for sanitization of hands. Plasma Med. 2016;6(3–4):235–45.
102. Ulmer M, Lademann J, Patzelt A, Knorr F, Kramer A, Koburger T, Assadian O, Daeschlein G, Lange-Asschenfeldt B. New strategies for preoperative skin antisepsis. Skin Pharmacol Physiol. 2014;27(6):283–92.
103. Lange-Asschenfeldt B, Marenbach D, Lang C, Patzelt A, Ulrich M, Maltusch A, Terhorst D, Stockfleth E, Sterry W, Lademann J. Distribution of bacteria in the epidermal layers and hair follicles of the human skin. Skin Pharmacol Physiol. 2011;24:305–11.
104. Kamel C, McGahan L, Polisena J, Mierzwinski-Urban M, Embil JM. Preoperative skin antiseptic preparations for preventing surgical site infections: a systematic review. Infect Control Hosp Epidemiol. 2012;33(6):608–17.
105. Ouf SA, El-Adly AA, Mohamed AAH. Inhibitory effect of silver nanoparticles mediated by atmospheric pressure air cold plasma jet against dermatophyte fungi. J Med Microbiol. 2015;64:1151–61.
106. Shapourzadeh A, Rahimi-Verki N, Atyabi SM, Shams-Ghahfarokhi M, Jahanshiri Z, Irani S, Razzaghi-Abyaneh M. Inhibitory effects of cold atmospheric plasma on the growth, ergosterol biosynthesis, and keratinase activity in Trichophyton rubrum. Arch Biochem Biophys. 2016;608:27–33.
107. Rahimi-Verki N, Shapoorzadeh A, Razzaghi-Abyaneh M, Atyabi SM, Shams-Ghahfarokhi M, Jahanshiri Z, Gholami-Shabani M. Cold atmospheric plasma inhibits the growth of

Candida albicans by affecting ergosterol biosynthesis and suppresses the fungal virulence factors in vitro. Photodiagn Photodyn Ther. 2016;13:66–72.
108. Xiong ZL, Roe J, Grammer TC, Graves DB. Plasma treatment of onychomycosis. Plasma Process Polym. 2016;13:588–97.
109. Habib M, Hottel TL, Hong L. Antimicrobial effects of non-thermal atmospheric plasma as a novel root canal disinfectant. Clin Plasma Med. 2014;2:17–21.
110. Li YL, Sun K, Ye GP, Liang YD, Pan H, Wang GM, Zhao YJ, Pan J, Zhang J, Fang J. Evaluation of cold plasma treatment and safety in disinfecting 3-week root canal enterococcus faecalis biofilm in vitro. J Endod. 2015;41:1325–30.
111. Pignata C, DÁngelo D, Fea E, Gilli G. A review on microbiological decontamination of fresh produce with nonthermal plasma. J Appl Microbiol. 2017;122:1438–55.
112. Pierdzioch P, Hartwig S, Herbst SR, Raguse JD, Dommisch H, Abu-Sirhan S, Wirtz HC, Hertel M, Paris S, Preissner S. Cold plasma: a novel approach to treat infected dentin—a combined ex vivo and in vitro study. Clin Oral Investig. 2016;20:2429–35.
113. Wang GM, Sun PP, Pan H, Ye GP, Sun K, Zhang J, Pan J, Fang J. Inactivation of Candida albicans on polymethyl methacrylate and enhancement of the drug susceptibility by cold Ar/$O_2$ plasma jet. Plasma Chem Plasma Process. 2016;36:383–96.
114. Preissner S, Wirtz HC, Tietz AK, Abu-Sirhan S, Herbst SR, Hartwig S, Pierdzioch P, Schmidt-Westhausen AM, Dommisch H, Hertel M. Bactericidal efficacy of tissue tolerable plasma microrough titanium dental implantats: an in-vitro-study. J Biophotonics. 2016;9:637–44.
115. Maisch T, Shimizu T, Li YF, Heinlin J, Karrer S, Morfill G, Zimmermann JL. Decolonisation of MRSA, S. aureus and E. coli by cold-atmospheric plasma using a porcine skin model in vitro. PLoS One. 2012;7(4):e34610.
116. Köck R, Becker K, Cookson B, van Gemert-Pijnen JE, Harbarth S, Kluytmans J, Mielke M, Peters G, Skov RL, Struelens MJ, Tacconelli E, Witte W, Friedrich AW. Systematic literature analysis and review of targeted preventive measures to limit healthcare-associated infections by meticillin-resistant Staphylococcus aureus. Euro Surveill. 2014;19(29):20860.
117. Li X, Farid M. A review on recent development in non-conventional food sterilization technologies. J Food Engin. 2016;182:33–45.
118. Mok C, Lee T, Puligundla P. Afterglow corona discharge air plasma (ACDAP) for inactivation of common food-borne pathogens. Food Res Int. 2015;69:418–23.
119. Shaw A, Shama G, Iza F. Emerging applications of low temperature gas plasmas in the food industry. Biointerphases. 2015;10:029402.
120. Surowky B, Schlueter O, Knorr D. Interactions of non-thermal atmospheric pressure plasma with solid and liquid food systems: a review. Food Eng Rev. 2015;7:82–108.
121. Abdi S, Dorranian D, Mohammadi K. Effect of oxygen on decontamination of cumin seeds by atmospheric pressure dielectric barrier discharge plasma. Plasma Med. 2016;6(3–4):339–47.
122. Afshari R, Hosseini H. Non-thermal plasma as a new food preservation method, its present and future prospect. Winter. 2014;5(1):116–20.
123. Al-Bukhaiti WQ, Noman A, Mahdi A. Characteristics and applications of cold atmospheric plasma—review. Int J Agricult Innov Res. 2016;5(2):257–61.
124. Amini M, Ghoranneviss M. Black and green tea decontamination by cold plasma. Res J Microbiol. 2016;11:42–6.
125. Dey A, Rasane P, Choudhury A, Singh J, Maisnam D, Rasane P. Cold plasma processing: a review. J Chem Pharmac Sci. 2016;9(4):2980–4.
126. Georgescu N, Apostol L, Gherendi F. Inactivation of Salmonella enterica serovar typhimurium on egg surface, by direct and indirect treatments with cold atmospheric plasma. Food Control. 2017;76:52–61.
127. Grabowski M, Strzelczak A, Dąbrowski W. Low pressure cold plasma as an alternative method for black pepper sterilization. J Life Sci. 2014;8:931–9.
128. Gurol C, Ekinci FY, Aslan N, Korachi M. Low temperature plasma for decontamination of E. coli in milk. Int J Food Microbiol. 2012;157(1):1–5.
129. Han L, Ziuzina D, Heslin CM, Boehm D, Patange A, Millan-Sango D, Valdramidis V, Cullen P, Bourke P. Controlling microbial safety challenges of meat using high voltage atmospheric cold plasma. Front Microbiol. 2016;7:977.

130. Hertwig C, Reineke K, Ehlbeck J, Knorr D, Schlüter O. Decontamination of whole black pepper using different cold atmospheric pressure plasma applications. Food Control. 2015;55:221–9.
131. Korachi M, Aslan N. Low temperature atmospheric plasma for microbial decontamination. Microbial pathogens and strategies for combating them. J Sci Educ Technol. 2013;1:453–9.
132. Korachi M, Ozen F, Asian N, Vannini L, Guerzoni ME, Gottardi D, Ekinci FY. Biochemical changes to milk following treatment by a novel, cold atmospheric plasma system. Int Dairy J. 2015;42:64–9.
133. Misra NN, Segat A, Cullen PJ. Atmospheric-pressure non-thermal plasma decontamination of foods. In: Rai VR, editor. Advances in food biotechnology. Wiley-Blackwell; 2015.
134. Moritz M, Wiacek C, Koethe M, Braun PG. Atmospheric pressure plasma jet treatment of salmonella enteritidis inoculated eggshells. Int J Food Microbiol. 2017;245:22–8.
135. Niemira BA. Cold plasma decontamination of foods. Annu Rev Food Sci Technol. 2012;3:125–42.
136. Noriega E, Shama G, Laca A, Díaz M, Kong MG. Cold atmospheric gas plasma disinfection of chicken meat and chicken skin contaminated with Listeria innocua. Food Microbiol. 2011;28(7):1293–300.
137. Pasquali F, Stratakos AC, Koidis A, Berardinelli A, Cevoli C, Ragni L, Mancusi R, Manfreda G, Trevisani M. Atmospheric cold plasma process for vegetible leaf decontamination: A feasibility study on radicchio (red chicory, Cichorium intybus L.). Food Control. 2016;60:552–9.
138. Perni S, Liu DW, Shama G, Kong MG. Cold atmospheric plasma decontamination of the pericarps of fruit. J Food Prot. 2008;71(2):302–8.
139. Perni S, Shama G, Kong MG. Cold atmospheric plasma disinfection of cut fruit surfaces contaminated with migrating microorganisms. J Food Prot. 2008;71(8):1619–25.
140. Puligundla P, Lee T, Mok C. Inactivation effect of dielectric barrier discharge plasma against foodborne pathogens on the surfaces of different packaging materials. Innovative Food Sci Emerg Technol. 2016;36:221–7.
141. Schnabel U, Niquet R, Andrasch M, Jakobs M, Schlüter O, Katroschan KU, Weltmann KD, Ehlbeck J. Broccoli: Antimicrobial efficacy and influences to sensory and storage properties by microwave plasma-processed air treatment. Plasma Med. 2016;6(3–4):375–88.
142. Smet C, Noriega E, Rosier F, Walsh J, Valdramidis V, Impe van J. Influence of food intrinsic factors on the inactivation efficacy of cold atmospheric plasma: impact of osmotic stress, suboptimal pH and food structure. Innovative Food Sci Emerg Technol 2016 38B: 393–406.
143. Smet C, Noriega E, Rosier F, Walsh J, Valdramidis V, van Impe J. Impact of food model (micro)structure on the microbial inactivation efficacy of cold atmospheric plasma. Int J Food Microbiol. 2017;240:47–56.
144. Song AY, YA O, Roh SH, Kim JH, Min SC. Cold oxygen plasma treatment for the improvement of the physicochemical and biodegradable properties of polylactic acid films for food packing. J Food Sci. 2016;81:E86–96.
145. Stoica M, Alexe P, Mihalcea L. Atmospheric cold plasma as new strategy for foods processing - an overview. Innov Rom Food Biotechnol. 2014;15:1–8.
146. Ulbin-Figlewicz N, Brychcy E, Jarmoluk A. Effect of low-pressure cold plasma on surface microflora of meat and quality attributes. J Food Sci Technol. 2015;52:1228–32.
147. Ulbin-Figlewicz N, Jarmoluk A, Marycz K. Antimicrobial activity of low-pressure plasma treatment against selected foodborne bacteria and meat microbiota. Ann Microbiol. 2015;65:1537–46.
148. Wan ZF, Chen Y, Pankaj SK, Keener KM. High voltage atmospheric cold plasma treatment of refrigerated chicken eggs for control of Salmonella Enteritidis contamination on egg shell. LTW Food Sci Technol. 2017;76:124–30.
149. Ziuzina D, Misra NN, Cullen PJ, Keener K, Mosnier JP, Vilaró I, Gaston E, Bourke P. Demonstrating the potential of industrial scale in-package atmospheric cold plasma for decontamination of cherry tomatoes. Plasma Med. 2016;6(3–4):387–412.
150. Ziuzina D, Patil S, Cullen PJ, Keener KM, Bourke P. Atmospheric cold plasma inactivation of Escherichia coli, Salmonella enterica serovar Typhimurium and Listeria monocytogenes inoculated on fresh produce. Food Microbiol. 2014;42:109–16.

151. Ziuzina D. Patil., Cullen PJ, Keener KM, Bourke P. Atmospheric cold plasma inactivation of Escherichia coli in liquid media inside a sealed package. J Appl Microbiol. 2013;114:778–87.
152. Ouf SA, Mohamed AAH, El-Sayed WS. Fungal decontamination of fleshy fruit washes by double atmospheric pressure cold plasma. Clean Soil Air Water. 2015;44:134–42.
153. Jahid IK, Han N, Zhang CY, Ha SD. Mixed culture biofilms of Salmonella typhimurium and cultivable indigenous microorganisms on lettuce show enhanced resistance of their sessile cells to cold oxygen plasma. Food Microbiol. 2015;46:383–94.
154. Lee H, Kim JE, Chung MS, Min SC. Cold plasma treatment for the microbiological safety of cabbage, lettuce, and dried figs. Food Microbiol. 2015;51:74–80.
155. Min SC, Roh SH, Boyd G, Sites JE, Uknalis J, Fan XT, Niemira BA. Inactivation of Escherichia coli O157:H7 and aerobic microorganisms in Romaine lettuce packaged in a commercial polyethylene terephthalate container using atmospheric cold plasma. J Food Prot. 2017;80:35–43.
156. Min SC, Roh SH, Niemira BA, Sites JE, Boyd G, Lacombe A. Dielectric barrier discharge atmospheric cold plasma inhibits Escherichia coli O157:H7, Salmonella, Listeria monocytogenes, and Tulane virus in Romaine lettuce. Int J Food Microbiol. 2016;237:114–20.
157. Song AY, YJ O, Kim JE, Bin Song K, DH O, Min SC. Cold plasma treatment for microbial safety and preservation of fresh lettuce. Food Sci Biotechnol. 2015;24:1717–24.
158. Cui HY, Ma CX, Li CZ, Lin L. Enhancing the antibacterial activity of thyme oil against Salmonella on eggshell by plasma-assisted process. Food Control. 2016;70:183–90.
159. Cui HY, Ma CX, Lin L. Synergistic antibacterial efficacy of cold nitrogen plasma and clove oil against Escherichia coli O157:H7 biofilms on lettuce. Food Control. 2016;66:8–16.
160. Cui HY, Wu J, Li CZ, Lin L. Promoting anti-listeria activity of lemongrass oil on pork loin by cold nitrogen plasma assist. J Food Saf. 2017;37:e12316.
161. Segat A, Misra NN, Cullen PJ, Innocente N. Effect of atmospheric pressure cold plasma (ACP) on activity and structure of alkaline phosphatase. Food Bioprod Process. 2016;98:181–8.
162. Amini M, Ghoranneviss M. Effects of cold plasma treatment on antioxidants activity, phenolic contents and shelf life of fresh and dried walnut (Juglans regia L.) cultivars during storage. LWT Food Science and Technology. 2016;73:178–84.
163. Bosch ten L, Pfohl K, Avramidis G, Wieneke S, Viöl W, Karlovsky P. Plasma-based degradation of mycotoxins produced by fusarium, aspergillus and alternaria species. Toxins. 2017;9:97.
164. Dasan BG, Boyaci IH, Mutlu M. Inactivation of aflatoxigenic fungi (Aspergillus spp.) on granular food model, maize, in an atmospheric pressure fluidized bed plasma system. Food Control. 2016;70:1–8.
165. Devi Y, Thirumdas R, Sarangapani C, Deshmukh RR, Annapure US. Influence of cold plasma on fungal growth and aflatoxins production on groundnuts. Food Control. 2017;77:187–91.
166. Kim JE, YJ O, Won MY, Lee KS, Min SC. Microbial decontamination of onion powder using microwave-powered cold plasma treatments. Food Microbiol. 2017;62:112–23.
167. Ouf SA, Basher AH, Mohamed AAH. Inhibitory effect of double atmospheric argon cold plasma on spores and mycotoxin production of Aspergillus niger contaminating date palm fruits. J Sci Food Agric. 2015;95:3204–10.
168. Sohbatzadeh F, Mirzanejhad S, Shokri H, Nikpour M. Inactivation of Aspergillus flavus spores in a sealed package by cold plasma streamers. J Theor Appl Phys. 2016;10:99–106.
169. Won MY, Lee SJ, Min SC. Mandarin preservation by microwave-powered plasma treatment. Innovative Food Sci Emerg Technol. 2017;39:25–32.
170. Yong HI, Lee H, Park S, Park J, Choe W, Jung S, Jo C. Flexible thin-layer plasma inactivation of bacteria and mold survival in beef jerky packaging and its effects on the meat's physicochemical properties. Meat Sci. 2017;123:151–8.
171. Hojnik N, Cvelbar U, Tavčar-Kalcher G, Walsh JL, Križaj I. Mycotoxin decontamination of food: Cold atmospheric pressure plasma versus "classic" decontamination. Toxins. 2017;9(5):151.
172. Karlovsky P, Suman M, Berthiller F, Meester JD, Eisenbrand G, Perrin I, Oswald IP, Speijers G, Chiodini A, Recker T, Dussort P. Impact of food processing and detoxification treatments on mycotoxin contamination. Mycotoxin Res. 2016;32(4):179–205.

173. Park BJ, Takatori K, Sugita-Konishi Y, Kim IH, Lee MH, Han DW, Chung KH, Hyun SO, Park JC. Degradation of mycotoxins using microwave-induced argon plasma at atmospheric pressure. Surf Coat Technol. 2007;201:5733–7.
174. Shi H, Ileleji K, Stroshine RL, Keener K, Jensen JL. Reduction of aflatoxin in corn by high voltage atmospheric cold plasma. Food Bioprocess Technol. 2017;10:1042–52.
175. Siciliano I, Spadaro D, Prelle A, Vallauri D, Cavallero MC, Garibaldi A, Gullino ML. Use of cold atmospheric plasma to detoxify hazelnuts from aflatoxins. Toxins (Basel). 2016;8(5):125.
176. Puligundla P, Mok C. Potential applications of nonthermal plasmas against biofilm-associated micro-organisms in vitro. J Appl Microbiol. 2017;122:1134–48.
177. Bauer A, Ni Y, Bauer S, Paulsen P, Modic M, Walsh JL, Smulders FJM. The effects of atmospheric pressure cold plasma treatment on microbiological, physical-chemical and sensory characteristics of vacuum packaged beef loin. Meat Sci. 2017;128:77–87.
178. Han L, Boehm D, Amias E, Milosavljevic V, Cullen PJ, Bourke P. Atmospheric cold plasma interactions with modified atmosphere packaging inducer gases for safe food preservation. Innov Food Sci Emerg Technol. 2016;38:384–92.
179. Han SH, Suh HJ, Hong KB, Kim SY, Min SC. Oral toxicity of cold plasma-treated edible films for food coating. J Food Sci. 2016;81:T3052–7.
180. Rothrock MJ, Zhuang H, Lawrence KC, Bowker BC, Gamble GR, Hiett KL. In-package inactivation of pathogenic and spoilage bacteria associated with poultry using dielectric barrier discharge cold plasma treatments. Curr Microbiol. 2017;74:149–58.
181. Wang JM, Zhuang H, Hinton A, Zhang JH. Influence of in-package cold plasma treatment on microbiological shelf life and appearance of fresh chicken breast fillets. Food Microbiol. 2016;60:142–6.
182. Wang JM, Zhuang H, Zhang JH. Inactivation of spoilage bacteria in package by dielectric barrier discharge atmospheric cold plasma-treatment time effects. Food Bioprocess Technol. 2016;9:1648–52.
183. Calvo T, Alvarez-Ordonez A, Prieto M, Gonzalez-Raurich M, Lopez M. Influence of processing parameters and stress adaptation on the inactivation of listeria monocytogenes by non-thermal atmospheric plasma (NTAP). Food Res Int. 2016;89:631–7.
184. Misra NN, Pankaj SK, Segat A, Ishikawa K. Cold plasma interactions with enzymes in foods and model systems. Trends Food Sci Technol. 2016;55:39–47.
185. Thirumdas R, Sarangapani C, Annapure US. Cold plasma: a novel non-thermal technology for food processing. Food Biophys. 2015;10:1–11.
186. Bussler S, Ehlbeck J, Schlueter O. Pre-drying treatment of plant related tissues using plasma processed air: Impact on enzyme activity and quality attributes of cut apple and potato. Innov Food Sci Emerg Technol. 2017;40:78–86.
187. Shaer ME, Mobasher M, Abdelghany A. Effect of gliding arc plasma on plant nutrient content and enzyme activity. Plasma Med. 2016;6(3–4):209–18.
188. Khani MR, Shokri B, Khajeh K. Studying the performance of dielectric barrier discharge and gliding arc plasma reactors in tomato peroxidise inactivation. J Food Eng. 2017;197:107–12.
189. Thirumdas R, Kadam D, Annapure US. Cold plasma: an alternative technology for the starch modification. Food Biophys. 2017;12:129–39.
190. Pankaj SK, Bueno-Ferrer C, Misra NN, O'Neill L, Tiwari BK, Bourke P, Cullen PJ. Dielectric barrier discharge atmospheric air plasma treatment of high amylase corn starch films. LWT Food Sci Technol. 2015;63:1076–83.
191. Thirumdas R, Deshmukh RR, Annapure US. Effect of low temperature plasma on the functional properties of basmati rice flour. J Food Sci Technol. 2016;53(6):2742–51.
192. Thirumdas R, Trimukhe A, Deshmukh RR, Annapure US. Functional and rheological properties of cold plasma treated rice starch. Carbohydr Polym. 2017;157:1723–31.
193. Sarangapani C, Devi Y, Thirumdas R, Annapure US, Deshmukh RR. Effect of low-pressure plasma on physico-chemical properties of paraboiled rice. LWT Food Sci Technol. 2015;63:452–60.
194. Bahrami N, Bayliss D, Chope G, Penson S, Perehinec T, Fisk ID. Cold plasma: A new technology to modify wheat flour functionality. Food Chem. 2016;202:247–53.

195. Segat A, Misra NN, Cullen PJ, Innocente N. Atmospheric pressure cold plasma (ACP) treatment of whey protein isolate model solution. Innovative Food Sci Emerg Technol. 2015;29:247–54.
196. Sahin O, Kaya M, Saka C. Plasma-surface modification on bentonite clay to improve the performance of adsorption of methylene blue. Appl Clay Sci. 2015;116:46–53.
197. Moghaddam MS, Heydari G, Tuominen M, Fielden M, Haapanen J, Makela JM, Walinder MEP, Claesson PM, Swerin A. Hydrophobisation of wood surfaces by combining liquid flame spray (LFS) and plasma treatment: dynamic wetting properties. Holzforschung. 2016;70:527–37.
198. Huynh A, Li T, Kovalenko M, Robinson RD, Fridman AA, Rabinovich A, Fridman G. Nonequilibrium plasma decontamination of corn steep liquor for ethanol production: $SO_2$ removal and disinfection. Plasma Med. 2016;6(3–4):219–34.
199. Buonopane GJ, Antonacci C, Lopez JL. Effect of cold plasma processing on botanicals and their essential oils. Plasma Med. 2016;6(3–4):315–24.
200. Gholami A, Safa NN, Khoram M, Hadian J, Ghomi H. Effect of low-pressure radio frequency plasma on ajwain seed germination. Plasma Med. 2016;6(3–4):389–96.
201. Holc M, Junkar I, Primc G, Iskra J, Titan P, Mlakar SG, Kovac J, Mozetic M. Improved sprout emergence of garlic cloves by plasma treatment. Plasma Med. 2016;6(3–4):325–38.
202. Hayashi N, Ono R, Nakano R, Shiratani M, Tashiro K, Kuhara S, Yasuda K, Hagiwara H. DNA microarray analysis of plant seeds irradiated by active oxygen species in oxygen plasma. Plasma Med. 2016;6(3–4):459–71.
203. Brar J, Jiang J, Oubarri A, Ranieri P, Fridman AA, Fridman G, Miller V, Peethambaran B. Non-thermal plasma treatment of flowing water: a solution to reduce water usage and soil treatment cost without compromising yield. Plasma Med. 2016;6(3–4):413–27.
204. Peethambaran B, Han J, Kermalli K, Jiaxing J, Fridman G, Balsamo R, Fridman AA, Miller V. Nonthermal plasma reduces water consumption while accelerating arabidopsis thaliana growth and fecundity. Plasma Med. 2015;5(2–4):87–98.
205. Haertel B, Backer C, Lindner K, Musebeck D, Schulze C, Wurster M, von Woedtke T, Lindequist U. Effects of physical plasma on biotechnological processes in mycelia of the cultivated lingzhi or reishi medicinal mushroom Ganoderma lucidum (Agaricomycetes). Int J Med Mushrooms. 2016;18(6):521–31.
206. Leclaire C, Lecoq E, Orial G, Clement F, Bousta F. Fungal decontamination by cold plasma: an innovating process for wood treatment. Braga: COST Action IE0601 / ESWM—Int Conf; 2008; 5–7. https://www.researchgate.net/publication/264845493_Fungal_decontamination_by_cold_plasma_an_innovating_process_for_wood_treatment.
207. Zahoranova A, Henselova M, Hudecova D, Kalinakova B, Kovacik D, Medvecka V, Cernak M. Effect of cold atmospheric pressure plasma on the wheat seedlings vigor and on the inactivation of microorganisms on the seed surface. Plasma Chem Plasma Process. 2016;36:397–414.
208. Kordas L, Pusz W, Czapka T, Kacprzyk R. The effect of low-temperature plasma on fungus colonization of winter wheat grain and seed quality. Pol J Environ Stud. 2015;24:433–8.
209. Stepczynska M. Surface modification by low temperature plasma: sterilization of biodegradable materials. Plasma Process Polym. 2016;13:1080–8.
210. Li L, Li JG, Shen MC, Zhang CL, Dong YH. Cold plasma treatment enhances oilseed rape seed germination under drought stress. Sci Rep. 2015;5:13033.
211. Mohamed AAH, Al Shariff SM, Ouf SA, Benghanem M. Atmospheric pressure plasma jet for bacterial decontamination and property improvement of fruit and vegetable processing wastewater. J Phys D Appl Phys. 2016;49:195401.
212. Benidris E, Ghezzar MR, Ma A, Ouddane B, Addou A. Water purification by a new hybrid plasma-sensitization-coagulation process. Sep Purif Technol. 2017;178:253–60.
213. Ikawa S, Tani A, Nakashima Y, Kitano K. Physicochemical properties of bactericidal plasma-treated water. J Phys D Appl Phys. 2016;49:425401.
214. Rashmei Z, Bornasi H, Ghoranneviss M. Evaluation of treatment and disinfection of water using cold atmospheric plasma. J Water Health. 2016;14(4):609–16.

215. Tian Y, Ma RN, Zhang Q, Feng HQ, Liang YD, Zhang J, Fang J. Assessment of the physicochemical properties and biological effects of water activated by non-thermal plasma above beneath the water surface. Plasma Process Polym. 2015;12:439–49.
216. Zhou RW, Zhou RS, Zhuang JX, Zong ZC, Zhang XH, Liu DP, Bazaka K, Ostrikov K. Interaction of atmospheric-pressure air microplasmas with amino acids as fundamental processes in aqueous solution. PLoS One. 2016;11:e0155584.
217. Brisset JL, Fanmoe J, Hnatiuc E. Degradation of surfactant by cold plasma treatment. J Environml Chem Eng. 2016;4:385–7.
218. Malik MA, Ghaffar A, Malik SA. Water purification by electrical discharges. Plasma Sources Sci Technol. 2001;10:82–91.
219. Okumura T, Saito Y, Takano K, Takahashi K, Takaki K, Satta N, Fujio T. Inactivation of bacteria using discharge plasma under liquid fertilizer in a hydroponic culture system. Plasma Med. 2016;6(3–4):247–54.
220. El-Sayed WS, Ouf SA, Mohamed AAH. Deterioration to extinction of wastewater bacteria by non-thermal atmospheric pressure air plasma as assessed by 16S rDNA-DGGE fingerprinting. Front Microbiol. 2015;6:1098.
221. Arnó J, Bevan JW. Detoxification of trichloroethylene in a low-pressure surface wave plasma reactor. Environ Sci Technol. 1996;30(8):2427–31.
222. Attri P, Yusupov M, Park JH, Lingamdinne LP, Koduru JR, Shiratani M, Choi EH, Bogaerts A. Mechanism and comparison of needle-type non-thermal direct and indirect atmospheric pressure plasma jets on the degradation of dyes. Sci Rep. 2016;6:34419.
223. Vanraes P, Ghodbane H, Davister D, Wardenier N, Nikiforov A, Verheust YP, Van Hulle SWH, Hamdaoui O, Vandamme J, Dume JV, Surmont P. Removal of several pesticides in a falling water film DBD reactor with activated carbon textile: energy efficiency. Water Res. 2017;116:1–12.
224. Lai ACK, Cheung ACT, Wong MML, Li WS. Evaluation of cold plasma inactivation efficacy against different airborne bacteria in ventilation duct flow. Build Environ. 2016;98:39–46.
225. Zhou P, Yang Y, Lai ACK, Huang GS. Inactivation of airborne bacteria by cold plasma in air duct flow. Build Environ. 2016;106:120–30.
226. Alva E, Pacheco M, Colin A, Sanchez V, Pacheco J, Valdivia R, Soria G. Nitrogen oxides and methane treatment by non-thermal plasma. J Phys Conf Ser. 2015;591(1):012052.
227. Karatrum O, Deshusses MA. A comparative study of dilute VOCs treatment in a non-thermal plasma reactor. Chem Eng J. 2016;294:308–15.
228. Machado MM, Machado MM, Dutra ARD, Moecke EHS, Cubas ALV. Construction of a corona discharge plasma reactor for elimination of volatile organic compounds. Quim Nova. 2015;38:128–31.
229. Veerapandian SKP, Leys C, De Geyter N Morent R. Abatement of VOCs using packed bed non-thermal plasma reactors: a review. Catalysts. 2017;7:113.
230. Ye SY, Liang JL, Song XL, Luo SC, Liang JY. Modelling intrinsic kinetics in a rector of corona discharge coupled with $TiO_2$-activated carbon fibre for ethylene degradation and ozone regulation. Biosyst Eng. 2016;150:123–30.
231. Assadi AA, Bouzaza A, Wolbert D. Comparative study between laboratory and large pilot scales for VOC's removal from gas streams in continuous flow surface discharge plasma. Chem Eng Res Design. 2016;106:308–14.
232. Blumberg A, Blumberg D, Pubule J, Romagnoli F. Cost-benefit analysis of plasma-based technologies. Energy Pro. 2015;72:170–4.
233. Dam TN, Dung DV. Treatment exhaust gas from engine by plasma at atmospheric pressure. Proc 3rd Int Conf on green technology and Sustainable Development 2016; 228–31.
234. Harling AM, Demidyuk V, Fischer SJ, Whitehead JC. Plasma-catalysis destruction of aromatics for environmental clean-up: effect of temperature and configuration. Appl Catal B Environ. 2008;82:180–9.
235. Huang JY, Dang XQ, Qin CH, Shu Y, Wang HC, Zhang F. Toluene decomposition using adsorption combined with plasma-driven catalysis with gas circulation. Environ Prog Sustain Energy. 2016;35:386–94.

236. Jiang LY, Li H, Chen JM, Zhang D, Cao SL, Ye JX. Combination of non-thermal plasma and biotricking filter for chlorobenzene removal. J Chem Technol Biotechnol. 2016;91:3079–87.
237. Nguyen DB, Lee WG. Effects of ambient gas on cold atmospheric plasma discharge in the decomposition of trifluoromethane. RSC Adv. 2016;6:26505–13.
238. Schiavon M, Schiorlin M, Torretta V, Brandenburg R, Ragazzi M. Non-thermal plasma assisting the biofiltration of volatile organic compounds. J Clean Prod. 2017;148:498–508.
239. Stasiulaitiene I, Martuzevicius D, Abromaitis V, Tichonovas M, Baltrusaitis J, Brandenburg R, Pawelec A, Schwock A. Comparative life cycle assessment of plasma-based and traditional exhaust gas treatment technologies. J Clean Prod. 2016;112:1804–12.
240. Bussler S, Steins V, Ehlbeck J, Schlueter O. Impact of thermal treatment versus cold atmospheric plasma processing on the techno-functional protein properties from Pisum Sativum "Salamanca". J Food Eng. 2015;167:166–74.
241. Park JH, Kim M, Shiratani M, Cho AE, Choi EH, Attri P. Variation in structure of proteins by adjusting reactive oxygen and nitrogen species generated from dielectric barrier discharge jet. Sci Rep. 2016;6:35883.
242. Choi S, Attri P, Lee I, Oh J, Yun JH, Park JH, Choi EH, Lee W. Structural and functional analysis of lysozyme after treatment with dielectric barrier discharge plasma and atmospheric pressure plasma jet. Sci Rep. 2017;7(1):1027.
243. Kousal J, Shelemin A, Kylioan O, Slavinska D, Biederman H. In-situ monitoring of etching of bovine serum albumin using low-temperature atmospheric plasma jet. Appl Surf Sci. 2017;392:1049–54.
244. Recek N, Primc G, Vesel A, Mozetic M, Avila J, Razado-Colambo I, Asensio MC. Degradation of albumin on plasma-treated polystyrene by soft X-ray exposure. Polymers. 2016;8:244.
245. Zhang H, ZM X, Shen J, Li X, Ding LL, Ma J, Lan Y, Xia WD, Cheng C, Sun Q, Zhang Z, Chu PK. Effects and mechanism of atmospheric-pressure dielectric barrier discharge cold plasma on lactate dehydrogenase (LDH) enzyme. Sci Rep. 2015;5:10031.
246. Arfaoui M, Behary N, Mutel B, Perwuelz A, Belhacene K, Dhulster P, Mamede AS, Froidevaux R. Activity of enzymes immobilized on plasma treated polyester. J Mol Catal B Enzym. 2016;134:261–72.
247. Liu CJ, Li MY, Wang JQ, Zhou XT, Guo QT, Yan JM, Li YZ. Plasma methods for preparing green catalysts: Current status and perspective. Chin J Catal. 2016;37:340–8.
248. Pan YX, Cong HP, Men YL, Xin S, Sun ZQ, Liu CJ, Yu SH. Peptide self-assembled biofilm with unique electron transfer flexibility for highly efficient visible-light-driven photocatalysis. ACS Nano. 2015;9:11258–65.
249. Bussler S, Herppich WB, Neugart S, Schreiner M, Ehlbeck J, Rohn S, Schlueter O. Impact of cold atmospheric pressure plasma on physiology and flavonol glycoside profile of peas (Pisum sativum "Salamanca"). Food Res Int. 2015;76:132–41.
250. Zhang JJ, Jo JO, Huynh DL, Mongre RK, Ghosh M, Singh AK, Lee SB, Mok YS, Hyuk P, Jeong DK. Growth-inducing effects of argon plasma on soybean sprouts via the regulation of demethylation levels of energy metabolism-related genes. Sci Rep. 2017;7:41917.
251. Yan DY, Xiao HJ, Zhu W, Nourmohammadi N, Zhang LG, Bian K, Keidar M. The role of aquaporins in the anti-glioblastoma capacity of the cold plasma-stimulated medium. J Phys D Appl Phys. 2017;50:055401.
252. Bartis EAJ, Luan PS, Knoll AJ, Graves DB, Seong J, Oehrlein GS. A comparative study of biomolecule and polymer surface modifications by a surface microdischarge. Eur Phys J D. 2016;70(25):1–19.
253. Stoleru E, Dumitriu RP, Munteanu BS, Zaharescu T, Tanase EE, Mitelut A, Ailiesei GL, Vasile C. Novel procedure to enhance PLA surface properties by chitosan irreversible immobilization. Appl Surf Sci. 2016;367:407–17.
254. Bastekova K, Guselnikova O, Postnikov P, Elashnikov R, Kunes M, Kolska Z, Svorcik V, Lyutakov O. Spatially selective modification of PLA surface: from hydrophobic to hydrophilic or to repellent. Appl Surf Sci. 2017;397:226–34.
255. Stoleru E, Zaharaescu T, Hitruc EG, Vese A, Ioanid EG, Coroaba A, Safrany A, Pricope G, Lungu M, Schick C, Vasile C. Lactoferrin-immobilized surfaces onto functionalized PLA

assisted by the gamma-rays and nitrogen plasma to create materials with multifunctional properties. ACS Appl Mater Interfaces. 2016;8:31902–15.
256. Pankaj SK, Bueno-Ferrer C, O'Neill L, Tiwari BK, Bourke P, Cullen PJ. Characterization of dielectric barrier discharge atmospheric air plasma treated chitosan films. J Food Process Preserv. 2017;41:e12889.
257. Irimia A, Ioanid GE, Zaharescu T, Coroaba A, Doroftei F, Safrany A, Vasile C. Comparative study on gamma irradiation and cold plasma pretreatment for a cellulosic substrate modification with phenolic compounds. Radiat Phys Chem. 2017;130:52–61.
258. Memon H, Kumari N. Study of multifunctional nanocoated cold plasma treated polyester cotton blended curtains. Surf Rev Lett. 2016;23:1650036.
259. Primc G, Tomasic B, Vesel A, Mozetic M, Razic SE, Gorjanc M. Biodegradability of oxygen-plasma treated cellulose textile functionalized with ZnO nanoparticles as antibacterial treatment. J Phys D Appl Phys. 2016;49:324002.
260. Sousa S, Gaiolas C, Costa AP, Baptista C, Amaral ME. Cold plasma treatment of cotton and viscose fabrics impregnated with essential oils of Lavandula angustifolia and Melaleuca alternifolia. Cellul Chem Technol. 2016;50:711–9.
261. Karam L, Casetta M, Chihib NE, Bentiss F, Maschke U, Jama C. Optimization of cold nitrogen plasma surface modification process for setting up antimicrobial low density polyethylene films. J Taiwan Inst Chem Eng. 2016;64:299–305.
262. Pan H, Wang GM, Pan J, Ye GP, Sun K, Zhang J, Wang J. Cold plasma-induced surface modification of heat-polymerized acrylic resin and prevention of early adherence of Candida albicans. Dent Mater J. 2015;34:529–36.
263. Qian K, Pan H, Li YL, Wang GM, Zhang J, Pan J. Time-related surface modification of denture base acrylic resin treated by atmospheric pressure cold plasma. Dent Mater J. 2016;35:97–103.
264. Kredl J, Kolb JF, Schnabel U, Polak M, Weltmann KD, Fricke K. Deposition of antimicrobial copper-rich coatings on polymers by atmospheric pressure jet plasmas. Materials (Basel). 2016;9:274.
265. Ibis F, Oflaz H, Ercan UK. Biofilm inactivation and prevention on common implant material surfaces by nonthermal dbd plasma treatment. Plasma Med. 2016;6(1):33–45.
266. Guastaldi FPS, Yoo D, Marin C, Jimbo R, Tovar N, Zanetta-Barbosa D, Coelho PG. Plasma treatment maintains surface energy of the implant surface and enhances osseointegration. Int J Biomaterials. 2013:354125.
267. Rezaei F, Shokri B, Sharifian M. Atmospheric-pressure DBD plasma-assisted surface modification of polymethyl methacrylate: a study on cell growth/proliferation and antibacterial properties. Appl Surf Sci. 2016;360:641–51.
268. Joslin JM, McCall JR, Bzdek JP, Johnson DC, Hybertson BM. Aqueous plasma pharmacy: preparation methods, chemistry, and therapeutic applications. Plasma Med. 2016;6(2): 135–77.
269. Treshchalov A, Tsarenko S, Avarmaa T, Saar R, Lohmus A, Vanetsev A, Ilmo Sildos I. He/$H_2$ pulsed-discharge plasma as a tool for synthesis of surfactant-free colloidal silver nanoparticles in water. Plasma Med. 2016;6(1):85–100.
270. Ingels R, Graves DB. Improving the efficiency of organic fertilizer and nitrogen use via air plasma and distributed renewable energy. Plasma Med. 2015;5(2–4):257–70.
271. Pierdzioch P, Hartwig S, Herbst SR, Raguse JD, Dommisch H, Abu-Sirhan S, Wirtz HC, Hertel M, Paris S, Preissner S. Cold plasma: a novel approach to treat infected dentin—a combined ex vivo and in vitro study. Clin Oral Investig. 2016;20:2429–35.

# Application in Veterinary Medicine

# 15

Claudia Bender, Axel Kramer, and Matthias B. Stope

## 15.1 Introduction

**For the application of cold atmospheric plasmas (CAP) on animals, there are at present two indications: treatment of mainly chronic wounds, as well as the (supportive) treatment of superficial infections and parasitoses.**

Since the efficacy of CAP was also proven regarding the direct application to tumors [1–7], the use in the field of veterinary medicine appears perceptively conceivable.

## 15.2 Applications for Wound Treatment

### 15.2.1 Causes of Delayed Wound Healing and Resulting Targets for CAP

On the one hand, systemic factors inhibit wound healing in terms of reduced immune response, blood vessel disorder with reduced oxygen supply to the wound, reduced energy supply due to metabolic disease or lack of nutrition, lack of coagulation

C. Bender (✉)
Tierarztpraxen Dr. Claudia Bender in Karrin and Lubmin, Kröslin, Germany
e-mail: Bender@Tierarztpraxis-karrin.de

A. Kramer
Institute for Hygiene and Environmental Medicine, University Medicine Greifswald, Greifswald, Germany
e-mail: kramer@uni-greifswald.de

M. B. Stope
Department of Urology, University Medicine Greifswald, Greifswald, Germany
e-mail: matthias.stope@uni-greifswald.de



H.-R. Metelmann et al. (eds.), *Comprehensive Clinical Plasma Medicine*,
https://doi.org/10.1007/978-3-319-67627-2_15

factors, protein building blocks or vitamins, anemia, drugs (particularly cytostatics, corticoids, anticoagulants, and thyrostatic agents) and hormonal diseases including diabetes mellitus, hyperadrenocorticism, and hypothyroidism. On the other hand, wound healing is prevented or inhibited by local factors in the form of foreign bodies, dead tissue (necrosis), critical colonization or infection, pressure, hypothermia or dehydration. This can lead to the so-called dormant state of the chronic wound, either by a single or in the summation of different partial factors. However, even the acute wound cannot heal as long as it is critically colonized or infected [8–11].

Chronic wounds can be identified by the following properties [12, 13]:

- Because the healing process consumes energy, an energy input is required for healing. The center of chronic wounds is hypoxic and hypothermic, the deficient energy supply in the tissue inhibits wound healing.
- Increased tissue temperature (>38°C), increased partial pressure of oxygen (for aerobic energy supply) and increased blood flow (for the transport of energy-efficient substrates and removal of metabolic slag) promote wound healing.
- Damaged cells within the wound and necrotic tissue inhibit wound healing.
- Critical colonization / biofilm formation or infection prevents wound healing.
- Endotoxin absorption or binding is an adjuvant for wound healing.
- The existence of induced currents as well as the distribution of ions, on which the electrical signals are based on, is of high importance for the control of cell migration and cell division at the wound edge [14].
- In chronic wounds, all causes inhibiting healing must be eliminated as far as possible. Even then the healing of the wound often stagnates; in this case wound healing can be initiated or promoted by biochemical or physically initiated perforation of the so-called dormant stage [12].

The following influences have already demonstrated supportive effects for wound healing in the individual application:

- Induced currents and the electrical signals on the basis of the distribution of ions and electric fields [14, 15],
- Slightly elevated temperature [16],
- Antiseptic treatment for infected and critically colonized wounds, and experimental application for aseptic wounds [8, 9].

CAP treatment does cover all the listed properties. Therefore the hypothesis, that CAP is a new option for the treatment of chronic wounds in particular, was established and systematically verified. In addition to the fact that the energy supply and the elimination of damaged cells in wounds is also promoted by CAP, the decisive novelty was discovered (in contrast to the sole antiseptic treatment) in the interaction of antiseptic and debriding effects, induction of apoptosis and activation of resorptive inflammation, the dormant stage of the chronic wound is broken, and the wound is healed by passing through intermediate stage of the acute inflammation (Fig. 15.1).

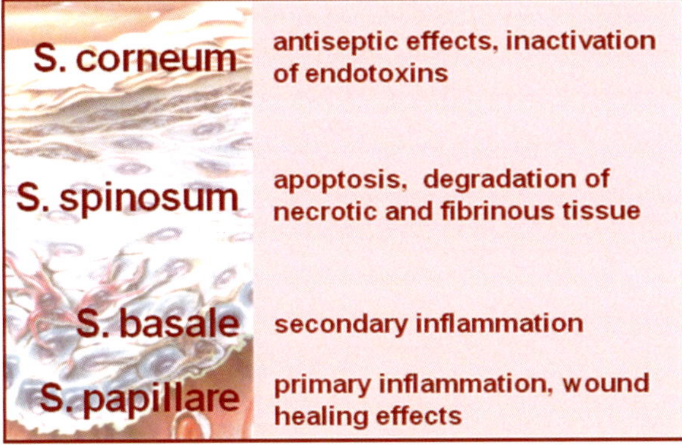


**Fig. 15.1** Targets of CAP in wound treatment

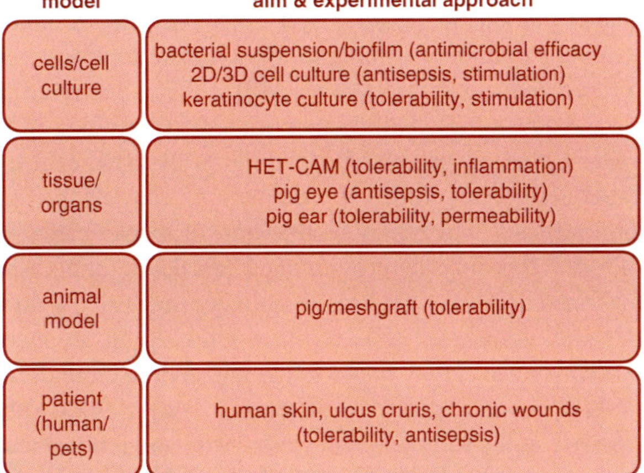


**Fig. 15.2** Hierarchy for the pre-clinical investigation procedure of CAP

### 15.2.2 Results of the Preclinical Test for the Suitability of CAP for Wound Treatment

**The synergistic potential of antiseptic and biofilm-inhibiting efficacy, endotoxin inactivation** [17]**, induction of apoptosis and inflammation, up-regulation of wound healing factors and tolerance to wounds makes CAP a promising option for the treatment of chronic wounds in particular.**

In model systems relevant for wound healing, the applicability of CAP with regard to antiseptic action and compatibility has been verified (Fig. 15.2).

*In vitro* CAP surpasses the microbicidal effect of the established wound antiseptics chlorhexidine digluconate, PVP-iodine and polihexanide [18, 19]. Furthermore, CAP is able to inactivate endotoxins [20]. In the 3-D epidermis model, *P. aeruginosa*, *S. aureus*, and *S. epidermidis* are inactivated without affecting the structure of the epidermis and carrying the bacteria into the depths [12, 21]. When used on monospecies biofilms of *P. aeruginosa, S. aureus, S. epidermidis* and *C. albicans*, as well as multispecies biofilms of saliva, CAP surpasses the efficiency of established antiseptics, whereas the efficacy is increased by the addition of 1% oxygen to CAP [22–29]. At the same time, the effect of antiseptics is reinforced by CAP [30]. Due to the microbicidal mechanism of action of CAP, no resistance has been induced in *S. aureus* biofilms [31]. From the range of test organisms, *P. aeruginosa* and *S. aureus* are considered to be relevant animal pathogens for which multiresistances are being described in increasing numbers. Both can infect a variety of animals, including mammals, as "broad host range pathogens" [32, 33]. *C. albicans* is also capable of infecting various animal species [34] and is especially pathogenic on reptiles [35, 36]. The microbicidal efficacy demonstrated in vitro could be confirmed on the eye and on the skin as well as on wounds [37–41] and oral mucosa [42].

The muscosal compatibility of CAP was first examined in the hen's egg test on the chorioallantoic membrane (HET-CAM) because compatible antiseptics are tolerated without irritation or without inhibition of wound healing in this model [43, 44], both for eye and wound antiseptics [45]. CAP is tolerated by the CAM comparable to wound antiseptics. At the same time, the promotion of blood circulation and angiogenesis were detectable. Depending on the treatment time, tissue processes can be generated in the form of contraction, coagulation and inflammation-associated angiogenesis, which may be relevant for the activation of secondary wound healing [43, 44]. Possibly the programmed cell death (apoptosis) induced by CAP, as demonstrated in *in vitro* systems, plays a decisive role [7, 46–51]. It is conceivable that in this way disordered cells of the wound region are inactivated and the state of the dormant stage is thus transformed into an acute inflammatory state [52, 53].

In a further study, an increased leukocyte-endothelium interaction with an increase in the rolling leukocyte fraction and leukocytes adhered to the vessel endothelium as a precursor of diapedesis into the surrounding tissue was detected by intravital microscopy. This indicates an increased local inflammatory and immunological response of the organism to the stimulus CAP [44]. CAP is also tolerated by the ear as well as by the freshly enucleated eye of slaughter pigs without histological changes [38, 54, 55].

In cell culture the proliferation of keratinocytes is promoted. In conformity with this, the up regulation of the following factors promoting the healing of the wound was demonstrated by CAP: Vascular Endothelial Growth Factor A (VEGF-A), Heparin-binding Epidermal Growth Factor (HBEGF), Granulocyte Macrophage Colony Stimulating Factor (GM-CSF), Prostaglandin endoperoxides synthase 2 (PTGS2) and Interleukin-6 (IL-6) [56].

With dermal aseptic wound degree IIa and with complete skin loss grade III in the pig, the wound healing time did not differ from the control, and no increased inflammatory responses and no cell abnormalities were observed, which means CAP did not cause wound healing delay [21]. In further animal experimental applications, the animal species mouse, rat and pig have shown a very good compatibility for CAP [57–60].

There was also no evidence for side effects on human skin [55, 61]. Similarly, no sensitization was inducible [62]. CAP only penetrates into the upper cell layers of the human stratum corneum [61]. Likewise in tumor tissue, the penetration depth does not exceed 60 μm [6], which corresponds to two to three cell diameters. This does not lead to any systemic risks. No mutagenic potency was detectable in accordance [63, 64].

In conclusion to the studies outlined in Fig. 15.2, a treatment time of max. 5 s/cm$^2$ of wound surface for the continuous mode of the plasma source was derived for the plasma source tested by us (KinPen09, neoplas tools GmbH Greifswald, Germany) [43, 44].

### 15.2.3 Compatibility of CAP for Humane Chronic Wounds

**Since the mammalian organism has numerous possibilities for the enzymatic and non-enzymatic detoxification of oxygen and nitrogen radicals and the lifetime of the CAP components as well as the penetration depth are uncritical, it is not to be expected that the superficial treatment of wounds with CAP is associated with long-term risks.**

No adverse reactions were observed in 8 trials (n = 260 patients) of treatment in chronic wounds [37, 39, 41, 65–69]. Even though previous data indicate no carcinogenic potential of CAP treatment, further systematic studies are necessary.

### 15.2.4 Results of Wound Treatment with CAP on Animals

**The clinical course of cure after the use of CAP on chronic wounds of different pet species (dog, cat, guinea pig) confirmed the hypothesis that by using CAP on chronic wounds, the healing process is initiated via the intermediate stage of acute inflammation. Even acute wounds can benefit from treatment with CAP.**

The efficacy of CAP with the Plasma-Jet kINPen09 using argon as carrier gas (5 l/min) on eight chronic wounds (Table 15.1) and 12 wound healing disorders (Table 15.2) previously treated unsuccessfully with conventional methods were examined in off-label healing experiments [43]. Prior to the application of CAP, the wound margins were excised and the wounds cleaned with sterile saline solution. Treatment with CAP was usually performed twice a week. The treatment time per square centimeter was 5 s. Simultaneously, the adjacent skin was treated as well. Due to the fact that CAP has no remanent antiseptic effect, wound antiseptics with

**Table 15.1** Successful treatment of chronic wounds of dogs (D) and cats (C) with CAP

| No. | Species | Duration (month) of the chronic wounds | Locali-sation | Pretreatments | Underlying disease | Treatment period with CAP (weeks) | Complete wound closure, observation | Heeling after weeks |
|---|---|---|---|---|---|---|---|---|
| 1 | D | ~60 | Nose | Surgery ointments, antiseptics | No | 14 | Yes | 10.5 |
| 2 | C | ~24 | Left foreleg | Autologous skin graft, antiseptics, antibiotics, ointments, wound dressings | Diabetes mellitus | 14 | Yes | 14 |
| 3 | D | ~36 | Left foreleg | Ointments, wound dressings, antiseptics | No | 5.5 | Yes | 7.5 |
| 4 | D | Lifelong | Face, ears | Immunosupressants, diet, antiseptics, antibiotics | Pemphigus foliaceus | 10 | Yes | 14 |
| 5 | C | 2 | Back | Antibiotics, ointments | Flea bite allergy | 3 | Yes | 3 |
| 6 | D | 6 | Right heel | Ointments, wound dressings | Paraplegia, bedsore | 4 | Yes | 4 |
| 7 | D | 0.75 | Left armpit | Antibiotics, ointments, powder, prednisolone | Juvenile cellulitis, pemanent treatment with prednisolon | 4 | Yes | 7 |
| 8 | D | 48 | Elbow | Repeated sore revision, antibiotics | No | 2.5 | No, reduction of the wound size, formation of granulation tissue | |

remanent efficacy and good tissue tolerability have been administered between the applications of CAP [43, 70, 71]. After treatment with CAP, the wounds were antiseptically treated daily with 0.02% polihexanide in Ringer or 0.05% polihexanide in Lipofundin® MCT 10% or with Octenilin® wound rinse solution. Afterwards, wound dressings were applied as wound protectors, and these were changed daily. The combination of polihexanide with lipofundin further improves the already low cytotoxicity of polihexanide with antiseptic efficacy still guaranteed [72, 73]. Wound healing was assessed using the following criteria:

- Visually noticeable change of the wound image with formation of an exudative wound with clean granulation tissue.
- Measurable reduction of the wound area within 1 week.
- Wound closure.

**Table 15.2** Successful treatment of wound healing disorders of different causes of dogs (D), cats (C) and a guinea pig (GP) with CAP

| No. | Species | Kind of wound healing disorder | Localisation | Pretreatment | Underlying disease | Treatment period with CAP (weeks) | Complete wound closure, observation | Heeling after weeks |
|---|---|---|---|---|---|---|---|---|
| 1 | D | Purulent suture dehiscence | Right hind-quaters | Surgery, ointment, antiseptics | No | 14 | Yes | 10.5 |
| 2 | C | Purulent suture dehiscence | Left hindlimb | Antiseptics, antibiotics ointments, wound dressings | No | 3 | Yes | 3.5 |
| 3 | D | Suture dehiscence | Right hindlimb | Ointments, wound dressings, antiseptics | No | 3 | Yes | 3.5 |
| 4 | C | Seroma formation in suture | Abdoma | Antibiotics, ointments | No | 1 | Yes | 1 |
| 5 | GP | Seroma formation in suture | Right abdominal wall | Antiseptic lavage | No | 1 | Yes | 1 |
| 6 | C | Fat necrosis, suspicion of snake bite | Lower abdomen | Antibiotics, wound irrigation | No | 5 | Yes | ca. 8 |
| 7 | D | Chronic inflammation and wound due to Demodicosis | All four paws | Antiseptics, ointments, lavage | Demodikosis | 2 | Yes | 2 |

(continued)

**Table 15.2** (continued)

| No. | Species | Kind of wound healing disorder | Localisation | Pretreatment | Underlying disease | Treatment period with CAP (weeks) | Complete wound closure, observation | Heeling after weeks |
|---|---|---|---|---|---|---|---|---|
| 8 | C | Tissue necrosis after skin tear by footfall, purulent suture dehiscence | Right hind paw | Antiseptics, suture, antibiotics | No | 6 | Yes | 8 |
| 9 | D | Suture dehiscence after removal of a mast cell tumor including the regional lymph node | Popliteal | Wound revision and renew suture | No | 5,5 | Yes | 5.5 |
| 10 | D | Pyoderma | Back | Antiseptics, antibiotics | Tumor of the maxilla (suspected squamous cell carcinoma) | 1 | Yes | 1 |
| 11 | D | Suture dehiscence after toe amputation, complicated by multiresitant *E. Coli* | Right hind paw | Antibiotics antiseptics, wound dressings | Squamous cell carcinoma | 4 | Yes | 4 |
| 12 | D | Suture dehiscence after thumb claw amputation, complicated by multiresistant *E. Coli* | Right forepaw | Antibiotics, antiseptics, wound dressings | Squamous cell carcinoma | 6 | Yes | 6 |

In cases when the therapy with CAP could not be carried out up to the closure of the wound due to the animal owners, the positive change in the wound pattern and a measurable reduction in the wound area were regarded as success.

The results of the accelerated appearance of the inflammatory phase, improved granulation, epithelialization and neovascularization [7, 74], which were obtained previously in animal experiments, were confirmed in the treatment of the domestic animals. In addition, even large-area wounds had only a slight scarring after complete epithelialization. With the gas flow, the CAP also reaches deep wound areas such as caverns and cavities, which is important in the treatment of abscess and seroma caves or after resection of larger tissue parts. The coagulation and coagulation-promoting plasma effects here [43, 75] apparently led to reduced exudate accumulation in the wound cavity, with the contraction-promoting effect [44] supporting the wound closure. Both on the wounds and on healthy skin, CAP was tolerated without recognizable side effects. The gas flow of the plasma jet can lead to tickling in sensitive areas such as the face and auditory canal. Sedation was not necessary in any case.

## 15.3 Options for Use of CAP in Infections, Parasitoses and Tumors

**The anti-bacterial, antiviral, acaricidal, antiprotozoal, anti-exudative and antitumoral effects open up new therapeutic possibilities.**

The anti-bacterial and anti-exudative effects [76, 77], which are also present in the hair follicles, are likely to be useful for the treatment of superficial infected skin diseases such as superficial pyodermia, pyotraumatic dermatitis (hotspot), intertrigo, talcum inflammation, acne and otitis externa [78].

On top of this, CAP is virucidal [79]. Human DNA viruses (adenoviridae, herpesviridae) as well as RNA viruses (respiratory viruses, caliciviridae, retroviruses) were similarly inactivated by CAP [80–82]. An antiviral effect could also be detected in an animal pathogenic feline calicivirus [83]. In the case of the following viral infections of pets, the use of CAP appears promising: feline calicivirus associated tongue ulcera, feline gingivitis stomatitis complex [84]. Due to the nonspecific mode of action, local effectiveness is to be assumed against other, non tested, viral species.

In conjunction with the antitumoral effect [1–6, 50, 51], use in canine papillomatosis, or concomitantly with surgical resection of an equine sarcoid or feline squamous cell carcinoma are examples for promising application areas.

Plasma operates acaricidal [85, 86]. Due to the efficacy against demodex mites [86] in combination with the effect of CAP [76] in the hair follicles, the use in localized demodicosis or in support of severe and generalized forms of demodicosis appears to bc succcssful and was proven successfully in first case at a dog [70].

Also *S. japonicum* cercariae [82] and leishmania [87] are killed by CAP; in the case of the cutaneous manifestation of canine leishmaniasis supportive application of CAP would be conceivable. On the other hand, it appears questionable to reach manifested cercariae with CAP.

**Conclusion**

The transition from the chronic wound to resorptive inflammation [88] with the promotion of cell proliferation and differentiation as well as microcirculation and increased leukocyte-endothelial interaction [89] is presumably due to the electric field [90] in combination with the radicals contained in CAP with activation of the respiratory burst and the redox-coupled wound healing [17]. The increased leucocyte-endothelial interaction reflects an increased local inflammatory and immunological response of the organism to the stimulus of the CAP. The clinical course of cure is initiated after the application of CAP in chronic wounds, via the intermediate stage of acute inflammation. So far, no undesirable side effects have been observed in wound treatment with CAP, therefore CAP can be used in combination with remanent antiseptics for the treatment of chronic wounds on animals [70]. Apparently the combination with a remanent antiseptic is necessary on at least critically colonized or infected wounds because no adequate results have been achieved with the use of CAP alone in chronic ulcers in human medicine without remanent antiseptics [91].

## References


1. Babington P. Use of cold atmospheric plasma in the treatment of cancer. Biointerphases. 2015;10(2):029403.
2. Graves DB. Reactive species from cold atmospheric plasma: implications for cancer therapy. Plasma Proc Polym. 2014;11:1120–7.
3. Keidar M, Shashurin A, Volotskova O, Stepp MA, Srinivasan P, Sandler A, Trink B. Cold atmospheric plasma in cancer therapy. Phys Plasmas. 2013;20:057101.
4. Keidar M, Walk R, Shashurin A, Srinivasan P, Sandler A, Dasgupta S, Ravi R, Guerrero-Preston R, Trink B. Cold plasma selectivity and the possibility of a paradigm shift in cancer therapy. Br J Cancer. 2011;105:1295–301.
5. Keidar M. Plasma for cancer treatment. Plasma Sourc Sci Technol. 2015;24(033001):20. 5; 10: 029403.
6. Partecke LI, Evert K, Haugk J, Döring F, Normann L, Diedrich S, Weiss F, Evert M, Hübner NO, Günther C, Heidecke C, Kramer A, Bussiahn R, Weltmann K, Pati O, Bender C, Bernstorff W. Tissue tolerable plasma (TTP) induce apoptosis in the human pancreatic cancer cell line Colo-357 in vitro and in vivo. BMC Cancer. 2012;12(1):473.
7. Yan D, Sherman JH, Keidar M. Cold atmospheric plasma, a novel promising anti-cancer treatment modality. Oncotarget. 2017;8(9):15977–95.
8. Kramer A, Assadian O, Below H, Willy C. Wound antiseptics today—an overview. In: Willy C, editor. Antiseptics in surgery—update 2013. Berlin: Lindqvist; 2013. p. 85–111.
9. Kramer A, Dissemond J, Kim S, Willy C, Mayer D, Papke R, Tuchmann F, Assadian O. Consensus on wound antisepsis: update 2018. Skin Pharmacol Physiol 2017;31(1):28-58. doi: https://doi.org/10.1159/000481545.

10. Schlüter B, KÖnig W. Microbial pathogenicity and host defense mechanisms: crucial parameters of posttraumatic infectitons. Thorac Cardiovasc Surg. 1990;38(6):339–47.
11. Thomson PD. Immunology, microbiology, and the recalcitrant wound. Ostomy Wound Manage. 2000;46(1A suppl):77S–82S.
12. Kramer A, Hübner NO, Assadian O, Below H, Bender C, Benkhai H, Bröker B, Ekkernkamp A, Eisenbeiß W, Hammann A, Hartmann B, Heidecke CD, Hinz P, Koban I, Koch S, Kocher T, Lademann J, Lademann O, Lerch MM, Maier S, Matthes R, Müller G, Partecke I, Rändler C, Weltmann KD, Zygmunt M. Chancen und Perspektiven der Plasmamedizin durch Anwendung von gewebekompatiblen Atmosphärendruckplasmen (Tissue Tolerable Plasmas, TTP). GMS Krankenhaushyg Interdiszip. 2009;4(2):Doc10.
13. Kramer A, Hübner NO, Weltmann KD, Lademann J, Ekkernkamp A, Hinz P, Assadian O. Polypragmasia in the therapy of infected wounds—conclusions drawn from the perspectives of low temperature plasma technology for plasma wound therapy. GMS Krankenhaushyg Interdiszip. 3(1):Doc13. (20080311).
14. Daeschlein G, Assadian O, Kloth LC, Kramer A. Antibacterial activity of positive and negative polarity low-voltage pulsed current (LVPC) on six typical gram-positive and gram-negative bacterial pathogens of chronic wounds. Wound Repair Regen. 2007;15(3):399–403.
15. Tai G, Reid B, Cao L, Zhao M. Electrotaxis and wound healing: experimental methods to study electric fields as a directional signal for cell migration. Methods Mol Biol. 2009;571:77–97.
16. Mercer JB, Nielsen SP, Hoffmann G. Improvement of wound healing by water-filtered infrared-A (wIRA) in patients with chronic venous stasis ulcers of the lower legs including evaluation using infrared thermography. GMS Krankenhaushyg Interdiszip. 2008;6:Doc11.
17. Sen CK, Roy S. Redox signals in wound healing. Biochim Biophys Acta. 2008;1780(11):1348–61.
18. Matthes R, Bekeschus S, Bender C, Koban I, Hübner NO, Kramer A. Pilot-study on the influence of carrier gas and plasma application (open resp. delimited) modifications on physical plasma and its antimicrobial effect against Pseudomonas aeruginosa and Staphylococcus aureus. GMS Krankenhhyg Interdiszip. 2012;7(1):Doc02.
19. Matthes R, Lührman A, Holtfreter S, Kolata J, Radke D, Hübner NO, Assadian O, Kramer A. Antibacterial activity of cold atmospheric pressure argon plasma against 78 genetically different (meca, luk-p, agr or capsular polysaccharide type) staphylococcus aureus strains. Skin Pharmacol Physiol. 2016;29(2):83–91.
20. Shintani H, Shimizu N, Imanishi Y, Sekiya T, Tamazawa K, Taniguchi A, Kido N. Inactivation of microorganisms and endotoxins by low temperature nitrogen gas plasma exposure. Biocontrol Sci. 2007;12(4):131–43.
21. Kramer A, Lademann J, Bender C, Sckell A, Hartmann B, Münch S, Hinz P, Ekkernkamp A, Matthes R, Koban I, Partecke I, Heidecke CD, Masur K, Reuter S, Weltmann KD, Assadian O. Suitability of tissue tolerable plasmas (TTP) for the management of chronic wounds. Clin Plasma Med. 2013;1:11–8.
22. Fricke K, Koban I, Tresp H, Jablonowski L, Schröder K, Kramer A, Weltmann KD, von Woedtke T, Kocher T. Atmospheric pressure plasma: a high-performance tool for the efficient removal of biofilms. PLoS One. 2012;7(8):1–8.
23. Gorynia S, Koban I, Matthes R, Welk A, Gorynia S, Hübner NO, Kocher T, Kramer A. In vitro efficacy of cold atmospheric pressure plasma on S. sanguinis biofilms in comparison of two test models. GMS Hyg Inf Contr. 2013;8(1):Doc01.
24. Hübner NO, Matthes R, Koban I, Rändler C, Müller G, Bender C, Kindel E, Kocher T, Kramer A. Efficacy of chlorhexidine, polihexanide and tissue-tolerable plasma against Pseudomonas Aeruginosa biofilms grown on polystyrene and silicone materials. Skin Pharmacol Physiol. 2010;23(Suppl):28–34.
25. Koban I, Holtfreter B, Hübner NO, Matthes R, Sietmann R, Kindel E, Weltmann KD, Welk A, Kramer A, Kocher T. Antimicrobial efficacy of non-thermal plasma in comparison to chlorhexidine against dental biofilms on titanium discs in vitro–proof of principle experiment. J Clin Periodontol. 2011;38(10):956–65.
26. Koban I, Matthes R, Hübner NO, Welk A, Meisel P, Holtfreter B, Sietmann R, Kindel E, Weltmann KD, Kramer A, Kocher T. Treatment of Candida albicans biofilms with low-tem-

perature plasma induced by dielectric barrier discharge and atmospheric pressure plasma jet. New J Phys. 2010;12:073039.
27. Matthes R, Bender C, Schlüter R, Koban I, Bussiahn R, Reuter S, Lademann J, Weltmann KD, Kramer A. Antimicrobial efficacy of two surface barrier discharges with air plasma against in vitro biofilms. PLoS One. 2013;8(7):e70462.
28. Matthes R, Jablonowski L, Koban I, Quade A, Hübner NO, Schlueter R, Weltmann KD, Woedtke v T, Kramer A, Kocher T. In vitro treatment of Candida Albicans biofilms on denture base material with volume dielectric barrier discharge plasma (VDBD) compared with common chemical antiseptics. Clin Oral Invest. 2015;19:2319–26.
29. Matthes R, Koban I, Bender C, Masur K, Kindel E, Weltmann KD, Kocher T, Kramer A, Hübner NO. Antimicrobial efficacy of an atmospheric pressure plasma jet against biofilms of Pseudomonas aeruginosa and Staphylococcus epidermidis. Plasma Proc Polym. 2013;10(2):161–6.
30. Koban I, Geisel MH, Holtfreter B, Jablonowski L, Hübner NO, Matthes R, Masur K, Weltmann KD, Kramer A, Kocher T. Synergistic effects of nonthermal plasma and disinfecting agents against dental biofilms in vitro. ISRN Dent. 2013;2013:573262.
31. Matthes R, Assadian O, Kramer A. Repeated applications of cold atmospheric pressure plasma does not induce resistance in Staphylococcus aureus embedded in biofilms. GMS Hyg Infect Contr. 2014;9(3):Doc17.
32. Hernandez-Divers SJ. Pulmonary candidiasis caused by Candida albicans in a Greek tortoise (Testudo graeca) and treatment with intrapulmonary amphotericin B. J Zoo Wildl Med. 2001;32:352–9.
33. Sung JM, Lloyd DH, Lindsay JA. Staphylococcus aureus host specificity: comparative genomics of human versus animal isolates by multi-strain microarray. Microbiology. 2008;154(7):1949–59.
34. Nett J, Andes D. Candida albicans biofilm development, modeling a host-pathogen interaction. Curr Opin Microbiol. 2006;9(4):340–5.
35. Friedrich A, Friedrich R, Heckers K, Rütten M, Steinmetz HW. Candida-Dermatitis bei einer Spornschildkröte (Geocholone sulcata). Tierärztl Prax Kleint. 2010;5:328–32.
36. Rahme LG, Ausubel FM, Cao H, Drenkard E, Goumnerov BC, Lau GW, Mahajan-Miklos S, Plotnikova J, Tan MW, Tsongalis J, Walendziewicz CL, Tompkins RG. Plants and animals share functionally common bacterial virulence factors. Proc Natl Acad Sci USA. 2000;97(16):8815–21.
37. Brehmer F, Haenssle HA, Daeschlein G, Ahmed R, Pfeiffer S, Görlitz A, Simon D, Schön MP, Wandke D, Emmert S. Alleviation of chronic venous leg ulcers with a hand-held dielectric barrier discharge plasma generator (PlasmaDerm(®) VU-2010): results of a monocentric, two-armed, open, prospective, randomized and controlled trial (NCT01415622). J Eur Acad Dermatol Venereol. 2015;29:148–55.
38. Hammann A, Hübner NO, Bender C, Ekkernkamp A, Hartmann B, Hinz P, Kindel E, Koban I, Koch S, Kohlmann T, Lademann J, Matthes R, Müller G, Titze R, Weltmann KD, Kramer A. Antiseptic efficacy and tolerance of tissue-tolerable plasma compared with two wound antiseptics on artificially bacterially contaminated eyes from commercially slaughtered pigs. Skin Pharmacol Physiol. 2010;23(6):328–32.
39. Isbary G, Heinlin J, Shimizu T, Zimmermann JL, Morfill G, Schmidt HU, Monetti R, Steffes B, Bunk W, Li Y, Klaempfl T, Karrer S, Landthaler M, Stolz W. Successful and safe use of 2 min cold atmospheric argon plasma in chronic wounds: results of a randomized controlled trial. Br J Dermatol. 2012;167:404–10.
40. Lademann J, Richter H, Schanzer S, Patzelt A, Thiede G, Kramer A, Weltmann KD, Hartmann B, Lange-Asschenfeldt B. Comparison of the antiseptic efficacy of tissue-tolerable plasma and an octenidine hydrochloride-based wound antiseptic on human skin. Skin Pharmacol Physiol. 2012;25(2):100–6.
41. Ulrich C, Kluschke F, Patzelt A, Vandersee S, Czaika VA, Richter H, Bob A, Hutten J, Painsi C, Hüge R, Kramer A, Assadian O, Lademann J, Lange-Asschenfeldt B. Clinical use of

cold atmospheric pressure argon plasma in chronic leg ulcers: a pilot study. J Wound Care. 2015;24:196–203.
42. Preissner S, Kastner I, Schütte E, Hartwig S, Schmidt-Westhausen AM, Paris S, Preissner R, Hertel M. Adjuvant antifungal therapy using tissue tolerable plasma on oral mucosa and removable dentures in oral candidiasis patients: a randomised double-blinded split-mouth pilot study. Mycoses. 2016;59:467–75.
43. Bender C, Matthes R, Kindel E, Kramer A, Lademann J, Weltmann KD, Eisenbeiß W, Hübner NH. The irritation potential of nonthermal atmospheric pressure plasma in the HET-CAM. Plasma Proc Polym. 2010;7(3–4):318–26.
44. Bender C, Partecke LI, Kindel E, Döring F, Lademann J, Heidecke CD, Kramer A, Hübner NO. The modified HET-CAM as a model for the assessment of the inflammatory response to tissue tolerable plasma. Toxicol In Vitro. 2011;25:530–7.
45. Kramer A, Behrens-Baumann W. Prophylactic use of topical anti-infectives in ophthalmology. Ophthalmologica. 1997;211(Suppl 1):68–76.
46. Arndt S, Landthaler M, Zimmermann JL, Unger P, Wacker E, Shimizu T, Li YF, Morfill GE, Bosserhoff AK, Karrer S. Effects of cold atmospheric plasma (cap) on ß-defensins, inflammatory cytokines, and apoptosis-related molecules in keratinocytes in vitro and in vivo. PLoS One. 2015;10(3):e0120041.
47. Arndt S, Unger P, Wacker E, Shimizu T, Heinlin J, Li YF, Thomas HM, Morfill GE, Zimmermann JL, Bosserhoff AK, Karrer S. Cold atmospheric plasma (cap) changes gene expression of key molecules of the wound healing machinery and improves wound healing in vitro and in vivo. PLoS One. 2013;8(11):e79325.
48. Arndt S, Wacker E, Li YF, Shimizu T, Thomas HM, Morfill GE, Karrer S, Zimmermann JL, Bosserhoff AK. Cold atmospheric plasma, a new strategy to induce senescence in melanoma cells. Exp Dermatol. 2013;22:284–9.
49. Choi JY, Joh HM, Park J-M, Kim MJ, Chung TH, Kang TH. Non-thermal plasma-induced apoptosis is modulated by ATR- and PARP1-mediated DNA damage responses and circadian clock. Oncotarget. 2016;7:32980.
50. Kim SJ, Chung TH. Cold atmospheric plasma jet-generated RONS and their selective effects on normal and carcinoma cells. Sci Rep. 2016;6:20332.
51. Xu D, Luo X, Xu Y, Cui Q, Yang Y, Liu D, Chen H, Kong MG. The effects of cold atmospheric plasma on cell adhesion, differentiation, migration, apoptosis and drug sensitivity of multiple myeloma. Biochem Biophys Res Commun. 2016;473(4):1125–32.
52. Chang JW, Kang SU, Shin YS, Kim KI, Seo SJ, Yang SS, Lee JS, Moon E, Baek SJ, Lee K, Kim CH. Non-thermal atmospheric pressure plasma induces apoptosis in oral cavity squamous cell carcinoma: involvement of DNA-damage-triggering sub-G1 arrest via the ATM/p53 pathway. Arch Biochem Biophys. 2014;545:133–40.
53. Weiss M, Gümbel D, Hanschmann EM, Mandelkow R, Gelbrich N, Zimmermann U, Walther R, Ekkernkamp A, Sckell A, Kramer A, Burchardt M, Lillig CH, Stope MB. Cold atmospheric plasma treatment induces anti-proliferative effects in prostate cancer cells by redox and apoptotic signaling pathways. PLoS One. 2015;10:e0130350.
54. Lademann J, Richter H, Alborova A, Humme D, Patzelt A, Kramer A, Weltmann KD, Hartmann B, Ottomann C, Fluhr JW, Hinz P, Hübner G, Lademann O. Risk assessment of the application of a plasma-jet in dermatology. J Biomed Opt. 2009;14(5):054025.
55. Lademann O, Richter H, Patzelt A, Alborova A, Humme D, Weltmann KD, Hartmann B, Hinz P, Kramer A, Koch S. Application of a plasma-jet for skin antisepsis: analysis of the thermal action of the plasma by laser scanning microscopy. Laser Phys Lett. 2010;7(6):458–62.
56. Barton A, Wende K, Lena Bundscherer L, Hasse S, Schmidt A, Bekeschus S, Weltmann KD, Lindequist U, Masur K. Nonthermal plasma increases expression of wound healing related genes in a keratinocyte cell line. Plasma Med. 2013;3(1–2):125–36.
57. Chakravarthy K, Dobrynin D, Fridman G, Friedman G, Murthy S, Fridman A. Cold spark discharge plasma treatment of in flammatory bowel disease in an animal model of ulcerative colitis. Plasma Med. 2001;1(1):3–19.

58. Dobrynin D, Wu A, Kalghatgi S, Park S, Shainsky N, Wasko K, Dumani E, Ownbey R, Joshi S, Sensenig R, Brooks AD. Live pig skin tissue and wound toxicity of cold plasma treatment. Plasma Med. 2011;1(1):93–108.
59. Ermolaeva SA, Varfolomeev AF, Chernukha MY, Yurov DS, Vasiliev MM, Kaminskaya AA, Moisenovich MM, Romanova JM, Murashev AN, Selezneva II, Shimizu T, Sysolyatina EV, Shaginyan IA, Petrov OF, Mayevsky EI, Fortov VE, Morfill GE, Naroditsky BS, Gintsburg AL. Bactericidal effects of non-thermal argon plasma in vitro, in biofilms and in the animal model of infected wounds. J Med Microbiol. 2011;60(1):75–83.
60. Yu Y, Tan M, Chen H, Wu Z, Xu L, Li J, Cao J, Yang Y, Xiao X, Lian X, Lu X, Tu Y. Non-thermal plasma suppresses bacterial colonization on skin wound and promotes wound healing in mice. J Huazhong Univ Sci Technol Med Sci. 2011;31(3):390–4.
61. Fluhr JW, Sassning S, Lademann O, Darvin ME, Schanzer S, Kramer A, Richter H, Sterry W, Lademann J. In vivo skin treatment with tissue tolerable plasma influences skin physiology and antioxidant profile in human stratum corneum. Exp Dermatol. 2012;21(2):130–4.
62. van der Linde J, Liedtke KR, Matthes R, Kramer A, Heidecke CD, Partecke LI. Repeated cold atmospheric plasma application to intact skin causes no sensitization in a standardized murine model. Plasma Med. https://doi.org/10.1615/PlasmaMed.2017019167.
63. Boxhammer V, Li YF, Köritzer J, Shimizu T, Maisch T, Thomas HM, Schlegel J, Morfill GE, Zimmermann JL. Investigation of the mutagenic potential of cold atmospheric plasma at bactericidal dosages. Mut Res Genet Toxicol Environ. 2013;753:23–8.
64. Kluge S, Bekeschus S, Bender C, Benkhai H, Sckell A, Below H, Stope MB, Kramer A. Investigating the mutagenicity of a cold argon-plasma jet in an HET-MN model. PLoS One. 2016;11(9):e0160667.
65. Heinlin J, Maisch T, Zimmermann JL, Shimizu T, Holzmann T, Simon M, Heider J, Landthaler M, Morfill G, Karrer S. Contact-free inactivation of Trichophyton rubrum and Microsporum canis by cold atmospheric plasma treatment. Future Microbiol. 2013;8:1097–106.
66. Heinlin J, Zimmermann JL, Zeman F, Bunk W, Isbary G, Landthaler M, Maisch T, Monetti R, Morfill G, Shimizu T, Steinbauer J, Stolz W, Karrer S. Randomized placebo-controlled human pilot study of cold atmospheric argon plasma on skin graft donor sites. Wound Repair Regen. 2013;21:800–7.
67. Isbary G, Morfill G, Schmidt HU, Georgi M, Ramrath K, Heinlin J, Karrer S, Landthaler M, Shimizu T, Steffes B, Bunk W, Monetti R, Zimmermann JL, Pompl R, Stolz W. A first prospective randomized controlled trial to decrease bacterial load using cold atmospheric argon plasma on chronic wounds in patients. Br J Dermatol. 2010;163:78–82.
68. Isbary G, Shimizu T, Zimmermann JL, Thomas HM, Morfill GE, Stolz W. Cold atmospheric plasma for local infection control and subsequent pain reduction in a patient with chronic post-operative ear infection. New Microbes New Infect. 2013;1:41–3.
69. Kisch T, Schleusser S, Helmke A, Mauss KL, Wenzel ET, Hasemann B, Mailaender P, Kraemer R. The repetitive use of non-thermal dielectric barrier discharge plasma boosts cutaneous microcirculatory effects. Microvasc Res. 2016;106:8–13.
70. Bender C, Kramer A. Therapy of wound healing disorders in pets with atmospheric pressure plasma. Tierärztl Umschau. 2016;71:262–8.
71. Bender C, Kramer A. Options of antiseptic wound treatment in veterinary practice with special consideration of tissue compatibility. Kleintierpraxis. 2017;62(6):372–94.
72. Müller G, Koburger T, Kramer A. Interaction of polyhexamethylene biguanide hydrochloride (PHMB) with phosphatidylcholine containing o/w emulsion and consequences for microbicidal efficacy and cytotoxicity. Chem Biol Interact. 2013;201:58–64.
73. Müller G, Kramer A, Schmitt J, Harden D, Koburger T. Reduced cytotoxicity of polyhexamethylene biguanide hydrochloride (PHMB) by egg phosphatidylcholine while maintaining antimicobial efficacy. Chem Biol Interact. 2011;190:171–8.
74. Nastuta AV, Topala I, Grigoras C, Pohoata V, Popa G. Stimulation of wound healing by helium atmospheric pressure plasma treatment. J Phys D Appl Phys. 2011;44:105204.
75. Raiser J, Zenker M. Argon plasma coagulation for open surgical and endoscopic applications: state of the art. J Phys D Appl Phys. 2006;39:3520–3.

76. Lademann O, Kramer A, Richter H, Patzelt A, Meinke M, Roewert-Huber J, Czaika V, Weltmann KD, Hartmann B, Koch S. Antisepsis of the follicular reservoir by treatment with tissue-tolerable plasma (TTP). Laser Phys Lett. 2011;8:313.
77. Lange-Asschenfeldt B, Marenbach D, Lang C, Patzelt A, Ulrich M, Maltusch A, Terhorst D, Stockfleth E, Sterry W, Lademann J. Distribution of bacteria in the epidermal layers and hair follicles of the human skin. Skin Pharmacol Physiol. 2011;24:305–11.
78. Horstmann C. Localisation and typing of multiresistant staphylcocci in dogs and their owners. Tierärztl Fakultät: Diss Ludwig-Maximilians-Univ München; 2012.
79. Weiss M, Daeschlein G, Kramer A, Burchardt M, Brucker S, Wallwiener D, Stope MB. Virucide properties of cold atmospheric plasma for future clinical applications. J Med Virol. 2017;89:952–9.
80. Puligundla P, Mok C. Non-thermal plasmas (NTPs) for inactivation of viruses in abiotic environment. Res J Biotechnol. 2016;11(6):91–6.
81. Volotskova O, Dubrovsky L, Keidar M, Bukrinsky M. Cold atmospheric plasma inhibits HIV-1 replication in macrophages by targeting both the virus and the cells. PLoS One. 2016;11(10):e0165322.
82. Wang XQ, Wang FP, Chen W, Huang J, Bazaka K, Ostrikov K. Non-equilibrium plasma prevention of Schistosoma japonicum transmission. Sci Rep. 2016;6:35353.
83. Aboubakr HA, Williams P, Gangal U, Youssef MM, El-Sohaimy SA, Bruggeman PJ, Goyal SM. Virucidal effect of cold atmospheric gaseous plasma on feline calicivirus, a surrogate for human norovirus. Appl Environ Microbiol. 2015;81(11):3612–22.
84. Lommer MJ, Verstraete FJM. Concurrent oral shedding of feline calicivirus and feline herpesvirus 1 in cats with chronic gingivostomatitis. Oral Microbiol Immunol. 2003;18:131–4.
85. Bender C, Kramer A. Efficacy of tissue tolerable plasma (TTP) against Ixodes ricinus. GMS Hyg Infect Control. 2014;9(1):Doc04.
86. Daeschlein G, Scholz S, Arnold A, von Woedtke T, Kindel E, Niggemeier M, Weltmann KD, Jünger M. In-vitro activity of atmospheric pressure plasma jet (APPJ) against clinical isolates of Demodex folliculorum. IEEE Trans Plasma Sci. 2010;38(10):2969–73.
87. Pournaseh Y, Irani S, Amin M. Cold atmospheric plasma jet against Leishmania major in vitro study. Bas Res J Med Clin Sci. 2015;4(3):90–4.
88. Tipa RS, Kroesen GMW. Plasma-stimulated wound healing. IEEE Trans Plasma Sci. 2011;39:2978–9.
89. Bender C, Pavlovic D, Wegner A, Hinz P, Ekkernkamp A, Kramer A, Sckell A. Intravital fluorescence microscopy for the assessment of microcirculation and leucoyte-endothel interaction after application of tissue tolerable plasma in the HET-CAM. In: Mikikian M, Rabat H, Robert E, Pouvesle JM (eds) Book of Abstracts 4th Int Conf Plasma Medicine, Orleans, 2012; p. 86.
90. Rajnicek AM, Foubister LE, McCaig CD. Growth cone steering by a physiological electric field requires dynamic microtubules, microfilaments and Rac-mediated filopodial asymmetry. J Cell Sci. 2006;119:1736–45.
91. Assadian O, Ousey K, Daeschlein G, Kramer A, Parker C, Tanner J, Leaper D. Effects of atmospheric low temperature plasma on bacterial reduction in chronic wounds and wound size reduction. Br J Dermatol. (In rev).

# Part III

# Investigating Physical Plasma: New Horizons

# Side Effect Management

# 16

Georg Bauer, David B. Graves, Matthias Schuster, and Hans-Robert Metelmann

## 16.1 Introduction

The area of medical applications of cold atmospheric plasma (CAP) is including skin disinfection, tissue regeneration, chronic wounds and cancer treatment. Clinical studies are encouraging and generally conclude that CAP is well-tolerated and causes no severe side effects or complications [1–3]. Understanding the effects of CAP as well as its unexpected low side effects requires an analysis of the biological chemistry of CAP constituents. Of particular interest thereby are reactive oxygen and nitrogen species (ROS and RNS), as well as the sophisticated control systems of cells directed towards ROS and RNS. This knowledge may help to avoid the emergence of side effects at high doses of CAP or when its composition is changed. Cellular control systems directed towards ROS and RNS have evolved as (1) cells are using ROS and RNS for multiple biological functions, (2) ROS and RNS have intra- and intercellular signaling functions, (3) ROS and RNS are used for antimicrobial and antioncogenic defence mechansims, (4) and organisms are also confronted with exogenous sources of ROS and RNS [4–7].

An impressive example of the multiple modes of ROS and RNS action and its control becomes overt when the interactions between Helicobacter pylori (H. pylori) and human tissue are studied [8]. The analysis of this interaction

G. Bauer (✉)
Institute of Virology, Medical Center and Faculty of Medicine, University of Freiburg, Freiburg, Germany
e-mail: georg.bauer@uniklinik-freiburg.de

D. B. Graves
Department of Chemical and Biomolecular Engineering, University of California at Berkeley, Berkeley, CA, USA

M. Schuster • H.-R. Metelmann
Department of Oral and Maxillofacial Surgery/Plastic Surgery, University Medicine Greifswald, Greifswald, Germany



H.-R. Metelmann et al. (eds.), *Comprehensive Clinical Plasma Medicine*,
https://doi.org/10.1007/978-3-319-67627-2_16

demonstrates the role of ROS and RNS for the (1) defence towards the bacteria, (2) induction of mutagenesis after chronic infection with H. pylori; (3) establishment of the transformed state of cells and (4) mechanisms counteracting and eliminating transformed cells. It also shows the role of the protective functions of catalase and SOD for H. pylori and the malignant cells.

The take-home lesson from this scenario for other applications, such as CAP treatment, is the necessity to study the quality of ROS/RNS, their site of application, their dose, the length of time of application and the strength as well as the dynamics of counteracting antioxidative systems. This then may allow to evaluate the potential benefit or risk from the application of ROS/RNS.

Cold atmospheric plasma supplies UV radiation, free electrons and ROS and RNS such as superoxide anions ($O_2\bullet^-$), hydroperoxide radicals ($HO_2\bullet$), hydrogen peroxide ($H_2O_2$), hydroxyl radicals ($\bullet OH$), singlet oxygen ($^1O_2$), nitrogen monoxide ($\bullet NO$), nitrogen dioxide ($\bullet NO_2$), nitrite ($NO_2^-$), nitrate ($NO_3^-$), peroxynitrite ($ONOO^-$), hypochlorite anion ($OCl^-$) and dichloride anion radicals ($Cl_2\bullet^-$) [9–17]. These species show divergent free diffusion path lengths, different reactivities and multiple modes of interactions [9, 17].

## 16.2 Biological Effects of CAP and Risk Assessment

When CAP is allowed to *directly* interact with enzymes or DNA, its damaging and mutagenic potential is easily demonstrated and light is shed on the underlying mechanisms [18, 19]. However, though showing the strong reactivity of CAP, these data cannot be directly translated into risk assessment, mainly for two reasons: (1) only few CAP-derived species can indeed enter cells. These are essentially (i) NO that passes the cell membrane, and (ii) $H_2O_2$ that enters the cells through aquaporins. Other reactive species like singlet oxygen, peroxynitrite, hydroxyl radicals and hypochlorite can be expected to react with the extracellular matrix or the cell membrane, rather than to enter the cell. (2) Multiple antioxidative defence systems of cells will counteract intruding CAP constituents and their reaction products. In line with these assumptions, no genotoxic risk by CAP treatment above the dose range used for the treatment of chronic wound has been demonstrated when the hypoxantine-guanine phosphoribosyl transferase-1 (HPRT1) mutation assay, the test systems for micronuclei formation and colony formation had been applied [20–22]. Boxhammer et al. [20] showed that whereas 30 s treatment with their CAP device caused inactivation of E. coli by 5 log steps, even 120 s of treatment did not cause detectable genotoxicity. In the study by Kluge et al. [21], using a cold argon plasma jet (kinPenMed), a dose of CAP tenfold above the usual dose used for the treatment of chronic wounds did not cause genotoxic effects. A study by Wende et al. [23] demonstrated that higher dose ranges of CAP applied to HaCaT keratinocytes may cause single strand breaks, but no double strand breaks. Importantly, the single strand breaks were only detected immediately after treatment and were no longer detected at 24 h after treatment. This important finding demonstrates that the defence system of the cells is also efficient at the level of repair, in cooperation with prevention and interception, following the concept of protection against oxidative stress as originally outlined by Sies [4]. A study by Isbary et al. [24] showed that CAP treatment of ex vivo skin samples up to 2 min was tolerable for the skin and did not lead to double strand breaks, in line with the findings presented by Wende et al. [23]. The absence of genotoxic effect after CAP treatment at the indicated doses is in perfect agreement with the observations that CAP did not induce a long term oncogenic effect in an animal model [25, 26] and human studies [26].

It is predictable that glutathione should be one of the central and determining molecules involved in the intracellular defence towards CAP-derived ROS and RNS, either through its potential for direct interaction, or as essential cofactor for glutathione peroxidase and phospholipid hydroperoxide glutathione peroxidase. These enzymes protect cells against the damaging effects of lipid peroxidation. The interaction between CAP and glutathione has been carefully studied by Ke and Huang [27] and Klinkhammer et al. [28]. It is reasonable to assume that the intracellular glutathione level, in interaction with other intracellular antioxidant defence mechanisms like catalase, glutathione peroxidase and peroxiredoxin, lowers the level of intruding molecules from CAP to a level where damaging effects are abolished and only physiological signaling functions are remaining. Therefore, cells are definitely sensing CAP treatment. They then respond with an upregulation of antioxidant defence systems, but potentially also with proliferation. In the case of skin cells or immune cells, these proliferation-stimulating effects can even contribute to the beneficial effects of CAP treatment on wound healing [25, 29–36].

There is a general consensus that CAP treatment at appropriate doses that are used under defined conditions is free of risks and does not cause severe side effects [2, 3, 33, 37]. Several clinical studies demonstrate the efficacy and safety of CAP treatment [1, 26, 38–45]. In line with these results, Schuster et al. [46] summarized the findings on CAP treatment of 20 patients suffering from advanced head and neck cancer and contaminated ulcerations. They reported mainly very mild reactions in a few cases.

Though more studies are required in the expanding field of plasma medicine, the existing data and concepts are encouraging and should allow to define strategies for prevention of side effects in future applications. This is especially important as different CAP devices and non-standardized CAP compositions are going to be used.

The following sections suggest a rational approach for side effect evaluation and management.

## 16.3 Approach for Side Effect Evaluation and Management

### 16.3.1 CAP Treatment of Infected Tissues

Conditions for efficient bacterial decontamination of chronic wounds by cold atmospheric plasma without negative side effects on the regenerating tissue have been established by many researchers [1, 2, 15]. The removal of biofilms as well as individual bacteria is essential for wound healing. It acts in concert with beneficial effects of plasma on the wound healing process. Bacterial decontamination through application of CAP also represents an early and essential step during palliative cancer treatment. It has been shown to be very efficient. In several cases, this treatment seemed to be followed by a CAP-mediated antitumor effect [47, 48]. An analysis on 20 patients suffering from advanced head and neck cancer and contaminated ulcerations showed mainly very mild reactions in a few cases [46].

Successful decontamination of infected cancer ulcerations and wounds by cold atmospheric plasma [1, 2, 47], without harming nonmalignant tissue, indicates that the effect of plasma on bacteria must be more complex and sophisticated than comparable direct antimicrobial effects of chemical disinfectants or radiation. Otherwise a certain degree of damage of the tissue would be expected, especially in the case of regenerating tissue in a healing wound. A reflection on the dose of CAP applied for treating a chronic wound and on the ROS/RNS species within CAP or generated after CAP/liquid interaction might give an explanation for the observed effects. It also might help to determine the parameters required to avoid unwanted side effects. Figure 16.1 shows two conceivable alternative modes of action of CAP, determined

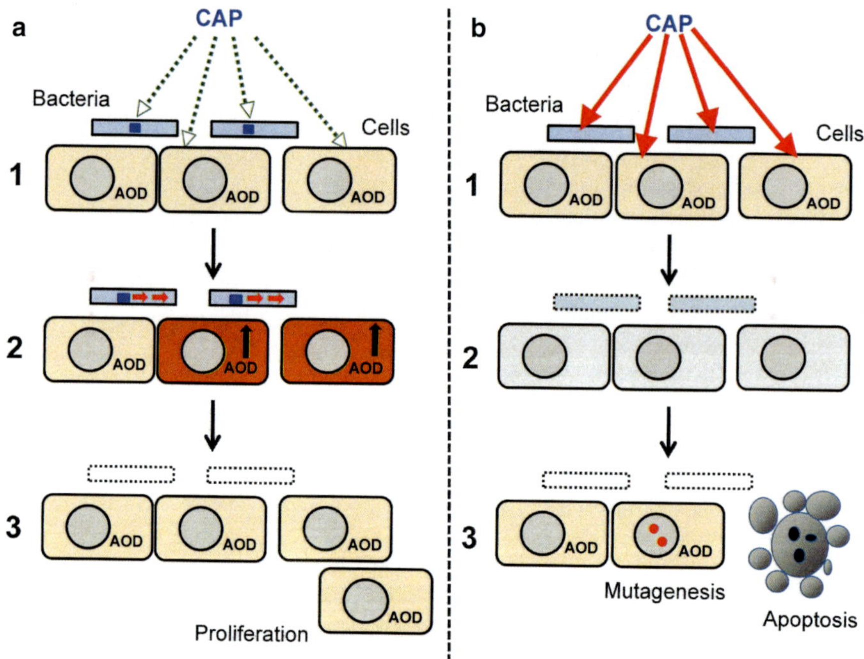


**Fig. 16.1** Antibacterial treatment with CAP. (**a**) A relatively low dose of CAP triggers a specific target response in bacteria. The target response and not CAP itself cause the antibacterial effect. Therefore the required dose of CAP is low, but specific CAP constituents such as singlet oxygen are required. CAP is sensed by the tissue and causes induction of a protective antioxidant defence (AOD). Therefore mutagenic effects are avoided and cell proliferation is possibly induced. (**b**) High doses of CAP have a direct damaging effect on bacteria but also can cause depletion of the antioxidant defence of tissue, leading to mutagenesis and cell death

by its dose and effectiveness of compounds. The dose applied in Fig. 16.1a is assumed to be too low to cause (1) a direct destruction of bacteria and (2) a sustained negative effect on healthy tissue. The mechanism underlying the indirect damaging effect of CAP on bacteria is assumed to trigger a cascade of effects within the bacteria that specifically damage the bacteria. In this way they cause their elimination. In this scenario, CAP would be the selective trigger that induces a strong, but locally restricted damaging effect in the target structure bacterium. This damaging effect would depend on the metabolism of the bacteria. As the required dose for the initial triggering effect of CAP may be reasonably low, the surrounding tissue would not be negatively affected. As the cells seem to sense the applied CAP constituents (those that are triggering the specific effect in bacteria as well as those that are accompanying), the upregulation of their natural antioxidant defense system will prevent ROS/RNS-related damages within the cells. $H_2O_2$ may be one of the central molecules involved in this scenario [32, 49]. $H_2O_2$ may enter the cells through aquaporins, but its concentration can be expected to be minimized by the intracellular antioxidant systems to the level of biological signaling functions [5, 6]. As low concentrations of $H_2O_2$ regulate fine-tuned proliferation control, cells in the regenerating wound may be stimulated by this process. They thus contribute to the success of treatment [30, 49, 50]. Though the exact mechanism of CAP-mediated killing of bacteria is still a matter of scientific debate, the combination of several experimental findings allow to establish circumstantial evidence for the model presented under Fig. 16.1a. Wu et al. have shown that CAP-mediated effects on bacterial killing are mainly due to singlet oxygen contained in or generated by CAP [51], as scavenging of singlet oxygen largely abrogated the antibacterial effect. This finding is in perfect agreement with data that show the very efficient antibacterial potential of singlet oxygen [52, 53]. According to Dahl et al. [52] singlet oxygen-dependent bacterial killing was about 3–4 orders of magnitude more effective as bacterial killing by $H_2O_2$. Even extremely radiation-resistant bacteria like Deinococcus radiodurans were highly sensitive to singlet oxygen-dependent inactivation [54]. The report on the inactivation of bacterial respiratory chain enzymes by singlet oxygen [55] might be the clue for the understanding of the remarkable inactivation of bacteria by singlet oxygen. It therefore seems to be likely that the damaging effect of singlet oxygen on bacteria is not based on general destruction of bacterial components by singlet oxygen (which would require a large number of hits), but that the site-directed inactivation of central elements of the ATP generating system by a relatively low dose of singlet oxygen causes a strong subsequent effect on bacterial survival through depletion of their ATP-generating system. Based on direct measurements of singlet oxygen action directed towards mammalian cells [56], it may be concluded that the singlet oxygen doses required for decontamination of bacteria are not sufficient to harm nonmalignant cells. This conclusion, that fits the actual findings for CAP-based contamination, is also substantiated by the fact that singlet oxygen generated by photosensitizers is effective towards bacteria-induced dental caries without affecting the tissue in the mouth [57]. It becomes obvious from Fig. 16.1b, that a dose of CAP that is sufficiently high to directly damage bacteria might do this at the price of damaging effects on the tissue. A high dose of CAP can be predicted to cause an initial depletion of cellular antioxidants (especially glutathione in its reduced form) which can be expected to be followed by mutagenesis and/or induction of apoptosis or necrosis.

Therefore, efficient management of, or outright prevention of side effects during the antibacterial treatment of chronic wounds, ulcers and tumors appears to require a combination of the right dose and the right composition of CAP. These two aspects then meet the requirements for the triggering function of CAP for induction of a damaging effect in the bacteria without negatively affecting the healthy tissue. It seems that the concentration of singlet oxygen in CAP as well as the potential of other CAP constituents to generate singlet oxygen after interaction [17] might be one of the most crucial factors for this determination. The concentration of $H_2O_2$ might also be important for predictions of the side effects. However, further experimental work along these lines and a thorough investigation of the properties and characteristics of various CAP-generating devices to be use is highly recommended.

In order to avoid mutagenic effects after CAP treatment due to damaging doses of certain CAP constituents, it seems reasonable to reflect on those constituents that may enter tissues and cause depletion of the antioxidant defence and subsequent mutagenesis. The effect of CAP on GSH in solution and its mutagenic effect on isolated DNA are obvious. However, hazardous biological effects require defined CAP constituents to enter target cells and act inside, being faced with a strong and flexible biological antioxidant defence system. As shown in Fig. 16.2, CAP constituents like singlet oxygen, hydroxyl radicals or peroxynitrite have little or no chance to enter a cell, as they will react with reaction partners in the cell membrane. If the concentration of these ROS/RNS is sufficiently high and the counterbalance by glutathione peroxidase/GSH is insufficient, this may trigger the onset of apoptosis. By contrast, both hydrogen peroxide and nitric oxide may easily enter cells, the former through aquaporins and the latter readily passes the membrane. These compounds or their reaction products can be expected to be counteracted by the antioxidant system in several ways. Only if the cellular antioxidant status is lowered by the insult or in defined local situations, the reactions outlined in Fig. 16.2 have a chance to contribute to mutagenesis, damage or signaling. Based on a rich literature, hydroxyl radical formation based on Fenton chemistry of $H_2O_2$ or decomposition of peroxynitrous acid might be one driving force for mutagenesis, provided it occurs at the right site, i.e. in the nucleus. In addition, the intracellular generation of singlet oxygen might lead to mutagenesis as well. A deeper understanding of these processes and the chance to modulate the composition of CAP may be instrumental to avoid damaging and mutagenic effects of CAP and to develop further improvement of treatment in the future.

### 16.3.2 Treatment of Tumors with CAP

CAP has been shown to trigger a strong apoptosis or necrosis-inducing effect on tumor cells in vitro and on tumors in vivo [48, 58–73], reviewed in Keidar et al. [74–76], Schlegel et al. [77], Tanaka et al. [78]; Barekzi and Laroussi [79]; Laroussi [80, 81];

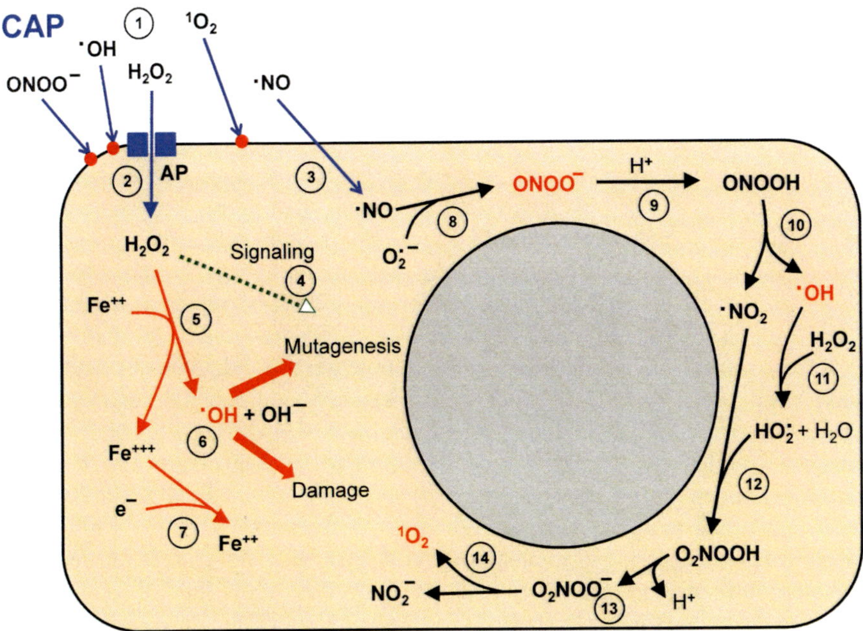


**Fig. 16.2** Intracellular effects of CAP. CAP-derived species like peroxynitrite, hydroxyl radicals and singlet oxygen have no chance to enter the cell as they react with extracellular matrix or the cell membrane (#1). $H_2O_2$ enters the cells through aquaporins (AP) (#2). NO passes the membrane directly (#3). $H_2O_2$ may contribute to intracellular signaling (#4) or may be the source for hydroxyl radicals after Fenton reaction (#5–#7). The reaction between NO and superoxide anions yields peroxynitrite (#8) that may lead to the generation of hydroxyl radicals (#9, #10). Reactions #11–#14 lead to the generation of singlet oxygen. In case the antioxidant defence system of the cells does not remove hydroxyl radicals, peroxynitrite or singlet oxygen, these species may cause damage. If these species are produced within the nucleus and not counteracted by the antioxidant defence, mutagenesis may be induced

Laroussi et al. [82]; Graves [10]; Ratovitski et al. [83], Yan et al. [84]; Gay-Mimbrera et al. [85], Babington et al. [86]. The review of CAP treatment of tumor cells in vitro and in vivo by Keidar et al. [74–76], Schlegel et al. [77], Barekzi and Laroussi [79]; Laroussi [80, 81]; Graves [10]; Ratovitski et al. [83], Yan et al. [84]; Gay-Mimbrera et al. [85], Babington et al. [86] leads to the common theme that anticancer effects of CAP i) have the potential to be selective with respect to the malignant phenotype of target cells, i) seem to be mediated or at least initiated by CAP-derived reactive oxygen/nitrogen species (ROS/RNS) and iii) are amplified by intracellular ROS. A selective action of precisely defined doses of CAP towards tumor cells has been established in many publications by direct comparison of tumor and corresponding nonmalignant cells. Whereas the tumor cells were responsive to CAP treatment, the nonmalignant control cells showed no apoptosis induction or only a marginal effect [62, 65, 74, 76, 87–90]), reviewed in Schlegel et al. [77]; Utsumi et al. [91]; Ishaq et al. [92]. These findings are the inspiring basis for the further development of CAP-based tumor therapy [47, 48, 93].

However, it is also important to realize that sufficiently high doses of CAP may cause induction of apoptosis or necrosis in nonmalignant cells as well [23, 35, 49, 94, 95]. These investigations will help to determine the limit of CAP application in order to prevent unwanted damage to nonmalignant tissue during tumor treatment. Importantly, the study of CAP effects on immune cells [95] presented the unexpected finding that nonmalignant immune cells (CD4+ T helper cells and monocytes) reacted more sensitively to CAP treatment than corresponding leukemic cells. This finding points to the need for more information on the mode of interaction between defined constituents of CAP with immune cells, in order to avoid unwanted side effects on the immune system and to establish an efficient antitumor effect through CAP-based tumor treatment.

Recent work strongly indicates that tumor treatment by radiation, chemotherapy and photodynamic therapy can only be successful, when the initial treatment triggers immunogenic cell death (defined by the release of DAMPS) [96, 97] or immunogenic modulation [98]. These processes may be mechanistically linked. They cause the induction of a response that is mediated by attracted antigen presenting cells (APC) and is finalized by activated specific cytotoxic T cells. Importantly, CAP-mediated triggering of immunogenic cell death and parallel activation of antigen presenting cells has been directly demonstrated [99, 100]. These findings are in line with the recent finding that a CAP-induced antitumor effect in vivo also affects an untreated tumor at a distant side of the animal [73]. These findings show that CAP is an efficient and selective inducer of immunogenic cell death. Immunogenic cell death then results in a T cell response that is fully effective even in the absence of plasma treatment. Importantly, this provoked T cell response might be instrumental to target migrating tumor cells as well as metastatic tumor cells at distant locations from the clinically overt tumor.

The potential interaction between CAP-dependent selective apoptosis induction in tumor cells, that is related to immunogenic cell death and HOCl-mediated immunogenic modulation and the subsequently established T cell response has been recently summarized by Bauer [101] (Fig. 16.3). This model is based on

1. the protection of tumor cells against exogenous ROS/RNS through membrane-associated catalase and the constitutive expression of NOX1 by tumor cells, related to the establishment of ROS/RNS apoptosis-inducing signaling [102–104];
2. abrogation of this protection through CAP-derived singlet oxygen [17, 101] or singlet oxygen generated in PAM [105],
3. subsequent reactivation of intercellular signaling through the HOCl and the NO/peroxynitrite signaling pathway,
4. influx of $H_2O_2$ through aquaporins,
5. subsequent induction of immunogenic cell death and provocation of a cytotoxic T cell response,
6. enhancement of the cytotoxic T cell response through modification of tumor cell proteins by HOCl [106, 107].
7. NO-mediated processes, triggered by T cell activity, leading to the inactivation of protective catalase [101, 104].

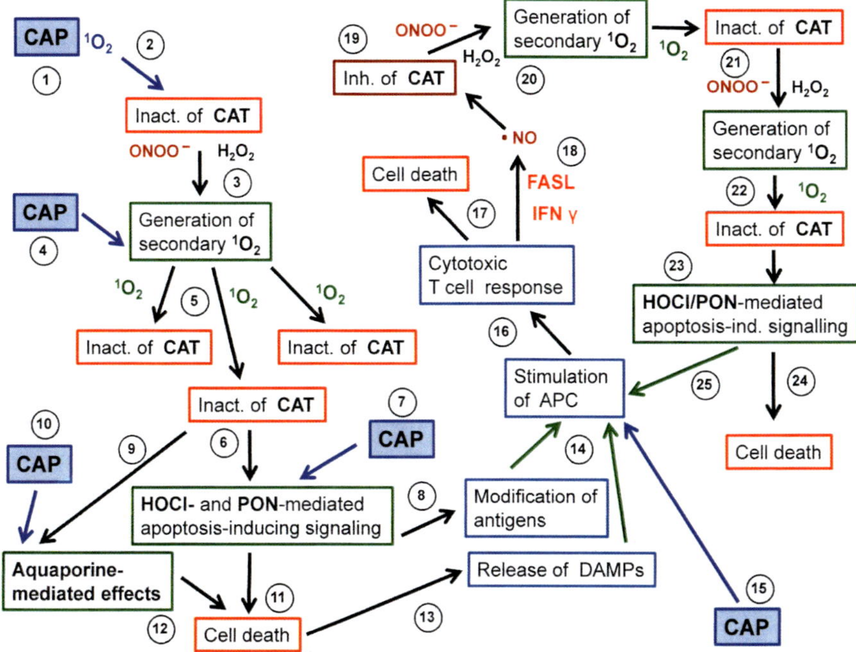


**Fig. 16.3** CAP may act at different sites during tumor treatment. Singlet oxygen from CAP (#1) causes local inactivation of membrane-associated catalase of tumor cells (#2) and thus allows the generation of secondary singlet oxygen, based on the interaction between free peroxynitrite and $H_2O_2$ (#3). This leads to the inactivation of more catalase molecules (#5) and finally HOCl and/or peroxynitrite (PON)-dependent apoptosis-inducing signaling is reactivated (#6). This signaling causes tumor cell death (#11), but also modifies tumor antigens (#8) and makes them more attractive for antigen presenting cells (APC) (#14). This effect acts in line with classical immunogenic cell death that is characterized by the release of Damage-associated molecular patterns (DAMPS) (#13) and the stimulation of APCs. As shown by Fridman, Lin and Miller [99, 100], CAP causes release of DAMPs that stimulate APCs. In parallel, the inactivation of catalase allows extracellular $H_2O_2$ to enter the tumor cells through aquaporins (#9) and thus to enhance apoptosis, as suggested by Keidar, Yan and colleagues [112, 113]. The cytotoxic T cell response resulting from the stimulation of APCs (#16) causes tumor cell death (even at sites distant of treatment) (#17). In addition, interferon gamma and FAS ligand derived from T cells induces NOS (#18) and thus causes NO-dependent inhibition of catalase (#19), which leads to the generation of secondary singlet oxygen (#20) and reactivation of intercellular apoptosis-inducing signaling through reactions #21–#23. This interplay establishes mutual enhancement between ROS/RNS signaling and immunological effects directed towards tumor cells. Importantly, CAP might act on many distinct steps along this scheme (#1, #4, # 7, #10, #15). This may cause enhancement or inhibition of treatment and even might cause unwanted side effects

The model shown in Fig. 16.3 takes into account that CAP may get involved with this complex process at distinct points, such as (1) inactivation of catalase; (2) generation of secondary singlet oxygen; (3) intercellular ROS/RNS signaling, (4) aquaporin-mediated effects, (5) stimulation of immune cells. Potential CAP effects at these different stages are not necessarily due to the same molecular species. For example, singlet oxygen seems to be centrally involved in the inactivation of protective catalase, whereas CAP-derived $H_2O_2$ and peroxynitrite may contribute to the generation of secondary singlet oxygen and to intercellular apoptosis-inducing ROS/RNS signaling. There may be different optimal doses for distinct ROS/RNS from CAP for enhancement of wanted effects, as well as for preventing negative effects that disturb this balanced interaction. The elucidation of these requirements will be a challenge for those colleagues that modulate the composition of plasma and for the studies that are focused on the determination of optimal therapeutic effects and avoidance of side effects that otherwise might interfere with therapy or damage nonmalignant tissue.

Based on our present knowledge, a tumor might be treated with two different strategies (Fig. 16.4). As shown in Fig. 16.4a, local application of a *nonselective high dose of CAP* specifically to the site of tumor would cause cell death of the tumor in focus and some adjacent nonmalignant tissue. The resultant immunogenic cell death would preferentially trigger a tumor specific T cell response, mediated by APCs. However, the high concentrations of CAP-derived ROS and ROS set free during execution of cell death might lead to the modification of antigens on nonmalignant cells and thus cause the induction of potential autoimmune processes [108, 109]. This theoretically conceivable unwanted side effect seems to be much less likely when CAP treatment causes selective induction of cell death in tumor cells through triggering the reactivation of ROS/RNS-dependent apoptosis-inducing signaling after inactivation of protective catalase (Fig. 16.4b). This scenario is based on signal amplification by the target cells [17, 101, 110, 111], and therefore seems to require doses that are nontoxic to nonmalignant tissue. This approach should lead to immunogenic cell death preferentially in tumor cells. It thus would cause the desired highly specific cytotoxic T cell response directed towards the tumor itself and bear the chance to reach distant metastatic tumor clones as well.

## Conclusions

The present use of CAP for skin disinfection, tissue regeneration, treatment of chronic wounds and cancer shows a surprisingly low incidence of unwanted side effects. The reason for this finding seems to be based on specific signaling functions of CAP-derived ROS/RNS, their extracellular application and the provoked cellular antioxidant systems. An evidence-based analysis allows to propose a model in which CAP is not a direct effector of antimicrobial or antitumor action, but rather triggers a singlet oxygen-mediated switch-on effect on the specific target, leading to energy depletion in bacteria and to reactivation of intercellular ROS/RNS-dependent apoptosis signaling in tumor cells. As these final processes are strictly restricted to the specific targets due to the biochemistry of the switch-on mechanism and its consequent reactions. As normal tissue is devoid of the required target structure to allow switch on by singlet oxygen, it is neither harmed nor affected. This explains the lack of severe side effects of CAP treatment, provided the optimal doses and the adequate composition of CAP are applied. It is suggested that those reports that demonstrate damaging effects of CAP in model experiments or show nonselective effects in tumor cell treatment might be extremely useful to define the borderline between beneficial and detrimental

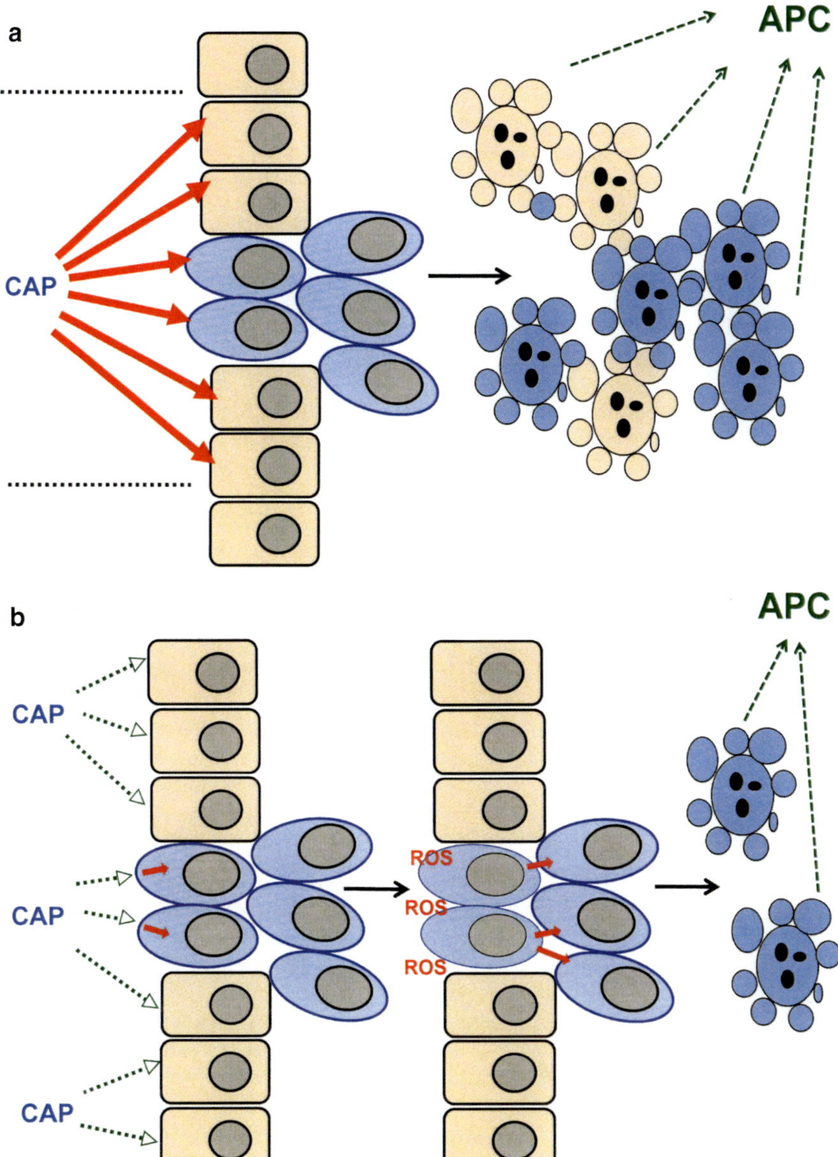


**Fig. 16.4** Different modes of tumor treatment by CAP. (**a**) Site-specific treatment of tumors with high concentrations of CAP may cause cell death of tumor cells as well as of adjacent nonmalignant tissue. ROS/RNS-dependent modifications of tumor cell proteins may be instrumental for the induction of a specific T cell response, whereas modifications of proteins from nonmalignant cells might trigger autoimmune processes. (**b**) Treatment of tumors with CAP doses that are not damaging per se but trigger a damaging response selectively in the tumor cells, will lead to selective cell death of tumor cells that may cause specific stimulation of immune effects directed towards tumor cells

effects of CAP. Further work is required to experimentally verify or falsify these conclusions and to work out more biochemical details that may be instrumental for further optimization of CAP-dependent medical applications.

## References


1. Isbary G, Morfill G, Schmidt HU, Georgi M, Ramrath K, Heinlein J, Karrer S, Landthaler M, Shimizu T, Steffes B, Bunk W, Monetti R, Zimmermann JL, Pompl R, Stolz W. A first prospective randomized controlled trial to decrease bacterial load using cold atmospheric argon plasma on chronic wounds in patients. Br J Dermatol. 2010;163:78–82.
2. Von Woedtke T, Metelmann H-R, Weltmann KD. Clinical plasma medicine: state and perspectives of in vivo application of cold atmospheric plasma. Contrib Plasma Phys. 2014; 54:104–17.
3. Lademann J, Richter H, Alborov A, Hume D, Patzelt A, Kramer A, Weltmann K-D, Hartmann B, Ottomann C, Fluhr JW, Hinz P, Hübner G, Lademann O. Risk assessment of the application of a plasma jet in dermatology. J Biomed Opt. 2009;14:054025. https://doi.org/10.1117/1.3247156.
4. Sies H. Strategies of antioxidant defense. FEBS J. 1993;215:213–9. https://doi.org/10.1111/j.1432-1033.1993.tb18025.x.
5. Sies H. Role of metabolic $H_2O_2$. Generation, redox signaling and oxidative stress. J Biol Chem. 2014;289:8735–41.
6. Sies H. Hydrogen peroxide as a central redox signaling molecule in physiological oxidative stress: Oxidative eustress. Redox Biol. 2017;11:613–8.
7. Bauer G, Chatgilialoglu C, Gebicki JL, Gebicka L, Gescheidt G, Golding BT, Goldstein S, Kaizer J, Merenyi G, Speier G, Wardman P. Biologically relevant small radicals. Chimia. 2008; 62:1–9.
8. Bauer G. Helicobacter and reactive oxygen species. In: Gracia-Sancho J, Salvadó J, editors. Gastrointestinal tissue. Oxidative stress and dietary antioxidants. Cambridge: Academic; 2017. p. 81–96.
9. Graves DB. The emerging role of reactive oxygen and nitrogen species in redox biology and some implications for plasma applications to medicine and biology. J Phys D Appl Phys. 2012;45(26):263001.
10. Graves DB. Reactive species from cold atmospheric plasma: implications for cancer therapy. Plasma Process Polym. 2014;11:1120–7.
11. Graves DB. Oxy-nitroso shielding burst model of cold atmospheric plasma therapeutics. Clin Plasma Med. 2014;2:38–49.
12. Jablonowski H, Bussiahn R, Hammer MU, Weltman DK, von Woedtke T, Reuter S. Impact of plasma jet vacuum ultraviolet radiation on reactive species generation in bio-relevant liquids. Phys Plasmas. 2015;22:122008.
13. Sousa JS, Niemi K, Cox LJ, Algwari QT, Gans T, O'Connell D. Cold atmospheric pressure plasma jets as sources of singlet delta oxygen for biomedical applications. J Appl Phys. 2011;109:123302.
14. Schmidt-Bleker A, Bansemer R, Reuter S, Weltmann K-D. How to produce an NOx-indstead of Ox-based chemistry with a cold atmospheric plasma jet. Plasma Process Polym. 2016. https://doi.org/10.1002/ppap.201600062.
15. Wende K, Williams P, Dalluge J, Van Gaens W, Akoubakr H, Bischof J, von Woedtke T, Goyal SM, Weltmann K-D, Bogaerts A, Masur K, Bruggeman PJ. Identification of biologically active liquid chemistry induced by nonthermal atmospheric pressure plasma jet. Biointerphases. 2015;10:029518. https://doi.org/10.1116/1.4919710.
16. Gianella M, Reuter S, Aguila AL, Ritchie GAD, van Helden JPH. Detection of $HO_2$ in an atmospheric pressure plasma jet using optical feedback cavity-enhanced absorption spectroscopy. New J Phys. 2016;18:113027.

17. Bauer G, Graves DB. Mechanisms of selective antitumor action of cold atmospheric plasma-derived reactive oxygen and nitrogen species. Plasma Process Polym. 2016;13:1157–78.
18. Lackmann J-W, Baldus S, Steinborn E, Edengeiser E, Kogelheide F, Langklotz S, Schneider S, Leichert LIO, Benedikt J, Awakowicz P, Bandow JE. A dielectric barrier discharge terminally inactivates RNase A by oxidizing sulfur-containing amino acids and breaking structural disulfide bonds. J Phys D Appl Phys. 2015;48:494003. https://doi.org/10.1088/0022-3727/48/49/494003.
19. O'Connell D, Cox LJ, Hyland WB, McMahon SJ, Reuter S, Graham WG, Gans T, Currell FJ. Cold atmospheric pressure plasma jet interactions with plasmid DNA. Appl Phys Lett. 2011;98:043701. https://doi.org/10.1063/1.3521502.
20. Boxhammer V, Li YF, Köritzer J, Shimizu T, Maisch T, Thomas HM, Schlegel J, Morfill GE, Zimmermann JL. Investigation of the mutagenic potential of cold atmospheric plasma at bactericidal dosages. Mutat Res. 2013;753:23–8.
21. Kluge S, Bekeschus S, Bender C, Benkhai H, Schkell A, Below H, Stope MB, Kramer A. Investigating the mutagenicity of a cold argon-plasma jet in an HET-MEN model. PLoS One. 2016;11(9):e0160667. https://doi.org/10.1371/journal.pone.0160667.
22. Wende K, Bekeschus S, Schmidt A, Jatsch L, Hasse S, Weltmann KD, Masur K, von Woedtke T. Risk assessment of a cold argon plasma jet in respect to its mutagenicity. Mutat Res Genet Toxicol Environ Mutagen. 2016;798–799:48–54.
23. Wende K, Straßenburg S, Haertel B, Harms M, Holtz S, Barton A, Masur K, von Woedtke T, Lindequist U. Atmospheric pressure plasma jet treatment evokes transient oxidative stress in HaCat keratinocytes and influences cell physiology. Cell Biol Int. 2014;38:412–25.
24. Isbary G, Köritzer J, Mitra A, Li Y-F, Shimizu T, Schroeder J, Schlegel J, Morfill GE, Stolz W, Zimmermann JL. Ex vivo human skin experiments for the evaluation of safety of new cod atmospheric plasma devices. Clin Plasma Med. 2013;1:36–44. https://doi.org/10.1016/j.cpme.2012.10.0001.
25. Schmidt A, von Woedtke T, Stenzel J, Lindner T, Polei S, Vollmar B, Bekeschus S. One year follow-up risk assessment in SKH-1 Mice and wounds treated with an argon plasma jet. Int J Mol Sci. 2017;18:868. https://doi.org/10.3390/ijms18040868.
26. Metelmann HR, Vu TT, Do HT, Le TNB, Hoang THA, Phi TTT, Luong TML, Doan VT, Nguyen TTH, Nguyen THM, Nguyen TL, Le DQ, Le TKX, von Woedtke T, Bussiahn R, Weltmann KD, Khalili R, Podmelle F. Scar formation of laser skin lesions after cold atmospheric pressure plasma (CAP) treatment: a clinical long term observation. Clin Plasma Med. 2013;1:30–5. https://doi.org/10.1016/j.cpme.2012.12001.
27. Ke Z, Huang Q. Assessment of damage of glutathione by glow discharge plasma at the gas-solultion interface through Raman spectroscopy. Plasma Process Polym. 2013;10:181–8.
28. Klinkhammer C, Verlackt C, Smilowicz D, Kogelheide F, Bogaerts A, Metzler-Nolte N, Stapelmann K, Havenith M, Lackmann J-W. Elucidation of plasma-induced chemical modifications on glutathione and glutathione disulfide. Sci Rep. 2017;7(1):13828.
29. Arndt S, Unger P, Wacker E, Shimizu T, Heinlin J, Li Y-F, Thomas HM, Morfill GE, Zimmermann JL, Bosserhoff A-K, Karrer S. Cold atmospheric plasma (CAP) changes gene expression of key molecules of the wound healing machinery and improves wound healing in vitro and in vivo. PLoS One. 2013;8:e79325.
30. Hasse S, Tran D, Hahn O, Kindler S, Metelmann H-R, von Woedtke T, Masur K. Induction of proliferation of basal epidermal keratinocytes by cold atmospheric-pressure plasma. Clin Exp Dermatol. 2016;41:202–9.
31. Schmidt A, Wende K, Bekeschus S, Bundscherer L, Barton A, Ottmüller K, Weltmann K-D, Masur K. Non-thermal plasma treatment is associated with changes in transcriptome of human epithelial skin cells. Free Radic Res. 2013;47:577–92. https://doi.org/10.3109/10715762.2013.804623.
32. Bekeschus S, von Woedtke T, Kramer A, Weltmann KD, Masur K. Cold physical plasma treatment alters redox balance in human immune cells. Plasma Med. 2013;3:267–78.
33. Bekeschus S, Schmidt A, Weltmann KD, von Woedtke T. The plasma jet kINpen—a powerful tool for wound healing. Clin Plasma Med. 2016;4:19–28.

34. Stoffels E, Roks AJM, Deelman LE. Delayed effects of cold atmospheric plasma on vascular cells. Plasma Process Polym. 2008;5:599–605. https://doi.org/10.1002/ppap.200800028.
35. Bekeschus S, Iseni S, Reuter S, Masur K, Weltmann KD. Nitrogen shielding of an argon plasma jet and its effects on human immune cells. IEEE Trans Plasma Sci. 2015;43:776–81. https://doi.org/10.1109/TPS.205.2393379.
36. Schmidt A, Dietrich S, Steuer A, Weltmann KD, von Woedtke T, Masur K, Wende K. Non-thermal plasma activates human keratinocytes by stimulation of antioxidant and phase II pathways. J Biol Chem. 2015;290:6731–50.
37. Weltmann K-D, Kindel E, Brandenburg R, Meyer C, Bussiahn R, Wilke C, von Woedtke T. Atmospheric pressure plasma jet for medical therapy: plasma parameters and risk estimation. Contrib Plasma Phys. 2009;49:634–40. https://doi.org/10.1002/ctpp.200910067.
38. Isbary G, Zimmermann JL, Shimizu T, Li Y-F, Morfill GE, Thomas HM, Steffes B, Heinlin J, Karrer S, Stolz W. Non-thermal plasma-More than five years of clinical experience. Clin Plasma Med. 2013;1:19–23.
39. Isbary G, Shimizu T, Zimmermann JL, Heinlin J, Al-Zaabi S, Rechfeld M, Morfill GE, Karrer S, Stolz W. Randomized placebo-controlled clinical trial shoed cold atmospheric argon plasma relieved acute pain and accelerated healing. Clin Plasma Med. 2014;2:50–5.
40. Emmert S, Brehmer F, Hänßle H, Helmke A, Mertens N, Ahmed R, Simon D, Wandke D, Maus-Friedrichs W, Däschlein g SMP, Viöl W. Atmospheric pressure plasma in dermatology: ulcus treatment and much more. Clin Plasma Med. 2013;1:24–9. https://doi.org/10.1016/j.cpme.2012.11.002.
41. Heinlin J, Isbary G, Stolz W, Zeman F, Landthaler M, Morfill G, Shimizu T, Zimmermann JL, Karrer S. A randomized two-sided placebo-controlled study on the efficacy and safety of atmosperic non-thermal argon plasma for pruritus. J Eur Acad Dermatol Venereol. 2013;27:324–31. https://doi.org/10.1111/j.1468-3038.2011.04395.x.
42. Heinlin J, Zimmermann JL, Zeman F, Bunk W, Isbary G, Landthaler M, Maisch T, Monetti R, Morfill G, Shimizu T, Steinbauer J, Stolz W, Karrer S. Randomized placebo-controlled human pilot study of cold atmospheric argon plasma on skin graft donor site. Wound Repair Regen. 2013;21:800–7. https://doi.org/10.1111/wrr.12078.
43. Klebes M, Lademann J, Philipp S, Ulrich C, Patzelt A, Ulmer M, Kluschke F, Kramer A, Weltmann KD, Serry W, Lange-Asschenfeldt B. Effects of tissue-tolerable plasma on psoriasis vulgaris treatment compared to conventional local treatment: a pilot study. Clin Plasma Med. 2014;2:22–7.
44. Brehmer F, Haenssle HA, Daeschlein G, Ahmed R, Pfeiffer S, Görlitz A, Simon D, Schön MP, Wandke D, Emmert S. Allevation of chronic venous leg ulcers with a hand-held dielectric barrier discharge plasma generator (PlasmaDerm® VU-2010): results of a monocentric, two-armed, open, prospective, randomized and controlled trial (NCT01415622). J Eur Acad Dermatol Venereol. 2015;29:148–55. https://doi.org/10.1111/jdv.12490.
45. Ulrich C, Kluschke F, Patzelt A, Vandersee S, Czaika VA, Richter H, Bob A, von Hutten J, Painsi C, Hügel R, Kramer A. Clinical use of cold atmospheric pressure argon plasma in chronic leg ulcers: a pilot study. J Wound Care. 2015;24:196, 198–200, 202–203.
46. Schuster M, Rana A, Hauschild A, Seebauer C, Bauer G, Metelmann P, Rutkowski R, Shojaei RK, von Woedtke T. Why are there no side effects in plasma treatment of oral cancer? Clin Plasma Med. 2018 (in press).
47. Metelmann H-R, Nedrelow DS, Seebauer C, Schuster M, von Woedtke T, Weltman K-D, Kindler S, Metelmann PH, Finkelstein SE, von Hoff DD, Podmelle F. Head and neck cancer treatment and physical plasma. Clin Plasma Med. 2015;3:17–23.
48. Schuster C, Seebauer R, Rutkowski A, Hauschild F, Podmelle C, Metelmann B, Metelmann T, von Woedtke S, Hasse S, Weltmann K-D, Metelmann H-R. Visible tumor surface response to physical plasma and apoptotic cell kill in head and neck cancer. J Craniomaxillofac Surg. 2016;44:1445–52.
49. Bekeschus S, Masur K, Kolata J, Wende K, Schmidt A, Bundscherer L, Barton A, Kramer A, Bröker B, Weltmann K-D. Human mononuclear cell survival and proliferation is modu-

lated by cold atmospheric plasma jet. Plasma Process Polym. 2013;10:706–13. https://doi.org/10.1002/ppap.2013.300008.

50. Bekeschus S, Kolata J, Winterbourn C, Kramer A, Turner R, Weltmann K-D, Bröker B, Masur K. Hydrogen peroxide: a central player in physical plasma-induced oxidative stress in human blood cells. Free Radic Res. 2014;48:542–9. https://doi.org/10.3109/10715762.2014.892937.
51. Wu H, Sun P, Feng H, Zhou H, Wang R, Liang Y, Lu J, Zhu W, Zhang J, Fang J. Reactive oxygen species in a nonthermal plasma microjet and water system: generation, conversion and contributions to bacteria inactivation–an analysis by electron spin resonance spectroscopy. Plasma Process Polym. 2012;9:417–24.
52. Dahl TA, Middenand WR, Hartman PE. Pure singlet oxygen cytotoxicity for bacteria. Photochem Photobiol. 1987;46:345–52.
53. Maisch T, Baier J, Franz B, Maier M, Landthaler M, Szeimies R-M, Bäumler W. The role of singlet oxygen and oxygen concentration in photodynamic inactivation of bacteria. Proc Natl Acad Sci U S A. 2007;104:7223–8.
54. Schafer M, Schmitz C, Horneck G. High sensitivity of Deinococcus radiodurans to photodynamically-produced singlet oxygen. Int J Radiat Biol. 1998;74:249–53.
55. Tatsuzawa H, Maruyama T, Misawa N, Fujimori K, Hori K, Sano Y, Kambayashi Y, Nakano M. Inactivation of bacterial respiratory chain enzymes by singlet oxygen. FEBS Lett. 1998;439:329–33.
56. Dahl TA. Direct exposure of mammalian cells to pure endogenous singlet oxygen (1-delta-$GO_2$). Photochem Photobiol. 1993;57:248–54.
57. Nagata JY, Hioka N, Kimura E, Batistela VR, Terada RSS, Graciano AX, Baesso ML, Hayacibara MF. Antibacterial photodynamic therapy for dental caries: evaluation of the photosensitizer used and light source properties. Photodiagn Photodyn Ther. 2012;9:122–31.
58. Vandamme M, Pesnel S, Barbosa E, Dozias S, Sobilo J, Lerondel S, Le Pape A, Pouvesle J-M. Antitumor effect of plasma treatment on U87 glioma xenografts: preliminary results. Plasma Process Polym. 2010;7:264–73.
59. Vandamme M, Robert E, Lerondel S, Sarron V, Ries D, Dozias S, Sobilo J, Gosset D, Kieda C, Legrain B, Pouvesle J-M, Le Pape A. ROS implication in a new antitumor strategy based on nonthermal plasma. Int J Cancer. 2012;130:2194–85.
60. Tanaka H, Ishikawa K, Nakamura K, Kajiyama H, Komo H, Kikkawa T, Hori M. Plasma-activated medium selectively kills glioblastoma brain tumor cells by down-regulating a survival signaling molecule, AKT kinase. Plasma Med. 2011;1:265–77. https://doi.org/10.1615/PlasmaMed.2012006275.
61. Walk RM, Snyder JA, Srinivasan P, Kirsch J, Diaz SO, Blanco FC, Shashuin A, Keidar M, Sandler AD. Cold atmospheric plasma for the ablative treatment of neuroblastoma. J Pediatr Surg. 2013;48:67–73.
62. Wang M, Holmes B, Cheng X, Zhu W, Keidar M, Zhang LG. Cold atmospheric plasma for selectively ablating metastatic breast cancer cells. PLoS One. 2013;8:e73741.
63. Cheng X, Sherman J, Murphy W, Ratovitski E, Canady J, Keidar M. The effect of tuning cold plasma composition on glioblastoma cell viability. PLoS One. 2014;9:e98652.
64. Chang JW, Kang SU, Shin YS, Kim KI, Seo SJ, Yang SS, Lee JS, Moon E, Lee K, Kim CH. Non-thermal atmospheric pressure plasma inhibits thyroid papillary cancer cell invasion via cytoskeletal modulation, altered mmp-2/−9/upa activity. PLoS One. 2014;9:e92198.
65. Guerrero-Preston R, Ogawa T, Uemura M, Shumulinsky G, Valle BL, Pirini F, Ravi R, Sidransky D, Keidar M, Trink B. Cold atmospheric plasma treatment selectively targets head and neck squamous cell carcinoma cells. Int J Mol Med. 2014;34:941–6.
66. Von Behr M, Masur K, Hackbarth C, Bekeschus S, Wende K, Kantz L, Heidecke C-D, von Bernstorff PLI. Effects of tissue tolerable plasma in combination with gemcitabine on pancreatic cancer cells. Pancreatology. 2015;15:S36–7.
67. Ishaq M, Han ZJ, Kumar S, Evans MOM, Ostrikov K. Atmospheric plasma- and TRAIL-induced apoptosis in TRAIL-resistant colorectal cancer cells. Plasma Process Polym. 2015;12:574–82.

68. Hattori N, Yamada S, Torii K, Takeda S, Nakamura K, Tanaka H, Kajiyama H, Kanda M, Fujii T, Nakayama G, Sugimoto H, Koike M, Nomoto S, Fujiwara M, Mizuno M, Hori M, Kodera Y. Effectiveness of plasma treatment on pancreatic cancer cells. Int J Oncol. 2015;47:1655–62.
69. Ikeda J-I, Tsuruta Y, Nojima S, Sakakita H, Hori M, Ikehara Y. Anti-cancer effects of non-equilibrium atmospheric pressure plasma on cancer-initiating cells in human endometrioid adenocarcinoma cells. Plasma Process Polym. 2015;12:1370–6.
70. Weiss M, Gümbel D, Hanschmann E-M, Mandelkow R, Gelbrich N, Zimmermann U, Walther R, Ekkernkamp A, Sckell A, Kramer A, Burchardt M, Lillig CH, Stope MB. Cold atmospheric plasma treatment induces anti-proliferative effects in prostate cancer cells by redox and apoptotic signaling pathways. PLoS One. 2015;10:e0130350. https://doi.org/10.1371/journal.pone0130350.
71. Bekeschus S, Wende K, Hefny MM, Rödder K, Jablonowski H, Schmidt A, von Woedtke T, Weltmann K-D, Benedikt J. Oxygen atoms are critical in rendering THP-1 leukaemia cells susceptible to cold physical plasma-induced apoptosis. Sci Rep. 2017;7:2791.
72. Duan J, Lu X, He G. The selective effect of plasma-activated medium in an in vitro co-culture of liver cancer and normal cells. J Appl Phys. 2017;121:013302.
73. Mizuno K, Yonetamari K, Shirakawa Y, Akiyama T, Ono R. Anti-tumor immune response induced by nanosecond pulsed streamer discharge in mice. J Phys D Appl Phys. 2017;50:12LT01.
74. Keidar M, Walk R, Shashurin A, Srinivasan P, Sandler P, Sandler A, Dasgupta S, Ravi R, Guerrero-Preston R, Trink B. Cold plasma selectivity and the possibility of a paradigm shift in cancer therapy. Br J Cancer. 2011;105:1295–301.
75. Keidar M, Shashurin A, Volotskova O, Stepp MA, Srinivasan P, Sandler A, Trink B. Cold atmospheric plasma in cancer therapy. Phys Plasmas. 2013;20:057101. https://doi.org/10.1063/1.4801516.
76. Keidar M. Plasma for cancer treatment. Plasma Sources Sci Technol. 2015;24:033001.
77. Schlegel J, Köritzer J, Boxhammer V. Plasma in cancer treatment. Clin Plasma Med. 2013;1:2–7.
78. Tanaka H, Mizuno M, Ishikawa K, Takeda K, Nakamura K, Utsumi F, Kajiyama H, Kano H, Okazaki Y, Toyokuni S, Maruyama S, Kikkawa F, Hori M. Plasma medical Science for Cancer therapy: toward cancer therapy using nonthermal atmospheric pressure plasma. IEEE Trans Plasma Sci. 2014;42:3760–4. https://doi.org/10.1109/TPS.014.2353659.
79. Barekzi N, Laroussi M. Effects of low temperature plasmas on cancer cells. Plasma Process Polym. 2013;10:1039–50.
80. Laroussi M. From killing bacteria to destroying cancer cells: 20 years of plasma medicine. Plasma Process Polym. 2014;11:1138–41.
81. Laroussi M. Low-temperature plasma jet for biomedical applications: a review. IEEE Trans Plasma Sci. 2015;43:703–12.
82. Laroussi M, Mohades S, Barekzi N. Killing adherent and nonadherent cancer cells with the plasma pencil. Biointerphases. 2015;10:029401.
83. Ratovitski EA, Heng X, Yan D, Sherman JH, Canady J, Trink B, Keidar M. Anti-Cancer Therapies of 21st century: novel approach to treat human cancers using cold atmospheric plasma. Plasma Process Polym. 2014;11:1128–37.
84. Yan DY, Sherman JH, Keidar M. Cold atmospheric plasma, a novel promising anti-cancer treatment modality. Oncotarget. 2017;8:15977–95.
85. Gay-Mimbrera J, Garcia MC, Tejera BI, Rodero-Serrano A, Garcia-Nieto AV, Ruano J. Clinical and biological principles of cold atmospheric plasma application in skin cancer. Adv Ther. 2016;33:894–909.
86. Babington P, Rajjoub K, Canady J, Siu A, Keidar M, Sherman JH. Use of cold atmospheric plasma in the treatment of cancer. Biointerphases. 2015;10:029403.
87. Kaushik N, Kumar N, Kim CH, Kaushik NK, Choi EH. Dielectric barrier discharge plasma efficiently delivers an apoptotic response in human monocytic lymphoma. Plasma Process Polym. 2014;11:1175–87. https://doi.org/10.1002/ppap.201400102.

88. Siu A, Volotskova O, Cheng X, Khaisa SS, Bian K, Murad F, Keidar M, Sherman JH. Differential effects of cold atmospheric plasma in the treatment of malignant glioma. PLoS One. 2015;10:e0126313. https://doi.org/10.1371/journal.pone.0126313.
89. Kim SJ, Chung TH. Cold atmospheric plasma jet-generated RONS and their selective effects on normal and carcinoma cells. Sci Rep. 2016;6:20332. https://doi.org/10.1038/srep.20332.
90. Zucker SN, Zirnheld J, Bagati A, DiSanto TM, Des Soye B, Wawrzyniak JA, Eternadi K, Nikiforov M, Berezney R. Preferential induction of apoptotic cell death in melanoma cells as compared with normal keratinocytes using a non-thermal plasma torch. Cancer Biol Ther. 2012;13:1299–306. https://doi.org/10.4161/cbt.21787.
91. Utsumi F, Kajiyama H, Nakamura K, Tanaka H, Hori M, Kikkawa F. Selective cytotoxicity of indirect nonequilibrium atmospheric pressure plasma against ovarian clear-cell carcinoma. Springerplus. 2014;3:398–16. https://doi.org/10.1186/2193-1801-3-398.
92. Ishaq M, Evans M, Ostrikov K. Effect of atmospheric gas plasmas on cancer cell signaling. Int J Cancer. 2013;134:1517–28. https://doi.org/10.1002/ijc.28323.
93. Metelmann H-R, Seebauer C, Miller V, Fridman A, Bauer G, Graves DB, Pouvesle J-M, Rutkowski R, Schuster M, Bekeschus S, Wende K, Masur K, Hasse S, Gerlin T, Hori M, Tanaka H, Choi EH, Weltmann K-D, Metelmann PH, Von Hoff DD, von Woedtke T. Clinical experience with cold plasma in the treatment of locally advanced head and neck cancer. Clin Plasma Med. 2018;9:6–13.
94. Hirst AM, Simms MS, Mann VM, Maitland NJ, O'Connell D, Frame FM. Low temperature plasma treatment induces DNA damage leading to necrotic cell death in primary prostate epithelial cells. Br J Cancer. 2015;112:1536–45. https://doi.org/10.1038/bjc.2025.113.
95. Bundscherer L, Bekeschus S, Tresp H, Hasse S, Reuter S, Weltmann K-D, Lindequist U, Masur K. Viability of human blood leucocytes compared with their respective cell lines after plasma treatment. Plasma Med. 2013;3:71–80.
96. Apetoh L, Tesnier A, Ghiringhelli F, Kroemer G, Zitvogel L. Interactions between dying tumor cells and the innate immune system determine the efficiency of conventional antitumor therapy. Cancer Res. 2008;68:4026–30.
97. Kroemer G, Galluzzi L, Kepp O, Zitvogel L. Immunogenic cell death in cancer therapy. Annu Rev Immunol. 2013;31:51–72.
98. Hodge JW, Garnett CT, Farsaci B, Palena C, Tsang K-Y, Ferrone S, Gameiro SR. Chemotherapy-induced immunogenic modulation of tumor cells enhances killing by cytotoxic T lymphocytes and is distinct from immunogenic cell death. Int J Cancer. 2013;133: 624–37.
99. Lin A, Truong B, Pappas A, Kirifides L, Oubarri A, Chen S, Lin S, Dobrynin D, Fridman G, Fridman A, Sang N, Miller V. Uniform nanosecond pulsed dielectric barrier discharge plasma enhances anti-tumor effects by induction of immunogenic cell death in tumors and stimulation of macrophages. Plasma Process Polym. 2015;12:1392–9.
100. Miller V, Lin A, Fridman A. Why target immune cells for plasma treatment of cancer. Plasma Chem Plasma Process. 2016;36:259–68.
101. Bauer G. Signal amplification by tumor cells: clue to the understanding of the antitumor effects of cold atmospheric plasma and plasmaactivated medium. IEEE Trans Rad Plasma Med Sci. 2017;1(6):1–12.
102. Heinzelmann S, Bauer G. Multiple protective functions of catalase against intercellular apoptosis-inducing ROS signaling of human tumor cells. Biol Chem. 2010;391:675–93.
103. Bauer G. Targeting extracellular ROS signaling of tumor cells. Anticancer Res. 2014;34: 1467–82.
104. Bauer G. Increasing the endogenous NO level causes catalase inactivation and reactivation of intercellular apoptosis signaling specifically in tumor cells. Redox Biol. 2015;6:353–71.
105. Bauer G. Targeting the protective catalase of tumor cells with cold atmospheric plasma-treated medium (PAM). Anticancer Agents Med Chem. 2017. https.//doi.org/ 10.2174/18715 20617666170801103708.

106. Chiang CLL, Ledermann JA, Rad AN, Katz DR, Chain BM. Hypochlorous acid enhances immunogenicity and uptake of allogeneic ovarian tumor cells by dendritic cells to cross-prime tumor-specific T cells. Cancer Immunol Immunother. 2006;55:1384–95.
107. Biedron R, Konopinski MK, Marcinkiewicz J, Jozefowski S. Oxidation by neutrophil-derived HOCl increases immunogenicity of proteins by converting them into ligands of several endocytic receptors involved in antigen uptake by dendritic cells and macrophages. PLoS One. 2015;10:e01123293.
108. Griffiths HR. Is the generation of neo antigenic determinants by free radicals central to the development of autoimmune rheumatoid disease? Autoimmun Rev. 2008;7:544–9. https://doi.org/10.1016/j.autorev.2008.04.013.
109. Kurien BT, Scotfield RH. Autoimmunity and oxidatively modified autoantigens. Autoimmun Rev. 2008;7:567–73. https://doi.org/10.1016/j.autorev.2008.04.019.
110. Riethmüller M, Burger N, Bauer G. Singlet oxygen treatment of tumor cells triggers extracellular singlet oxygen generation, catalase inactivation and reactivation of intercellular apoptosis-inducing signaling. Redox Biol. 2015;6:157–68.
111. Bauer G. Autoamplificatory singlet oxygen generation sensitizes tumor cells for intercellular apoptosis-inducing signaling. Mech Ageing Dev. 2017. https://doi.org/10.1016/j.mad.2017.11.005.
112. Yan DY, Talbot A, Nourmohammadi N, Sherman JH, Cheng XQ, Keidar M. Toward understanding the selective anticancer capacity of cold atmospheric plasma—a model based on aquaporins. Biointerphases. 2015;10:040801.
113. Yan DY, Xiao H, Zhu W, Nourmohammadi N, Zhang LG, Bian K, Keidar M. The role of aquaporins in the anti-glioblastoma capacity of the cold plasma-stimulated medium. J Phys D Appl Phys. 2017;50:055401.

# Perspectives in Dental Implantology 17

Lukasz Jablonowski, Rutger Matthes, Kathrin Duske,
and Thomas Kocher

## 17.1 Plasma in Dental Implantology

### 17.1.1 Aspects of Implants and Peri-Implantitis (Implant-Associated Inflammation)

The use of implants belongs to the standard repertoire of possible treatment options in dental practice and is growing in popularity due to decreasing costs. In recent years, implantation numbers have continued to rise (approximately 14 millions worldwide). Similar to teeth, implants can also be affected by infection and inflammation, which may lead to bone destruction. In approximately 20% of the patients and 10% of the implants, peri-implantitis [1] occurs. In a Swedish study, it was reported that implant loss occurs in 4.2% of patients after 9 years, which corresponds to 2% of the implants [2].

Peri-implantitis is an inflammation of the implant bed with a loss of bone tissue caused by bacteria embedded in a biofilm (Fig. 17.1). The biofilm increases the survival capacity of the bacteria against the immune defense and intensifies the inflammatory reaction of the surrounding tissue, which can subsequently lead to bone resorption (Fig. 17.2). Similar to periodontitis, bacterial deposits first cause a reversible inflammatory reaction, which affects the mucosa (peri-mucositis) and subsequently leads to an irreversible, progressive destruction of the surrounding

L. Jablonowski (✉) • R. Matthes • T. Kocher
Unit of Periodontology, Department of Restorative Dentistry, Periodontology, Endodontology, Preventive Dentistry and Pedodontics, University Medicine Greifswald, Greifswald, Germany
e-mail: lukasz.jablonowski@uni-greifswald.de; rmatthes@uni-greifswald.de; kocher@uni-greifswald.de

K. Duske
Department of Orthodontics, School of Dentistry "Hans Moral", University Medicine Rostock, Rostock, Germany
e-mail: kathrin.duske@med.uni-rostock.de



H.-R. Metelmann et al. (eds.), *Comprehensive Clinical Plasma Medicine*,
https://doi.org/10.1007/978-3-319-67627-2_17

bone (peri-implantitis). This is reflected in increased probing depth and bleeding on probing. Commonly occurring and inflammatory associated gram-negative anaerobes are *Prevotella intermedia, Porphyromonas gingivalis, Actinobacillus actinomycetemcomitans, Bacteroides forsythus, Treponema denticola, Prevotella nigrescens, Peptostreptococcus micros* and *Fusobacterium nucleatum* [3].

The treatment of peri-implantitis infected dental implants is a challenge for the treating dentist. If the implant is not removed, the affected implant must be cleaned and disinfected in order to facilitate the healing process and re-osseointegration.

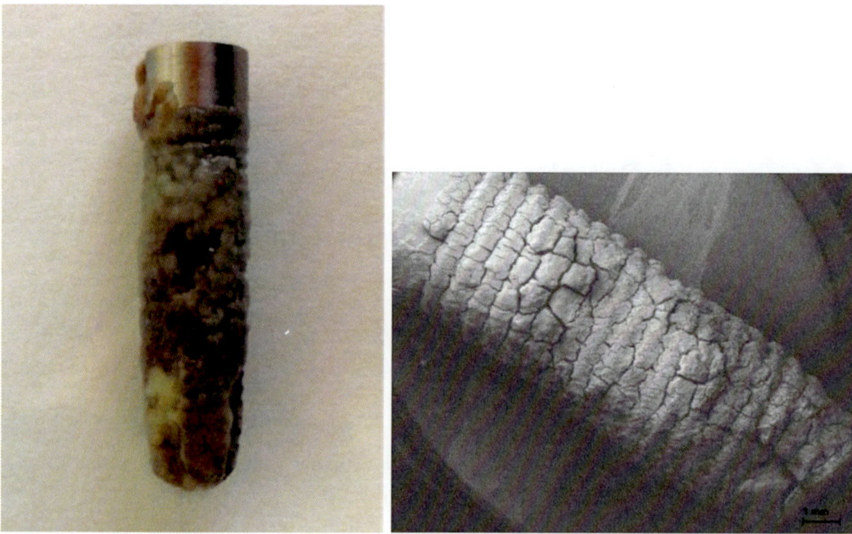

**Fig. 17.1** Pictures from reflected light microscope and scanning electron micrograph (Dental School, University Medicine Greifswald, Germany) of an explanted implant affected by peri-implantitis. A dense biofilm covering the entire implant surface is clearly visible

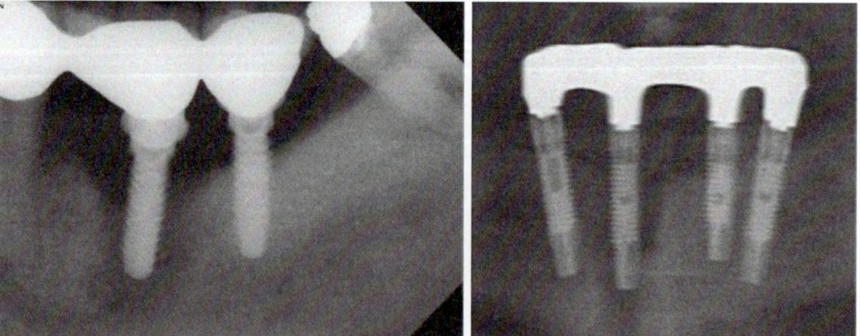

**Fig. 17.2** X-ray images (Dental School, University Medicine Greifswald, Germany) of two mandibles with two or four implants. Due to peri-implant inflammation, there is clear bone loss around the first implant (picture left) and the second implant (picture right)

**Similar to periodontitis in natural teeth, peri-implantitis at implants is a bacterial disease that causes inflammation which in turn leads to bone destruction. If untreated, peri-implantitis can lead to implant loss.**

### 17.1.2 Non-Surgical Peri-Implantitis Therapy

A non-surgical treatment, which predictably leads to a successful resolution of peri-implantitis, as performed in periodontitis, does not currently exist. Reversible conditions can only be achieved for peri-mucositis treatment. By means of suitable mechanical cleaning methods and/or antibacterial solutions and early diagnosis, further progress of the inflammation and the manifestation of peri-implantitis can be prevented [4]. Due to the complex shape, the screw threads and the microrough titanium surface, cleaning methods such as those used in teeth are currently unsuitable.

**A safe, predictable and non-invasive treatment option currently exists only for peri-mucositis.**

### 17.1.3 Surgical Peri-Implantitis Therapy

The surgical peri-implantitis procedure includes the removal of the granulation tissue in the peri-implant area and the subsequent decontamination of the implant surface with disinfection rinses and mechanical methods. The aim of the treatment is bone regeneration and the re-osseointegration of the exposed implant part. None of the current procedures leads to a predictable success of the treatment [5]. For the re-attachment of bone cells to previously bacterially contaminated implant surfaces, it is important that the surface is free from vital bacteria and dead bacteria residues [6]. The use of cold plasma could contribute to re-osseointegration.

**For the surgical treatment of peri-implantitis, there are currently no recommended protocols that are promising or should be preferred.**

Cold atmospheric pressure plasma (CAP) showed antimicrobial effects, antioxidant effects, immunomodulatory effects, as well as the possibility of biocompatible surface modifications like influencing cell adhesion or antibacterial coatings [7–13], and also had wound healing properties [14–16]. This mix promises new therapeutic approaches for dental implantology. Reading the literature it must be noted that there is not only a single plasma device, but there exist many different plasma sources with different physical set-ups and gas mixtures which result in a great variability of the physical effects, which in turn may have very different biological effects.

Against the background of the findings reported so far reported and the combinable effects for disinfection, surface functionalization and possible wound-healing stimulation properties of plasma, the use of atmospheric pressure plasmas is conceivable in the field of implantology both for prevention and treatment of peri-implantitis.

### 17.1.4 Antimicrobial Effect of Cold Plasma

Medical plasma will usually be generated by using the working gases helium, argon or mixtures of these with oxygen or nitrogen as well as air [17, 18].

**The antimicrobial effect of the different plasmas (different working gases and energy transfer used) are mainly caused by the excited and ionized gas species and subsequently by their produced reactive species after contact with the surrounding air at the working place or after contact with the treated substrate, as well as caused by emitted ultraviolet radiation.** Especially, reactive oxygen and nitrogen species seem to play the key role in inactivating microorganisms [19, 20]. Therefore, the reactive components generate oxidative stress and destabilize or destroy lipid and polysaccharide structures by oxygenation processes and radical chain reactions on microbial membrane and cell walls or organic substrates [19].

**It should be noted that the distance between the exit point of the plasma or the location of the plasma formation toward the sample with the biofilm influences the effectiveness of the plasma. Usually the plasma effect decreases rapidly with increasing distance.**

### 17.1.5 Disinfection of Microbially Contaminated Implants

**The antimicrobial effect of plasma was often investigated and confirmed** [7, 8, 13, 21–23].

*In-vitro*-results showed that the single use of cold plasma [24, 25] or with an additional mechanical pre-treatment [26] can lead to a sterile surface under specific conditions and properties.

The study of Duske et al. [26] demonstrated that neither the sole mechanical treatment nor the sole plasma treatment led to sterile surfaces. However, after the combined mechanical and plasma treatment the biofilm-coated discs were sterile (Fig. 17.3). This was confirmed by subsequent cultivation of treated discs with seeded osteoblastic cells on the disc surface for a period of 5 days in cell culture media, with the result that osteoblastic cells could spread over the specimen surface but no microbial regrowth was detectable.

To our knowledge there is only one currently published *in-vivo*-study (in beagle dogs), which investigated CAP as a new therapy option for treating peri-implantitis [27]. This study showed promising results between the two investigated groups (scaling with subsequent chlorhexidine treatment alone or with additional cold atmospheric plasma); the bone level was significantly higher and the detection of

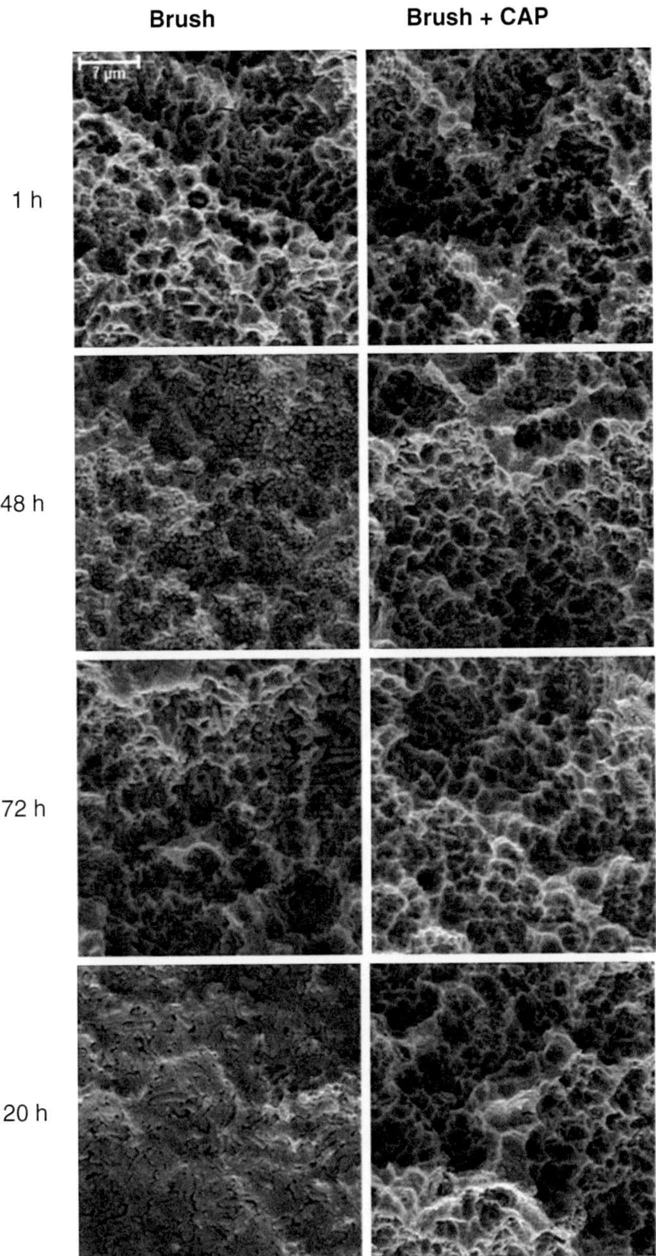


**Fig. 17.3** Cleaning of a rough implant surface with a brush or a combination of brush and subsequent plasma treatment. After 1 h of incubation, the brushed surface seemed to be devoid of bacteria, but on closer inspection it was found that the brush left some vital bacteria on the surface. After 48 h, a biofilm had formed, which further matured into a dense biofilm after 120 h. The combined treatment with a brush and plasma always achieved a sterile surface, because vital bacteria were killed and microbial residues were removed by the final plasma treatment. Thus no microbial regrowth is shown

*Porphyromonas gingivalis* and *Tannerella forsythia* had decreased after 3 months of plasma treatment [27]. However, that study did not include plasma treatment combined with an efficient mechanical pre-treatment such as air polishing, which could further improve the results [28].

**A combination of plasma and mechanical treatment opens up new possibilities for the decontamination of implant surfaces.**

Further, to reduce treatment time and to increase the antimicrobial effect of CAP, some studies investigated the combination of different antimicrobials such as sodium hypochloride and chlorhexidine, which can lead to increased efficiency [22, 27, 29, 30]. Combined application of conventional mechanical and antiseptic treatment with CAP should be further investigated to find the optimal treatment regime.

Cold plasma is suited as a new adjuvant therapy to inactivate and to remove microorganisms from implant surfaces, because beside their antimicrobial effect, plasma will not or virtually not destroy the implant surface. Also, the gaseous plasma flow could spread along the implant and could reach difficult-to-access areas (deeper regions, screw threads). This feature could be an important advantage of plasma compared to sole mechanical treatment and antiseptic rinse and therefore become a helpful adjuvant therapeutical option to improve peri-implantitis treatment.

However, it is also known that plasma can etch synthetic materials and organic substances [24, 31]. The etching effect depends on the working gas used and the energy input. For example, with increasing oxygen content in the inert gas for plasma ignition the etching effect can be increased. It was shown that especially carbon-carbon (C-C) and carbon-hydrogen (C-H) bonds were oxidized and the number of chemical oxygen rich groups increased [32]. This effect could also be helpful in eliminating microbial biofilms [24, 33]. However, if the etching effect is efficient enough in removing biofilms, then the plasma will probably be unsuited to treat living human tissue, because the energy input could be too high.

### 17.1.6 Modification of Implant Surfaces by Cold Plasma Treatment

Generally, plasma can influence the chemical properties of metallic and ceramic implant materials [7, 34–36] and it leaves the surface without any chemical residues [37] or topographical changes [38].

Different studies about implant surface treatment with plasma demonstrated the ability of plasma to change the surface hydrophilicity, which was reflected in the change of the water contact angle (WCA). After plasma treatment, the WCA was reduced and formerly hydrophobic surfaces (WCA > 90°) became hydrophilic or the hydrophilicity of hydrophilic surfaces was significantly increased [37, 39–41]

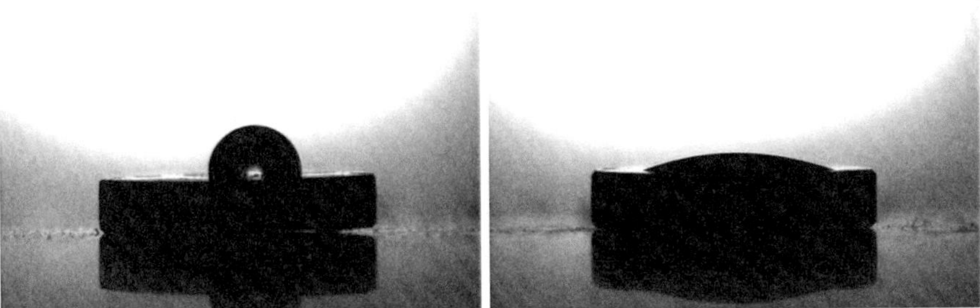

**Fig. 17.4** Untreated implant surface (image left) and plasma-treated implant surface (image right) with water droplets for contact angle measurement. A plasma treatment leads to a reduced water-surface contact angle; the hydrophilicity of the implant surface increases

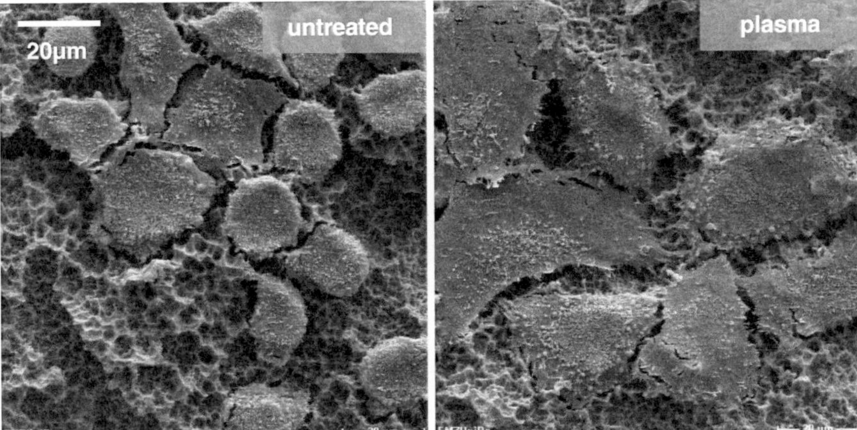


**Fig. 17.5** Osteoblasts (osteosarcoma cells, MG63) after 1 h of cell cultivation on untreated rough titanium implant surface (image left) and mechanically-plasma-treated implant surface (image right). After plasma treatment, the cells cultivated on the titanium surface are much flatter and wider with more pronounced filopodia than cells on the untreated implant surface

(Fig. 17.4). The formation of reversible polar groups (e.g., -OH, -COOH, -$NH_2$) on the treated surface could be the cause of the increase in hydrophilization [42]. It was observed that the adhesion of cells was closely related to the WCA and the surface energy of a material. Hydrophilicity also supports primary adhesion of proteins, which in turn can stimulate the cell adhesion [43, 44]. Concurrently, **In vitro studies show that the decrease of WCA results in a cell-adhesive effect by plasma-treated surfaces** [37, 39, 44–46]. As a result, the cells become flatter and cover more surface area of the substrate after CAP treatment (Fig. 17.5). This aspect is important after the insertion of dental implants. A rapid attachment of cells and complete covering of the surface with cells closes the access to the implant for bacteria more quickly. The "race for the surface" described by Gristina [47], which means the competition between bacteria and human cells directly after implantation, may be supported in favor of the cells by plasma.

A further specific application of CAP could be the surface functionalization of abutments. An abutment is the connecting part between an implant and the prosthetic restoration (i.e., the visible crown). It breaks through the oral mucosa to the mouth cavity and peri-implant soft tissue seals the abutment. Abutments often have to be adapted to the implant in the dental laboratory before being screwed on the implant and can be contaminated in the dental laboratory. Dirt as a foreign material inhibits the colonization of the abutment surface by cells of the surrounding tissue. Similar to the biofilm removal effect by CAP, plasma can also contribute to the cleaning of the surface of the abutment and thus promote wound healing after implantation [48]. Canullo et al. [49] showed that titanium abutments after CAP treatment with argon enhanced cell adhesion, even at the early stage of soft tissue healing, compared to the untreated control abutments and abutments treated with a steam pressure device. Here, plasma also seems to promote collagen fiber orientation [50]. In a clinically examined *in-vivo* study for 2 years it was documented that implants with CAP treated abutments exhibited a lower microbial load and significantly lower bone loss than the controls [51, 52]. Inflammatory response of soft tissue to plasma-treated abutments seems to be comparable to non-plasma-treated abutments [53].

**Ceramic and metallic implant surfaces can be hydrophilized by CAP, which leads to a cell-adhesive effect.**

### 17.1.7 Study About Possible Side Effect of CAP on Oral Mucosa

For an intraoral application of plasma, it is important to know that it does not cause irreversible damage to the oral mucosa during application. The plasma sources can differ significantly, especially regarding temperature or UV radiation. There is a lack of dental-relevant investigations. The *in-vivo* study of Liu et al. [54] also investigated its side effects on oral mucosa. In this study, three rabbits were treated per group and observed for a maximum of 5 days. The results suggested that no intense mucosal membrane irritation responses occurred [54]. However, possible carcinogenic effects after an extended or repeated CAP application were not investigated. Since peri-implantitis is not a life-threatening disease, no treatment-related side effects with carcinogenic potential could be accepted. Thus, the question of safety of peri-implantitis with CAP treatment needs to be investigated and clarified before clinical introduction.

**While the advantages of plasma are extensively described, studies to exclude possible undesirable side effects are rare and desirable to ensure patient´s and operators' safety.**

### 17.1.8 Conclusion and Outlook

The use of CAP in the field of implantology for the prevention and treatment of peri-implantitis is reasonable against the background of diverse effects of decontamination, disinfection, surface functionalization and possibly wound-healing-stimulation properties of plasma. To functionalize the surfaces of implant materials with the aim of shortening the healing time [34, 36] or of optimizing wound healing in the abutment area [51] in daily practice in the foreseeable future, could be possible with suitable CAP devices. The oral use of plasma technology for peri-implant therapy as an additional method seems very promising [26]. However, further *in-vivo* studies will be necessary [27] to ensure patient safety.

**The plasma treatment of implant surfaces shows antimicrobial effects, modifies the implant surface to improves cell adhesion, and thus also the healing or integration of the implant into the tissue. Plasma has promising properties for the development of a new treatment option for peri-implantitis therapy.**

## References


1. Mombelli A, Müller N, Cionca N. The epidemiology of peri-implantitis. Clin Oral Implants Res. 2012;23(6):67–76. https://doi.org/10.1111/j.1600-0501.2012.02541.x.
2. Derks J, Hakansson J, Wennstrom JL, Tomasi C, Larsson M, Berglundh T. Effectiveness of implant therapy analyzed in a Swedish population: early and late implant loss. J Dent Res. 2015;94:44S–51S. https://doi.org/10.1177/0022034514563077.
3. Bobia F, Pop RV. Periimplantitis. Aetiology, diagnosis, treatment. A review from the literature. Curr Health Sci J. 2010;36:171–5.
4. Renvert S, Roos-Jansaker A-M, Claffey N. Non-surgical treatment of peri-implant mucositis and peri-implantitis: a literature review. J Clin Periodontol. 2008;35(Suppl. 8):305–15. https://doi.org/10.1111/j.1600-051X.2008.01276.x.
5. Claffey N, Clarke E, Polyzois I, Renvert S. Surgical treatment of peri-implantitis. J Clin Periodontol. 2008;35(Suppl. 8):316–32. https://doi.org/10.1111/j.1600-051X.2008.01277.x.
6. Persson LG, Ericsson I, Berglundh T, Lindhe J. Osseintegration following treatment of peri-implantitis and replacement of implant components. An experimental study in the dog. J Clin Periodontol. 2001;28:258–63. https://doi.org/10.1034/j.1600-051x.2001.028003258.x.
7. Duske K, Wegner K, Donnert M, Kunert U, Podbielski A, Kreikemeyer B, et al. Comparative in vitro study of different atmospheric pressure plasma jets concerning their antimicrobial potential and cellular reaction. Plasma Process Polym. 2015b;12(10):1050–60. https://doi.org/10.1002/ppap.201400176.
8. Koban I, Holtfreter B, Hübner N, Matthes R, Sietmann R, Kindel E, et al. Antimicrobial efficacy of non-thermal plasma in comparison to chlorhexidine against dental biofilms on titanium discs in vitro - proof of principle experiment. J Clin Periodontol. 2011b;38:956–65. https://doi.org/10.1111/j.1600-051X.2011.01740.x.
9. Monetta T, Scala A, Malmo C, Bellucci F. Antibacterial activity of cold plasma-treated titanium alloy. Plasma Med. 2011;1:205–14. https://doi.org/10.1615/PlasmaMed.v1.i3-4.30.

10. Nebe B, Finke B, Hippler R, Meichsner J, Podbielski A, Schlosser M, Bader R. Physical plasma processes for surface functionalization of implants for orthopedic surgery. Hyg Med. 2013;38:192–7.
11. de Queiroz JDF, de Sousa Leal AM, Terada M, Agnez-Lima LF, Costa I, de Souza Pinto NC, de Medeiros Batistuzzo SR. Surface modification by argon plasma treatment improves antioxidant defense ability of CHO-k1 cells on titanium surfaces. Toxicol In Vitro. 2014;28:381–7. https://doi.org/10.1016/j.tiv.2013.11.012.
12. Walschus U, Hoene A, Patrzyk M, Finke B, Polak M, Lucke S, et al. Serum profile of pro- and anti-inflammatory cytokines in rats following implantation of low-temperature plasma-modified titanium plates. J Mater Sci Mater Med. 2012;23:1299–307. https://doi.org/10.1007/s10856-012-4600-z.
13. Wiegand C, Beier O, Horn K, Pfuch A, Tölke T, Hipler U, Schimanski A. Antimicrobial impact of cold atmospheric pressure plasma on medical critical yeasts and bacteria cultures. Skin Pharmacol Physiol. 2014;27:25–35. https://doi.org/10.1159/000351353.
14. Bender CP, Hübner N, Weltmann K, Scharf C, Kramer A. Tissue tolerable plasma and polihexanide: are synergistic effects possible to promote healing of chronic wounds? In Vivo and In Vitro results. In: Machala Z, Hensel K, Akishev Y, editors. Plasma for bio-decontamination, medicine and food security. Dordrecht: Springer Netherlands (NATO Science for Peace and Security Series A: Chemistry and Biology); 2012. p. 321–34.
15. Isbary G, Heinlin J, Shimizu T, Zimmermann J, Morfill G, Schmidt H, et al. Successful and safe use of 2 min cold atmospheric argon plasma in chronic wounds: results of a randomized controlled trial. Br J Dermatol. 2012;167:404–10. https://doi.org/10.1111/j.1365-2133.2012.10923.x.
16. Jacofsky MC, Lubahn C, McDonnell C, Seepersad Y, Fridman G, Fridman AA, Dobrynin D. Spatially resolved optical emission spectroscopy of a helium plasma jet and its effects on wound healing rate in a diabetic murine model. Plasma Med. 2014;4:177–91. https://doi.org/10.1615/PlasmaMed.2015012190.
17. Chen W, Huang J, Du N, Liu X, Wang X, Lv G, et al. Treatment of enterococcus faecalis bacteria by a helium atmospheric cold plasma brush with oxygen addition. J Appl Phys. 2012;112:013304. https://doi.org/10.1063/1.4732135.
18. Xiong Z, Cao Y, Lu X, Du T. Plasmas in tooth root canal. IEEE Trans Plasma Sci. 2011;39:2968–9. https://doi.org/10.1109/TPS.2011.2157533.
19. Bourke P, Zuizina D, Han L, Cullen P, Gilmore BF. Microbiological Interactions with cold plasma. J Appl Microbiol. 2017;123(2):308–24. https://doi.org/10.1111/jam.13429.
20. Li Y, Sun K, Ye G, Liang Y, Pan H, Wang G, et al. Evaluation of cold plasma treatment and safety in disinfecting 3-week root canal enterococcus faecalis biofilm in vitro. J Endod. 2015;41:1325–30. https://doi.org/10.1016/j.joen.2014.10.020.
21. Idlibi AN, Al-Marrawi F, Hannig M, Lehmann A, Rueppell A, Schindler A, et al. Destruction of oral biofilms formed in situ on machined titanium (Ti) surfaces by cold atmospheric plasma. Biofouling. 2013;29:369–79. https://doi.org/10.1080/08927014.2013.775255.
22. Matthes R, Jablonowski L, Koban I, Quade A, Hübner N, Schlueter R, et al. In vitro treatment of Candida albicans biofilms on denture base material with volume dielectric barrier discharge plasma (VDBD) compared with common chemical antiseptics. Clin Oral Investig. 2015:1–8. https://doi.org/10.1007/s00784-015-1463-y.
23. Rupf S, Lehmann A, Hannig M, Schafer B, Schubert A, Feldmann U, Schindler A. Killing of adherent oral microbes by a non-thermal atmospheric plasma jet. J Med Microbiol. 2010;59:206–12. https://doi.org/10.1099/jmm.0.013714-0.
24. Fricke K, Koban I, Tresp H, Jablonowski L, Schroder K, Kramer A, et al. Atmospheric pressure plasma: a high-performance tool for the efficient removal of biofilms. PLoS One. 2012a;7:e42539. https://doi.org/10.1371/journal.pone.0042539.
25. Rupf S, Idlibi AN, Marrawi FA, Hannig M, Schubert A, von Mueller L, et al. Removing biofilms from microstructured titanium ex vivo: a novel approach using atmospheric plasma technology. PLoS One. 2011;6:e25893. https://doi.org/10.1371/journal.pone.0025893.
26. Duske K, Jablonowski L, Koban I, Matthes R, Holtfreter B, Sckell A, et al. Cold atmospheric plasma in combination with mechanical treatment improves osteoblast growth on

biofilm covered titanium discs. Biomaterials. 2015a;52:327–34. https://doi.org/10.1016/j.biomaterials.2015.02.035.
27. Shi Q, Song K, Zhou X, Xiong Z, Du T, Lu X, Cao Y. Effects of non-equilibrium plasma in the treatment of ligature-induced peri-implantitis. J Clin Periodontol. 2015;42:478–87. https://doi.org/10.1111/jcpe.12403.
28. Matthes R, Duske K, Kebede TG, Pink C, Schlüter R, Woedtke T, et al. Osteoblast growth, after cleaning of biofilm-covered titanium discs with air-polishing and cold plasma. J Clin Periodontol. 2017;44(6):672–80. https://doi.org/10.1111/jcpe.12720.
29. Du T, Shi Q, Shen Y, Cao Y, Ma J, Lu X, et al. Effect of modified nonequilibrium plasma with chlorhexidine digluconate against endodontic biofilms in vitro. J Endod. 2013;39:1438–43. https://doi.org/10.1016/j.joen.2013.06.027.
30. Zhou X, Xiong Z, Cao Y, Lu X, Liu D. The antimicrobial activity of an atmospheric-pressure room-temperature plasma in a simulated root-canal model infected with enterococcus faecalis. IEEE Trans Plasma Sci. 2010;38:3370–4. https://doi.org/10.1109/TPS.2010.2078522.
31. Fricke K, Steffen H, von Woedtke T, Schroeder K, Weltmann K. High rate etching of polymers by means of an atmospheric pressure plasma jet. Plasma Process Polym. 2011;8:51–8.
32. Fricke K, Tresp H, Bussiahn R, Schröder K, Woedtke T, Weltmann K. On the use of atmospheric pressure plasma for the bio-decontamination of polymers and its impact on their chemical and morphological surface properties. Plasma Chem Plasma Process. 2012b;32:801–16. https://doi.org/10.1007/s11090-012-9378-8.
33. Jablonowski L, Fricke K, Matthes R, Holtfreter B, Schlüter R, Woedtke T, et al. Removal of naturally grown human biofilm with an atmospheric pressure plasma jet: an in-vitro study. J Biophotonics. 2017;10(5):718–26. https://doi.org/10.1002/jbio.201600166.
34. Coelho PG, Giro G, Teixeira HS, Marin C, Witek L, Thompson VP, et al. Argon-based atmospheric pressure plasma enhances early bone response to rough titanium surfaces. J Biomed Mater Res. 2012;100A:1901–6. https://doi.org/10.1002/jbm.a.34127.
35. Danna NR, Beutel BG, Tovar N, Witek L, Marin C, Bonfante EA, et al. Assessment of atmospheric pressure plasma treatment for implant osseointegration. Biomed Res Int. 2015;2015:761718. https://doi.org/10.1155/2015/761718.
36. Shon W, Chung SH, Kim H, Han G, Cho B, Park Y. Peri-implant bone formation of non-thermal atmospheric pressure plasma-treated zirconia implants with different surface roughness in rabbit tibiae. Clin Oral Impl Res. 2014;25:573–9. https://doi.org/10.1111/clr.12115.
37. Duske K, Koban I, Kindel E, Schröder K, Nebe B, Holtfreter B, et al. Atmospheric plasma enhances wettability and cell spreading on dental implant metals. J Clin Periodontol. 2012;39:400–7. https://doi.org/10.1111/j.1600-051X.2012.01853.x.
38. Lee J-H, Kim Y-H, Choi E-H, Kim K-M, Kim K-N. Air atmospheric-pressure plasma-jet treatment enhances the attachment of human gingival fibroblasts for early peri-implant soft tissue seals on titanium dental implant abutments. Acta Odontol Scand. 2015;73:67–75. https://doi.org/10.3109/00016357.2014.954265.
39. Koban I, Duske K, Jablonowski L, Schröder K, Nebe B, Sietmann R, et al. Atmospheric plasma enhances wettability and osteoblast spreading on dentin in vitro: proof-of-principle. Plasma Process Polym. 2011a;8:975–82. https://doi.org/10.1002/ppap.201100030.
40. Lai J, Sunderland B, Xue J, Yan S, Zhao W, Folkard M, et al. Study on hydrophilicity of polymer surfaces improved by plasma treatment. Appl Surf Sci. 2006;252:3375–9. https://doi.org/10.1016/j.apsusc.2005.05.038.
41. Ritts AC, Li H, Yu Q, Xu C, Yao X, Hong L, Wang Y. Dentin surface treatment using a non-thermal argon plasma brush for interfacial bonding improvement in composite restoration. Eur J Oral Sci. 2010;118:510–6. https://doi.org/10.1111/j.1600-0722.2010.00761.x.
42. Favia P, d'Agostino R. Plasma treatments and plasma deposition of polymers for biomedical applications. Surf Coat Technol. 1998;98:1102–6. https://doi.org/10.1016/S0257-8972(97)00285-5.
43. Duewelhenke N, Eysel P. Serumfreie Kultivierung von Osteoprogenitorzellen und Osteoblasten zur Testung von Biomaterialien. Orthopade. 2007;36:220–6. https://doi.org/10.1007/s00132-007-1057-8.

44. Wei J, Igarashi T, Okumori N, Igarashi T, Maetani T, Liu B, Yoshinari M. Influence of surface wettability on competitive protein adsorption and initial attachment of osteoblasts. Biomed Mater. 2009;4:045002. https://doi.org/10.1088/1748-6041/4/4/045002.
45. Finke B, Luethen F, Schroeder K, Mueller PD, Bergemann C, Frant M, et al. The effect of positively charged plasma polymerization on initial osteoblastic focal adhesion on titanium surfaces. Biomaterials. 2007;28:4521–34. https://doi.org/10.1016/j.biomaterials.2007.06.028.
46. Satriano C, Marletta G, Guglielmino S, Carnazza S. Cell adhesion to ion- and plasma-treated polymer surfaces: the role of surface free energy. In: Mittal KL, editor. Contact angle, wettability and adhesion. Leiden, Boston: VSP; 2006. p. 471–86. http://gateway.isiknowledge.com/gateway/Gateway.cgi?GWVersion=2&SrcAuth=ResearchSoft&SrcApp=EndNote&DestLinkType=FullRecord&DestApp=WOS&KeyUT=000242465600028.
47. Gristina A. Biomaterial-centered infection: microbial adhesion versus tissue integration. Science. 1987;237:1588–95. https://doi.org/10.1126/science.3629258.
48. Canullo L, Micarelli C, Lembo-Fazio L, Iannello G, Clementini M. Microscopical and microbiologic characterization of customized titanium abutments after different cleaning procedures. Clin Oral Implants Res. 2014a;25:328–36. https://doi.org/10.1111/clr.12089.
49. Canullo L, Penarrocha-Oltra D, Marchionni S, Bagan L, Penarrocha-Diago M, Micarelli C. Soft tissue cell adhesion to titanium abutments after different cleaning procedures: preliminary results of a randomized clinical trial. Med Oral Patol Oral Cir Bucal. 2014b;19:e177–83.
50. Garcia B, Camacho F, Peñarrocha D, Tallarico M, Perez S, Canullo L. Influence of plasma cleaning procedure on the interaction between soft tissue and abutments: a randomized controlled histologic study. Clin Oral Implants Res. 2017;28(10):1269–77. https://doi.org/10.1111/clr.12953.
51. Canullo CLL, Penarrocha D, Micarelli C, Massidda O, Bazzoli M. Hard tissue response to argon plasma cleaning/sterilisation of customised titanium abutments versus 5-second steam cleaning: results of a 2-year post-loading follow-up from an explanatory randomised controlled trial in periodontally healthy patients. Eur J Oral Implantol. 2013;6(3):251–60.
52. Canullo L, Tallarico M, Peñarrocha-Diago M, Garcia B, Peñarrocha D. Plasma of argon cleaning treatment on implant abutments in periodontally healthy patients: five years post-loading results of an RCT. Clin Oral Implants Res. 2016a;27(Suppl. 13):47. https://doi.org/10.1111/clr.45_12957.
53. Canullo L, Dehner JF, Penarrocha D, Checchi V, Mazzoni A, Breschi L. Soft tissue response to titanium abutments with different surface treatment: preliminary histologic report of a randomized controlled trial. Biomed Res Int. 2016b;2016:2952530. https://doi.org/10.1155/2016/2952530.
54. Liu D, Xiong Z, Du T, Zhou X, Cao Y, Lu X. Bacterial-killing effect of atmospheric pressure nonequilibrium plasma jet and oral mucosa response. J Huazhong Univ Sci Technolog. 2011;31(6):852–6.

# 18 Perspectives in Orthodontics

Philine H. Metelmann and Karl-Friedrich Krey

## 18.1 Introduction

The subject of Orthodontics and Dentofacial Orthopedics deals with the prevention, diagnosis and treatment of abnormalities and malfunctions in the dentofacial and stomatognathic system as a specialty field of dentistry.

"Plasma orthodontics" is a new emerging area of Plasmamedicine which is why at present only few specific research results are available. However, the great potential of cold atmospheric pressure plasma (CAP) that has already been demonstrated in other dental disciplines, can also be applied to certain aspects of orthodontics.

Thanks to the invention of compact CAP-sources with hand-held units, Plasmamedicine was able to enter the field of dentistry. Modern plasmajet-devices create a fine, needle-shaped plasma-effluent of about 10 mm that is very suitable for treating intraoral areas and surfaces that are otherwise hard to reach.

Possible applications of CAP in orthodontics mainly derive from the following three properties of CAP:

- antimicrobial efficacy
- surface conditioning
- wound healing

P. H. Metelmann (✉) • K.-F. Krey
Department of Orthodontics, Center for Dental, Oral and Craniomandibular Sciences, University Medicine Greifswald, Greifswald, Germany
e-mail: metelmannp@uni-greifswald.de; kreyk@uni-greifswald.de



H.-R. Metelmann et al. (eds.), *Comprehensive Clinical Plasma Medicine*,
https://doi.org/10.1007/978-3-319-67627-2_18

## 18.2 Antimicrobial Efficacy

### 18.2.1 Special Aspects of Oral Hygiene during Orthodontic Treatment

**Sufficient oral hygiene is one of the basic prerequisites for a successful orthodontic therapy.** Although the orthodontic straightening of teeth can simplify oral hygiene in the long term by treating malocclusions such as crowding, there is an increased risk of plaque accumulation during the active treatment phase.

Physiologically, more than 700 different bacterial species can be detected in the oral cavity [1]. Orthodontic appliances change the balance of this ecosystem by providing altered physio-chemical conditions and an enlarged surface for the adhesion of normal oral microflora [2].

Several studies have shown that fixed orthodontic treatment devices, such as multi-bracket-appliances, enhance the intraoral plaque retention [3, 4]. After 1 month in situ, metal brackets are already multicolonized with different bacterial species, including cariogenic and periodontal pathogenic organisms [5].

Even removable orthodontic devices serve as reservoirs for microorganisms: after 1 week of intensive wearing time, Streptococcus mutans colonies can be found on their acrylic baseplates [6].

These changes in the oral flora and the development of biofilms increase the risk of gum disease (gingivitis) and decalcifications of the tooth (white spots, caries) during active orthodontic treatment [7–10], emphasizing the importance of thorough oral hygiene.

A study by Ren et al. [11] underlines the need for improved antimicrobial measures in orthodontic therapy: 15% of all orthodontic patients develop dental complications that require professional care. This high treatment demand generates costs of US$ 500 million a year in the US health care system, turning a deficient biofilm control in orthodontics into a problem of public health. The authors therefore conclude, that "Improved preventive measures and antimicrobial materials are urgently required to prevent biofilm-related complications of orthodontic treatment from overshadowing its functional and esthetic advantages."

**Plasmamedicine as a supporting and preventive measure would be a useful addition to current oral hygiene regimes**.

### 18.2.2 CAP as an Effective Instrument for Oral Hygiene

CAP is a promising tool for antimicrobial use in the oral cavity, as it is effective in destroying biofilms and can disinfect tooth surfaces [12–14].

Studies have also demonstrated the antimicrobial efficacy of CAP on polymethylmethacrylate (PMMA) [15]—the basic material of many orthodontic treatment appliances—and on various metals, such as titanium [16, 17] (Fig. 18.1).

However, since oral infections are polymicrobial, (future) research needs to evaluate the effect of CAP on every pathogen involved in dental plaque formation [18].

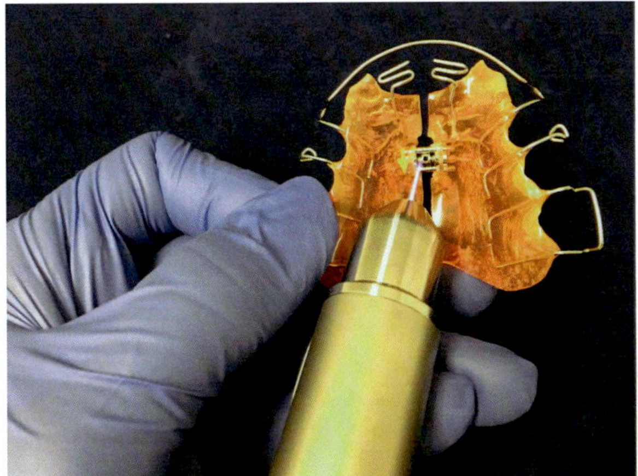

**Fig. 18.1** Antimicrobial efficacy of CAP on removable orthodontic appliances. CAP is effective in destroying biofilms on acrylic baseplates and could therefore be a useful addition to current oral hygiene regimes. (Plasma source pictured: kinPen med, Neoplas tool, Greifswald, Germany)

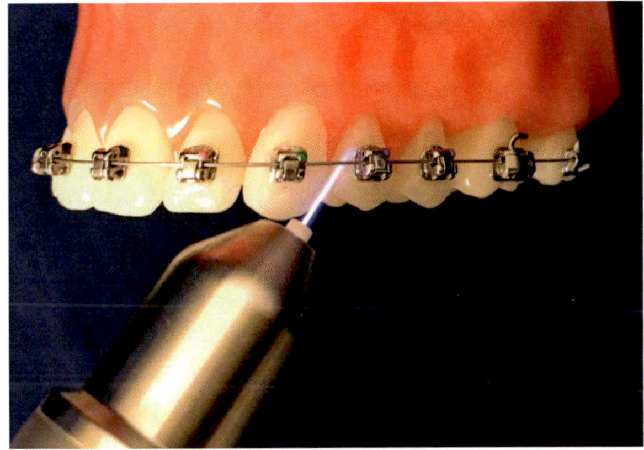

**Fig. 18.2** Antimicrobial efficacy of CAP on teeth and fixed orthodontic multi-bracket appliances. The needle-shaped plasma-effluent can reach surfaces that are otherwise hardly accessible for proper hygiene. (Plasma source pictured: kinPen med, Neoplas tool, Greifswald, Germany; Bracket system pictured: Damon, Ormco, Orange, USA)

Cariogenic bacteria like Streptococcus mutans and Lactobacillus acidophilus are sensitive to CAP treatment. The great potential of CAP in caries prevention can be demonstrated with a 99.9999% cell reduction in less than 15 s of plasma irradiation for S. mutans and within 5 min for L. acidophilus [19].

Furthermore, Porphyromonas gingivalis, a periodontal pathogenic bacterium, can be deactivated using CAP [20].

CAP and its combination with other antiseptics are also a promising approach to control Candida albicans [21]. Orthodontic appliances are considered as a predisposition to the proliferation of Candida albicans in the oral cavity [22], especially in immunosuppressed patients [23].

**Using CAP as an antimicrobial agent in orthodontics could be beneficial in various areas and treatment phases: Since CAP remains in gaseous medium it can reach surfaces that are otherwise nearly inaccessible for proper hygiene** (Fig. 18.2).

Most importantly, CAP has the ability to eliminate biofilms on teeth, gums and appliances without having toxic effects on the oral epithelium [14].

The application of CAP induces micromorphological changes of bacteria embedded in biofilm. After plasma treatment microbial remnants, cells with perforated cell walls, and only a few intact microorganisms can be detected via electron microscopy. This observation suggests that CAP is suitable for the reduction of biofilms, yet no complete removal can be achieved [12]. Several studies therefore recommend CAP as a supporting antimicrobial agent, for example in connection with mechanical cleaning by air-water spray [16, 24]. The latter is available at every dentist's treatment chair.

Since some biological effects of CAP are mediated by liquids, plasma-enhanced antimicrobial fluids are investigated intensively [25, 26]. There is evidence that plasma supports the benefits of common mouthwash-agents like chlorhexidine, octenidine and $H_2O_2$ and thus may reduce the amount needed [27]. Future research will have to focus on synergistic effects between CAP and established antimicrobial agents.

## 18.3 Surface Conditioning

### 18.3.1 Aspects of Orthodontic Adhesive Systems

Fixed "multibracket orthodontic appliances" function based on the principle of a metal wire that is ligated to the teeth via anchoring elements ("brackets"). The shape of the wire defines an ideal arch form on which the teeth align.

Nowadays, most brackets are bonded to the teeth using composite adhesives. This material by itself does not establish a chemical bond with enamel. The main force of bonding is provided by micromechanical interlocking at the enamel-adhesive interface. Hence, in order to create a micro-retentive surface for the composite to infiltrate into, the enamel must be conditioned with acid, which causes porosities in the hard substance. Ever since the concept of etching enamel with orthophosphoric acid was introduced by Buonocore in 1955 [28], there has been discussion concerning the loss of enamel due to bonding and debonding of attachments. Approximately 55.6 μm of enamel are lost as a result of etching, bracket placement and subsequent removal and "clean-up" [29]. Also, the permanent loss of fluoride-rich surface enamel may make teeth more susceptible to decalcification during orthodontic treatment [30]. For these reasons, the establishment of a high bond strength on non-etched enamel is a desirable scenario, yet also challenging—due to the lack of mechanical interlocking on the limited surface area.

### 18.3.2 CAP for Improving Adhesive Properties

The application of CAP on enamel does not substantially change the surface morphology, but increases the surface energy by deliberately incorporating free radicals. This enhances the penetration ability allowing for a more intimate interaction of enamel and adhesive in a primary chemical bonding [31, 32]. CAP treatment also increases the surface polarity, transforming enamel into a more hydrophilic state. The underlying mechanisms of this conditioning are under discussion: Possibly, the replacement of carbon groups with new oxygen-containing polar moieties is responsible for increased hydrophilicity [33]. A better wettability may have a positive effect on the retention of hydrophilic adhesives [34]. Teixeira et al. [32] studied the influence of CAP on the mechanical properties of enamel and sealant bond strength. They report that CAP application to non-etched enamel significantly enhances the microshear bond strength, leading to values comparable with the etched control.

**Therefore, owing to its ability to modify and functionalize surfaces without compromising the morphology, CAP presents the potential to optimize orthodontic bonding techniques** [35, 36].

Further research—especially in vivo studies and clinical evaluation—will show if CAP can be considered as a valid substitute for conventional acid etching procedures (Fig. 18.3).

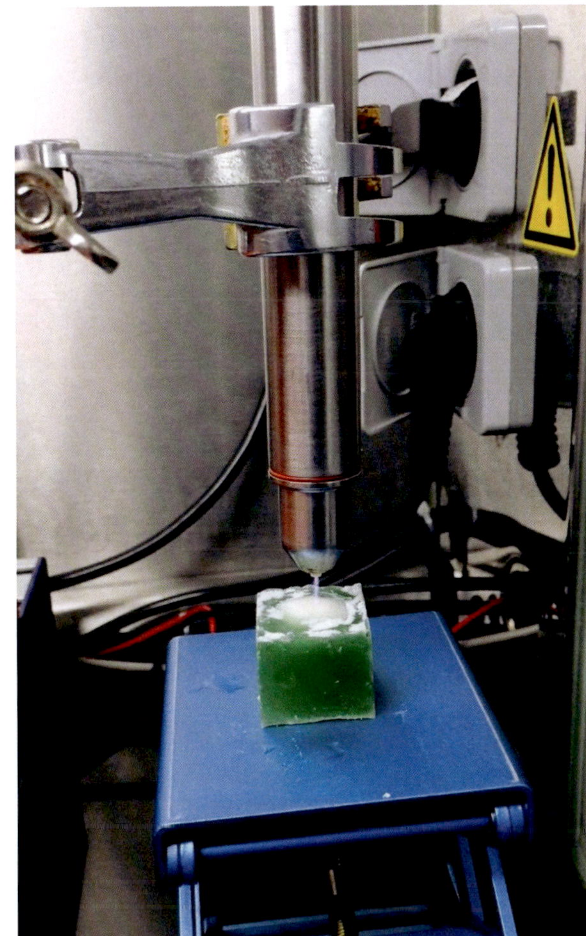

**Fig. 18.3** Surface conditioning with CAP. Bovine teeth embedded in resin are used in preliminary examinations to test the effect of CAP on the bond strength of orthodontic attachments. (Plasma source pictured: kinPen med, Neoplas tool, Greifswald, Germany)

## 18.4 Wound Healing

Orthodontic therapy makes use of directional forces to achieve the desired tooth movements. Following Newton's law of motion, forces are always accompanied by equal and opposite forces (actio = reactio). That is why, in order to avoid unwanted reciprocal movements, proper anchorage is necessary. Enossal anchorage provided by metallic implants, plate systems or mini-screws on the palate or alveolar process, are recently gaining widespread acceptance [37, 38]. After inserting temporary anchorage devices (TADs) the mucosal wound created may cause complications such as pain and swelling. Excellent oral hygiene and compliance are crucial to avoid infections of the surrounding area and consequent loss of the TAD [39, 40]. Nowadays, the use of special brushes and antibacterial mouthwash solutions are means of choice to prevent infections. However, in a proof-of-principle-experiment Koban et al. [17] treated dental biofilms on titanium discs with plasma and found that CAP is more efficient than chlorhexidine-solution in vitro. In a comparable case—the peri-implant inflammation of osseointegrated implants—the application of CAP showed good results in vivo [41]. Consequently, CAP could be a valuable support for disinfecting the mucosal junction [42] and antibacterial treatment of the TAD [16].

One more promising indication for intraoral CAP treatment is to promote gingival tissue healing [43, 44]. Accidental mucosal traumas due to orthodontic appliances and wires often lead to unscheduled consultations in the orthodontic practice [45]. Adding symptomatic relief to the simple elimination of the cause would increase patient satisfaction.

**The further development of plasma devices to treat peri-implant mucositis and promote intraoral wound-healing may thus be helpful for both oral surgery and orthodontics.**

## References

1. Aas JA, Paster BJ, Stokes LN, Olsen I, Dewhirst FE. Defining the normal bacterial flora of the oral cavity. J Clin Microbiol. 2005;43(11):5721–32.
2. Pathak A, Sharma D. Biofilm associated microorganisms on removable oral orthodontic appliances in children in the mixed dentition. J Clin Pediatr Dent. 2013;37(3):335–40.
3. Erbe C, Hornikel HS, Schmidtmann I, Wehrbein H. Quantity and distribution of plaque in orthodontic patients treated with molar bands. J Orofac Orthop. 2011;72(1):13–20.
4. Liu H, Sun J, Dong Y, Lu H, Zhou H, Hansen BF, Song X. Periodontal health and relative quantity of subgingival porphyromonas gingivalis during orthodontic treatment. Angle Orthod. 2011;81(4):609–15.
5. Andrucioli MCD, Nelson-Filho P, Matsumoto MAN, Saraiva MCP, Feres M, De Figueiredo LC, Martins LP. Molecular detection of in-vivo microbial contamination of metallic orthodontic brackets by checkerboard DNA-DNA hybridization. Am J Orthod Dentofac Orthop. 2012;141(1):24–9.
6. Lessa FCR, Enoki C, Ito IY, Faria G, Matsumoto MAN, Nelson-Filho P. In-vivo evaluation of the bacterial contamination and disinfection of acrylic baseplates of removable orthodontic appliances. Am J Orthod Dentofacial Orthop. 2007;131(6):705.e11–7.

7. Rego RO, Oliveira CA, dos Santos-Pinto A, Jordan SF, Zambon JJ, Cirelli JA, Haraszthy VI. Clinical and microbiological studies of children and adolescents receiving orthodontic treatment. Am J Dent. 2010;23(6):317–23.
8. Martignon S, Ekstrand KR, Lemos MI, Lozano MP, Higuera C. Plaque, caries level and oral hygiene habits in young patients receiving orthodontic treatment. Commun Dent Health. 2010;27(3):133–8.
9. van Gastel J, Quirynen M, Teughels W, Coucke W, Carels C. Longitudinal changes in microbiology and clinical periodontal parameters after removal of fixed orthodontic appliances. Eur J Orthod. 2011;33(1):15–21.
10. Tufekci E, Dixon JS, Gunsolley J, Lindauer SJ. Prevalence of white spot lesions during orthodontic treatment with fixed appliances. Angle Orthod. 2011;81(2):206–10.
11. Ren Y, Jongsma MA, Mei L, van der Mei HC, Busscher HJ. Orthodontic treatment with fixed appliances and biofilm formation—a potential public health threat? Clin Oral Investig. 2014;18(7):1711–8.
12. Rupf S, Lehmann A, Hannig M, Schafer B, Schubert A, Feldmann U, Schindler A. Killing of adherent oral microbes by a non-thermal atmospheric plasma jet. J Med Microbiol. 2010;59(2):206–12.
13. Hoffmann C, Berganza C, Zhang J. Cold atmospheric plasma: methods of production and application in dentistry and oncology. Med Gas Res. 2013;3:21.
14. Delben JA, Zago CE, Tyhovych N, Duarte S, Vergani CE. Effect of atmospheric-pressure cold plasma on pathogenic oral biofilms and in vitro reconstituted oral epithelium. PLoS One. 2016;11(5):e0155427.
15. Matthes R, Jablonowski L, Koban I, Quade A, Hübner N, Schlueter R, Weltmann K, von Woedtke T, Kramer A, Kocher T. In vitro treatment of candida albicans biofilms on denture base material with volume dielectric barrier discharge plasma (VDBD) compared with common chemical antiseptics. Clin Oral Investig. 2015;19(9):2319–26.
16. Idlibi AN, Al-Marrawi F, Hannig M, Lehmann A, Rueppell A, Schindler A, Jentsch H, Rupf S. Destruction of oral biofilms formed in situ on machined titanium (ti) surfaces by cold atmospheric plasma. Biofouling. 2013;29(4):369–79.
17. Koban I, Holtfreter B, Hübner N, Matthes R, Sietmann R, Kindel E, Weltmann K, Welk A, Kramer A, Kocher T. Antimicrobial efficacy of non-thermal plasma in comparison to chlorhexidine against dental biofilms on titanium discs in vitro–proof of principle experiment. J Clin Periodontol. 2011;38(10):956–65.
18. Ranjan R, Krishnamraju P, Shankar T, Gowd S. Nonthermal plasma in dentistry: an update. J Int Soc Prev Commun Dent. 2017;7(3):71–5.
19. Yang B, Chen J, Yu Q, Li H, Lin M, Mustapha A, Hong L, Wang Y. Oral bacterial deactivation using a low-temperature atmospheric argon plasma brush. J Dent. 2011;39(1):48–56.
20. Mahasneh A, Darby M, Tolle SL, Hynes W, Laroussi M, Karakas E. Inactivation of porphyromonas gingivalis by low-temperature atmospheric pressure plasma. Plasma Med. 2011;1(3–4):191–204.
21. Fricke K, Koban I, Tresp H, Jablonowski L, Schröder K, Kramer A, Weltmann K, von Woedtke T, Kocher T. Atmospheric pressure plasma: a high-performance tool for the efficient removal of biofilms. PLoS One. 2012;7(8):e42539.
22. Addy M, Shaw W, Hansford P, Hopkins M. The effect of orthodontic appliances on the distribution of candida and plaque in adolescents. Br J Orthod. 1982;9(3):158–63.
23. Hibino K, Wong RW, Haegg U, Samaranayake LP. The effects of orthodontic appliances on candida in the human mouth. Int J Paediatr Dent. 2009;19(5):301–8.
24. Rupf S, Idlibi AN, Marrawi FA, Hannig M, Schubert A, von Mueller L, Spitzer W, Holtmann H, Lehmann A, Rueppell A. Removing biofilms from microstructured titanium ex vivo: a novel approach using atmospheric plasma technology. PLoS One. 2011;6(10):e25893.
25. von Woedtke T, Haertel B, Weltmann K, Lindequist U. Plasma pharmacy–physical plasma in pharmaceutical applications. Pharmazie. 2013;68(7):492–8.

26. Jablonowski H, Hänsch MAC, Dünnbier M, Wende K, Hammer MU, Weltmann K, Reuter S, von Woedtke T. Plasma jet's shielding gas impact on bacterial inactivation. Biointerphases. 2015;10(2):029506.
27. Koban I, Geisel MH, Holtfreter B, Jablonowski L, Hübner N, Matthes R, Masur K, Weltmann K, Kramer A, Kocher T. Synergistic effects of nonthermal plasma and disinfecting agents against dental biofilms in vitro. ISRN Dent. 2013;2013:573262. https://doi.org/10.1155/2013/573262.
28. Buonocore MG. A simple method of increasing the adhesion of acrylic filling materials to enamel surfaces. J Dent Res. 1955;34(6):849–53.
29. Fitzpatrick DA, Way DC. The effects of wear, acid etching, and bond removal on human enamel. Am J Orthod. 1977;72(6):671–81.
30. Legler L, Retief D, Bradley E, Denys F, Sadowsky P. Effects of phosphoric acid concentration and etch duration on the shear bond strength of an orthodontic bonding resin to enamel: an in vitro study. Am J Orthod Dentofac Orthop. 1989;96(6):485–92.
31. Lehmann A, Rueppell A, Schindler A, Zylla I, Seifert HJ, Nothdurft F, Hannig M, Rupf S. Modification of enamel and dentin surfaces by non-thermal atmospheric plasma. Plasma Process Polym. 2013;10(3):262–70.
32. Teixeira HS, Coelho PG, Duarte S, Janal MN, Silva N, Thompson VP. Influence of atmospheric pressure plasma treatment on mechanical proprieties of enamel and sealant bond strength. J Biomed Mater Res Part B. 2015;103B:1082–91.
33. Chen M, Zhang Y, Driver MS, Caruso AN, Yu Q, Wang Y. Surface modification of several dental substrates by non-thermal, atmospheric plasma brush. Dent Mater. 2013;29(8):871–80.
34. Metelmann PH, Quooß A, von Woedtke T, Krey K. First insights on plasma orthodontics-application of cold atmospheric pressure plasma to enhance the bond strength of orthodontic brackets. Clin Plasma Med. 2016;4(2):46–9.
35. Gu M, Yu Q, Tan J, Li H, Chen M, Wang Y, Dong X. Improving bond strength of ground and intact enamel to mild self-etch adhesive by plasma treatment. Clin Plasma Med. 2016;4(1):29–33.
36. Šantak V, Vesel A, Biščan M, Milošević S. Surface treatment of human hard dental tissues with atmospheric pressure plasma jet. Plasma Chem Plasma Process. 2017;2(37):401–13.
37. Göllner P. Skeletal anchorage in orthodontics–basics and clinical application. J Orofac Orthop. 2007;68(6):443–61.
38. Motoyoshi M. Clinical indices for orthodontic mini-implants. J Oral Sci. 2011;53(4):407–12.
39. Park H, Jeong S, Kwon O. Factors affecting the clinical success of screw implants used as orthodontic anchorage. Am J Orthod Dentofac Orthop. 2006;130(1):18–25.
40. Hoste S, Vercruyssen M, Quirynen M, Willems G. Risk factors and indications of orthodontic temporary anchorage devices: a literature review. Aust Orthod J. 2008;24(2):140–8.
41. Shi Q, Song K, Zhou X, Xiong Z, Du T, Lu X, Cao Y. Effects of non-equilibrium plasma in the treatment of ligature-induced peri-implantitis. J Clin Periodontol. 2015;42(5):478–87.
42. Duske K, Jablonowski L, Koban I, Matthes R, Holtfreter B, Sckell A, Nebe JB, von Woedtke T, Weltmann KD, Kocher T. Cold atmospheric plasma in combination with mechanical treatment improves osteoblast growth on biofilm covered titanium discs. Biomaterials. 2015;52:327–34.
43. Metelmann H, Nedrelow DS, Seebauer C, Schuster M, von Woedtke T, Weltmann K, Kindler S, Metelmann PH, Finkelstein SE, Von Hoff DD. Head and neck cancer treatment and physical plasma. Clin Plasma Med. 2015;3(1):17–23.
44. Lee J, Choi E, Kim K, Kim K. Effect of non-thermal air atmospheric pressure plasma jet treatment on gingival wound healing. J Phys D. 2016;49(7):075402.
45. Ozcelik O, Haytac MC, Akkaya M. Iatrogenic trauma to oral tissues. J Periodontol. 2005; 76(10):1793–7.

# Perspectives in Dental Caries

# 19

Stefan Rupf

## 19.1 Dental Caries

Caries is an opportunistic infection disease that leads to the destruction of the hard substances and tissues of the teeth. Caries is also nowadays the most prevalent chronic disease one of the most important causes of acute pain and of tooth loss and [1]. As a result, caries is of great importance both epidemiologically and economically [2], although the prevalence as well as the severity of caries in temporary and permanent dentition are lower in many countries around the world [3, 4]. In addition, caries is the cause of infections in the jawbone and the facial area. The most important path of infection is the route through the toothpulp, which is connected to the bone via blood vessels and nerves [5].

Caries is characterized as a demineralization process [6] which is caused by microbial biofilms on the tooth surface [7, 8]. The most important source of acid formation in the biofilm is the metabolism of low molecular weight carbohydrates. If the biofilm has contact with the root cement or the dentin, the proteolytic activity of the microorganisms is important besides the demineralizing. The tooth surfaces are so-called "non-shedding surfaces" [9, 10]. As a result, the disease process is irreversible apart from initial stages [11]. Caries is not caused by only one bacterial species. In addition to the frequently mentioned mutans streptococci, many other acid-tolerant and acid-producing streptococci, lactobacilli and numerous other bacteria and fungi are also known to be involved in the caries process [12]. In all stages of the disease the caries process is influenced, however, by physiological remineralization. It can proceed very fast, or stagnate over a long time [13]. The saliva as a

S. Rupf
Clinic of Operative Dentistry, Periodontology and Preventive Dentistry,
Saarland University Hospital, Homburg, Germany
e-mail: stefan.rupf@uks.eu



H.-R. Metelmann et al. (eds.), *Comprehensive Clinical Plasma Medicine*,
https://doi.org/10.1007/978-3-319-67627-2_19

protein-buffered, supersaturated mineral solution and the pellicle layer as a mediator between solid and liquid phase play are important in the demin-remin-processes [14, 15].

## 19.2 Caries Prevention and Caries Therapy

Caries preventive measures must be suitable to prevent the formation of lesions in the tooth hard substances or to stop a progression of initial carious defects. The most important intervention points are the regular reduction of biofilms by oral hygiene, the increase of the resistance of the tooth surfaces by fluorides, the closure of predilection sites by sealing and a reduction in the availability of low molecular weight carbohydrates for the biofilm by nutritional counselling [16–18].

If caries lesions occur, the main goal is their arrest. Early clinical caries infections are treated by fluoridation and caries infiltration [19]. If open lesions occur in the dentin, filling therapy is necessary in most cases. By filling carious defects, the cariogenic biofilms are removed in the defect and the function of the tooth is restored. A large proportion of the fillings and sealants as well as nearly all infiltration treatments are based on materials containing methacrylates. These materials are adhesively attached to the enamel and dentin by microretention [20, 21].

## 19.3 Enamel and Dentin

Enamel and dentin are different in their composition. Enamel has a prismatic structure and consists of 96% of hydroxyapatite, water and a small amount of organic substances. The enamel surface displays amphiphilic characteristic. Dentin contains 20% of water and 30% of organic matter. From the pulp to the enamel-dentin border, the dentin is traversed by fluid-filled tubules. Caused by intrapulpal pressure, a steady flow of fluid through the dentin is seen in the peripheral direction [22]. The mineralized dentin surrounding the tubules is stabilized by a collagen network. Dentin surfaces are hydrophilic [23]. The hydroxyapatites of the enamel and dentin are dissolved by the abrasion and by acid attack at a pH of less than 5.5. Above all fluorides can reduce the solubility of the tooth hard substances [9, 10, 24].

Differences of composition, structure and surface properties of tooth substances cause high demands on the coupling of restorative materials to tooth surfaces. The most effective method to ensure adhesion to enamel is the etching technique [25]. The use of phosphoric acid dissolves crystallites in the center and the base of the enamel prisms to different extents, resulting in a micro-structured surface. The attachment of hydrophobic filling materials to the hydrophilic dentin surface makes the application of adhesive systems necessary. The superficial dentin layer is etched by phosphoric or an organic acid and the collagen network is exposed as well as the dentinal tubules are opened. By means of hydrophilic components of the adhesive system, the crosslinking of the methacrylates with the collagen network is achieved and a surface suitable for the attachment of hydrophobic composite materials is created. Typically, adhesive systems are classified as "etch-and-rinse" or "self-etch" adhesives. Depending on the adhesive system used, either phosphoric acid is used which is removed by rinsing after a few seconds or organic acids which remain on the tooth surface and are neutralized by reaction with the so called "smear layer", a mixture of hydroxyapatite and organic tooth or microbial material. While "etch-and-rinse" systems provide predominantly safe adhesion to, the "self-etch" adhesives exhibit lower enamel adhesion, but are advantageous for the dentin adhesion of composite materials [26].

## 19.4 Perspectives for the Use of Cold Atmospheric Plasmas for Caries Prevention and Caries Therapy

The use of cold atmospheric plasmas for caries therapy was proposed at the beginning of the millennium [27, 28]. In recent years, numerous *in vitro* studies and some animal experiments have been carried out. *In vivo* studies are not available up to now [29]. Conclusions for the principal applicability of cold atmospheric plasmas for caries prevention and therapy can, however, be drawn from the available results of experimental studies.

## 19.5 Suface Disinfection and Biofilm Reduction

Microbial biofilms are the cause of the caries process [8]. The frequent oral hygiene is essential for biofilm control. Here, biofilms are removed from the tooth surfaces, initiation or progression of the disease process is prevented. The use of cold atmospheric plasmas to support oral hygiene has not been discussed yet. However, the effect of cold plasmas against biofilms of cariogenic bacteria, *Candida* fungi and oral biofilms has already been successfully investigated [30–41] (Fig. 19.1).

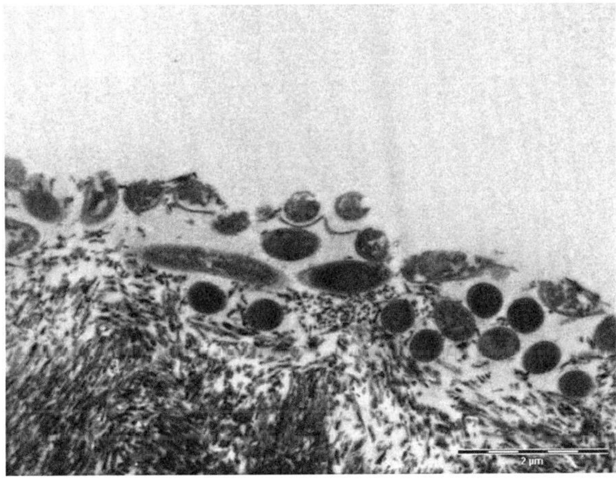


**Fig. 19.1** Transmission electron microscopic image of a biofilm consisting of oral bacteria on enamel. After plasma treatment (1 s/mm$^2$, T: 35 °C) the microorganisms are disintegrated or bleached

An established method of caries prevention is fissure sealing [17]. By this technique the caries susceptible occlusal fissure is made inaccessible to biofilms. Typically, acid etching techniques and low-viscosity methacrylates are used. There are few data suggesting an improvement in enamel-sealant interaction. On the one hand, the wettability of the enamel is increased after plasma application [42, 43], on the other hand, potential-free plasmas do not yet appear optimal, because the fissure ground is not reached by the plasma. Investigations are, however, still pending.

## 19.6 Disinfection of Dentin

The dentin is destroyed during the caries process by microbial acids and enzymatic proteolysis. Current therapeutic strategies promote the incomplete caries removal in order to reduce the trauma of the pulp through the preparation and at the same time to preserve a maximum of tooth substance. However, the leaving of caries softened infected dentin requires disinfecting measures accompanying filling therapy. There are conclusions from *in vitro* studies and an *ex vivo* study that it is possible to clean dentin tubules infiltrated by bacteria using cold atmospheric plasma [36, 44, 45] (Fig. 19.2).

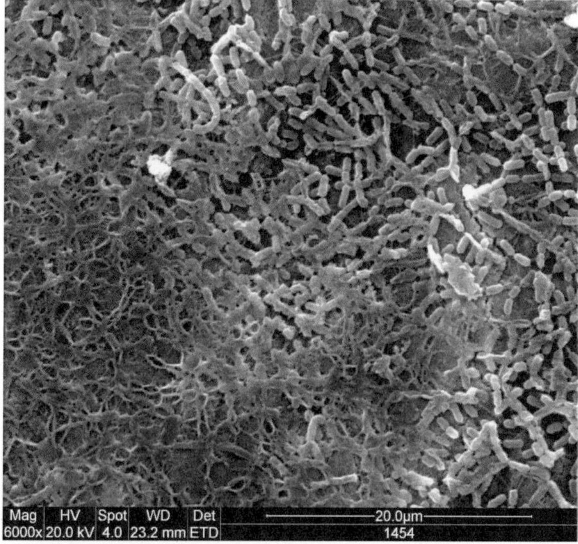


**Fig. 19.2** Scanning electron microscopic micrograph of a bacterial biofilm after plasma treatment (1 s/mm$^2$, T: 35 °C). The bacteria on the left side are disintegrated. On the right, untreated, side the bacteria appear intact

## 19.7 Improvement of Tooth-Composite Interaction Zone (Fig. 19.3)

In various *in vitro* studies it was demonstrated that the tooth-composite interaction zone in the dentin is influenced by the treatment with cold atmospheric plasma. The adhesion force of the composite to the dentin was found to be increased [46, 47]. At the same time, the tooth-composite interaction zone proved to be thicker after the application of cold atmospheric plasma [48, 49]. It was also demonstrated, that cold atmospheric is a suitable method to increase the tensile-shear bond strength between endodontic post and composite [50]. *In vivo* studies have not been carried out so far.

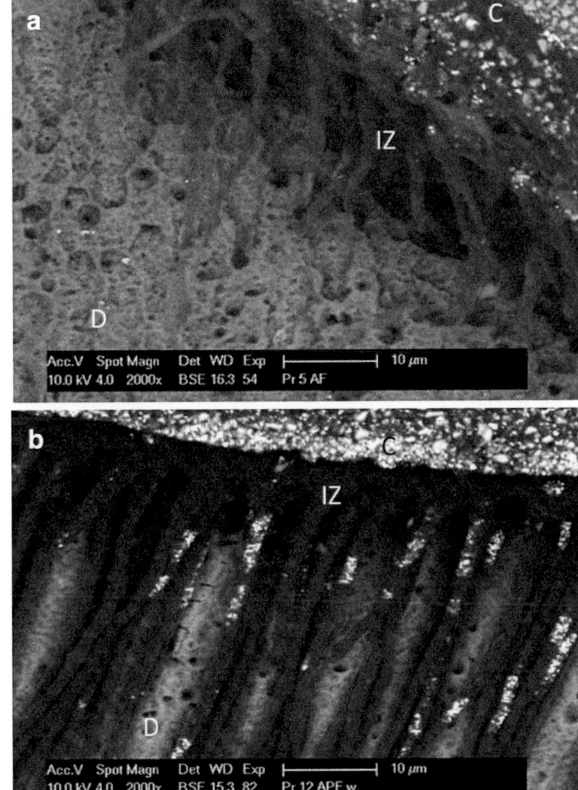


**Fig. 19.3** Dentin (D)-composite (C) interaction pattern. (**a**) Interaction zone (IZ) after artificial thermo-mechanical aging, (**b**) Dentin (D)-composite (C) interaction zone (IZ) after additional plasma treatment. The tooth-composite interaction zone appears to be more pronounced and more intensively interlaced

## 19.8 Reaction of the Pulp

Only sparse data are available in this field. In a histological study in rat molars, no influence of the plasma treatment could be determined in addition to preparation and adhesive filling therapy [51].

Problems for the application of cold atmospheric plasma for caries prevention and caries therapy

- Slim fissures and narrow cavities are challenging for potential-free atmospheric plasmas. In particular, the most interesting bottom of fissures or cavities is difficult to treat.
- The permanent presence of high humidity in the oral cavity and the salivary flow are influencing the treatment effectivity. In dental practice saliva, aerosols and dusts are permanently removed from the operation field by suction. In dental practice saliva, aerosols and dusts are permanently removed from the operation field by suction. Clinical data or appropriate simulations are missing up to date.
- The teeth have surface areas that are difficult to reach using cold atmospheric plasma jets, e.g. interdental spaces or the gingival crevice. Instrumental modifications are required here.

**Conclusion**

Fundamental questions are still the subject of intensive research in the field of caries prevention and therapy supported by cold atmospheric plasma. From today's perspective, cold atmospheric plasma provides promising potential as an adjunctive measure for the disinfection of the carious dentin and for the improvement of the tooth-composite filling interaction zone.

## References

1. GBD 2015 Disease and Injury Incidence and Prevalence Collaborators. Global, regional, and national incidence, prevalence, and years lived with disability for 310 diseases and injuries, 1990–2015: a systematic analysis for the Global Burden of Disease Study 2015. Lancet. 2016;388(10053):1545–602.
2. Listl S, Galloway J, Mossey PA, Marcenes W. Global economic impact of dental diseases. J Dent Res. 2015;94(10):1355–61.
3. Micheelis W, Schiffner U. The Fifth German Oral Health Study (Fünfte Deutsche Mundgesundheitsstudie, DMS V). Köln: Deutscher Zahnärzteverlag DÄV; 2016.
4. Steiner M, Menghini G, Marthaler TM, Imfeld T. Changes in dental caries in Zurich schoolchildren over a period of 45 years. Schweiz Monatsschr Zahnmed. 2010;120:1084–104.
5. Robertson DP, Keys W, Rautemaa-Richardson R, Burns R, Smith AJ. Management of severe acute dental infections. BMJ. 2015;350:h1300. https://doi.org/10.1136/bmj.h1300.
6. Nyvad B, Crielaard W, Mira A, Takahashi N, Beighton D. Dental caries from a molecular microbiological perspective. Caries Res. 2013;47:89–102.
7. Hannig C, Hannig M. The oral cavity-a key system to understand substratum-dependent bioadhesion on solid surfaces in man. Clin Oral Investig. 2009;13:123–39.
8. Marsh PD. Dental plaque as a microbial biofilm. Caries Res. 2004;38:204–11.

9. Hannig C, Hannig M. Natural enamel wear—a physiological source of hydroxylapatite nanoparticles for biofilm management and tooth repair? Med Hypotheses. 2010a;74:670–2.
10. Hannig M, Hannig C. Nanomaterials in preventive dentistry. Nat Nanotechnol. 2010b;5:565–9.
11. Pretty IA, Ellwood RP. The caries continuum: opportunities to detect, treat and monitor the re-mineralization of early caries lesions. J Dent. 2013;41(Suppl 2):S12–21.
12. Beighton D. The complex oral microflora of high-risk individuals and groups and its role in the caries process. Community Dent Oral Epidemiol. 2005;33:248–55.
13. Takahashi N, Nyvad B. The role of bacteria in the caries process: ecological perspectives. J Dent Res. 2011;90:294–303.
14. Hannig C, Berndt D, Hoth-Hannig W, Hannig M. The effect of acidic beverages on the ultrastructure of the acquired pellicle—an in situ study. Arch Oral Biol. 2009;54:518–26.
15. Siqueira WL, Custodio W, McDonald EE. New insights into the composition and functions of the acquired enamel pellicle. J Dent Res. 2012;91:1110–8.
16. Kumar S, Tadakamadla J, Johnson NW. Effect of Toothbrushing Frequency on Incidence and Increment of Dental Caries: A Systematic Review and Meta-Analysis. J Dent Res. 2016;95:1230-1236.
17. Anneli Ahovuo-Saloranta, Helena Forss, Tanya Walsh, Anne Nordblad, Marjukka Mäkelä, Helen V Worthington, Pit and fissure sealants for preventing dental decay in permanent teeth. Cochrane Database of Systematic Reviews. 2017;7:CD001830.
18. Pitts NB, Zero DT, Marsh PD, Ekstrand K, Weintraub JA, Ramos-Gomez F, Tagami J, Twetman S, Tsakos G, Ismail A. Dental caries. Nat Rev Dis Primers. 2017;3:17030.
19. Meyer-Lueckel H, Paris S. When and How to Intervene in the Caries Process. Oper Dent. 2016;41:S35-S47.
20. Heintze SD, Rousson V, Hickel R. Clinical effectiveness of direct anterior restorations—a meta-analysis. Dent Mater. 2015;31:481–95.
21. Mante FK, Ozer F, Walter R, Atlas AM, Saleh N, Dietschi D, Blatz MB. The current state of adhesive dentistry: a guide for clinical practice. Compend Contin Educ Dent. 2013;(34 Spec 9): 2–8.
22. Pioch T, Staehle HJ, Schneider H, Duschner H, Dörfer CE. Effect of intrapulpal pressure simulation in vitro on shear bond strengths and hybrid layer formation. Am J Dent. 2001;4:319–23.
23. Mount GJ, Hume WR. Preservation and restoration of tooth structure. Mosby; 1998.
24. Robinson C. Fluoride and the caries lesion: interactions and mechanism of action. Eur Arch Paediatr Dent. 2009;10:136–40.
25. Buonocore MG. A simple method of increasing the adhesion of acrylic filling materials to enamel surfaces. J Dent Res. 1955;34:849–53.
26. Cardoso MV, de Almeida Neves A, Mine A, Coutinho E, Van Landuyt K, De Munck J, Van Meerbeek B. Current aspects on bonding effectiveness and stability in adhesive dentistry. Aust Dent J. 2011;56(Suppl 1):31–44.
27. Sladek REJ, Stoffels E, Walraven R, Tielbeek PJA, Koolhoven RA. Plasma treatment of dental cavities: a feasibility study. IEEE Trans Plasma Sci. 2004;32:1540–3.
28. Stoffels E, Flikweert AJ, Stoffels WW, Kroesen GMW. Plasma needle: a non-destructive atmospheric plasma source for fine surface treatment of (bio)materials. Plasma Sources Sci Technol. 2002;11:383–8.
29. Cha S, Park YS. Plasma in dentistry. Clin Plasma Med. 2014;2:4–10.
30. Fricke K, Koban I, Tresp H, Jablonowski L, Schroder K, Kramer A, et al. Atmospheric pressure plasma: a high-performance tool for the efficient removal of biofilms. PLoS One. 2012;7:e42539.
31. Goree J, Liu B, Drake D, Stoffels E. Killing of S. mutans bacteria using a plasma needle at atmospheric pressure. IEEE Trans Plasma Sci. 2006;34:1317–21.
32. Gorynia S, Koban I, Matthes R, Welk A, Gorynia S, Hübner NO, Kocher T, Kramer A. In vitro efficacy of cold atmospheric pressure plasma on S. sanguinis biofilms in comparison of two test models. GMS Hyg Infect Control. 2013;8(1):Doc01.

33. Idlibi AN, Al-Marrawi F, Hannig M, Lehmann A, Rueppell A, Schindler A, Jentsch H, Rupf S. Destruction of oral biofilms formed in situ on machined titanium (Ti) surfaces by cold atmospheric plasma. Biofouling. 2013;29:369–79.
34. Koban I, Matthes R, Hubner NO, Welk A, Meisel P, et al. Treatment of Candida albicans biofilms with low-temperature plasma induced by dielectric barrier discharge and atmospheric pressure plasma jet. New J Phys. 2010;12:073039.
35. Koban I, Holtfreter B, Hübner NO, Matthes R, Sietmann R, Kindel E, Weltmann KD, Welk A, Kramer A, Kocher T. Antimicrobial efficacy of non-thermal plasma in comparison to chlorhexidine against dental biofilms on titanium discs in vitro - proof of principle experiment. J Clin Periodontol. 2011;38:956–65.
36. Rupf S, Lehmann A, Hannig M, Schäfer B, Schubert A, Feldmann U, Schindler A. Killing of adherent oral microbes by a non-thermal atmospheric plasma jet. J Med Microbiol. 2010;59:206–12.
37. Rupf S, Idlibi AN, Marrawi FA, Hannig M, Schubert A, et al. Removing biofilms from microstructured titanium ex vivo: a novel approach using atmospheric plasma technology. PLoSOne. 2011;6:e25893.
38. Sladek REJ, Filoche SK, Sissons CH, Stoffels E. Treatment of Streptococcus mutans biofilms with a nonthermal atmospheric plasma. Lett Appl Microbiol. 2007;45:318–23.
39. Yamazaki H, Ohshima T, Tsubota Y, Yamaguchi H, Jayawardena JA, et al. Microbicidal activities of low frequency atmospheric pressure plasma jets on oral pathogens. Dent Mater J. 2011;30:384–91.
40. Yang B, Chen J, Yu Q, Li H, Lin M, et al. Oral bacterial deactivation using a low-temperature atmospheric argon plasma brush. J Dent. 2011;9:48–56.
41. Zhang X, Huang J, Liu X, Peng L, Guo L, Lv G, Chen W, Feng K, Yang S. Treatment of Streptococcus mutans bacteria by a plasma needle. J Appl Phys. 2009;105:063302.
42. Chen M, Zhang Y, Sky Driver M, Caruso AN, Yu Q, Wang Y. Surface modification of several dental substrates by non-thermal, atmospheric plasma brush. Dent Mater. 2013;29:871–80.
43. Lehmann A, Rueppell A, Schindler A, Zylla I-M, Seifert HJ, Nothdurft F, Hannig M, Rupf S. Modification of enamel and dentin surfaces by non-thermal atmospheric plasma. Plasma Processes Polym. 2013;10:262–70.
44. Pierdzioch P, Hartwig S, Herbst SR, Raguse JD, Dommisch H, Abu-Sirhan S, Wirtz HC, Hertel M, Paris S, Preissner S. Cold plasma: a novel approach to treat infected dentin-a combined ex vivo and in vitro study. Clin Oral Investig. 2016;20(9):2429–35.
45. Wang R, Zhou H, Sun P, Wu H, Pan J, Zhu W. The effect of an atmospheric pressure, DC non-thermal plasma microjet on tooth root canal, dentinal tubules infection and re-infection prevention. J Plasma Med. 2012;1:143–55.
46. Dong X, Ritts AC, Staller C, Yu Q, Chen M, Wang Y. Evaluation of plasma treatment effects on improving adhesive-dentin bonding by using the same tooth controls and varying cross-sectional surface areas. Eur J Oral Sci. 2013;121:355–62.
47. Ritts AC, Li H, Yu Q, Xu C, Yao X, et al. Dentin surface treatment using a non-thermal argon plasma brush for interfacial bonding improvement in composite restoration. Eur J Oral Sci. 2010;118:510–6.
48. Dong X, Chen M, Wang Y, Yu Q. A mechanistic study of plasma treatment effects on demineralized dentin surfaces for improved adhesive/dentin interface bonding. Clin Plasma Med. 2014;2:11–6.
49. Dong X, Li H, Chen M, Wang Y, Yu Q. Plasma treatment of dentin surfaces for improving self-etching adhesive/dentin interface bonding. Clin Plasma Med. 2015;3:10–6.
50. Yavirach P, Chaijareenont P, Boonyawan D, Pattamapun K, Tunma S, et al. Effects of plasma treatment on the shear bond strength between fiber-reinforced composite posts and resin composite for core build-up. Dent Mater J. 2009;6:686–92.
51. Rupf S, Georg M, Hannig M, Laschke M, Lehmann A, Rueppell A, Schindler A. Effect of cold atmospheric plasma treatment on dental pulp in rat molars. Orleans: Tagungsbeitrag ICPM4; 2012.

# 20 Perspectives in General Surgery

Lars Ivo Partecke, Sander Bekeschus, and Kim Rouven Liedtke

## 20.1 Introduction

The modern surgery of the twenty-first century has developed steadily, especially in tumour surgery. The use of multimodal therapy concepts, in particular, led to an ever-increasing radicalisation of the surgical resection of the tumours. Nevertheless, there are limitations in the surgical radicality of resection. This is true, for example, in the surgery of pancreatic carcinoma and the surgical treatment of peritoneal carcinomatosis. Remaining tumour cells are the cause of local tumour recurrence and the poor prognosis. Plasma medicine offers great opportunities in the future to further increase the radicality in the area of these residual micro-tumour cell clusters. This is noteworthy because the application of cold atmospheric plasma appears to produce very low local side effects and hardly any systemic side effects according to the latest results. Foreign materials (e.g., osteosynthesis material, joint replacement and hernia meshes) are increasingly implanted in all surgical disciplines. Here, in the future, modern plasma medicine can offer a therapeutic option for the prevention and treatment of bacterial infections and biofilms on the implants while simultaneously improving wound healing. From a surgical perspective, the application of thermal plasmas must be distinguished from the use of cold plasmas. While hot plasma has been used safely in the clinic for more than 40 years as argon plasma coagulation (APC), especially in endoscopy for cutting and coagulation, the investigation of the application of cold, and thus tissue-compatible, plasma is still largely at the stage of basic research. On the other hand, the plasma source type also plays an important role. While DBD plasmas offer advantages in extracorporeal and

L. I. Partecke (✉) • K. R. Liedtke
Department of Surgery, University of Greifswald, Greifswald, Germany
e-mail: partecke@uni-greifswald.de

S. Bekeschus
Leibniz Institute for Plasma Science and Technology|INP, ZIK Plasmatis, Greifswald, Germany



H.-R. Metelmann et al. (eds.), *Comprehensive Clinical Plasma Medicine*,
https://doi.org/10.1007/978-3-319-67627-2_20

dermatological applications due to the larger treatment area, a high degree of precision is required intraoperatively. Therefore, it seems sensible to resort to jet plasmas for the surgical application in the body.

The following overview provides a look at the practical application possibilities of cold atmospheric plasma in modern surgery.

### 20.1.1 Three possible applications of cold atmospheric plasma in modern surgery:

**First:** Direct primary tissue treatment by the surgeon as a supplement to the scalpel or electrometer or for direct haemostasis on tissue. Here, non-thermal plasma sources are used on the tissue surface in the "non-contact process". This results in significantly less necrosis formation and more possibilities for targeted local application.

**Second:** The supplemental treatment of tissue with non-thermal plasma after completing the actual surgical tumour resection to increase local radicality without negatively affecting the healthy tissue. By producing apoptosis and avoiding necrosis, the adverse local tissue inflammation is considerably reduced, and the surrounding healthy tissue is spared.

**Third:** Ex vivo or in vivo treatment of surgical implants by cold plasma for the treatment of biofilms and bacterial infections as well as for surface modification is an important area of application in plasma medicine.

## 20.2 Surgical Applications of Non-Thermal Plasmas

There are several interesting approaches that make a surgical application of non-thermal plasma conceivable. Due to the different plasma sources and an as yet non-standardised nomenclature, many statements can initially only be made for individual devices. Here, research is needed in studies and analyses to characterise the plasmas and make them comparable to each other. An excerpt of current research on possible applications of non-thermal plasma in surgery is given below.

### 20.2.1 Possible Applications in Tumour Surgery

The use of non-thermal plasmas in multimodal tumour surgery as a fourth treatment option alongside chemotherapy and irradiation offers great opportunities. Non-thermal, tissue-compatible plasma takes effect via the reactive oxygen and nitrogen species (ROS and RNA) formed, UV radiation and electric fields. Here, it preferentially induces apoptosis in tumour cells and acts very precisely at the site of its application when using jet plasmas. Interestingly, the plasma effect can be achieved both by direct application and by the indirect application via plasma-treated fluids.

Fundamental research has already laid a good foundation for the development of targeted, surgically controlled tumour treatment with non-thermal plasma in humans:

1. The CE-certified plasma jet kINPen Med showed a penetration depth of approx. 60 μm in tumour tissue depending on the application duration [1]. At the same time, the intra-abdominal, serosa-coated organs (especially the intestine) exhibited high compatibility *in vivo* experiments in murines compared to directly-applied plasma [2].
2. Healthy tissue tolerates the non-thermal plasma considerably better than malignant degenerative tissue. In the case of targeted dosage of the non-thermal plasma with a correspondingly lowered application time, cell death is induced by apoptosis in tumour cells, and necrosis formation with a corresponding inflammation reaction can be avoided.
3. In a combined application of chemotherapy and plasma, synergistic effects could be demonstrated, which on the one hand, significantly reduce the systemic side effects of the chemotherapeutic agent via a dose adjustment, and on the other hand, could additionally protect the healthy tissue locally [3].

In the supplementary surgical treatment of gastrointestinal carcinomas, two very promising therapeutic approaches are obtained.

1. Local treatment of resection limits to increase (surgical) radicality, e.g., during the resection of pancreatic carcinomas in the retroperitoneal space and around the large visceral vessels (e.g., *arteria mesenterica superior* and *arteria hepatica*) or after liver resections.
2. Application of indirect plasma in fluids for flushing the abdomen after surgical resection of an extensive peritoneal carcinomatosis in order to also increase the radicality of microscopic tumour cell residues and scattered tumour cells with high systemic and local compatibility.

### 20.2.2 Possible Applications for Blood Clotting

Surgical measures are associated with tissue trauma and bleeding. APC has been used for many years in surgery for haemostasis [4]. Although the process is fast, simple, and low in side effects, it is associated with local thermal tissue damage. Because of its wound healing-promoting quality, the use of non-thermal plasmas in vessel and organ injury presents a possible field of application. *Fridman et al.* showed that plasma application leads to painless blood coagulation without tissue damage. A treatment period of 15 s stopped the bleeding of a wound made to the *vena saphena magna* in the murine animal experiment [5]. A 30 s lasting application resulted in a stable haemostasis on the human spleen [6]. In both cases, an FE-DBD plasma was used. As a cause, *Fridman et al.* postulated that body's own blood coagulation was possibly supported by a physical fibrinogen activation. However, the exact mechanism of action is still unclear. In addition, the direct activation of platelets seems to support coagulation. While APC acts immediately and is very effective in the coagulation cascade and is independent of any anticoagulants or gene defects, non-thermal plasma is not yet conceivable as an intraoperative alternative because of the comparatively long latency until the blood coagulation occurs and the still unclear mode of action. The painless and simple application without induction of necrosis justifies further research initiatives in this field.

**Key point 1**

NTP leads to tissue-protective, scar-free blood coagulation by supporting the body's own coagulation.

## 20.2.3 Implants in Surgery

The implantation of foreign material is always a risk for the patient. Possible complications include, in particular, immunological defence reactions, accelerated material wear as well as bacterial colonisation. In particular, the bacterial colonisation of synthetic material is a major problem, since the systemic antibiotic therapy is usually only inadequately effective and a haematogenic spread of the pathogens to colonise other organs can lead to sepsis formation with a fatal outcome. This usually necessitates the disassembly of the implant. Revision interventions are accompanied by significantly higher tissue trauma. In addition to the individual burden, the economic impact is a considerable burden on the social systems [7, 8].

For these reasons, an improvement in biocompatibility is a desirable goal of implantology. Biocompatibility describes a state in which the implant is accepted by the body without an immune reaction and is largely integrated into the tissue. This can positively influence the healing process. In order to ensure high biocompatibility, the ideal implant has to satisfy the following two requirements in addition to corresponding biomechanical stability and function: First, it must be integrated rapidly into the surrounding physiological tissue without any major tissue reaction, and second, the surface texture of the material should prevent colonisation by pathogenic germs. The application of non-thermal plasmas in numerous studies shows a significant antimicrobial effect on biofilms [9] and ensures a complex modification of the implant surface [10, 11]. In addition, non-thermal plasma treatment enables a prior coating of the implants with heatable proteins or medication [12]. This way, the biocompatibility can also be significantly improved.

### 20.2.3.1 Material Modification in Vascular Surgery

In vascular surgery, stents and bypasses are used for arterial recanalisation in vascular occlusions. As a bypass, an endogenous vein or a vascular prosthesis made of synthetic material can be selected. A feared complication is the infection of the bypass, as septic seam breakage can result in bleeding which is difficult to control. *Martins et al.* showed that the hydrophilicity could be significantly improved by plasma treatment of polycaprolactone while maintaining the mechanical properties [13]. Based on this, *de Valence et al.* showed an increased affinity of muscle cells to the implant *in vitro*, which is expected to allow a faster engraftment of the bypass *in vivo*. Furthermore, it was shown in the animal model that an existing plasma treatment significantly improves subsequent vascularisation *in vivo* [14]. *Chong et al.* demonstrated a faster and more uniform endothelialisation of synthetic bypasses after plasma treatment *in vitro* [15]. Corresponding results were confirmed by *Loya et al.* for metal stents used in cardiology [16]. The advantage of rapid, uniform endothelialisation of vascular implants is the reduction of thrombosis risk with the correspondingly shorter necessity of medicinal anticoagulation. Plasma vacuum chambers were used in all three studies, and although the last two studies were only carried out in static *in vitro* systems, the results are extremely promising and deserve special attention in the future.

**Key point 2**
According to initial studies, NTP treatment accelerates the incorporation of synthetic bypass materials and reduces the risk of postoperative complications such as infections and thromboses.

#### 20.2.3.2 Material Modification in Bone Surgery

In traumatology during the operative treatment of a fracture, as well as in orthopaedics during the implantation of a replacement joint prosthesis, the use of materials made of titanium plays a major role. *Seon et al.* showed a higher hydrophilicity on titanium implants *in vitro* after non-thermal plasma treatment, which resulted, among other things, in improved cell adhesion and cell proliferation [17]. Hauser *et al.* confirm the increased hydrophilicity in the modification in their experiments in a low-temperature high-vacuum plasma reactor and could also detect a significantly more homogeneous coating of collagen on treated titanium implants [18]. Hydroxyapatite coated, plasma-treated titanium implants, as described by Tan et al. *in vitro*, promote bone mineralisation for up to 3 weeks [19]. *Ferraz et al.*, however, could not demonstrate a superiority of non-thermal plasma treated titanium implants in bone mineralisation *in vivo* [20]. However, the early phase of engraftment remained unobserved so that the situation in this clinically particularly critical phase requires further research. *Testrich et al.* investigated the durability of the implant modification and found that even after 360 days, titanium implants coated with ethylenediamine polymerised via non-thermal plasmas had a 55% higher affinity for cells [21], which could significantly improve the engraftment of the implants. In order to prevent loosening of implants (e.g., hip joint endoprostheses), bone cement is often used for anchoring in the bone. In the investigation of the influence of plasma-mediated surface modification, *Seker et al.* showed that no change in the interaction of implant surfaces and bone cement could be demonstrated by a previous plasma treatment [22] so that no negative effects in clinical use are to be expected in this regard.

**Key point 3**
NTP treatment of titanium implants leads to stable, long-lasting modifications of the surface, which should result in improved engraftment by increasing the hydrophilicity and collagen affinity.

### 20.2.4 Further Possible Applications in Traumatology/Orthopaedics

In contrast to joint replacement, the osteosynthesis material should not frequently be removed after complete fracture healing. A too close interaction between bone tissue and metal is a hindrance and causes damage upon material removal. In addition, screws can break, so that the channel must be drilled to recover it. In these screw channels, non-thermal plasma could produce positive, bone stabilising effects via its proliferation-inducing effect. Thus, *Steinbeck et al.* showed that the direct plasma-cell interaction *in vitro* results in an increased rate of division as well as an accelerated differentiation of osteoblasts and chondroblasts [23]. The proliferation and differentiation of the chondroblasts here is of particular interest. Excessive sports, poor posture and being overweight increase wear-related arthrosis significantly in old age. The development of an arthrosis is also facilitated by fractures with joint involvement since defects of the cartilage surface can only be treated unsatisfactorily with the current methods which can necessitate a joint replacement in the long term. At this point, there is an enormous need for research. The use of non-thermal plasma for tissue healing and differentiation could play a key role here, especially since an arthroscopically supported plasma application could be implemented in modern, minimally invasive surgery. In addition to trauma, destructive bone diseases such as osteoporosis or tumour metastases can also be responsible for fractures. Although tumour treatment is discussed elsewhere, the possibility is briefly mentioned here in the context of the surgical stabilisation of metastatically fractured vertebral bodies by the intraoperative use of non-thermal plasma to increase the radicality and at the same time promoting bone healing.

A traumatological emergency is presented by the open fracture. Through contact with pathogens of the outer world, the fracture is highly susceptible to infections. The mostly extensive soft tissue damage requires a large-area wound debridement and, in particularly severe cases, amputation is the only option. The reduction of the tissue surface to be debrided by treatment with non-thermal plasma promotes wound healing. In addition, the antibacterial effect of non-thermal plasma is useful for reducing the bacterial load [5]. Thus, it is conceivable in the future that an early plasma treatment, possibly already carried out at the scene of the accident, could be used to reduce the pathogen load and activate the endogenous tissue. These effects also qualify non-thermal plasma for the acute treatment of burns. *Lee et al.* showed an accelerated healing of burn wounds after plasma application by the promotion of an anti-inflammatory immune status in second-degree burns [24].

**Key point 4**

The antibacterial, wound healing-promoting effect and its easy, painless application make NTP a promising tool in acute and field surgery.

## 20.3 Outlook

Plasma medicine represents a growing, interdisciplinary field of medicine, in which physicochemical properties are to be exploited in a biomedical context. Surgery as a historically innovative special discipline [25] offers numerous application possibilities for plasma medicine and can lead to wider acceptance in the future. In order to achieve this, engineers, scientists and doctors must be in active dialogue and work in an application-oriented fashion. In addition to the development of appropriate control elements, the tasks of plasma medical research for the development of practical applications of non-thermal plasma in future clinical-operational routine include, in particular, the creation of risk profiles for the whole organism.

Tasks for plasma medical research:

1. Development of more convenient, sterilisable control elements with sufficiently wide jet plasma radiation of 5–10 mm for the direct plasma application.
2. Development and characterisation of ideal carrier fluids for indirect plasma application.
3. Extension of the design of endoscopic plasma applicators.
4. Creation of application-oriented risk profiles in animal experiments and long-term application studies.

## References

1. Partecke LI, Evert K, Haugk J, Doering F, Normann L, Diedrich S, Weiss FU, Evert M, Huebner NO, Guenther C, et al. Tissue tolerable plasma (TTP) induces apoptosis in pancreatic cancer cells in vitro and in vivo. BMC Cancer. 2012;12:473.
2. Doppstadt C, van der Linde J, Diedrich S, Evert K, Menges P, Matthes R, Partecke I, Weltmann K, Heidecke C. Untersuchung zur intraperitonealen Anwendung von Tissue Tolerable Plasma (TTP) auf den Darm der Maus. Z Gastroenterol. 2013;51(08):K347.
3. Masur K, von Behr M, Bekeschus S, Weltmann KD, Hackbarth C, Heidecke CD, von Bernstorff W, von Woedtke T, Partecke LI. Synergistic inhibition of tumor cell proliferation by cold plasma and gemcitabine. Plasma Process Polym. 2015;12(12):1377–82.
4. Raiser J, Zenker M. Argon plasma coagulation for open surgical and endoscopic applications: state of the art. J Phys D Appl Phys. 2006;39(16):3520–3.
5. Fridman G, Friedman G, Gutsol A, Shekhter AB, Vasilets VN, Fridman A. Applied plasma medicine. Plasma Process Polym. 2008;5(6):503–33.
6. Fridman G, Peddinghaus M, Balasubramanian M, Ayan H, Fridman A, Gutsol A, Brooks A. Blood coagulation and living tissue sterilization by floating-electrode dielectric barrier discharge in air. Plasma Chem Plasma Process. 2006;26(4):425–42.
7. Schierholz JM, Beuth J. Implant infections: a haven for opportunistic bacteria. J Hosp Infect. 2001;49(2):87–93.
8. Leaper DJ, Van Goor H, Reilly J, Petrosillo N, Geiss HK, Torres AJ, Berger A. Surgical site infection—a European perspective of incidence and economic burden. Int Wound J. 2004;1(4):247–73.
9. Bazaka K, Jacob MV, Crawford RJ, Ivanova EP. Plasma-assisted surface modification of organic biopolymers to prevent bacterial attachment. Acta Biomater. 2011;7(5):2015–28.

10. Briem D, Strametz S, Schroder K, Meenen NM, Lehmann W, Linhart W, Ohl A, Rueger JM. Response of primary fibroblasts and osteoblasts to plasma treated polyetheretherketone (PEEK) surfaces. J Mater Sci Mater Med. 2005;16(7):671–7.
11. Gomathi N, Sureshkumar A, Neogi S. RF plasma-treated polymers for biomedical applications. Curr Sci. 2008;94(11):1478–86.
12. Desmet T, Morent R, De Geyter N, Leys C, Schacht E, Dubruel P. Nonthermal plasma technology as a versatile strategy for polymeric biomaterials surface modification: a review. Biomacromolecules. 2009;10(9):2351–78.
13. Martins A, Pinho ED, Faria S, Pashkuleva I, Marques AP, Reis RL, Neves NM. Surface modification of electrospun polycaprolactone nanofiber meshes by plasma treatment to enhance biological performance. Small. 2009;5(10):1195–206.
14. Valence SD, Tille J-C, Chaabane C, Gurny R, Bochaton-Piallat M-L, Walpoth BH, Möller M. Plasma treatment for improving cell biocompatibility of a biodegradable polymer scaffold for vascular graft applications. Eur J Pharm Biopharm. 2013;85(1):78–86.
15. Chong DS, Turner LA, Gadegaard N, Seifalian AM, Dalby MJ, Hamilton G. Nanotopography and plasma treatment: redesigning the surface for vascular graft endothelialisation. Eur J Vasc Endovasc Surg. 2015;49(3):335–43.
16. Loya MC, Brammer KS, Choi C, Chen LH, Jin S. Plasma-induced nanopillars on bare metal coronary stent surface for enhanced endothelialization. Acta Biomater. 2010;6(12):4589–95.
17. Seon GM, Seo HJ, Kwon SY, Lee MH, Kwon BJ, Kim MS, Koo MA, Park BJ, Park JC. Titanium surface modification by using microwave-induced argon plasma in various conditions to enhance osteoblast biocompatibility. Biomater Res. 2015;19:13.
18. Hauser J, Kruger CD, Halfmann H, Awakowicz P, Koller M, Esenwein SA. Surface modification of metal implant materials by low-pressure plasma treatment. Biomed Tech (Berl). 2009;54(2):98–106.
19. Tan F, O'Neill F, Naciri M, Dowling D, Al-Rubeai M. Cellular and transcriptomic analysis of human mesenchymal stem cell response to plasma-activated hydroxyapatite coating. Acta Biomater. 2012;8(4):1627–38.
20. Ferraz EP, Sverzut AT, Freitas GP, Sa JC, Alves C Jr, Beloti MM, Rosa AL. Bone tissue response to plasma-nitrided titanium implant surfaces. J Appl Oral Sci. 2015;23(1):9–13.
21. Testrich H, Rebl H, Finke B, Hempel F, Nebe B, Meichsner J. Aging effects of plasma polymerized ethylenediamine (PPEDA) thin films on cell-adhesive implant coatings. Mater Sci Eng C Mater Biol Appl. 2013;33(7):3875–80.
22. Seker E, Kilicarslan MA, Deniz ST, Mumcu E, Ozkan P. Effect of atmospheric plasma versus conventional surface treatments on the adhesion capability between self-adhesive resin cement and titanium surface. J Adv Prosthodont. 2015;7(3):249–56.
23. Steinbeck MJ, Chernets N, Zhang J, Kurpad DS, Fridman G, Fridman A, Freeman TA. Skeletal cell differentiation is enhanced by atmospheric dielectric barrier discharge plasma treatment. PLoS One. 2013;8(12):e82143.
24. Lee OJ, HW J, Khang G, Sun PP, Rivera J, Cho JH, Park SJ, Eden JG, Park CH. An experimental burn wound-healing study of non-thermal atmospheric pressure microplasma jet arrays. J Tissue Eng Regen Med. 2016;10(4):348–57.
25. Riskin DJ, Longaker MT, Gertner M, Krummel TM. Innovation in surgery: a historical perspective. Ann Surg. 2006;244(5):686–93.

# Perspectives in Aesthetic Medicine

# 21

Fred Podmelle, Reem Alnebaari, Roya Khallil Shojaei, Ajay Rana, and Rico Rutkowski

## 21.1 Introduction

For many years, hot Argon gas plasma devices are in use in surgery, e.g. for the resection of soft tissues of large surface areas with minimal bleeding. Hemostasis with hot plasma is always associated with a profound black carbonization and therefore is unsuitable for aesthetic skin treatments. What is more interesting for aesthetic surgery, are the hand-held devices that can produce cold plasma at a normal temperature and atmospheric pressure. CAP-plasma does not cause carbonization, making it not suitable for clinically relevant hemostasis but it has antimicrobial and anti-inflammatory properties and can also accelerate the healing of superficial wounds through the promotion of cell proliferation [1–4]. The introduction of approved medical devices which generate cold plasma opened the doors for its aesthetic and surgical applications in 2013.

Anyhow, the indications of aesthetic medicine are elective, emotional and lacking medical necessity. This means that an even more careful assessment of the

F. Podmelle, M.D., D.D.S., D.A.L.M. (✉) • R. Alnebaari • R. K. Shojaei
Department of Oral and Maxillofacial Surgery/Plastic Surgery,
University Medicine Greifswald, Greifswald, Germany
e-mail: podmelle@uni-greifswald.de

A. Rana
Institute of Laser and Aesthetic Medicine (ILAMED), New Delhi, India

Department of Oral and Maxillofacial Surgery/Plastic Surgery,
University Medicine Greifswald, Greifswald, Germany

National Center of Plasma Medicine, Berlin, Germany

R. Rutkowski
Department of Oral and Maxillofacial Surgery/Plastic Surgery,
University Medicine Greifswald, Greifswald, Germany

National Center of Plasma Medicine, Berlin, Germany


H.-R. Metelmann et al. (eds.), *Comprehensive Clinical Plasma Medicine*,
https://doi.org/10.1007/978-3-319-67627-2_21

risk-benefit ratio should be carried out in aesthetic plasma medicine as well. Current published studies give cold physical plasma a mainly adjuvant role or a rescue function for aesthetic medicine at risk, where the medical indication is obvious.

## 21.2 Indication Area: Skin Lesions with Risk of Infection

The proven efficacy of physical plasma against bacteria, fungi, viruses and also parasites defines its indication area. The use of ablative lasers to remove larger areas of the skin compromises it. These lasers are used with the intention to smoothen and tighten the skin's appearance and to improve the blood flow which in turn improves the tissue regeneration (facial rejuvenation). In the aesthetic facial surgery, it is indicated to use the physical plasma as an infection prophylaxis when laser skin resurfacing is combined with a face lift (Fig. 21.1a–d). This is because the surgery-induced compromised immunity in the initial phases is due to the insufficient blood flow. It is therefore recommended to reduce the exposure time to a minimum until full tissue regeneration is reached by stimulated reepithelialization. This process is improved by using ointments with the active substances like Betulin [5].

This adjuvant role of physical plasma turns to a clinical induced procedure when these wounds are already contaminated. Ablative laser treatment at a certain skin depth induces a superficial second-degree burn. When it is done over a large skin area, it causes a risk of surgical site infection which mainly occurs from the resident flora [6]. According to the same publication, when performing laser skin resurfacing, the infection rates of non-fractionated laser were at 1.1% [7], 4.3% [8] and even 7.6% [9]. With the fractionated lasers the rates are less by 0.3–2.0% [10]. As pathogens there are predominately Herpes simplex-1 [11], followed by P. aeruginosa, S.

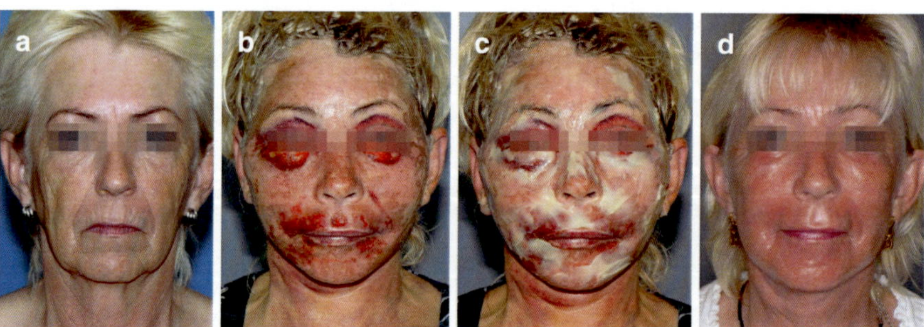


**Fig. 21.1** Patient with the diagnosis pre-aged face and a typical indication for physical plasma as an infection prophylaxis after an extensive aesthetic surgery combining a face lift with laser skin resurfacing, (**a**) Pre-operative situation, (**b**) Post-operative situation 3 days after intervention: surgical face lift and laser skin resurfacing with a $CO_2$-Laser. The laser treated periorabital and perioral regions show more profound lesions, (**c**) Prophylaxis of surgical site infection in combination with topical therapy to stimulate the repithelialisation, (**d**) Situation 4 weeks post-operatively [21]

aureus and S. epidermidis. Candida species are rarely seen as cause of wound infections. Postoperatively, a higher infection risk of S. aureus and P. aeruginosa would be seen, when closed dressings are used excessively [10]. Furthermore, infections could be caused by multi drug resistent bacteria, E. cloacae, Streptococci (severe progressive fasciitis) and also non-tuberculosis Mycobacteria [12–14].

After dermabrasio, e.g. to remove mutilating scars or to improve and smoothen the skin texture in the case of perioral lines (smokers' lines), similar observations and clinical risks are seen. Chemical peeling is often used to stimulate tissue regeneration. It could, however, pose a risk of contamination, especially when using closed dressings after applying the chemical peel on the desired areas. Such dressings could cause tissue destruction and possibly infection.

In the case of large surface epithelial lesions, decontamination and contamination prophylaxis are clinically indicated, for example after laser ablation, dermabrasio or chemical peeling.

## 21.3 Indication Area: Surgical Site Infections and Chronic Wounds

Extensive injuries can occur during an aesthetic surgery and not only through facial plastic surgeries but also extensive abdominoplasties, fat apron surgeries, liposuction and reduction plastic surgeries of the neck and extremities [15, 16]. Here, an imminent risk of wound infection is obvious. More commonly infections are caused by botulinum toxin for mimic muscle management or by implanted fillers. Fillers act to level out superficial tissue defects and to intensify contouring from an aesthetic point of view [17, 18]. When injecting fillers, e.g. for wrinkle treatment or for profiling, it can lead to a rejection of implanted materials or introduce pathogens into the tissues (Fig. 21.2a, b). Commonly, it is the combination of both, causing severe wounds that are difficult to treat. Physical plasma promotes wound healing, through its antimicrobial properties and stimulation of tissue proliferation. Achieving a secure wound closure can take several months and yet might not meet the desired aesthetic goals.

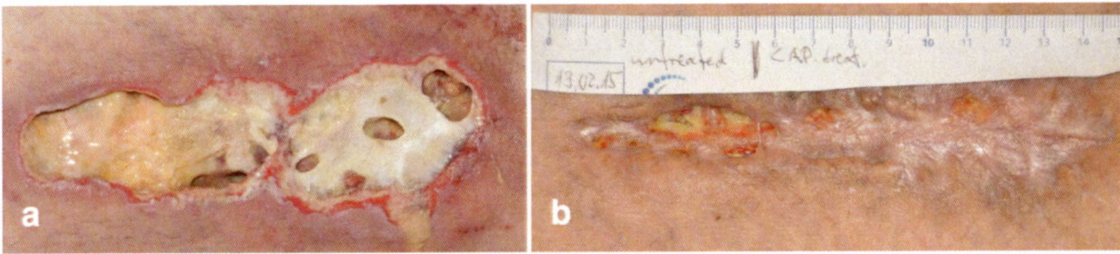


**Fig. 21.2** Exemplary patient with the diagnosis tissue infection close to the skin surface after a filler treatment for profile contouring which is the perfect task for physical plasma in order to decontaminate the wound and promote healing. (**a**) Initial situation, (**b**) Healing result after several weeks of cold plasma therapy (kINPen MED®, neoplas tools, Germany), the small lesion on the left side was left untreated to allow the drainage of wound secretion

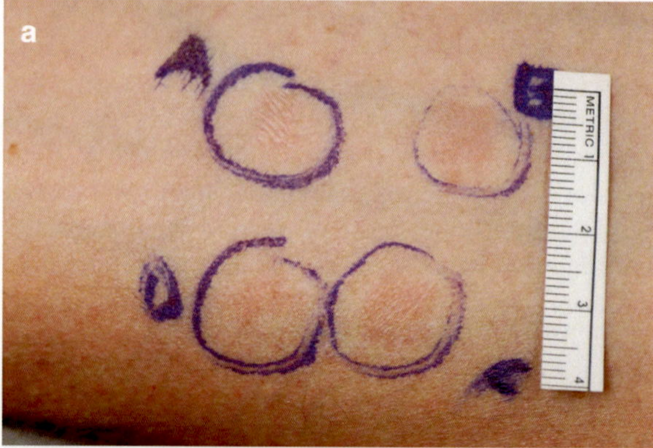


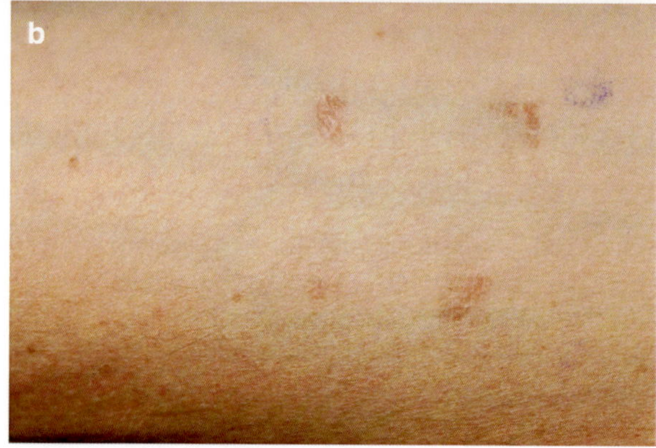


**Fig. 21.3** (**a**) Using a $CO_2$ Laser (Ultraplus, Lumenis, Germany) four skin lesions were placed on the forearm of a volunteer (single shot 20 W, 100 mJ, 200 pulses/min). Application of cold plasma (kINPen MED®, neoplas tools, Germany) (A) once for 10 s, (B) once for 30 s, (C) left untreated, (D) on three consecutive days for 10 s each. (**b**) After 10 days lesions A, B and D were less prominent than the untreated lesion (C). [20]; figure is reprinted with the kind permission of American Journal of Cosmetic Surgery)

## 21.4 Research Field: Improving Scars

Plasma applications are still in the development phase, when going beyond the adjuvant aesthetic plasma medicine. Case studies showed that an adjuvant physical plasma treatment of skin lesions after laser ablation, clearly leads to healing with aesthetically pleasing results and ideally with a normal skin complexion [19]. Three short plasma treatments on three consecutive days after an ablative laser treatment led to an improved aesthetic result in an intra individual comparison, when compared to a longer plasma treatment immediately after laser exposure. A single short plasma treatment on a laser skin lesion would disturb the healing process instead of promoting it (Fig. 21.3a, b). With regard to the literature on the promotion of wound healing, it is evident that a new indication area is emerging as an adjuvant measure to laser therapy.

## 21.5 Research Field: Active Ingredients Entering Skin

Current research is showing that physical plasma promotes the entry of chemical substances through the skin barrier and directly into the underlying tissues. A number of compounds can produce aesthetic results through plasma-assisted infiltration into the tissues. Figure 21.1c is a clinical example, showing how contamination prophylaxis using physical plasma can improve the infiltration of the active substance, in this case, Betulin, hence accelerating the re-epithelization of skin lesions. Despite having scientific foundations already laid for this treatment, there is a lack of clinical studies confirming its therapeutic effect.

Physical plasma increases the permeability of the skin to chemical substances and improve their penetration deeper into the tissues which can be used in aesthetic medicine.

## 21.6 Conceptual Idea: Skin Tightening

Moving away from the clinical practice, physical plasma can be solely used to smoothen and tighten the skin. Laboratory experiments demonstrated the tightening of the surface of a skin biopsy after a 10-min plasma exposure (Fig. 21.4a, b).

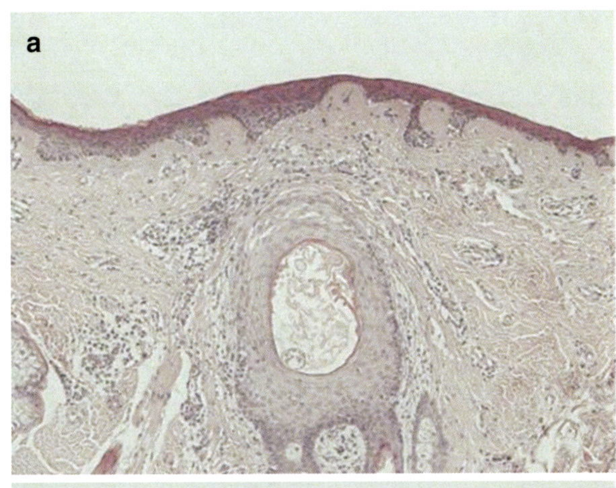


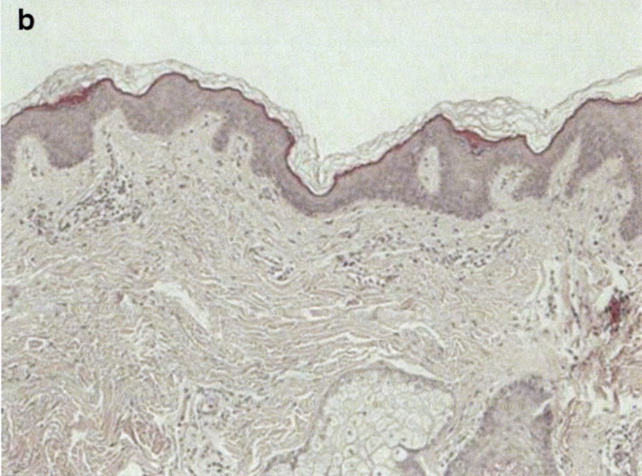


**Fig. 21.4** Two biopsies from adjacent areas of the skin after immediate removal (ex vivo) (**a**) The specimen was left for 10 min without a treatment or (**b**) after plasma treatment (kINPen MED®, neoplas tools, Germany). In comparison with HE-stained specimens (K. Evert, Institute of Pathology, University of Greifswald) a thinning and increase in the staining of the epithelium, a flattening of the upper and lower surfaces and removal of plaques is obvious were seen ([22]; Kindly permitted by K. Evert, Institute of Pathology, Greifswald University)

The interpretation of this finding is difficult because the biological reactions of an isolated skin sample are less predictable and mainly originate from the physical and chemical effects. In the literature, there are no clinical studies on the matter. Industrial statements from medical and non-medical plasma users or plasma device producers are not substantiated.

## 21.7 Outcome Research

Regarding risk assessment, it is important to take into consideration the lack of long-term experience in clinical plasma medicine, especially in its aesthetic applications. This applies to the stability of results achieved as well as a long-term absence of complex side effects. When it comes to the penetration of active substances into the skin, side effects from several sources are to be considered during in the monitoring phase. On one side, there are active substances which reach deeper tissue layers and on the other side, there is the effect of cold plasma itself. Currently, there is a small number of long-term studies regarding the stability of the aesthetic effects and absence of side effects, e.g. not at least the carcinogenesis risk [19].

## 21.8 Summary

The clinical application of cold plasma in aesthetic medicine is at present adjuvant and adds to the laser and scalpel to prevent or treat surgical site infections or chronic wounds as the nearly worst case in procedures without medical necessity. The combination of cold physical plasma with application of topical therapy is promising, especially since it improves the penetration ability of medicines and having better results. The plasma's sole mechanism of action could be used in the future to treat wrinkles but for this highly elective procedure without a medical indication to be established, studies are still at the beginning of the road.

## References


1. Daeschlein G, Scholz S, Arnold A, von Podewils S, Haase H, Emmert S, von Woedtke T, Weltmann KD, Jünger M. In vitro susceptibility of important skin and wound pathogens against low temperature atmospheric pressure plasma jet (APPJ) and dielectric barrier discharge plasma (DBD). Plasma Process Polym. 2012;9(4):380.
2. Fridman G, Friedman G, Gutsol A, Shekter AB, Vasilets VN, Fridman A. Applied plasma medicine. Plasma Process Polym. 2008;5:503.
3. Heinlin J, Isbary G, Stolz W, Morfill G, Landthaler M, Shimizu T. Plasma applications in medicine with a special focus on dermatology. J Eur Acad Dermatol Venereol. 2011;25:1.
4. Stoffels E, Sakiyama Y, Graves DB. Cold atmospheric plasma: charged species and their interactions with cells and tissue. IEEE Trans Plasma Sci. 2008;36:1441.
5. Metelmann HR, Brander JM, Schumann H, Bross F, Fimmers R, Böttger K, Scheffler A, Podmelle F. Accelerated reepithelialization by Triterpenes: proof of concept in the healing of surgical skin lesions. Skin Pharmacol Physiol. 2015;28:1–11.

6. Kramer A. Infektionsschutz in der Lasermedizin. In: Metelmann H-R, Hammes S, editors. Lasermedizin in der Ästhetischen Chirurgie. Heidelberg: Springer; 2015. p. 27.
7. Christian MM, Behroozan DS, Moy RL. Delayed infections following full-face $CO_2$ laser resurfacing and occlusive dressing use. Dermatol Surg. 2000;26(1):32.
8. Sriprachya-Anunt S, Fitzpatrick RE, Goldman MP, Smith SR. Infections complicating pulsed carbon dioxide laser resurfacing for photoaged facial skin. Dermatol Surg. 1997;23(7):527.
9. Manuskiatti W, Fitzpatrick RE, Goldman MP. Long-term effectiveness and side effects of carbon dioxide laser resurfacing for photoaged facial skin. J Am Acad Dermatol. 1999;40(3):401.
10. Metelitsa A, Alster TS. Fractionated laser skin resurfacing treatment complications: a review. Dermatol Surg. 2010;6(3):299.
11. Graber EM, Tanzi EL, Alster TS. Side effects and complications of fractional laser photothermolysis: experience with 961 treatments. Dermatol Surg. 2008;34(3):301.
12. Bellman B, Brandt FS, Holtmann M, Bebell WR. Infection with methicillin-resistant Staphylococcus aureus after carbon dioxide resurfacing of the face. Successful treatment with minocycline, rifampin, and mupirocin ointment. Dermatol Surg. 1998;24:279.
13. Culton DA, Lachiewicz AM, Miller BA, Miller MB, MacKuen C, Groben P, White B, Cox GM, Stout JE. Nontuberculous mycobacterial infection after fractionated $CO_2$ laser resurfacing. Emerg Infect Dis. 2013;19(3):365.
14. Willey A, Anderson RF, Azpiazu JL, Bakus AD, Barlow RJ, Dover JS, Garden JM, Kilmer SL, Landa N, Manstein D, Ross EV, Sadick N, Tanghetti EA, Yaghmai D, Zelickson BD. Complications of laser dermatologic surgery. Lasers Surg Med. 2006;38:1.
15. Hundeshagen G, Hundeshagen G, Assadov KF, Podmelle F. Facelift- und circum-occipital incision placement for fat extirpation of the neck in Madelung's disease—a two case report. J Craniomaxillofac Surg. 2014;42(2):175–9.
16. Podmelle F, Metelmann HR, Waite P. Endoscopic abdominoplasty providing a perforator fat flap for treatment of hemi-facial microsomia. J Craniomaxillofac Surg. 2012;40(8):665–7.
17. Funk W, Metelmann HR. Von Botulinumtoxin bis Kinnimplantat—Wie das Gesicht im Leben altert und was Sie dagegen tun können. Ästh Dermatol Kosmeteologie. 2011;5:6–12.
18. Podmelle F, Kaduk W, Metelmann HR. Individualästhetik in der Gesichtschirurgie. Faces. 2009;4:6.
19. Metelmann HR, Thom VT, Tung Do H, Binh Le TN, Anh Hoang TH, Trang Phi TT, Linh Luong TM, Tien Doan V, Huyen Nguyen TT, Minh Nguyen TH, Linh Nguyen T, Quyen Le D, Xuan Le TK, von Woedtke T, Bussjahn R, Weltmann KD, Khalili R, Podmelle F. Scar formation of laser skin lesions after cold atmospheric pressure plasma (CAP) treatment: a clinical long term observation. Clin Plasma Med. 2013;1:30–5.
20. Metelmann HR, von Woedtke T, Bussjahn R, Weltmann KD, Rieck M, Khalili R, Podmelle F, Waite PD. Experimental recovery of $CO_2$-laser skin lesions by plasma stimulation. Am J Cosmet Surg. 2012;29(1):52–6.
21. Metelmann HR, Podmelle F, Müller-Debus C, Funk W, Westermann U, Hammes S. Ästhetische Lasermedizin. MKG-Chirurg.
22. von Woedtke T, Metelmann HR. Editorial. Clin Plasma Med. 2013;1:1.

# Perspective in Pigmentation Disorders 22

Manish Adhikari, Anser Ali, Nagendra Kumar Kaushik, and Eun Ha Choi

## 22.1 Introduction

Pigmentation in all mammals including humans primarily determined by the distribution of melanin in body, which shows remarkable diversity in human population globally and is the most variable phenotype in human [1]. Pheomelanin is the typical biological form of melanin, a yellow–red pigment, whereas eumelanin is a brown-black pigment. Enzymes such as tyrosinase-related protein 1 and 2 regulate eumelanogenesis [2, 3]. Many signaling pathways help to produce melanin in cells, amongst which the cyclic adenosine monophosphate (cAMP) pathway is most studied [4, 5]. The cAMP stimulation results in the up-regulation of microphthalmia-associated transcription factor (MITF), tyrosinase, tyrosinase-related proteins-1 (Trp1) and tyrosinase-related proteins-2 (Trp2) [6–8]. Apart from haemoglobin, melanin is the main contributor to pigmentation in mammals [9]. Various genetic studies revealed that the average genetic variation due to differences between major continental groups is only 10–15% of the total genetic variation. Pigmentation in human is due to the presence of a complex group of biopolymers known as melanin which synthesized and stored in specialized cells known as melanocytes [10]. The variation in this trait is because of the natural selection but till date the evolutionary factors is not properly understood. Therefore, there is much advances in our knowledge about the pigmentary system, mainly using the animal models, and we correlate this it with studying pigmentation disorders in humans. The presence of melanin in melanocytes contributes in skin color and its deficiency results in skin

M. Adhikari • N. K. Kaushik • E. H. Choi (✉)
Department of Electrical and Biological Physics, Applied Plasma Medicine Center, Kwangwoon University, Seoul, Republic of Korea
e-mail: ehchoi@kw.ac.kr

A. Ali
Department of Zoology, Mirpur University of Science and Technology, Mirpur, AJK, Pakistan



H.-R. Metelmann et al. (eds.), *Comprehensive Clinical Plasma Medicine*,
https://doi.org/10.1007/978-3-319-67627-2_22

depigmentation disorder called as vitiligo. The repigmentation begins usually at the hair follicle opening in the skin and covers the whole skin area which is depigmented by vitiligo [11]. The follicular repigmentation of depigmented skin after treatment of external stimuli such as narrow band UVB (ultraviolet B) has been reported. The follicular repigmentation is characterized by the repigmentation of an unpigmented skin area [11–13]. Therefore, melanogenic stimuli may prove useful in stimulating the melanocytes for melanin synthesis which is important for tan skin color, black hair color and re-pigmentation of unpigmented skin area caused by imbalanced pigmentation such as vitiligo.

Melanin has a photo-screening ability, therefore provides skin photo-protection, prevents skin injury, absorbs and converts harmful UV-radiations into harmless heat [14]. Despite its advantages, hyper-pigmentations can cause skin problems such as age spots, melanoma, freckles, DNA damage, gene mutation, cancer and impaired immune system [15]. To avoid such abnormalities, reducing the melanin production could be an important.

Plasma is essentially an ionized gas commonly employed in physical sciences [16]. Plasma as an active ionized medium contain free radicals, free charges, excited molecules and energetic photons which can induce processes usually obtained through radiotherapy or chemical treatment [15]. When applied on tissue or cells, plasma is able to catalyze biochemical activities and regulate cellular processes such as differentiation, proliferation and apoptosis [17]. These biological effects of non-thermal plasma are due to augment of the reactive oxygen species (ROS) and reactive nitrogen species (RNS) [18]. Nonthermal plasma technology is fast growing due to its low temperature and vibrant composition. Applications of nonthermal plasma are reported in diabetic control, dental care, blood coagulation, cancer treatment and wound healing improvement ([16, 19–21]; Fridman et al. 2006). However, very little is known about the effect of nonthermal plasma on melanogenesis and so far only two reports are published. In first report, Kim et al. showed that plasma treatment to natural compound called naringin can increase its tyrosinase inhibition activity which is important enzyme required for melanin synthesis. Later, Ali et al. [22], synthesized new eugenol derivatives (ED) and reported new perspective on plasma treated compounds by regulating cellular melanogenesis with possibility to treat hypopigmentation and related skin disorders in future. In this book chapter, we review the biochemical and hormonal control of pigmentation that have been put forward to protect against UV radiation of sun and finally, in the last segment we review about the current state of our knowledge about disorders of hyperpigmentation and hypopigmentation among humans and its treatment using surgical, hormonal, immunological, antioxidative and cold atmospheric plasma treatment compounds.

## 22.2 Biology of Pigment Cells

Distribution and regulation of melanin pigment is different in the skin, hair and iris in humans. In the skin, the melanocytes present in the basal layer of the epidermis which transfer melanosomes to adjacent keratinocytes through their specialized dendritic structures, and the keratinocytes eventually migrate to the upper layers of the epidermis [23]. Melanosomes are aggregated over the nucleus of keratinocytes and protect the upper skin against ultraviolet radiation. In hair follicle, melanin produced at hair bulb. The melanin containing melanocytes transfer Melanosomes to precortical keratinocytes that migrate to form pigmented hair shaft [24]. Intercellular transfer of organelles is a key feature of body pigmentation [25]. The melanin formation in skin cells is continuous throughout the life and changed according to the climatic conditions and geographical location but melanogenesis in hair is only takes place during anagen phase of hair growth cycle that lasts on average 3–5 years. There are various other differences also which related to morphology of melanocytes and the microenvironment in which melanogenesis takes place [24]. Tobin and Paus 2001; Slominski et al. 2005). Dermal fibroblast plays a very key role in melanocyte pigmentation [26]. vitilEye color is determined by variations in a person's genes and is directly related to the amount and quality of melanin in the front layers of the iris. The gene responsible for eye color is OCA2 and HERC2 which is present on the region on chromosome 15. The OCA2 gene produced P protein which involved in maturation of Melanosomes and play a crucial role in the amount and quality of melanin that is present in the iris. HERC2 gene also known as intron 86 contains a segment of DNA that controls the expression of the OCA2 gene, turning it on or off as needed. Some other genes also play role in determining eye color include ASIP, IRF4, SLC24A4, SLC24A5, SLC45A2, TPCN2, TYR, and TYRP1.

The melanin act as concentrating hormone and work as an integrative peptide driving motivated behavior [27]. Skin color depends upon the size, number, shape, and distribution of melanosomes, as well as the chemical nature (level of activity) of their melanin content. Dermatologist differentiate skin types into six categories according to the level of sensitivity of skin due to the melanin presence (Table 22.1).

Both skin types have the same type of pigment cells or melanocytes. But, the pigment granules produced by melanocytes in dark pigmented skin are larger and more in amount as compared to those in light pigmented skin. When transported to epidermal cells (keratinocytes), pigment granules in dark skin (left side) persist inside the cells and many of them move towards the skin surface and some of the

**Table 22.1** Types of skin suggested by the dermatologists for common use

| Type of skin | Brief description |
|---|---|
| Type 1 | Very fair skin with red or blonde hairs. Always burns, never tans, mostly northern European peoples like Norway, Sweden and Finland |
| Type 2 | Fair skin, burns very easily but tans minimally |
| Type 3 | Sometimes burns but tans gradually |
| Type 4 | Minimum burning and always tans. White with medium pigmentation |
| Type 5 | Seldom burns, always tans. Medium to heavy pigmentation |
| Type 6 | Never burns but tans very quickly. African Americans, Africans, or dark-skinned individuals with heavy pigmentation |

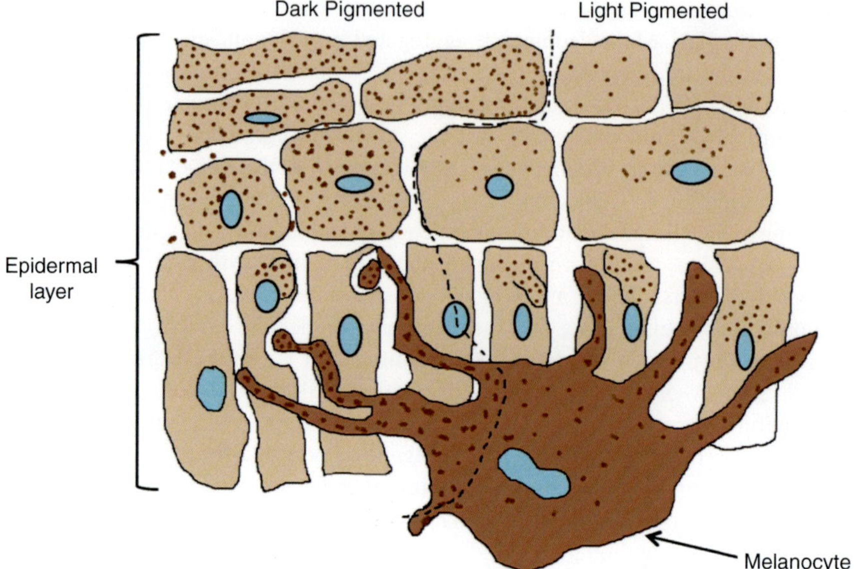


**Fig. 22.1** Distribution of melanin granules in dark pigmented skin (left panel) vs light pigmented skin (right panel)

granules "escape" into the spaces outside the cells. In contrast in lighter skin (right side) the small granules tend to make cluster over the top of the nucleus ('nuclear cap') where their function is to protect the DNA from sun damage. Only very few of them able to move outer skin cell layers and hence look like light pigment skin (Fig. 22.1).

## 22.3 Biochemical and Hormonal Control of Pigmentation

The embellishment of melanin pigment in the epidermal melanocyte primarily depends on the availability of three substances: -(a) the enzyme tyrosinase -a copper-protein complex attached to ultramicroscopic particles in the cytoplasm of the melanocyte; (b) a suitable substrate-usually tyrosine or DOPA; (c) molecular oxygen. Formation of melanin is alter or reduce if any one of the mentioned substance missing from the skin cells. Melanocytes begin to migrate from the neural crest as early as 2.5 weeks after post-fertilization. Melanin is mixture of biopolymers synthesized inside melanocytes present in the basal layer of the epidermis, the iris and the hair bulb. Within the melanocytes, melanin production takes place in the melanosomes which is lysosome-like structure where melanin granules are produced using tyrosine as the major substrate. Tyrosine (TYR) is the main enzyme for the synthesis of melanin and the process known as melanogenesis which comprises conversion of tyrosine into DOPA and subsequently to DOPA quinone using the enzyme tyrosine hydroxylase and DOPA oxidase respectively

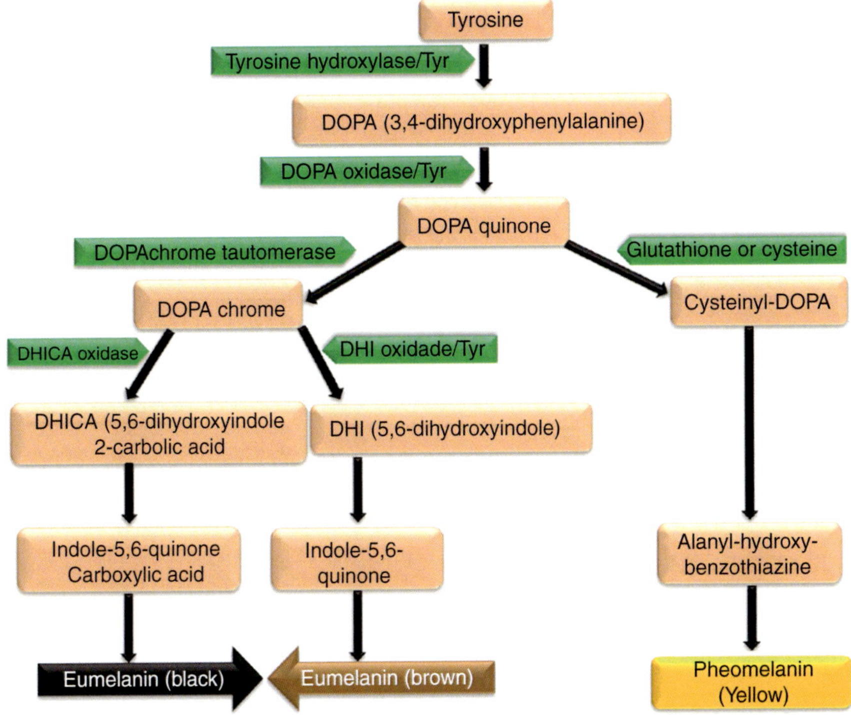


**Fig. 22.2** Melanin biosynthesis pathway

[28–30]. DOPA quinone is converted into DOPAchrome using enzyme DOPAchrome tautomerase which further subdivided into DHICA and DHI by catalytic reaction of DHICA oxidase and DHI oxidase [31, 32]. The final black color of the skin is formed by the conversion of indole-55,6-quinone carboxylic acid and is called eumelanin and brown pigment of skin is formed by cange of indole-5,6-quinone to eumelanin [32, 33]. DOPA quinone was also converted to cysteinyl-DOPA using the naturally present antioxidant enzyme Glutathione or cysteine which further changed to alanyl-hydroxy-benzothiazine and ultimately formed to pheomelanin which is responsible for yellow color of the skin (Fig. 22.2).

Eumelanin and pheomelanin play key roles in eye, hair, and skin color. Neuromelanin is the building block of color of certain distinctive regions of the brain. This coloration is independent of skin and hair type and abnormalities in neuromelanins is directly correlate with various neurodegenerative diseases, such as Parkinson's and Alzheimer's [34–37].

The total actions of tyrosine and DOPA in the pigmentary system strongly support an additional role for these melanin precursors as hormone like bio-regulators, and hence melanocytes regulate activities of these two precursors which affecting both metabolic consumption and production [24]. Cell surface proteins for these tyrosine (5 proteins) and DOPA (4 proteins) were detected and identified [38–40]. These proteins were neither adrenergic nor dopaminergic receptors. Melanogenesis-related proteins have the cysteine-rich sequences characteristic of peptide hormones, they may regulate melanocyte function through binding to proteins, acting at the translational or transcriptional levels [38].

One major factor of pigment phenotype of the skin is the melanocortin 1 receptor (MC1R), a G protein-coupled receptor that controls the quantity and quality of melanins produced [23, 41]. MC1R function is controlled by the agonists α-melanocyte-stimulating hormone (αMSH) and adrenocorticotropic hormone (ACTH) and by an antagonist, Agouti signaling protein (ASP). Activation of the MC1R by an agonist stimulates the expression of the melanogenic cascade and thus the synthesis of eumelanin (black and brown), whereas ASP can reverse those effects and elicit the production of pheomelanin (yellow). αMSH and ACTH can also up-regulate expression of the MC1R gene, thus acting in a positive feedback loop [42]. MC1R function controls the switch to produce eu- *versus* pheomelanin, but the mechanism(s) underlying that switch remains unknown. αMSH activate eumelanin and phaeomelanin by the activation of PI3K-AKT and ERK ½ pathways in the presence of ultraviolet radiation [43] (Fig. 22.3).

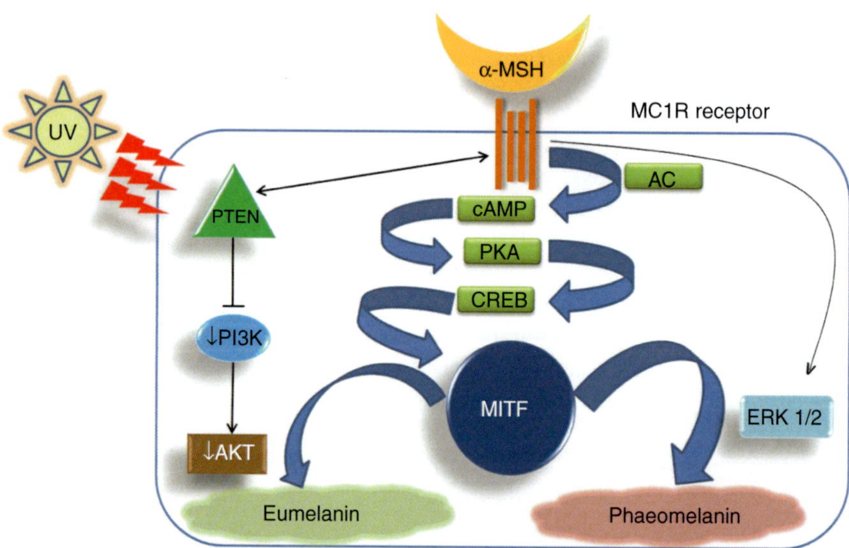


**Fig. 22.3** Activation of MC1R receptor within melanocyte triggers the cAMP and MAPK/ERK signalling pathways and interacts indirectly via PTEN with the PI3K pathway. (α-MSH - alpha-Melanocyte-stimulating hormone; AC – Adenylate Cyclase; cAMP – cyclic adenosine monophosphate; PKA – Protein kinase A; CREB - cyclic AMP responsive element binding protein; MITF - Microphthalmia Associated Transcription Factor; PTEN - Phosphatase and tensin homolog; PI3K - Phosphoinositide 3-kinase; ERK - Extracellular signal–regulated kinases

## 22.4 Function of Melanin

Melanin is located in many animal tissues, and in practically all living organisms, it is not surprising that melanin has a lot of different functions. Melanin has a very much high biomedical attention mostly due to its physiological photoprotective properties. Eumelanin present in the skin shows a very broad UV-visible absorption spectrum [44], and it is able to dissipate the absorbed energy from the sunlight radiation such as heat. This can contribute to thermoregulation of individuals having melanin pigment, which is especially important for cold-blooded animals who are unable to regulate their body temperature. Melanin prevents the skin from the potentially damaging effects of UV light and causing a moderate tan effect on the skin to increase the amount of photoprotective pigment [45]. Both eumelanin and pheomelanin are affected by the sunlight, and they form semiquinoid-type free radical species and then typical free radical species from water, but eumelanin is large enough to scavenge the originated species and quite stable. In contrast, pheomelanin has been shown to be rather photolabile under sunlight at physiological conditions, and it is involved in the high production of superoxide [46].

The people having pheomelanin pigment has the greater chance of having cutaneous skin cancer [47]. Melanins are quite reactive, and they display a series of complex structural and physicochemical properties Melanins are quite reactive, and they display a series of complex structural and physicochemical properties in addition to resistance to degradation. They show redox activity are outstanding stable radical, chelating agent, free radical scavenger, organic agents etc. [48]. It act as various other functions too which is mention in Fig. 22.4.

Apart from skin, melanin is also present in the iris, retinal pigment epithelium (RPE) and choroid which helps to protect retina from intense sunlight. Melanin in the RPE exhibits antioxidant properties, protecting components of RPE such as A2E from photooxidation [49]. This ability appears to decrease in humans as they grow older. Furthermore, melanin formation at RPE also may be implicated in the downregulation of rod outer segment phagocytosis. This may be related to foveal sparing in macular degeneration [50] because of the changes in the redox properties. Melanin may also function as a natural reservoir for divalent ions and as an ion exchanger, as well as an intracellular buffering system for calcium homeostasis in inner ear [51]. The function of neuromelanin in the human *substantia nigra* is a very interesting and intriguing issue, as other mammals have no neuromelanin in the brain. In a different strategy of mechanism of protection against physical attack some cephalopods have melanin kept in a sac to camouflage themselves. This form of melanin makes up the ink used by octopus, cuttlefish, and other cephalopods as a defense mechanism against marine predators. Melanin is also related to protective agent as it is considered a primitive form of immunity by conversion of phenol oxidases on phenols to form *o-quinone* intermediates and finally melanin [52, 53]. Melanin protects from oxidative stress and ROS, as it traps free radicals and protects microorganisms against oxidizing attacks, and ROS are part of the host mechanisms against invading microbes. Now a days, melanin also behaves as a semiconductor with interesting biophysical properties proposed for new biotechnological

Absorption of UV phototoxic and photosensitize
Thermo-regulation
Free radical quencher
Protection against lipid peroxidation
Camouflage and sexual appeal
Photoprotection photoageing
Protection from photocarcinogen
Regulation of Vitamin D synthesis
MELANIN

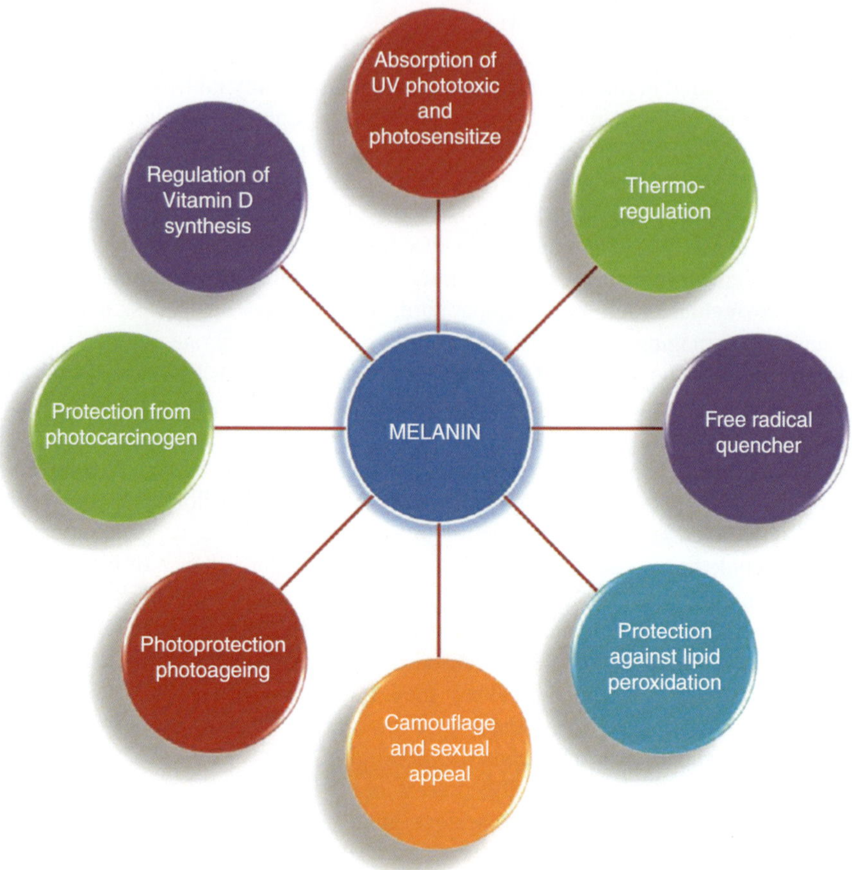

**Fig. 22.4** Functions of melanin pigment

applications. Synthetic dopamine melanin has been proposed for *in situ* formation of regular coatings [54]. Uniform flat melanin films can be obtained with dopamine or other similar precursors by spray deposition, and these thin films show a stacked planar structure with interesting electronic and optical properties [55] to be used as semiconductors in electrically qualified devices and other nanotechnological applications [56]. *Yarrowia lipolytica* is biotechnologically significant yeast, used for the synthesis of silver and gold nanostructures effective as paint-additives produce a dopa-melanin [57].

## 22.5 Measurement of Skin Pigmentation

There are various color match standardized techniques to measure skin pigmentation. The most accepted technique was Von Luschan's chromatic scale, where sample skin was compared with 36 small different colored ceramic tiles ranging from white to black [58]. After few decades, this technique was replaced by the introduction of EEL portable reflectance spectrometers (Evans Electroselenium Ltd.) with nine filters which showed high degree of sensitivity and selectivity. These spectrometers were improved in terms of objectivity and accuracy, measure percentage of light reflected from the skin at different wavelengths. The reflectance from the skin at each wavelength relative to that of a white standard (typically white magnesium carbonate). EEL portable reflectance spectrometers were replaced by Photovolt instrument which is refined form of the former having six filters with broader band transmittance. Results from both instruments were very hard to estimate, although conversion formulae were developed to overcome this issue [59, 60]. Presently, three techniques has been use based on reflectance technologies to study the pigmentation in the skin: tristimulus colorimetry, specialized narrow-band reflectometry, and diffuse reflectance spectroscopy. These modern instruments used to quantify skin pigmentation and offer significant advantages over traditional instruments in terms of reliability, sensitivity, portability and accuracy.

### 22.5.1 Tristimulus Colorimetry

Tristimulus colorimetry was developed in taken into manner analogues the way eye perceives color [61]. Photodiode array of this colorimeter perceive reflected light through three broad wavelength filters. Color parameters are then defined by the level of differences among the reflectance level of these three filters. Tristimulus colorimeters supports the Minolta Chroma Meter series which was made by Konica Minolta Sensing, Osaka, Japan, are usually able to report color values for a number of other color systems as well. By using tristimulus colorimeters, pigmentation is evaluated using L*, b*, or a combination of the three parameters and erythema (redness of the skin primarily due to hemoglobin) is typically evaluated using the a* parameter [62].

### 22.5.2 Specialized Narrow-Band Reflectometry

The approach for this kind of reflectometry was developed by [63], who specifically measure hemoglobin and melanin in the skin. Both form of hemoglobin i.e., deoxy-hemoglobin and oxy-hemoglobin absorbs light at lower wavelength of visible light, with absorption peaks in the green-yellow region of the spectrum (deoxy-hemoglobin absorption maxima, 555 nm; oxy-hemoglobin absorption maxima, 540 and 577 nm). Whereas, melanin absorbs light at all wavelength and its absorption decreases exponentially in 400–600 nm range and linear in 720–620 nm range [64]. Differences in spectral curves of hemoglobin and melanin suggested the reflectance of narrow-band light in the red spectrum that yield reasonable estimates of melanin content of the skin [63], by using the following equation:

$$M\left(\text{melanin index}\right) = \log_{10}\left(\frac{1}{\%\text{red reflectance}}\right)$$

The degree of skin redness or erythema can be estimated by subtracting the absorbance due to melanin from the absorbance of the green filter and is calculated as:

$$E\left(\text{erythema index}\right) = \log_{10}\left(\frac{1}{\%\text{green reflectance}}\right) - \log_{10}\left(\frac{1}{\%\text{red reflectance}}\right)$$

Various tristimulus colorimeter and narrow-band spectrometers that measures the melanin and erythema indices are commercially available which helps in carried out many comparative studies of hair and skin pigmentation [65].

### 22.5.3 Diffuse Reflectance Spectroscopy

The Diffuse reflectance spectroscopy (DRS) is considered as the most accurate and sensitive noninvasive method to measure skin pigmentation [62]. The advantage of DRS over the two methods which described before is that the DRS values are measured at high optical resolution throughout the visible spectrum. The incident light is delivered to the skin at the site of interest using fibre optic bundle and the reflectance from skin detected through an analyzer-detector system in the whole spectrum. Since, the received data is from full visible spectrum that means it is possible to separate the two major chromophores of the skin because of their different spectral properties. Amount of melanin presence in the skin can be calculated by DRS by the absorption spectrum in the region between 620 and 720 nm [66, 67] and hemoglobin content determined by absorbance of the skin at 560–580 nm [62]. The added advantage of new generation portable spectrometers is that they can be used to calculate all type of pigmentation measurements and can be determined by using appropriate formulae.

## 22.6 Human Exposure UV Radiation and Pigmentary System

Ultraviolet radiation (UVR) is most strongly correlated for skin pigmentation in humans compared with all other environmental factors measured [68]. Pigmentation has wide ranging effects on human body as it is one of the important factor in regulating the penetration of ultraviolet radiation [69]. Therefore, UV radiation from sun striking power in skin is estimated by the UV index number, which was first developed by Canadian scientists in 1992. Since, UV rays can penetrate clouds, clothes and even glass, UV index is an excellent 'guide' with lighter skin types and greater precautions are needed (Fig. 22.5).

Eumelanin which is responsible for the brown pigmentation in the body absorbs and scatters ultraviolet and visible light and prevent the formation of reactive

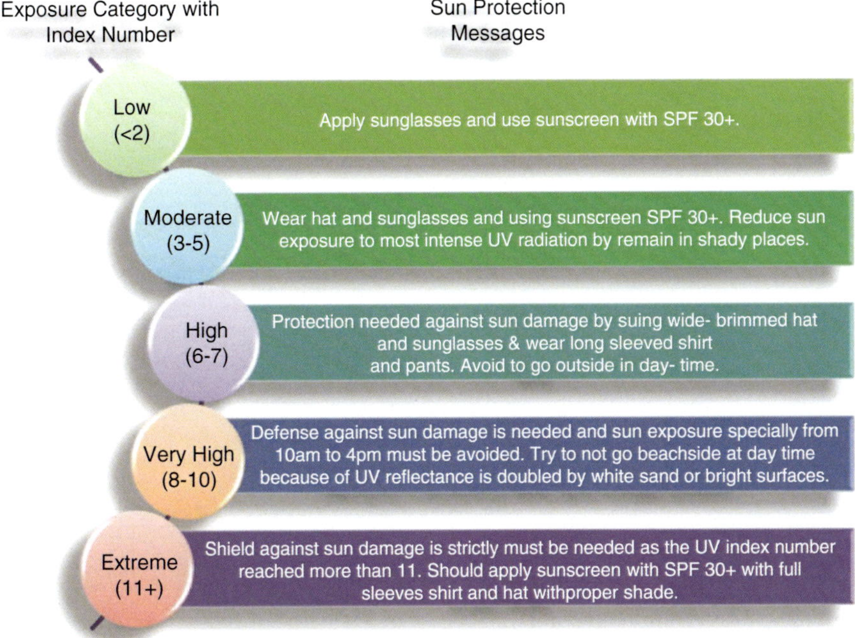


**Fig. 22.5** Protection from UV radiation on the basis of exposure to sun and index number with its protection methods

oxygen species inside the skin [70, 71]. Ultraviolet B (280–315 nm) is present abundant outside of tropical lattitudes which is necessary for the production and synthesis of cutaneous Vitamin $D_3$ in the skin [72–76]. The pre-vitamin D3 production is inversely proportional to skin pigmentation, the higher the eumelanin content, the lower the rate of pre-vitamin D3 production of skin [69, 75–79]. It is evident that low pigmented people residing the zone near the equator experience enough UVB through normal sun exposure on unprotected skin to produce physiologically adequate amounts of vitamin D.

The people with dark pigmented skin, these 'vitamin D safe zones' are smaller and shifted towards the equator because of the efficacious sunscreening action of eumelanin. People living at higher latitudes than 42° must supplement their diets with vitamin $D_3$-rich foods, in order to prevent vitamin D deficiency and its related diseases. Years of sun exposure may result in dark spots in light-skinned individuals and spotted as hyperpigmentation that results in patchy skin color or a blotchy complexion [80]. The extent of sun damage depends largely on a person's skin color and his or her history of long-term or intense sun exposure. To treat pigmentation problems due to sun damage in lighter-skinned individuals some recommendations are following in Fig. 22.6.

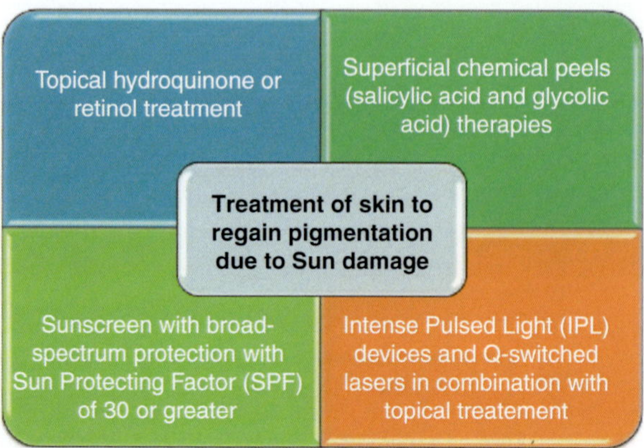


**Fig. 22.6** Recommended treatment methods to treat sun damaged skin due to ultraviolet radiation to regain normal skin pigmentation

## 22.7 Disorders of Pigmentation

Disorders of melanin pigment in the body can be characterized by decreased melanin production causing skin to get lighter (hypopigmentation) or by increased melanin production causing skin to get darker (hyperpigmentation). Skin disorders resulting in hypopigmentation may be acquired or congenital (present from birth). Acquired causes of hypopigmentation are more common than congenital causes of hypopigmentation. Collectively, the group of diseases is referred to as skin pigmentation disorders and is describing below in details.

## 22.8 Hypomelanosis

There are various skin disorders which is caused due to the non-presence or lesser presence of melanin pigment in the body. It may be arise due to the defects in embryological development of the melanocytes, defects in melanogenesis process, defects in biogenesis of Melanosomes, Melanosomes transport, survival of melanocytes and other pigmentary problems. The diseases associated with them are as follows.

### 22.8.1 Piebaldism

Piebaldism is very rare autosomal dominant disorder with congenital Hypomelanosis. This disorder is present only to hair and skin without its presence in neurological, ocular regions. The lesion caused due to the disease spread to the anterior part of trunk, abdomen, extremities and frontal part of scalp [81, 82]. In 90% cases the forelock is become white along with hairs and adjacent skins because of depigmentation. This disease gives "mosaic" like pattern because of hypo and hyper pigmentation in adjacent areas of skins. These patches are congenital, stable with time and do not repigment because of complete absent of melanocytes within the hair bulb and epidermis [81, 83].

Primarily, this disease caused due to the loss of function and dominant mutation of KIT gene which is located on chromosome 4 (4q12) [84, 85]. This gene is responsible for white spotting in humans and encodes for a tyrosine kinase receptor named as *c-kit*. This gene is present on cell surface of melanocyte, germ cells and hematopoetic stem cells [86]. This factor is involved in proliferation and survival of melanoblasts [87]. Recent studies revealed the identification of novel gene KIT mutation in chinese family suffered from Piebaldism [88]. The importance of *c-kit* pathway emphasized by treatment with new tyrosine kinase inhibitors in pigmentation disorders [89–91]. Dermabrasion and skin grafts are effective surgical techniques for treatment. Transplantation of melanocytes is another treatment option and many individuals have favorable responses to this therapy [92].

### 22.8.2 Waardenburg (WB) Syndrome

This skin disorder associated with congenital white patches with deafness. This disease distinguished in 4 types and is as follows.

WB syndrome 1 is an autosomal dominant disorder where clinical manifestations are highly variable. Symptoms are almost same as that of piebaldism that includes white forelock which is the most frequent manifestation (45% of cases) with neural tube defects in infants [93]. One third of the cases showed alopecia and hypopigmented patches also. Ocular manifestations, dystopia canthorum, Facial dysmorphia are the main clnical sign of WB syndrome 1 [94, 95]. Sensorineural deafness may be severe but usually stable with time, shown the absence of melanocytes in the vascular stria of cochlea in inner ear [96, 97].

WB1 and 3 result from loss of function mutations of PAX3 gene which is located in chromosome 2. PAX3 encrypts for a transcription factor with 4 functional domains. In patients, mutations have been described in each of these 4 domains presenting WB1 and WB3 syndrome [98–102]. PAX3 is also expressed at the lateral extremity of the neural plate showing the primitive streak and 2 bands of cells [103]. It is now established that PAX3 controls microphthalmia-associated transcription factor (MITF) [104]. MITF takes central role in melanogenesis by activates transcription of melanocyte proteins including tyrosinase and tyrosinase-related protein 1. It mediates survival of melanocytes via regulation of Bcl2 [105]. WS2 is genetically a heterogenic group and occurred due to mutations in MITF gene locatedin chromosome 3.

WB4 is an autosomal recessive disorder with dystopia canthorum, broad nasal root, white skin patches, or neonatal deafness symptoms [106]. This results from mutations in several different genes like endothelin-B receptor (EDNRB) gene and SOX10 gene [107]. Homozygous mutation in EDNRB gene results inWB4 [82, 108–110]. Heterozygote mutations of the transcription factor gene SOX10 also lead to WB4 [111]. Mutations in SOX10 also exhibit myelination deficiency in the central and peripheral nervous systems [112]. Transcription of MITF regulates with SOX10 along with PAX3 and plays a vital role in the survival of neural crest cells [113]. Structural myelin proteins genes overexpression coding for P0 due to mutation in SOX10 may explain the dysmyelination phenotype with an additional neurological disorder [112].

### 22.8.3 Oculocutaneous Albinism (OCA)

OCA type 1 is one of the two most common OCA present which is an autosomal recessive disorder characterized by non-pigmentation in hair, skin, and eyes. Forefront often shows Ocular manifestations symptoms like severe nystagmus, photophobia, reduced visual acuity etc. [114]. OCA type 1 divided into 2 types: type 1-A, with complete lack of tyrosinase activity because of production of an inactive enzyme, and type 1-B, with reduced activity of tyrosinase. In OCA1-A melanosomes are normally present within melanocytes and well-transferred to the keratinocytes.

OCA type 1 caused by mutation in the TYR gene [115, 116]. Mutation in this gene encodes albinism in mouse and it encodes tyrosinase and mutation in all four domain of tyrosinase occurred. OCA type 2 is the most common form of OCA which is autosomal recessive. Pigmentation is higher in black people and with time pigmented nevi, lentigos and freckles can be seen. Also, Ocular manifestations are also less severe, visual acuity and nystagmus tend to get better with time.

OCA type 3 is an autosomal recessive disorder and most common seen in African origin people in which skin and hairs are light brown and iris is gray or light brown in color. Ultrastructural analysis of melanocytes in OCA type 3 shows eumelanosomes and pheomelanosomes in all stages. OCA type 3 results from loss-of-function mutations of the tyrosinase related protein 1 (TYRP1) gene which is responsible for brown color in mouse [117, 118]. TYRP1 encodes for dihydroxyindol carboxylic acid oxidase which is a well-known melanogenic enzyme [119]. This enzyme is downstream of tyrosinase and necessary for eumelanin synthesis only but not pheomelanin synthesis and hence OCA3 associated with the abnormal presence of pheomelanin in black peoples.

OCA type 4 is rare form of recently known autosomal recessive form of OCA which results from mutations in membrane-associated transporter protein (MATP) gene (5p) which is human ortholog of *underwhite* gene in mouse and is same as OCA2 phenotypically. This protein predicted to span the membrane of melanosome 12 times and functions as a transporter [120].

### 22.8.4 Ocular Albinism (OA)

This disease is an X-linked recessive disorder and is the most frequent OA which is limited to eyes only. Ultrastructural analysis shows the presence of giant melanosomes called "macromelanosomes" within normal melanocytes. Which are present in skin, iris, and retina. Retinal pigment analysis suggested that the giant melanosomes may form by abnormal growth of single melanosomes rather than by the fusion of several organelles [121]. Treatment primarily involves protection of the skin and eyes from the sun. Sunscreen, long pants and sleeves, wide-brimmed hats, and sunglasses are all effective options for protection. Albinism does not usually affect lifespan. The prognosis is excellent and an individual's activity may be only limited by intolerance of the sun. Possible complications may include decreased vision, blindness, and skin cancer.

### 22.8.5 Hermansky-Pudlak Syndrome (HPS)

HPS is rare autosomal recessive disorder which has symptoms of bleeding and lysosomal ceroid storage [122]. Tyrosinase is absent from hair bulb and macromelanosomes is present within melanocytes and adjacent keratinocytes. Melanosomes with stage IV is very rare but with stages I to III are frequent [122]. Platlet counts is normal in bleeding case also but with the absence of dense bodies [123]. Ceroid substance comes from degradation of lipids and glycoproteins within lysosomes and its storage in HPS suggests a defect in mechanisms of elimination of lysosomes [117].

HPS type 1 is most common and results from mutation in HPS1 gene which is responsible for pale-ear phenotype in mouse model. HPS type 1 and 4 codes for cytosolic proteins that form lysosomal complex called biogenesis of lysosome-related organelles complex-3 (BLOC3) [124] which is involved in the mechanism different from that operated by AP3 complex. HPS type 2 includes immunodeficiency in its phenotype and results from mutations in AP3B1 gene which codes for beta-3A subunit of the AP3 complex in the pearl phenotype in mouse [125]. Additionally, CD1B surface protein binds the AP3 adaptor protein complex which shows defects in HPS2 patients results in repeat bacterial infections [126].

HPS type 3 results from mutation in HPS3 gene which is regularly occurring disease in Puerto rico. Mutation in HPS3 results in *cocoa* phenotype in mouse. HPS3 encodes cytoplasmic proteins of unknown function that can be involved in early stages of melanosome biogenesis and maturation [127]. HPS type 4 caused due to the mutation in HPS4 gene which stands for *light-ear* phenotype. This disease also involved in the formation of BLOC3 which has same function as of HPS1.

HPS type 5 and HPS 6 results from the mutations in HPS5gene and HPS6 gene. HPS5 mutation results in ruby eye 2 (ru2) and HPS6 mutation forms in ruby eye (ru) phenotype and both form a lysosomal complex called BLOC2 [128]. HPS type 7 caused by mutation in the DTNBP1 gene which forms sandy phenotype in mouse and encodes for dysbindin, a protein that binds to α- and β- dystrobrevins, components of the dystrophin-associated protein complex in muscle and nonmuscle cells and also important for normal platelet dense granule and melanosome biogenesis [129].

### 22.8.6 Chediak-Higashi Syndrome (CHS)

CHS is also a very rare autosomal recessive syndrome that associates a partial OCA and an immunodeficiency syndrome. Cutaneous pigmentation is usually not very decreased and hairs are blond or light brown, iris is pigmented, photophobia and nystagmus could be seen. This disease is characterized by the presence of giant melanosomes in melanocytes and giant inclusion bodies in most granulated cells. The key factor about this disease id the absence of natural killer cell cytotoxicity and decrease of neutrophil and monocyte migration and chemotaxis. The syndrome is due to the mutation in the CHS1 gene also called LYST. Mutation in this gene cause *beige* phenotype in mouse which encodes a large cytoplasmic protein of unknown function. CHS1 performs to function as an adapter protein that may put next to proteins that mediate intracellular membrane fusion reactions when both proteins interact [130].

### 22.8.7 Griscelli-Prunieras Syndrome (GS)

This syndrome is a very rare autosomal recessive disorder which relate with the defect of melanosome transport to nearby keratinocytes and hence results in hypopigmentation and neurological (GS1) or immunological (GS2) abnormalities whereas in GS3, only hypopigmentation is detected. Skin phenotype is common in all three types of GS and is characterized by silvery gray ear and a relative skin hypopigmentation. Patients with GS1 show neurological defects including developmental delay, hypotonia and mental retardation which is due to results from mutations in the MYO5A gene. This gene encodes for myosin 5a, molecular motor that binds with rab27a, and melanophilin, that allows the transport of the melanosomes on the actin fibers and the docking of the melanosomes at the extremities of the dendrites tips [131]. GS2 associates hypopigmentation and immunological abnormalities along with severe pyogenic infections with hemophagocytic syndrome. It comes with a mutation in RAB27A gene in mouse which result in the *ashen* phenotype, encodes and function as GTPase for melanosome transport [132]. GS3 expression is characteristic of hypopigmentation, results from mutation in the MLPH gene which results in *leaden* phenotype and encodes melanophilin thatact as same function as MYO5A (58). GS3 can also result from the deletion of the MYO5A F-exon, an exon with a tissue-restricted expression pattern [133]

### 22.8.8 Vitiligo

This disorder related to defect of survival of melanocytes and is an acquired cutaneous disorder of pigmentation, with a 1%–2% incidence worldwide. It is characterized by well-circumscribed, white cutaneous macules with absence of melanocytes. Latest studies reveal that it is an autoimmune disorder and relate to thyroid gland [134]. Many genes have been reported and published previously but none of them is convincing and promising till date. There are two large genome wide screens for generalized vitiligo linkage of an oligogenic auto immune susceptibility locus, termed AIS1 [135, 136] and also two new susceptibility loci have been found. Measures such as sun protection, concealers, topical steroids, phototherapy, depigmentation, and surgical grafting may improve the skin's appearance. Clinical trials of alternative treatments for vitiligo include *ginkgo biloba* only and the combination of folic acid and vitamin B-12, which have restored skin color in some individuals [137].

### 22.8.9 Tuberous Sclerosis

Tuberous Sclerosis complex (TSC) is congenital disease of high penetrance is characterized by the presence of hamartoma, which can affect mainly all the organs which affects skin, central nervous system, eyes, heart, and kidney mostly. It is also associated with multiple hepatic lipomatous tumours. [138] At later stages, brain and kidney malignant tumors pigmentary disorders can be observed. Almost in all cases Hypomelanotic macules are observed and described as white ash leaf-shaped macules [139]. Hypopigmented iris spots and leaf-shaped lesions of ocular fundus have been also reported [140, 141]. This disorder results from mutation in the TSC-1 gene and TSC-2 gene encoding for hamartin and tuberin, respectively [142, 143]. The exact function of these proteins is not known; however, both proteins interact directly with each other, and function together to regulate specific cellular processes [144]. Most patients with tuberous sclerosis have a normal life span. There is no proper treatment for tuberous sclerosis. Initial diagnosis and intervention can help individuals avoid or overcome developmental delays or progression of the disease. Seizures, a common complication, may respond to anti-seizure drugs. Complications of neurological, or brain, involvement are the most common cause of morbidity (sickness/hospitalization) and mortality (death). Kidney, or renal, complications are the next most frequent cause of morbidity and mortality.

## 22.9 Hypermelanosis

It is characterized by swirling streaks of hyperpigmented (darkened) skin. This disorder occurred may be due to the increase in tyrosine activity and hence results in more pigment formation within body. Some of the diseases which occurs due to hyperpigmentation are discussed below.

### 22.9.1 Café au lait macules

Café-au-lait is French for "coffee with milk" are hyperpigmented flat skin lesions ranging in color from tan to dark brown and ranging in size from 1 to 20-cm.

They can be found on any part of the body, but are commonly located on the thorax or trunk region. Microscopic examination reveals increased epidermal melanin pigment with normal number of melanocytes. Macromelanosomes that are a feature of cafe au lait macules of the neurofibromatosis are absent in sporadic cafe au lait macules. The occurrence of greater than six café-au-lait macules should raise the suspicion for the genetic disorder neurofibromatosis type 1 (NF1). Other genetic disorders associated with excessive café-au-lait macules include McCune-Albright syndrome, tuberous sclerosis, and Fanconi anemia. The macules are most frequently observed in childrens having dark pigmentation. Some of them are congenital, considered birthmarks, and some even fade or disappear with time. Café-au-lait macules usually do not require treatment, unless cosmetically necessary, in which case laser therapies and surgical removal is effective [145].

### 22.9.2 Neurofibromatosis (NF)

NF is an autosomal dominant disorder with a variable expressivity and affects approximately 1 in 3000 individuals, characterized by the presence of more than 6 cafe au lait spots, freckles in the axillary or inguinal regions, neurofibromas, Lisch nodules in the eyes, and bony defects. NF1 gene encode by a protein neurofibromin, a 327-kDa protein which presents homology with members of the GTPase-activating protein superfamily [146]. Neurofibromin involved in negative regulation of RAS oncogene [147] which showed tumor-suppressive activity. In NF1 patients, reduction in neurofibromin level in epidermis and hence pigmentation abnormalities occur. This was evidenced by neurofibromin level of cultured melanocytes by a mechanism independent NF1 gene transcription and translation, which might influence the degradation rate of the protein [148].

### 22.9.3 McCune-Albright Syndrome

McCune-Albright syndrome is a genetic disease that affects the bones and color (pigmentation) of the skin. This disease characterized by pigmented lesions, polyostotic fibrous dysplasia and endocrinologic abnormalities, including thyrotoxicosis, pituitary gigantism, precocious puberty and Cushing syndrome. The hallmark symptom of McCune-Albright syndrome is early puberty in girls. Menstrual periods may begin in early childhood, long before the breasts or pubic hair develop (which normally occur first). Puberty and menstrual bleeding may begin as early as 4 to 6 months in girls. This phenotype is associated with mutations in the GNAS1 gene [149, 150]. The mutation in α subunit of the G protein induces excess of endogenous cyclic adenosine monophosphate that causes constitutive activation of adenylyl cyclase which plays an essential role in melanogenesis and in melanosomes transport [4, 151]. There is no specific treatment for McCune-Albright syndrome. Drugs that block estrogen production, such as testolactone, have been tried with some success. Adrenal gland abnormalities (such as Cushing syndrome) may be treated with surgery to remove the adrenal glands. Gigantism and pituitary adenoma will need to be treated with medicines that block hormone production, or with surgery.

### 22.9.4 Melasma

An example of hyperpigmentation is melasma (also known as chloasma). This condition is characterized by brown to gray-brown patches, usually on the face. Most people get it on their cheeks, bridge of their nose, forehead, chin, and above their upper lip. It also can appear on other parts of the body that get lots of sun, such as the forearms and neck. Melasma can occur in pregnant women and is often called the "mask of pregnancy;" however, men can also develop this condition. However, it can develop after taking oral contraceptives, or anti-seizure medication (e.g. phenytoin [Dilantin]). Melasma sometimes goes away after pregnancy but has no specific symptoms but causes alarm due to its appearance. Available treatment therapies includes topical treatment with hydroquinone 3-percent or 4-percent, azelaic acid 20-percent cream, glycolic acid 10-percent peel and retinoids (e.g. tretinoin 0.05-percent or 0.1-percent cream, adapalene [Differin] 0.1-percent or 0.3-percent gel). Prevention of melasma may be aided by wearing sunscreen (at least SPF 30) and wide-brimmed hats [152].

### 22.9.5 Lentigens

Lentigens also called as Solar lentigines (singular, solar lentigo), or liver spots, are benign (noncancerous), hyperpigmented, flat skin lesions occurring on the sun-exposed areas of the body. They vary in color from light yellow to dark brown. The face, hands, forearms, chest, back, and shins are the most common areas of occurrence for solar lentigines. Caucasians and Asians are the most likely to develop solar lentigines and can be treated with lasers [153]. They are indicative of excess sun exposure (a risk factor for the development of skin cancer) and commonly appear when individuals are in their 30 s. When lentigens multiplies may be act as markr for the presence of a multisystem disorder. LEOPARD is a rare autosomal dominant disorder with high penetrance and variable expressivity. It shows lentigines, retardation of growth, ocular hypertelorism, pulmonary stenosis, electrocardiographic abnormalities, abnormal genitalia and deafness (sensorineural) [154, 155]. LEOPARD syndrome caused by mutations in the PTPN11 gene and is known as Noonan's syndrome [156]. Peutz-Jeghers syndrome is an autosomal dominant disorder described by lentiginosis of the buccal mucosa, digits, lips and hamartomatous polyps of the gastrointestinal tract and encodes the serine/threonine kinase STK11 gene [157, 158].

### 22.9.6 Freckles

Freckles, or ephelides, are small (one to two millimeter) flat skin lesions of uniform color and commonly found on the face, neck, chest, and arms, numbers from a few to hundreds. The gene for freckles is a recessive trait, which means both parents are carriers of the trait resulting in its appearance in offspring. Contrary to popular belief, freckles are not indicative of sun damage to the skin. Prevention of freckles may be accomplished with sunscreens, wide-brimmed hats, and long pants and sleeves. Undesired freckles can be treated similarly to solar lentigines with cryotherapy, hydroquinone, azelaic acid, glycolic acid peels, and laser therapy.

### 22.9.7 Leukomelanoderma

This is very rare autosomal recessive skin disorder. It is characterized by association of hypopigmented and hyperpigmented macules mostly on the back of the hands and feet. In this disease, an increase number of melanosomes in the melanocytes and the keratinocytes is resides within hyperpigmented macules, whereas a low density of DOPA (dihydroxyphenylalanine)- positive melanocytes is noted in hypopigmented lesions. In some areas, there are no visible melanocytes. The locus of the gene responsible for leukomelanoderma has recently been mapped to chromosome 1q21.3, and mutations were recognized in the DSRAD gene encoding double-stranded RNA-specific adenosine deaminase [159]. The pathogenesis of this disorder leading to these characteristic pigmentary troubles is, however, still unknown.

### 22.9.8 Melanoma

Melanoma is one of the most dangerous skin cancer that grows when unrepaired DNA damage to skin cells due to UV radiation or tanning beds and results in mutations that leads to the skin cells to multiply rapidly and form malignant tumors [160]. These tumors formed from the pigment-producing melanocytes present in the basal layer of the epidermis. Initially they resemble moles and some develop from moles. The majority of melanomas are black or brown, but they can also be skin-colored, pink, red, purple, blue or white. The survival time for metastatic melanoma patient is 8–9 months, and overall survival rate is less than 15% [161]. Conventional chemotherapy with the compound dacarbazine (DTIC) alone is associated with almost negligible survival response of 15% [162]. Immune studies (IFN-α and IL-2) shows some promising surviving rates but they showed intense toxicities and hence unfavorable for melanoma patients [163]. Molecular investigations suggested constant genetic patterns on each type of melanoma and 50–60% of them due to BRAF mutation [164, 165]. Deactivated tumor suppressor gene is also identifies in melanoma. In vitrostudies on various melanoma cell lines revealed that in melanoma transcriptional factors or cell cycle regulators, p16 and p14ARF are in activated

[166]. Melanoma at mucosal, acral and chronic sun damaged sites is due to the mutation in KIT genes [167], while uveal melanomas caused because of muataion in the α-subunit of G proteinof Gq family, GNAQ and GNA11 [168]. The cure of melanoma should be targeting signal molecules which is specific for definite type of melanoma. c-kit, RAS/RAF/MAPK/ERK pathway, MEK, PI3K pathways should be eligible for treatment in therapeutically manner. Treatment should also focus on targeting multiple coexistent aberrations in different pathways, and addressing the mechanisms that cause the tumor's tendency for growth and chemoresistance.

## 22.10 Treatment Options for Pigmentation Disorders

Multi-faceted approaches have been use in present treating scenario of treating skin pigmentation disorders. After getting detail about exact condition of the patient in case of pigmentation disorder, treatment regimen can be start at early as possible.

Many treatment modalities and therapeutic strategies are presently developed including chemical agents and physical therapies are now available to treat hypermelanosis and repigment hypomelanotic or amelanotic skin.

### 22.10.1 Wood's Light Investigation

This technique is performed in dark in which light source is from wood's lamp by which UV rays ranging from 320 to 400 nm is shone on to the skin of patients where melanin is in abundance. In pigmented skin, all the light were absorb and very little is reflect back and appears black, whereas less pigment skin (epidermal region), more light goes back and appear white. This method is useful when pigmentation is not apparent in visible light.

### 22.10.2 Phototherapy

Phototherapy also known as light therapy used to treat hyperpigmentation disorder with a special kind of light (narrowband ultraviolet B). other strategies used to treat skin disorder includes UV light A (UVA) phototherapy; photochemotherapy (oral and topical), such as psoralen plus UVA (PUVA) 308 nm excimer laser; and combination phototherapy.

### 22.10.3 Other Photochemotherapies

Phenylalanine plus UVA or Khellin (topical or systemic) plus UVA have also been proposed for the treatment of vitiligo. However, there has been conflicting reports regarding these treatment strategies, and reports suggested the hepatic toxicity due to excessive usage of khellin. For these reasons, these modalities were not suggested for the treatment of vitiligo.

### 22.10.4 IPL (Intense Pulsed Light)

IPL is also known as photofacial which is a noninvasive, no-downtime procedure to correct virtually any superficial blemish or hyperpigmentation. Nonerosive light has been use to addresses hyperpigmentation without harming healthy cells, allowing patients to resume their daily activities immediately. In this technique broad-spectrum light is use that reaches multiple layers of skin with brief flashes. This helps in skin natural healing process by warm the skin due to light flashes, as well as improves collagen growth underneath the skin. This multi-faceted approach take 30–60 min, makes skin look normal, smoother and more voluminous after treatment.

### 22.10.5 Fraxel Laser

This is FDA-approved fractional laser technology used for skin resurfacing, brighter, softer texturend pigmentation disorders without the nasty complications that tended to accompany it. This method is very new that creates thousands of microscopic treatment zones per square centimeter of skin, causing the natural healing process of the skin to stimulate melanin synthesis in case of depigmented disease and a regeneration of healthy skin cells with glowing texture.

### 22.10.6 Obagi Blue Peel

Obagi Blue Peel is a relatively simple, quick, in-office process considered to improve both the appearance and health of the skin by improving the pigmentation in skin. By mixing a low concentration (15–30%) of TCA (Trichloracetic Acid) in a blue solution, thin layers of damaged or depigmented cells can be removed from the skin.

### 22.10.7 Immunomodulators

Several previous studies reported various immunomodulatory drugs for the treatment of pigmentation disorders including levamisole, anapsos, isoprinosine, and suplatast, as repigmenting agents for the treatment of vitiligo. Nowadays, tacrolimus and pimecrolimus are used as an immune suppressant drugs which are known to possess additional anti-inflammatory action and are also used off-label for vitiligo treatment. Synergistic effects of these drugs with phototherapy are believed to produce a faster response but it also associated with an increased risk of skin infections and development of skin cancers when used for long term.

### 22.10.8 Corticosteroids

Steroid-induced repigmentation occurs within 5 months of treatment in a perifollicular way. They showed some side-effects too like steroid-induced acne, ecchymoses, rosacea, striae, dermal atrophy and telangiectasia. The mechanism of steroid-induced repigmentation is unknown, although several hypothesis are proposed, such as stimulation of melanocyte proliferation and migration and suppression of immunity-driven melanocyte destruction.

### 22.10.9 Surgical Therapy

This method targets to rebuild the epidermal (and perhaps follicular) compartment of the melanocyte population of the skin in patients with a total destruction of pigment cells and a lack of response to medical treatment [169, 170]. This option used in patients with persistent depigmentation caused by halo nevi, thermal burns, trauma, or piebaldism and in vitiligo patients, unlikely to respond to medical therapies [171–173]. Several methods are available including punch grafts; blister grafts; split-thickness grafts; and autologous transplantation of melanocyte suspensions, cultured melanocytes, or cultured epidermal grafts including melanocytes. Repigment of vitiligo leukotrichia has also been performed successfully by grafting of follicular melanocytes [174].

### 22.10.10 Antioxidant Therapy

The objective for this approach based on the hypothesis that vitiligo results from a deficiency of natural antioxidant mechanisms. Although till date not validated by a controlled clinical trial, ascorbic acid, tocopherol, selenium methionine and ubiquinone are widely used to arrest vitiligo spreading and to helps in repigmentation of skin.

### 22.10.11 Melagenina

Melagenina is a hydroalcoholic extract of the human placenta with α-lipoprotein as an active ingredient. Preliminary studies in Cuba claimed that 84% of vitiligo patients achieved total repigmentation but other laboratories have not been able to claim which was Cuban group said. Recently, an ointment was developed in Cuba by renowned Dr. Carlos Manuel Miyares and he made melagenina plus. They claimed this ointment that triggers the production of melanocytes which was made by mixing alcoholic extraction of the human placenta with Melagenina and calcium chloride.

### 22.10.12 Cold-Atmospheric Plasma

Cold-atmospheric plasma (CAP) is presently use in various dermatological diseases including vitiligo, scar reduction, wound healing and skin cancers like melanoma etc. Plasma treatment receives a lot of attention and opens a completely new unexplored area known as Plasma medicine. In the early stage of pigmentation disorders, plasma treatment seems to support the inflammation needed for skin recovery. CAP is now days used in cancer therapy, wound healing, MAPK signal pathway activation and anti-ageing therapy [175]. In later stages and in the hyperpigmentation disorder (melanoma), plasma treatment possibly shows better results compared to the control group in terms of avoiding different post-traumatic skin disorders. As the main result, plasma treatment in differentiated time related dosages shows superior aesthetic features from the beginning to the end of scar formation. The synergistic effects of nanoemulsion of some novel herbal compounds with cold-plasma also in its preliminary studies as better drug delivery system for the treatment of pigmentation disorder. Some natural compounds like naringin (flavonoid in citrus fruit) showed improved tyrosinase activity (83.3% activity increase in activity after 10 min plasma treatment) using μ-dielectric barrier discharge (μ-DBD) plasma source [2], hence can also prove potent candidate to treat hyper-pigmentation and related disorders in future. To understand the plasma treatment effect on eugenol derivatives circular dichroism (CD) study was performed. The CD spectrum for eugenol derivatives (ED) and plasma activated eugenol derivatives (PAED) showed changes in α-helix and β-sheets in mushroom tyrosinase.

These two derivatives reported to increase the melanin synthesis in B16F10 cells using cold atmospheric plasma through enhanced intracellular ROS and activation of cAMP pathway which in turn up-regulates the MITF and TRP1 expressions eventually triggering the melanin synthesis in cells [22].

Safety of the drug is the first requirement to test its any biological activity. Maximum concentration of 4b and 6a as safe dose for skin melanoma (B16F10), skin fibroblast (L929) and human skin epidermal keratinocyte (HaCaT) cells was determined as 42 μg/mL (Fig. 22.7).

The B16F10 cells were treated with 4b and 6a with or without plasma treatment in the absence or presence of MSH. The test compounds showed synergic effect and increase in melanin synthesis with plasma treatment and/or MSH addition. The cellular melanin content was detected as 125% and 156% with respect to normalized 100% control by the treatment of 4b (35 μg/mL) and 4b (35 μg/mL) + MSH, respectively (Fig. 22.8). This increase in melanin content was verified by visual test as shown in Fig. 22.9. Moreover, the melanin was increased to 125% and 143% and 188% with 4b (35 μg/mL), 10 min plasma treated 4b (35 μg/mL), and 4b (35 μg/mL) + MSH exposure, respectively (Fig. 22.8). Similar trend in melanin stimulation was observed with 6b compound with or without plasma treatment in the presence

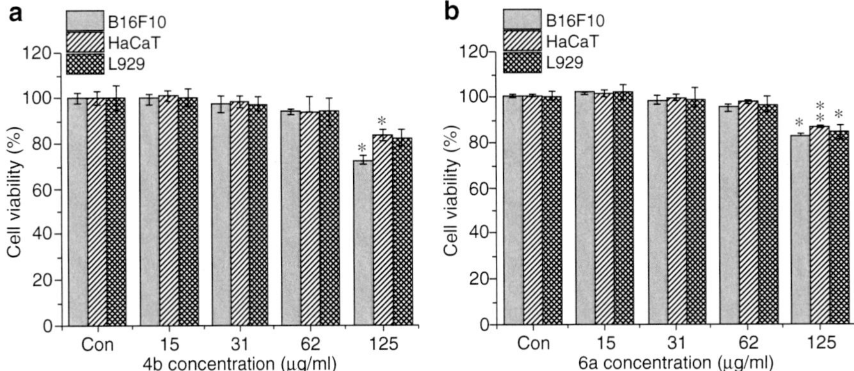


**Fig. 22.7** Cell viability measurement. The murine melanoma (B16F10), human skin keratinocyte (HaCaT), and murine skin fibroblast (L929) cells were incubated with different concentrations of (**a**) 4b and (**b**) 6a, and the cell viability was accessed by MTT assay. The data were expressed as a percentage of the control (normalized to 100%) from three independent experiments with mean ± standard deviation and were analyzed using Student's t-tests, $*p < 0.05$, $**p < 0.005$

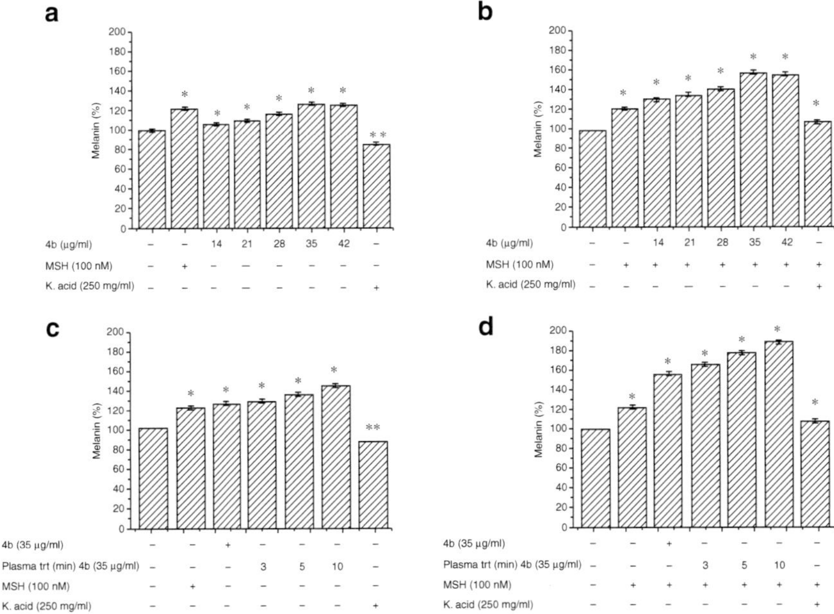


**Fig. 22.8** Intracellular melanin measurement. B16F10 cells were incubated with various concentrations of as-synthesized 4b in the (**a**) absence and (**b**) presence of α-MSH and melanin was detected. Moreover, B16F10 cells were also incubated with plasma-treated 4b in the (**c**) absence and (**d**) presence of α-MSH, except for the control containing only the media. All data were expressed as a percentage of the control (normalized to 100%) from three independent experiments with mean ± standard deviation and were analyzed using Student's t-tests, $*p < 0.05$, $**p < 0.005$

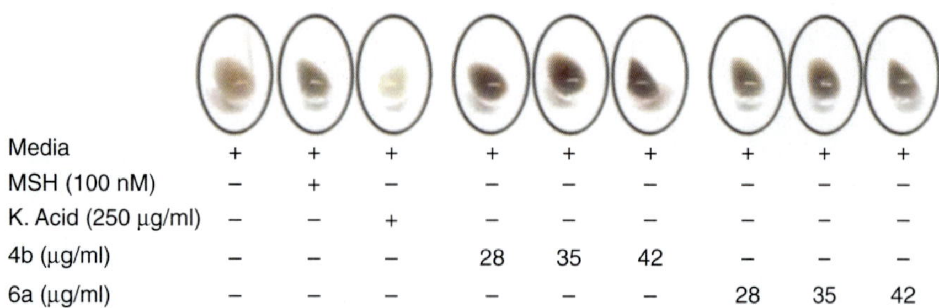


**Fig. 22.9** Images of melanoma B16F10 cell pallets. B16F10 cells were incubated with indicated concentrations of 4b and 6a for 24 h and then centrifuged to photograph the cell pellet. The cells grown with media only are shown as the control, while the cells grown with α-MSH and Kojic acid in media are shown as positive and negative controls, respectively

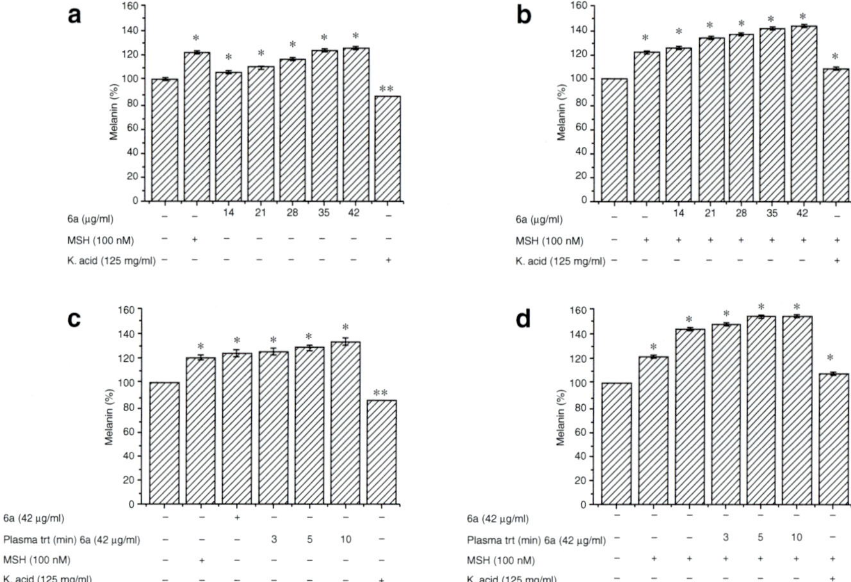


**Fig. 22.10** Intracellular melanin measurement. B16F10 cells were incubated with various concentrations of as-synthesized 6a in the (**a**) absence and (**b**) presence of α-MSH and melanin was detected. Moreover, B16F10 cells were also incubated with plasma-treated 6a in the (**c**) absence and (**d**) presence of α-MSH, except for the control containing only the media. All data were expressed as a percentage of the control (normalized to 100%) from three independent experiments with mean ± standard deviation and were analyzed using Student's t-tests, $*p < 0.05$, $**p < 0.005$

or absence of MSH (Fig. 22.10). To understand the mechanism of melanin activation by ED and PAED, the intracellular ROS and cAMP pathway was investigated.

The intracellular ROS was increased with the incubation of 4b and 6a compounds with B16F10 cells. Interestingly, more increase in intracellular ROS with PAED (4b, 6a) than ED (4b, 6a) was measured. However, 4b showed more increase in intracellular ROS than 6b with and without plasma treatment (Fig. 22.11).

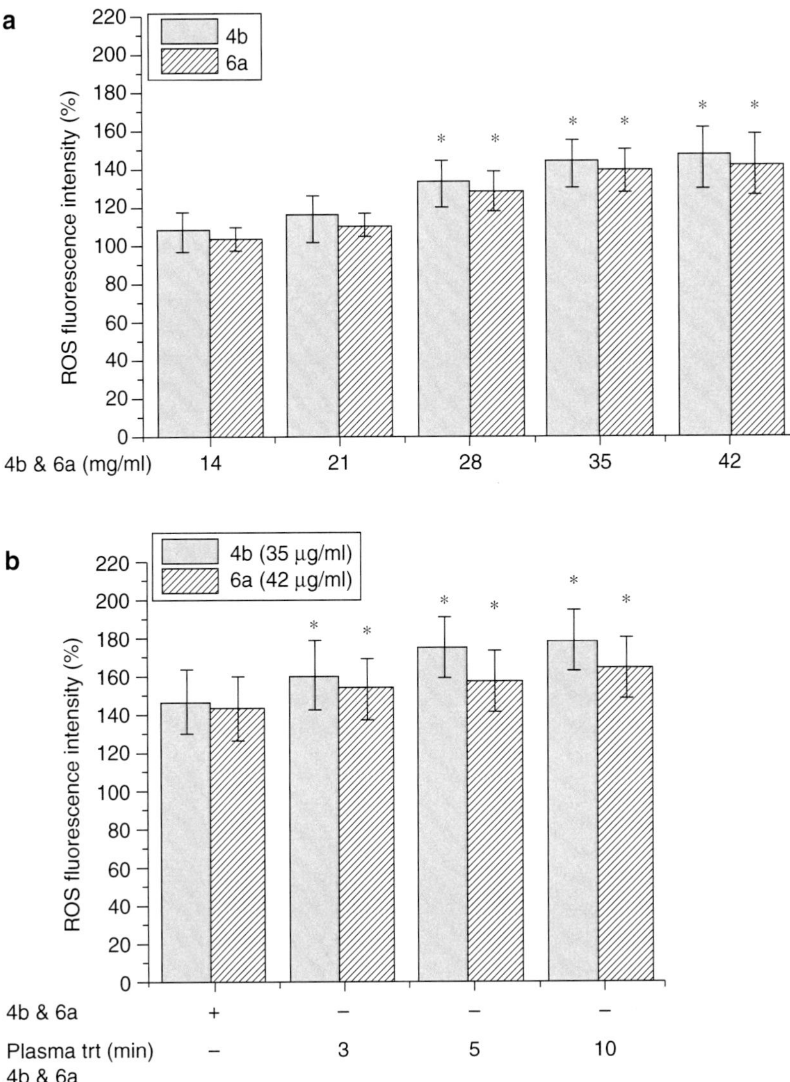


**Fig. 22.11** Intracellular ROS detection. The ROS detected from B16F10 cells, incubated with (**a**) assynthesized and (**b**) plasma-treated 4b and 6a compounds. The data were expressed as a percentage of the control (normalized to 100%) from three independent experiments with mean ± standard deviation and were analyzed using Student's t-tests, $^{*}p < 0.05$

To explore the mechanism further, cAMP level was quantified in B16F10 cells. The cAMP expression was increased with as synthesized 4b and 6a treatment. However, the cAMP expression was enhanced even more with plasma treated compounds (4b and 6a), and MSH treatment (Fig. 22.12). In general, the level of cAMP expression was higher for 4b than 6a at tested concentrations in the presence or absence of MSH. Moreover, western blot analysis showed higher expression of

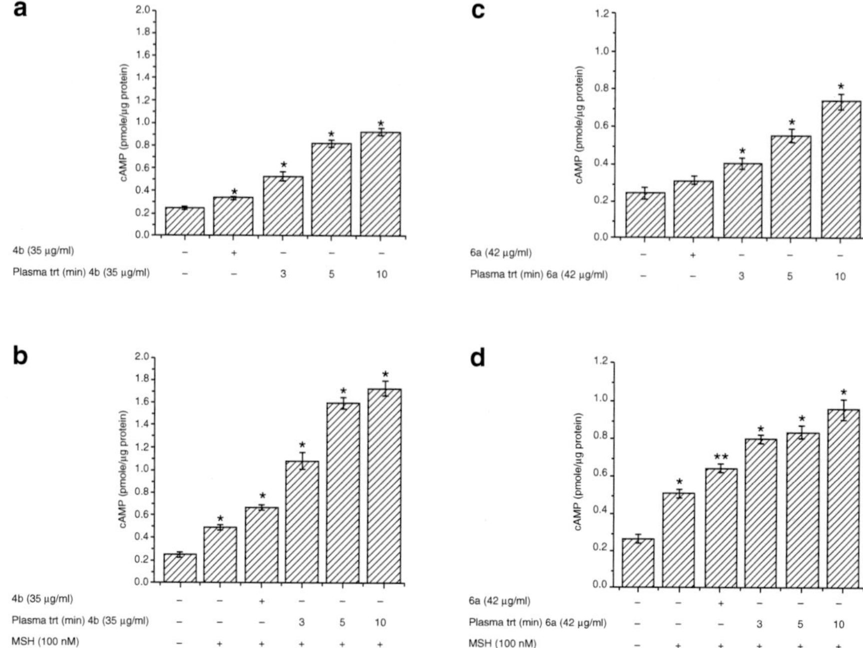


**Fig. 22.12** Analysis of cAMP expression in B16F10 cells incubated with (**a**) 4b with and without plasmatreatment, (**b**) 4b with and without plasma-treatment + α-MSH, (**c**) 6b with and without plasma-treatment, and (**d**) 6b with and without plasma-treatment + α-MSH as indicated in graph. The data from three independent experiments was expressed as mean ± standard deviation and was analyzed using Student's t-tests, $*p < 0.05$, $**p < 0.005$

MITF and TRP1 with ED and PAED (4b or 6a) treatment (Fig. 22.13). The MITF and TRP1 expression was more for PAED than ED (4b and 6a). However, no significant change in cellular tyrosinase expression was observed after incubation with ED and PAED.

The present results confirmed enhanced intracellular ROS with increasing concentration of test compound 4a and 6b (Fig. 22.11). The increased cellular ROS level activates the cAMP pathway, up-regulating the MITF and TRP1 expressions (Figs. 22.12 and 22.13), that eventually trigger the melanin synthesis in cells. Interestingly, higher expression of cAMP, MITF and TRP1 was observed for PAED than ED which could be the responsible for higher melanin synthesis in cells incubated with PAED (4b and 6a). Hence, this work confirmed that plasma activated eugenol derivatives (4b and 6a) have ability to increase their cellular melanogenic activity, suggesting important application to treat hypo-pigmentation and related disorders in future.

Interestingly, CAP itself in the form of plasma activated solutions (PAS) found to increase melanin content *in vitro* and *in vivo* animal models. The long term results

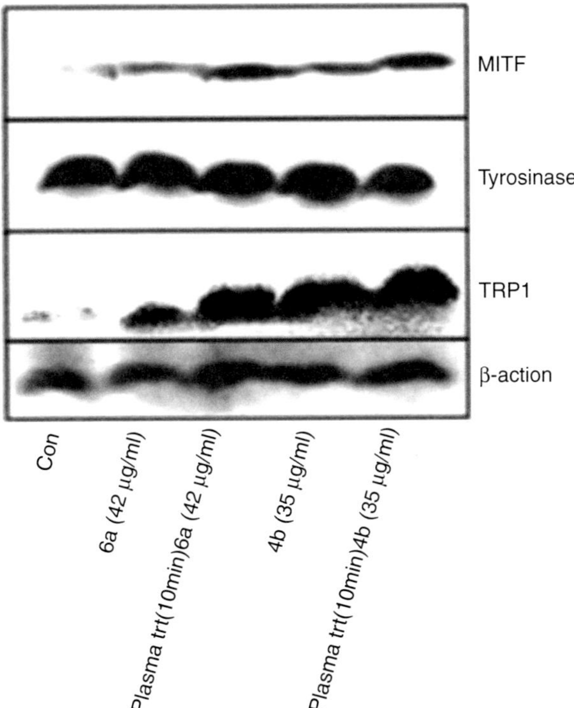


**Fig. 22.13** Analysis of MITF, tyrosinase and TRP1 expression in B16F10 cells. The cells were incubated with as-synthesized and plasma treated 4b and 6a compounds, and the expression of indicated proteins was checked by western blot technique

of these studies will certainly promising to go ahead preparing randomized clinical trials in plasma medicine and regulate melanogenesis which may help to control hyper or hypo pigmentation problems in future.

**Conclusion**

Skin pigmentation and its disorders till date remains in the crossroads of the laboratory and the clinics. Several mutations caused pigmentation disorder are phenotypically very intense but till now not fully characterized, however they give information about basic genetic and developmental mechanisms and provide crucial evidences about the process of photoprotection, cancer susceptibility and human evolution [176]. Technological advancement make targeted knockouts of certain genes responsible for pigmentation disorder that also spare embryonic lethality for vital genes showed elucidation of genetic regulators of pigmentation.

In this chapter an endeavor has been made to describe the mechanism of melanin formation and its correlation with the enzymatic process involved with experimental and clinical observation on melanin pigmentation. Presence of hypermelanin and hypomelanin causes malignancies in skin and likely to be most preventable. UVR is the most common known environmental carcinogen present which cause skin cancer in considerable fraction which is mainly caused because of sun-seeking activities in today's society. The role of pigmentation and the genetic diseases associated with them provide us the opportunities to improve our understanding of melanocytic contributions to pigmentation disorders. There are still many pigmentary disorders which is still completely unknown. Most of the skin diseases described showed the resembled symptoms to each other but the pathogenesis leading from altered gene to mutated protein to the clinical phenotype is still not clearly understood. According to the almost daily new research it is likely that our knowledge of the genes involved in pigmentary disorders will grow drastically in the near future. Through their aesthetical effect, pigmentary disorders are a recurrent therapeutic demand in dermatology. Cold-atmospheric plasma promisingly can be used to treat pigmentary disorder in future and may be used along with novel nanocompounds or natural products to increase their efficacy, for better drug delivery and hence available for treating skin syndromes. Although there are numerous therapeutic options are available but results are often difficult to obtained from them. The improved and better understanding of the molecular mechanisms responsible for these pigmentary changes and introduction of some new hormonal, immune enhancer medication will bring new therapeutic approaches for the pigmentary disorders.

**Conflict of Interest** The authors declare no conflict of interest.

**Funding** This work was supported by a grant from the National Research Foundation of Korea (NRF), which is funded by the Korean Government, Ministry of Science, ICT and Future Planning (MSIP), (NRF-2016K1A4A3914113) and Kwangwoon University in 2017.

## References

1. Deng L, Xu S. Adaptation of human skin color in various populations. Hereditas. 2017;15:155–61.
2. Kim HJ, Yong HI, Park S, Kim K, Kim TH, Choe W, Jo C. Effect of atmospheric pressure dielectric barrier discharge plasma on the biological activity of naringin. Food Chem. 2014;160:241–5.
3. Kobayashi T, Vieira WD, Potterf B, Sakai C, Imokawa G, Hearing VJ. Modulation of melanogenic protein expression during the switch from eu- to pheomelanogenesis. J Cell Sci. 1995;108:2301–9.
4. Busca R, Ballotti R. Cyclic AMP a key messenger in the regulation of skin pigmentation. Pigment Cell Res. 2000a;13:60–9.
5. Steingrímsson E, Copeland NG, Jenkins NA. Melanocytes and the microphthalmia transcription factor network. Annu Rev Genet. 2004;38:365–411.
6. Bertolotto C, Abbe P, Hemesath TJ, Bille K, Fisher DE, Ortonne JP, Ballotti R. Microphthalmia gene product as a signal transducer in cAMP-induced differentiation of melanocytes. J Cell Biol. 1998;142:827–35.
7. Yasumoto K, Yokoyama K, Takahashi K, Tomita Y, Shibahara S. Functional analysis of microphthalmia-associated transcription factor in pigment cell-specific transcription of the human tyrosinase family genes. J Biol Chem. 1997;272:503–9.

8. Yavuzer U, Keenan E, Lowings P. The Microphthalmia gene product interacts with the retinoblastoma protein in vitro and is a target for deregulation of melanocyte-specific transcription. Oncogene. 1995;10:123–34.
9. Verschoore M, Gupta S, Sharma VK, Ortonne JP. Determination of melanin and haemoglobin in the skin of idiopathic cutaneous hyperchromia of the orbital region (ICHOR): a study of Indian patients. J Cutan Aesthet Surg. 2012;5:176–82.
10. Solano F. Melanins: skin pigments and much more—types, structural models, biological functions, and formation routes. New J Sci. 2014;498276:1–28.
11. Nishimura EK. Melanocyte stem cells: a melanocyte reservoir in hair follicles for hair and skin pigmentation. Pigment Cell Melanoma Res. 2011;24:401–10.
12. Ortonne JP, et al. PUVA-induced repigmentation of vitiligo: scanning electron microscopy of hair follicles. J Invest Dermatol. 1980;74:40–2.
13. Staricco RG. Amelanotic melanocytes in the outer sheath of the human hair follicle and their role in the repigmentation of regenerated epidermis. Ann NY Acad Sci. 1963;100:239–55.
14. Paul M, Jennifer R. Radiative relaxation quantum yields for synthetic eumelanin. Photochem Photobiol. 2007;79:211–6.
15. Vandamme M. Antitumor effect of plasma treatment on U87 glioma xenografts: preliminary results. Plasma Process Polym. 2010;7:264–73.
16. Fridman A. Plasma chemistry. CambridgeCambridge University Press 2008. https://doi.org/10.1017/CBO9780511546075.
17. Graves DB. Low temperature plasma biomedicine: a tutorial review. Phys Plasmas. 2014;21:080901.
18. Lee A, Lin A, Shah K, Singh H, Miller V, Rao SG. Optimization of non-thermal plasma treatment in an in vivo model organism. PLoS One. 2016;11:e0160676.
19. Fathollah S, Mipour S, Mansouri P, Dehpour AR, Ghoranneviss M, Rahimi N, Naraghi ZS, Chalangari R, Chalangari KM. Investigation on the effects of the atmospheric pressure plasma on wound healing in diabetic rats. Sci Rep. 2016;6:19144.
20. Keidar M. Plasma for cancer treatment. Plasma Sources Sci Technol. 2015;24:33001.
21. Sladek REJ. Plasma treatment of dental cavities: a feasibility study. IEEE Trans Plasma Sci. 2004;32:2002–5.
22. Ali A, Ashraf Z, Kumar N, Rafiq M, Jabeen F, Park JH, Choi KH, Lee S, Seo SY, Choi EH, Attri P. Influence of plasma-activated compounds on melanogenesis and tyrosinase activity. Sci Rep. 2016;6:21779.
23. Rees JL. The melanocortin 1 receptor (MC1R): more than just red hair. Pigment Cell Res. 2000;13:135–40.
24. Slominski A, Paus R. Are l-tyrosine and l-dopa hormone-like bioregulators. J Theor Biol. 1990;143:123–38.
25. Tadokoro R, Takahashi Y. Intercellular transfer of organelles during body pigmentation. Curr Opin Genet Dev. 2017;45:132–8.
26. Wang Y, Viennet C, Robin S, Berthon JY, He L, Humbert P. Precise role of dermal fibroblasts on melanocyte pigmentation. J Dermatol Sci. 2017;S0923-1811(17):30082–8.
27. Diniz GB, Bittencourt JC. The melanin-concentrating hormone as an integrative peptide driving motivated behaviors. Front Syst Neurosci. 2017;11:32.
28. Hearing VJ, Tsukamoto K. Enzymatic control of pigmentation in mammals. FASEB J. 1991;5:2902–9.
29. Lerner AB, Fitzpatrick TB. Biochemistry of melanin formation. Physiol Rev. 1950;30:1–126.
30. Mason HS. The chemistry of melanin. III. Mechanism of the oxidation of dihydroxyphenylalanine by tyrosinase. J Biol Chem. 1948;172:83–98.
31. Pawelek JM, Korner AM. The biosynthesis of mammalian melanin. Am Sci. 1982;70:136–45.
32. Prota G. Melanins and melanogenesis. New York: Academic, 1992.
33. Prota G. The chemistry of melanins and melanogenesis. Fortsch Chem Organ Nat. 1995;64:93–148.

34. Hearing V. The melanosome: the perfect model for cellular responses to the environment. Pigment Cell Res. 2000;13:23–34.
35. Matsunaga J, Sinha D, Solano F, Santis C, Wistow G, Hearing V. Macrophage migration inhibitory factor (MIF)—its role in catecholamine metabolism. Cell Mol Biol. 1999;45:1035–40.
36. Rosengren E, Bucala R, Aman P, Jacobsson L, Odh G, Metz CN, Rorsman H. The immunoregulatory mediator macrophage migration inhibitory factor (MIF) catalyzes a tautomerization reaction. Mol Med. 1996;2:143–9.
37. Schallreuter KU, Lemke KR, Hill HZ, Wood JM. Thioredoxin reductase induction coincides with melanin biosynthesis in brown and black guinea pigs and in murine melanoma cells. J Invest Dermatol. 1994;103:820–4.
38. Slominski A, Paus R. Towards defining receptors for l-tyrosine and l-DOPA. Mol Cell Endocrinol. 1994;99:C7–C11.
39. Slominski A, Pruski D. L-DOPA binding sites in rodent melanoma cells. Biochem Biophys Acta. 1992;1139:324–8.
40. Slominski A. POMC gene expression in hamster and mouse melanoma cells. FEBS Lett. 1991;291:165–8.
41. Lin JY, Fisher DE. Melanocyte biology and skin pigmentation. Nature. 2007;445:843–50.
42. Herraiz C, Garcia-Borron JC, Jiménez-Cervantes C, Olivares C. MC1R signaling. Intracellular partners and pathophysiological implications. Biochim Biophys Acta. 2017;1863(10 Pt A):2448–61.
43. Haddadeen C, Lai C, Cho SY, Healy E. Variants of the melanocortin-1 receptor: do they matter clinically? Exp Dermatol. 2015;24:5–9.
44. Kollias N. The spectroscopy of human melanin pigmentation in melanin: its role in human photoprotection. Valdenmar; 1995. pp. 31–8.
45. de Gruijl FR. UV adaptation: pigmentation and protection against overexposure. Exp Dermatol. 2017;26:557–62.
46. Chedekel MR. Photochemistry and photobiology of epidermal melanins. Photochem Photobiol. 1982;35:881–5.
47. Mitra D, Luo X, Morgan A. An ultraviolet-radiation independent pathway to melanoma carcinogenesis in the red hair/fair skin. Nature. 2012;491:449–53.
48. Hill HZ. The function of melanin or six blind people examine an elephant. BioEssays. 1992;14:49–56.
49. Wang Z, Dillon J, Gaillard ER. Antioxidant properties of melanin in retinal pigment epithelial cells. Photochem Photobiol. 2006;82:474–9.
50. Sarangarajan R, Apte SP. Melanization and phagocytosis: implications for age related macular degeneration. Mol Vis. 2005;11:482–90.
51. Meyer zum Gottesberge AM. Physiology and pathophysiology of inner ear melanin. Pigment Cell Res. 1988;1:238–49.
52. Gonzalez-Santoyo I, Cordoba-Aguilar A. Phenoloxidase: a key component of the insect immune system. Entomol Exp Appl. 2012;142:1–16.
53. Nappi AJ, Vass E. Melanogenesis and the generation of cytotoxic molecules during insect cellular immune reactions. Pigment Cell Res. 1993;6:117–26.
54. Lee H, Dellatore SM, Miller WM, Messersmith PB. Mussel-inspired surface chemistry for multifunctional coatings. Science. 2007;318:426–30.
55. Abbas M, Amico FD, Morresi L, et al. Structural, electrical, electronic and optical properties of melanin films. Eur Phys J E Soft Matter. 2009;28:285–91.
56. Bothma JP, de Boor J, Divakar U, Schwenn PE, Meredith P. Device-quality electrically conducting melanin thin films. Adv Mater. 2008;20:3539–42.
57. Apte M, Girme G, Bankar A, RaviKumar A, Zinjarde S. 3,4-dihydroxy-L-phenylalanine-derived melanin from Yarrowia lipolytica mediates the synthesis of silver and gold nanostructures. J Nanobiotech. 2013;11:1–9.
58. Robins AH. Biological perspectives on human pigmentation. Cambridge, NY: Cambridge University Press; 1991.

59. Lees FC, Byard PJ. Skin colorimetry in Belize. I. Conversion formulae. Am J Phys Anthropol. 1978;48:515–22.
60. Lees FC, Byard PJ, Relethford JH. New conversion formulae for light-skinned populations using photovolt and E.E.L. reflectometers. Am J Phys Anthropol. 1979;51:403–8.
61. Hunter RS. Photoelectric tristimulus colorimetry with three filters. Circular of the National Bureau of Standards C429. J Opt Soc Am. 1942;32:509–38.
62. Stamatas GN, Zmudzka BZ, Kollias N, Beer JZ. Non-invasive measurements of skin pigmentation *in situ*. Pigment Cell Res. 2004;17:618–26.
63. Diffey BL, Oliver RJ, Farr PM. A portable instrument for quantifying erythema induced by ultraviolet radiation. Br J Dermatol. 1984;3:663–72.
64. Kollias N, Sayer RM, Zeise L, Chedekel MR. Photoprotection by melanin. J Photochem Photobiol B Biol. 1991;9:135–60.
65. Shriver MD, Parra EJ. Comparison of narrow-band reflectance spectroscopy and tristimulus colorimetry for measurements of skin and hair color in persons of different biological ancestry. Am J Phys Anthrop. 2000;112:17–27.
66. Kollias N, Baqer A. Spectroscopic characteristics of human melanin *in vivo*. J Invest Dermatol. 1985;85:38–42.
67. Kollias N, Baqer AH. Absorption mechanism of human melanin in the visible, 400-720 nm. J Invest Dermatol. 1987;89:384–8.
68. Chaplin G. Geographic distribution of environmental factors influencing human skin coloration. Am J Phys Anthropol. 2004;125:292–302.
69. Jablonski NG, Chaplin G. The evolution of human skin coloration. J Hum Evol. 2000;39:57–106.
70. Mason HS, Ingram DJE, Allen B. The free radical property of melanins. Arch Biochem Biophys. 1960;86:225–30.
71. Meredith P, Sarna T. The physical and chemical properties of eumelanin. Pigment Cell Res. 2006;19:572–94.
72. Fligge M, Solanki SK. The solar spectral irradiance since 1700. Geophys Res Lett. 2000;27:2157–60.
73. Kane RP. Mismatch between variations of solar indices, stratospheric ozone and UV-B observed at ground. J Atmos Sol Terr Phys. 2002;64:2063–74.
74. Kimlin MG. The climatology of vitamin D producing ultraviolet radiation over the United States. J Steroid Biochem Mol Biol. 2004;89-90:479–83.
75. Webb AR, Kline L, Holick MF. Influence of season and latitude on the cutaneous synthesis of vitamin D3: exposure to winter sunlight in Boston and Edmonton will not promote vitamin D3 synthesis in human skin. J Clin Endocrinol Metab. 1988;67:373–8.
76. Webb AR. Who, what, where and when–influences on cutaneous vitamin D synthesis. Prog Biophys Mol Biol. 2006;92:17–25.
77. Goor Y, Rubinstein A. Vitamin D levels in dark skinned people. Israel J Med Sci. 1995;31:237–8.
78. Holick MF. Photosynthesis of vitamin D in the skin: effect of environmental and life-style variables. Fed Proc. 1987;46:1876–82.
79. Skull SA, Ngeow JY, Biggs BA, Street A, Ebeling PR. Vitamin D deficiency is common and unrecognized among recently arrived adult immigrants from the Horn of Africa. Intern Med J. 2003;33:47–51.
80. Vashi NA, Wirya SA, Inyang M, Kundu RV. Facial hyperpigmentation in skin of color: special considerations and treatment. Am J Clin Dermatol. 2017;18:215–30.
81. Mosher DB, Fitzpatrick TB. Piebaldism. Arch Dermatol. 1988;124:364–5.
82. Spritz RA. Piebaldism, Waardenburg syndrome and related disorders of melanocyte development. Semin Cutan Med Surg. 1997;16:15–23.
83. Jimbow K, Fitzpatrick TB, Szabo G, Hori Y. Congenital circumscribed hypomelanosis: a characterization based on electron microscopic study of tuberous sclerosis, nevus depigmentosus, and piebaldism. J Invest Dermatol. 1975;64:50–62.

84. Ezoe K, Holmes SA, Ho L, et al. Novel mutations and deletions of the KIT (steel factor receptor) gene in human piebaldism. Am J Hum Genet. 1995;56:58–66.
85. Fleischman RA, Saltman DL, Stastny V, et al. Deletion of the c-kit protooncogene in the human developmental defect piebald trait. Proc Natl Acad Sci U S A. 1991;88:10885–9.
86. Grabbe J, Welker P, Dippel E, et al. Stem cell factor, a novel cutaneous growth factor for mast cells and melanocytes. Arch Dermatol Res. 1994;287:78–84.
87. Nishikawa S, Kusakabe M, Yoshinaga K, et al. *Inutero* manipulation of coat color formation by a monoclonal anti-c-kit antibody: two distinct waves of c-kit-dependency during melanocyte development. EMBO J. 1991;10:2111–8.
88. Wang R, Shu S, Zhang Y, Luo W, Zhang X. Identification of a novel KIT mutation in a Chinese family affected with piebaldism. Zhonghua Yi Xue Yi Chuan Xue Za Zhi. 2016;33:637–40.
89. Hasan S, Dinh K, Lombardo F, et al. Hypopigmentation in an African patient treated with imatinib mesylate: a case report. J Natl Med Assoc. 2003;95:722–4.
90. Raanani P, Goldman JM, Ben-Bassat I. Challenges in oncology. Case 3. Depigmentation in a chronic myeloid leukemia patient treated with STI-571. J Clin Oncol. 2002;20:869–70.
91. Robert C, Spatz A, Faivre S, et al. Tyrosine kinase inhibition and grey hair. Lancet. 2003;361:1056.
92. El Kouarty H, Dakhama BS. Piebaldism: a pigmentary anomaly to recognize: about a case and review of the literature. Pan Afr Med J. 2016;14:155.
93. Hart J, Miriyala K. Neural tube defects in Waardenburg syndrome: A case report and review of the literature. Am J Med Genet A. 2017;173(9):2472–7. https://doi.org/10.1002/ajmg.a.38325.
94. Hageman MJ, Delleman JW. Heterogeneity in Waardenburg syndrome. Am J Hum Genet. 1977;29:468–85.
95. Liu XZ, Newton VE, Read AP. Waardenburg syndrome type II: phenotypic findings and diagnostic criteria. Am J Med Genet. 1995;55:95–100.
96. Kaplan P, de Chaderevian JP. Piebaldism-Waardenburg syndrome: histopathologic evidence for a neural crest syndrome. Am J Med Genet. 1988;31:679–88.
97. Ortonne JP. Piebaldism, Waardenburg's syndrome, and related disorders. "Neural crest depigmentation syndromes?". Dermatol Clin. 1988;6:205–16.
98. Baldwin CT, Hoth CF, Macina RA, et al. Mutations in PAX3 that cause Waardenburg syndrome type I: ten new mutations and review of the literature. Am J Med Genet. 1995;58:115–22.
99. Baldwin CT, Lipsky NR, Hoth CF, et al. Mutations in PAX3 associated with Waardenburg syndrome type I. Hum Mutat. 1994;3:205–11.
100. Hoth CF, Milunsky A, Lipsky N, et al. Mutations in the paired domain of the human PAX3 gene cause Klein-Waardenburg syndrome (WS-III) as well as Waardenburg syndrome type I (WS-I). Am J Hum Genet. 1993;52:455–62.
101. Tassabehji M, Read AP, Newton VE, et al. Mutations in the PAX3 gene causing Waardenburg syndrome type 1 and type 2. Nat Genet. 1993;3:26–30.
102. Wollnik B, Tukel T, Uyguner O, et al. Homozygous and heterozygous inheritance of PAX3 mutations causes different types of Waardenburg syndrome mutations in the PAX3 gene causing Waardenburg syndrome type 1 and type 2. Am J Med Genet. 2003;122A:42–5.
103. Goulding MD, Lumsden A, Gruss P. Signals from the notochord and floor plate regulate the region-specific expression of two Pax genes in the developing spinal cord. Development. 1993;117:1001–16.
104. Watanabe A, Takeda K, Ploplis B, et al. Epistatic relationship between Waardenburg syndrome genes MITF and PAX3 mutations in PAX3 that cause Waardenburg syndrome type I ten new mutations and review of the literature mutations in PAX3 associated with Waardenburg syndrome type I mutations in the paired domain of the human PAX3 gene cause Klein-Waardenburg syndrome (WS-III) as well as Waardenburg syndrome type I (WS-I). Nat Genet. 1998;18:283–6.
105. McGill GG, Horstmann M, Widlund HR, et al. Bcl2 regulation by the melanocyte master regulator Mitf modulates lineage survival and melanoma cell viability. Cell. 2002;109:707–18.

106. Shah KN, Dalal SJ, Desai MP, et al. White forelock, pigmentary disorder of irides, and long segment Hirschsprung disease: possible variant of Waardenburg syndrome. J Pediatr. 1981;99:432–5.
107. Bogdanova-Mihaylova P, Alexander MD, Murphy RP, Murphy SM. Waardenburg syndrome: a rare cause of inherited neuropathy due to SOX10 mutation. J Peripher Nerv Syst. 2017;22(3):219–23. https://doi.org/10.1111/jns.12221.
108. Edery P, Attie T, Amiel J, et al. Mutation of the endothelin-3 gene in the Waardenburg-Hirschsprung disease (Shah-Waardenburg syndrome). Nat Genet. 1996;12:442–4.
109. McCallion AS, Chakravarti A. EDNRB/EDN3 and Hirschsprung disease type II. Pigment Cell Res. 2001;14:161–9.
110. Pingault V, Bondurand N, Lemort N, et al. A heterozygous endothelin 3 mutation in Waardenburg-Hirschsprung disease: is there a dosage effect of EDN3/EDNRB gene mutations on neurocristopathy phenotypes? J Med Genet. 2001;38:205–9.
111. Pingault V, Bondurand N, Kuhlbrodt K, et al. SOX10 mutations inpatients with Waardenburg-Hirschsprung disease. Nat Genet. 1998;18:171–3.
112. Chan KK, Wong CK, Lui VC, et al. Analysis of SOX10 mutations identified in Waardenburg-Hirschsprung patients: differential effects on target gene regulation. J Cell Biochem. 2003;90:573–85.
113. Paratore C, Goerich DE, Suter U, et al. Survival and glial fate acquisition of neural crest cells are regulated by an interplay between the transcription factor Sox10 and extrinsic combinatorial signaling. Development. 2001;128:3949–61.
114. Arveiler B, Lasseaux E, Morice-Picard F. Clinical and genetic aspects of albinism. Presse Med. 2017;46(7-8 Pt 1):648–54.
115. Barton DE, Kwon BS, Francke U. Human tyrosinase gene, mapped to chromosome 11 (q14-q21), defines second region of homology with mouse chromosome 7. Genomics. 1988;3:17–24.
116. Oetting WS, King RA. Molecular basis of albinism: mutations and polymorphisms of pigmentation genes associated with albinism. Hum Mutat. 1999;13:99–115.
117. Boissy RE, Nordlund JJ. Molecular basis of congenital hypopigmentary disorders in humans: a review. Pigment Cell Res. 1997;10:12–24.
118. Chintamaneni CD, Ramsay M, Colman MA, et al. Mapping the human CAS2 gene, the homologue of the mouse brown (b) locus, to human chromosome 9p22-pter. Biochem Biophys Res Commun. 1991;178:227–35.
119. Kobayashi T, Urabe K, Winder A, et al. Tyrosinase related protein 1 (TRP1) functions as a DHICA oxidase in melanin biosynthesis. EMBO J. 1994;13:5818–25.
120. Newton JM, Cohen-Barak O, Hagiwara N, et al. Mutations in the human orthologue of the mouse underwhite gene (uw) underlie a new form of oculocutaneous albinism, OCA4. Am J Hum Genet. 2001;69:981–8.
121. Incerti B, Cortese K, Pizzigoni A, et al. Oa1 knock-out: new insights on the pathogenesis of ocular albinism type 1. Hum Mol Genet. 2000;9:2781–8.
122. Schachne JP, Glaser N, Lee SH, et al. Hermansky-Pudlak syndrome: case report and clinicopathologic review. J Am Acad Dermatol. 1990;22:926–32.
123. Witkop CJ, Krumwiede M, Sedano H, et al. Reliability of absent platelet dense bodies as a diagnostic criterion for Hermansky-Pudlak syndrome. Am J Hematol. 1987;26:305–11.
124. Martina JA, Moriyama K, Bonifacino JS. BLOC-3, a protein complex containing the Hermansky-Pudlak syndrome gene products HPS1 and HPS4. J Biol Chem. 2003;278:29376–84.
125. Dell'Angelica EC, Shotelersuk V, Aguilar RC, et al. Altered trafficking of lysosomal proteins in Hermansky-Pudlak syndrome due to mutations in the beta 3A subunit of the AP-3 adaptor. Mol Cell. 1999;3:11–21.
126. Sugita M, Cao X, Watts GF, et al. Failure of trafficking and antigen presentation by CD1 in AP-3-deficient cells. Immunity. 2002;16:697–706.

127. Suzuki T, Li W, Zhang Q, et al. The gene mutated in cocoa mice, carrying a defect of organelle biogenesis, is a homologue of the human Hermansky-Pudlak syndrome-3 gene. Genomics. 2001;78:30–7.
128. Zhang Q, Zhao B, Li W, et al. Ru2 and Ru encode mouse orthologs of the genes mutated in human Hermansky-Pudlak syndrome types 5 and 6. Nat Genet. 2003;33:145–53.
129. Li W, Zhang Q, Oiso N, et al. Hermansky-Pudlak syndrome type 7 (HPS-7) results from mutant dysbindin, a member of the biogenesis of lysosome-related organelles complex 1 (BLOC-1). Nat Genet. 2003;35:84–9.
130. Tchernev VT, Mansfield TA, Giot L, et al. The Chediak-Higashi protein interacts with SNARE complex and signal transduction proteins. Mol Med. 2002;8:56–64.
131. Rogers SL, Karcher RL, Roland JT, et al. Regulation of melanosome movement in the cell cycle by reversible association with myosin V. J Cell Biol. 1999;146:1265–76.
132. Bahadoran P, Aberdam E, Mantoux F, et al. Rab27a: a key to melanosome transport in human melanocytes. J Cell Biol. 2001;152:843–50.
133. Menasche G, Ho CH, Sanal O, et al. Griscelli syndrome restricted to hypopigmentation results from a melanophilin defect (GS3) or a MYO5A F-exon deletion (GS1). J Clin Invest. 2003;112:450–6.
134. Ahluwalia J, Correa-Selm LM, Rao BK. Vitiligo: not simply a skin disease. Skin Med. 2017;15:125–7.
135. Alkhateeb A, Stetler GL, Old W, Talbert J, Uhlhorn C, Taylor M, et al. Mapping of an autoimmunity susceptibility locus (AIS1) to chromosome 1p31.3–p32.2. Hum Mol Genet. 2002;11:661–7.
136. Fain PR, Gowan K, LaBerge GS, et al. A genomewide screen for generalized vitiligo: confirmation of AIS1 on chromosome 1p31 and evidence for additional susceptibility loci. Am J Hum Genet. 2003;72:1560–4.
137. Rodrigues M, Ezzedine K, Hamzavi I, Pandya AG, Harris JE. Current and emerging treatments for vitiligo. J Am Acad Dermatol. 2017;77:17–29.
138. Calleja-Stafrace D, Vella C. Tuberous sclerosis associated with multiple hepatic lipomatous tumours. Images Paediatr Cardiol. 2016;18:1–4.
139. Hurwitz S, Braverman IM. White spots in tuberous sclerosis. J Pediatr. 1970;77:587–94.
140. Awan KJ. Leaf-shaped lesions of ocular fundus and white eyelashes in tuberous sclerosis. South Med J. 1982;75:227–38.
141. Gutman I, Dunn D, Behrens M, et al. Hypopigmented iris spot. An early sign of tuberous sclerosis. Ophthalmology. 1982;89:1155–9.
142. Sampson JR, Harris PC. The molecular genetics of tuberous sclerosis. Hum Mol Genet. 1994;3:1477–80.
143. van Slegtenhorst M, de Hoogt R, Hermans C, et al. Identification of the tuberous sclerosis gene TSC1 on chromosome 9q34. Science. 1997;277:805–8.
144. Benvenuto G, Li S, Brown SJ, et al. The tuberous sclerosis-1 (TSC1) gene product hamartin suppresses cell growth and augments the expression of the TSC2 product tuberin by inhibiting its ubiquitination. Oncogene. 2000;19:6306–16.
145. Zhang J, Li M, Yao Z. Molecular screening strategies for NF1-like syndromes with café-au-lait macules (review). Mol Med Rep. 2016;14:4023–9.
146. DeClue JE, Cohen BD, Lowy DR. Identification and characterization of the neurofibromatosis type 1 protein product. Proc Natl Acad Sci U S A. 1991;88:9914–8.
147. Basu TN, Gutmann DH, Fletcher JA, et al. Aberrant regulation of ras proteins in malignant tumour cells from type 1 neurofibromatosis patients. Nature. 1992;356:713–5.
148. Griesser J, Kaufmann D, Maier B, et al. Post-transcriptional regulation of neurofibromin level in cultured human melanocytes in response to growth factors. J Invest Dermatol. 1997;108:275–80.
149. Innamorati G, Valenti MT, Giacomello L, Dalle Carbonare L, Bassi C. GNAS mutations: drivers or co-pilots? Yet, promising diagnostic biomarkers. Trends Cancer. 2016;2:282–5.

150. Schwindinger WF, Francomano CA, Levine MA. Identification of a mutation in the gene encoding the alpha subunit of the stimulatory G protein of adenylyl cyclase in McCune-Albright syndrome. Proc Natl Acad Sci U S A. 1992;89:5152–6.
151. Passeron T, Bahadoran P, Bertolotto C, et al. Cyclic AMP promotes a peripheral distribution of melanosomes and stimulates melanophilin/Slac2-a and actin association. FASEB J. 2004;18:989–91.
152. Ogbechie-Godec OA, Elbuluk N. Melasma: an up-to-date comprehensive review. Dermatol Ther (Heidelb). 2017;7(3):305–18. https://doi.org/10.1007/s13555-017-0194-1.
153. Sardana K, Ghunawat S. Lasers for Lentigines, from Q-Switched to Erbium-Doped Yttrium Aluminium Garnet Micropeel, is There A Need to Reinvent the Wheel? J Cutan Aesthet Surg. 2015;8:233–5.
154. Ghosh SK, Majumdar B, Rudra O, Chakraborty S. LEOPARD syndrome. Dermatol Online J. 2015;21:13030/qt2d55s0t1.
155. Gorlin RJ, Anderson RC, Blaw M. Multiple lentigines syndrome. Am J Dis Child. 1969;117:652–62.
156. Digilio MC, Conti E, Sarkozy A, et al. Grouping of multiple-lentigines/LEOPARD and Noonan syndromes on the PTPN11 gene. Am J Hum Genet. 2002;71:389–94.
157. Jenne DE, Reimann H, Nezu J, et al. Peutz-Jeghers syndrome is caused by mutations in a novel serine threonine kinase. Nat Genet. 1998;18:38–43.
158. Mehenni H, Blouin JL, Radhakrishna U, et al. Peutz-Jeghers syndrome: confirmation of linkage to chromosome 19p13.3 and identification of a potential second locus, on 19q13.4. Am J Hum Genet. 1997;61:1327–34.
159. Miyamura Y, Suzuki T, Kono M, et al. Mutations of the RNA-specific adenosine deaminase gene (DSRAD) are involved in dyschromatosis symmetrica hereditaria. Am J Hum Genet. 2003;73:693–9.
160. Millet A, Martin AR, Ronco C, Rocchi S, Benhida R. Metastatic melanoma: insights into the evolution of the treatments and future challenges. Med Res Rev. 2017;37:98–148.
161. Balch CM, Gershenwald JE, Soong SJ, et al. Final version of 2009 AJCC melanoma staging and classification. J Clin Oncol. 2009;27:6199–206.
162. Lui P, Cashin R, Machado M, et al. Treatments for metastatic melanoma: synthesis of evidence from randomized trials. Cancer Treat Rev. 2007;33:665–80.
163. Eggermont AM, Schadendorf D. Melanoma and immunotherapy. Hematol Oncol Clin North Am. 2009;23:547–64.
164. Albino AP, Nanus DM, Mentle IR, et al. Analysis of ras oncogenes in malignant melanoma and precursor lesions: correlation of point mutations with differentiation phenotype. Oncogene. 1989;4:1363–74.
165. Tsao H, Goel V, Wu H, et al. Genetic interaction between NRAS and BRAF mutations and PTEN/MMAC1 inactivation in melanoma. J Invest Dermatol. 2004;122:337–41.
166. Sharpless E, Chin L. The INK4a/ARF locus and melanoma. Oncogene. 2003;22:3092–8.
167. Curtin JA, Busam K, Pinkel D, et al. Somatic activation of KIT in distinct subtypes of melanoma. J Clin Oncol. 2003;24:4340–6.
168. Van Raamsdonk CD, Bezrookove V, Green G, et al. Frequent somatic mutations of GNAQ in uveal melanoma and blue naevi. Nature. 2009;457:599–602.
169. Hartmann A, Brocker EB, Becker JC. Hypopigmentary skin disorders: current treatment options and future directions. Drugs. 2004;64:89–107.
170. Njoo MD, Westerhof W, Bos JD, et al. A systematic review of autologous transplantation methods in vitiligo. Arch Dermatol. 1998;134:1543–9.
171. Falabella R. Surgical therapies for vitiligo. Clin Dermatol. 1997;15:927–39.
172. Guerra L, Capurro S, Melchi F, et al. Treatment of stable vitiligo by timed surgery and transplantation of cultured epidermal autografts. Arch Dermatol. 2000;136:1380–9.

173. Yaar M, Gilchrest BA. Vitiligo: the evolution of cultured epidermal autografts and other surgical treatment modalities. Arch Dermatol. 2001;137:348–59.
174. Na GY, Seo SK, Choi SK. Single hair grafting for the treatment of vitiligo. J Am Acad Dermatol. 1998;38:580–4.
175. Keidar M, Walk R, Shashurin A, Srinivasan P, Sandler A, Dasgupta S, Ravi R, Guerrero-Preston R, Trink B. Cold plasma selectivity and the possibility of a paradigm shift in cancer therapy. Br J Cancer. 2011;105:1295–301.
176. Visscher MO. Skin color and pigmentation in ethnic skin. Facial Plast Surg Clin North Am. 2017;25:119–25.

# Perspectives in Immunology of Wound Healing

# 23

Kai Masur and Sander Bekeschus

## 23.1 Immunology: A General Introduction

From the outset of life, the struggle for habitats and food resulted in a "friend foe" recognition early from the development of life. This competition for scarce resources was an important step in the development of multicellular organisms, which resulted in a division of competencies and thus a distribution of tasks between the different cell types. With the occurrence of free oxygen in the earth's atmosphere, all living beings had to deal with this reactive molecule. In addition to the efficient use of oxygen for breathing, this has also led to the use of this highly reactive molecule as a weapon. In this context, the immune system developed, which comprises a complex network of organs, cells and molecules dissolved in the body fluids, all of which serve the defence of pathogens. A further task of the immune system consists, besides the combating of foreign organisms, also in the recognition of degenerated cells within the body, in order to eliminate them. This chapter will discuss the parallels between immune system responses and the effects of cold atmospheric pressure plasmas on cells and tissues.

## 23.2 The Immune System and Involved Cell Types

The defence mechanisms of the immune system are based not only on the functions of specialized cells, but begins with the purely mechanical protective function of the skin and mucosa, which is intended as a first barrier to prevent the penetration of

K. Masur, Ph.D. (✉)
Associated Research Group "Plasma Wound Healing", Centre for Innovation Competence (ZIK) Plasmatis, Greifswald, Germany
e mail: kai.masur@inp-greifswald.de

S. Bekeschus, Ph.D.
Young Research Group "Plasma Redox Effects", Centre for Innovation Competence (ZIK) Plasmatis, Greifswald, Germany



H.-R. Metelmann et al. (eds.), *Comprehensive Clinical Plasma Medicine*,
https://doi.org/10.1007/978-3-319-67627-2_23

microorganisms, parasites or foreign bodies. When the microorganisms have broken the first line of defence the cellular and non-cellular (humoral) processes of immune defence will be activated. In general, the immune cells are subdivided into the innate (non-specific) and acquired (specific) defences, which differ not only in their function, but also on exactly how the intruders are combated (Table 23.1).

The family tree of immune cells (depicted in Fig. 23.1) includes cells of the acquired immune system like B- and T-Lymphocytes and cells of the innate immune system like granulocytes and macrophages. Especially the phagocytes like

**Table 23.1** Cellular and humoral immune system as well as innate and acquired defence mechanisms

| | Cellular immunity | Humoral immunity |
|---|---|---|
| Innate immune system | NK-cells<br>Granulocytes<br>Monocytes/macrophages | Cytokines<br>Lysozyme<br>Interferons |
| Acquired immune system | B-lymphocytes<br>T-lymphocytes | Antibodies (Ab)<br>Immunoglobulin |

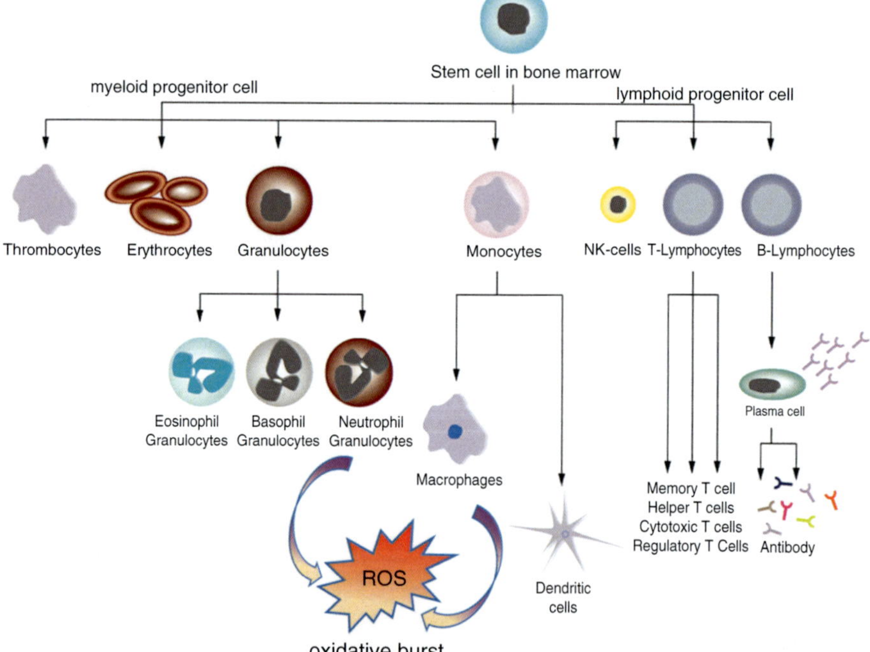


**Fig. 23.1** Presentation of the immune cell family tree. All human immune cells derive from stem cells of the bone marrow. After splitting into the lymphatic line (specific immune cells) and into the myeloid line (nonspecific immune cells), further steps of splitting and specialization follow. In particular, the neutrophil granulocytes and the macrophages are capable of generating reactive oxygen species (ROS)—a process called an oxidative burst

neutrophil granulocytes and macrophages are capable of generating endogenous reactive oxygen species (ROS), which are responsible for the oxidative burst. In addition to the NK cells, the so-called phagocytes, such as granulocytes and macrophages, are the first wave of defence, which patrols in tissue and encounters the first intruding microorganisms'. The cells of the innate immune defence are not specialized in the recognition of specific microorganisms, but recognize general surface markers and are therefore always prepared. In the case microorganisms have overcome the nonspecific part of the immune defence, cells of the acquired immune system come into play. These immune cells are activated due to the initial contact with the invading pathogens, leading to a maturation process and ultimately to increased proliferation of these specialized cells. Thus within a few days a large number of immunocompetent B- and T-cells can be formed, which then destroy the pathogens or begin the production of specific antibodies.

Both the innate as well as the specific immune system are supported by a large number of soluble substances, which are circulating through the blood and in other body fluids. These are primarily cytokines, interferons, enzymes and antibodies as well as free radicals. These soluble substances belong to the humoral defence (from "humor," Latin: liquid). Both the innate as well as the acquired immune system therefore contain cellular and humoral defence strategies, which mutually support each other.

## 23.3 Reactive Species in Immune Defence

The neutrophilic granulocytes and macrophages are the most important representatives of the innate defence system, which recognize debris (foreign bodies) or invaded microorganisms as foreign—and in a process designated as phagocytosis, they will take up and digest those particles and pathogens.

In most cases, the microorganisms that have penetrated are also recognized by the specific immune system, finally leading to the formation of antibodies (Ab), which in turn bind to these pathogens. Thereafter the Ab-labelled pathogens are recognized and absorbed by macrophages and granulocytes. This leads to an increased phagocytosis rate with additional activation of the macrophages or neutrophil granulocytes. The uptake of the Ab-labelled microorganisms leads to the activation of various enzymes and bio-active proteins, such as lysozyme and lactoferrin, which then attack the bacterial proteins in the phagocytic cells. The activation of further enzymes leads to the release of reactive oxygen species (ROS) in specific vesicles (lysosomes) by phagocytes—Table 23.2. After the absorption, the pathogen-bearing vesicles (phagosomes) are mixed with the enzyme and radical-loaded lysosomes, which ultimately leads to the killing of these pathogens. Therefore, macrophages triggering inflammation are called M1 macrophages, whereas those that counteract inflammation and trigger tissue repair are called M2 macrophages [1]. This difference is reflected in their metabolism; M1 macrophages have the unique ability to metabolize arginine to the "killer" molecule nitric oxide. But, other radicals and reactive oxygen species are also formed during these processes:

**Table 23.2** Overview of the major activities of activated phagocytes

| Effects in activated phagocytes | Released substances |
|---|---|
| Acidification | $H^+ \rightarrow pH < 4$ |
| Release of reactive oxygen species (ROS) | Hydrogen peroxide $H_2O_2$, superoxide $\cdot O_2^-$, hydroxyl radical $HO\cdot$, singlet-oxygen $^1O_2$ |
| Release of reactive nitrogen species (RNS) | Nitrogen monoxide NO |
| Induction of enzyme activities | Lysozyme, lactoferrin<br>NADPH-oxidase (NOX), superoxide-dismutase (SOD), myeloperoxidase (MPO) |

Therefore, macrophages as well as neutrophil granulocytes are able to eliminate microorganisms by secretion of endogenously formed reactive species such as hydrogen peroxide or hydroxyl radicals. In activated macrophages and neutrophil granulocytes, the MPO content can account for up to 5% of the total cell protein content.

It should also be noted that the activated phagolysosomes do possess the necessary enzymes such as catalase, superoxide dismutase or myeloperoxidase in order to break down the phagosomal contents after the uptake of pathogens. This process is supported by the so-called oxidative burst: the endogenous production of diverse ROS by macrophages and neutrophil granulocytes representing a significant part of the nonspecific defence. The central molecule in this defence mechanism is the enzyme NADPH oxidase, which is capable of generating large amounts of superoxide radicals $\cdot O_2^-$. The highly reactive $\cdot O_2^-$ as well as O—represent the starting point for the production of other ROS. One major source of ROS is the disproportionation catalysed by the enzyme superoxide dismutase resulting in the formation of hydrogen peroxide, which is considered a relatively stable reactive oxygen species—and a starting point for several other reactions. Both, in Fenton reaction ($H_2O_2$ reacts with $Fe^{2+}$ Ions) as well as in the catalytic decomposition of the $H_2O_2$, the hydroxyl radical $\cdot OH$ will be formed as a reaction product. The hydroxyl radical is capable of destroying a large number of biomolecules due to its high reactivity combined with a comparable long lifetime. Furthermore, the enzyme myeloperoxidase (MPO) catalyses the reaction of $H_2O_2$ with oxygen radicals as well as chloride ions forming large amounts of hypochlorous acid/hypochlorite ions ($HClO/ClO^-$), which are capable to oxygenise bacterial components (Fig. 23.2). All this highly reactive ROS result in the degradation of internalized pathogens.

The bactericidal effects of phagolysosomes differ with cell types. Phagolysosomes in dendritic cells have weaker bactericidal properties than those in macrophages and neutrophils. Furthermore, the subdivisions of macrophages generate different reactive species. Pro-inflammatory M1 macrophages produce more ROS and RNS than M2 macrophages. The phagolysosomes of M1 generate highly reactive nitric oxide (NO) by metabolizing arginine, while M2 produce ornithine out of arginine to foster cell proliferation and tissue repair [2].

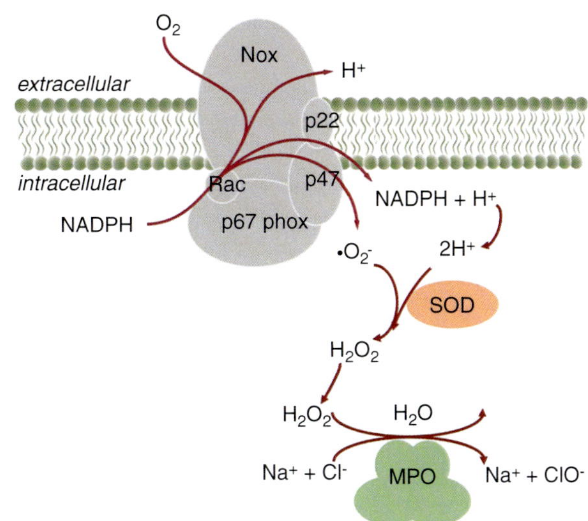


**Fig. 23.2** Overview of the generation of reactive species in phagocytes by redox enzymes. The main sources for reactive oxygen species are the enzymes NADPH oxidase (NOX), superoxide dismutase (SOD) and the myeloperoxidase (MPO), which are capable to form reactive oxygen species like $\cdot O_2^-$ and $H_2O_2$ as well as $ClO^-$ based on reactions which are depending on free oxygen $O_2$ and NAD(P)H. All highly reactive agents that can destroy biomolecules

## 23.4 Plasma Medicine, Cold Plasmas and Immune Cells

If one considers the repertoire of reactive oxygen species of the phagocytes, it is noticeable that these ROSs are identical to those identified in plasma medication as biologically active plasma components [3, 4]. Thus, it is not surprising that a plasma treatment of microorganisms is bactericidal, since other plasma components, such as UV radiation and ROS like hydroxyl radical HO·and $H_2O_2$ are also formed in relevant amounts. Together with acidification, this mixture of biological active agents can cause the killing of pathogens [5, 6]. On the other hand, it was shown that in human immune cells, hydrogen peroxide plays a central role in the mediation of plasma effects. However besides $H_2O_2$ other reactive oxygen species could also be identified, whose activity was not reduced by catalase [7].

Furthermore, it was found that not all immune cells have comparable sensitivities to treatment with cold plasma. It is known that lymphocytes have a lower tolerance limit to cold plasma, whereas macrophages have survived a longer plasma treatment without any damage. In addition, it was found that in principle the same intracellular signalling pathways were activated, but to a different extent or after different plasma treatment times [8]. Furthermore, adhesion molecules such as L-selectin, ICAM-1 and LFA-1alpha were shown to be downregulated by plasma treatment of lymphocytes [9], which also leads to immunomodulation of chilled plasma. On the other hand, the activation of heat shock proteins was only detected in the monocytes, displaying a protective mechanism completely lacking in lymphocytes [8].

Comparing those results with facts from immunology, it can be seen that the cells with endogenous ROS production are also more robust to a treatment with cold plasma. Thus, it can be stated that cold plasmas support and sometimes even imitate the function of the immune system. For this reason, it should be investigated further in the future whether cold plasma could be used to support an immune system that is affected by various diseases—ranging from type 2 diabetes to arteriosclerosis or neurodermatitis.

Also first data from clinical application of cold plasmas to treat chronic wounds provide hints that an activation of the immune systems is likely. In some case studies, wounds of otherwise incurable patients were treated with cold plasma by applying the Argon plasma jet kINPenMed® for 30–60 s/cm$^2$ [For more details please refer to Chapter IV 4.1 (kINPenMed®, neoplas tools.)]. In some cases a light swelling could be observed shortly after the plasma treatment—indicating a "turn on" of immune effects. In rare cases, patients had two wounds at two different legs. Figure 23.3 depicts the formerly incurable wounds one of these patients: a 71-year old male, who is suffering from chronic leg ulcers for almost 30 years. The wound on the right leg was treated with cold plasma and the remaining wound on the left leg just got the usual wound care. Besides the plasma treatment both wounds got

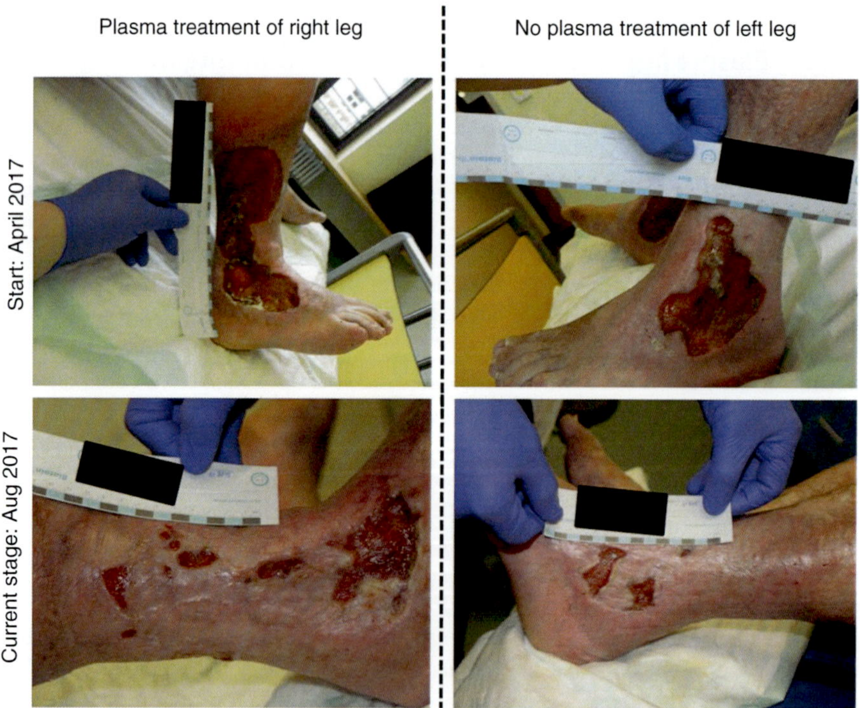


**Fig. 23.3** Two wounds of a 83-year old male patient. The upper row depicts the wounds at the beginning in April—left side plasma treated, right side not plasma treated. The pictures below display the current stage at the end of August 2017 of the plasma treated wound on the left side and the untreated wound to the right. Both formerly incurable wounds show wound healing effects—indicating that plasma treatment might have induced immunogenic effects

similar wound care—concerning bandages and rinsing solution, etc. The plasma treated wound displayed a significant improvement including a smaller wound size and a beginning of granulation after a few treatments. Surprisingly, 4 months after beginning of the plasma therapy the wound of the left leg—which was not plasma treated also showed improved healing—as shown in Fig. 23.3 lower right picture.

Since this patient was struggling with open incurable wounds for years, the application of plasma was causing wound healing by reducing the bacterial load, stimulating microcirculation and therefore increased the amount of oxygen und nutrition at the plasma treated area. There is a high likelihood that plasma mediated effects are responsible for the onset of wound healing, even in the untreated wounds—indicating a possible activation of the immune system. This type of plasma-based immunomodulation will be investigated more intensively in the future.

Cold plasmas contain biologically active components—mostly reactive oxygen species (ROS), which also play an essential role in natural processes such as immune defence. Furthermore, those plasma generated ROS act commonly with other plasma components such as UV radiation, mild heat and electrical fields. These effects mediate an improved microenvironment by generating bactericidal conditions and positively influencing microcirculation in the plasma treated areas—further promoting increase oxygen saturation and an improved supply with nutrition. Therefore, cold plasmas are useful to support wound healing by accelerating cell proliferation and triggering as well as imitating immune processes.

Furthermore, it has been observed that long-term plasma treatments lead to the induction of the programmed cell death (apoptosis). Depending on the treatment time, the respective tolerance threshold for reactive species (the antioxidative potential of a cell type) was exceeded, leading to increased oxidative stress and the activation of numerous apoptotic signalling pathways [8]. In the course of the plasma treatment, numerous cytokines and growth factors were found in immune cells as well as skin cells or fibroblasts [10]. In addition to a certain selectivity of the cold plasma against the different cell types, plasma could become an immune modulator through the release of messenger substances and signalling molecules. However, the temporary and locally acting ROS from cold plasma could also act as a chemoattractant for immune cells guiding them to the location of the treatment [11] or may be used to stimulate skin cell proliferation [12]. This local restriction combined with short-term effects of cold plasmas could become interesting for possible application as a future immune modulator.

A further aspect of the plasma-induced apoptosis of cells could play a role in cancer treatment. It has already been shown in many cases various tumour cell lines can be driven into apoptosis by cold plasma treatment [13–15]. Recent projects are working on combining this type of cancer treatment with an immune stimulation—also described in Chap. 24 of this book in more details. The activation of immune cells in order to fight cancer is described as "immunogenic cell death." Most of the agents normally inducing immunogenic cell death are targeting endoplasmic reticulum (ER), leading to ER stress and production of reactive oxygen species. In "Immunogenic cell death," phagocytes which are in contact with the plasma treated tumor cells will be able to fight the remaining tumor residues as activated immune cells subsequently [16].

## References

1. Mills CD. M1 and M2 macrophages: oracles of health and disease. Crit Rev Immunol. 2012;32(6):463–88.
2. Mills CD. Anatomy of a discovery: M1 and M2 macrophages. Front Immunol. 2015;6:212.
3. Tresp H, Hammer MU, Weltmann K-D, Reuter S. Effects of atmosphere composition and liquid type on plasma-generated reactive species in biologically relevant solutions. Plasma Med. 2013;3(1–2):45–55.
4. Tresp H, Hammer MU, Winter J, Weltmann KD, Reuter S. Quantitative detection of plasma-generated radicals in liquids by electron paramagnetic resonance spectroscopy. J Phys D Appl Phys. 2013;46(43):435401.
5. Arjunan KP, Clyne AM. Hydroxyl radical and hydrogen peroxide are primarily responsible for dielectric barrier discharge plasma-induced angiogenesis. Plasma Process Polym. 2011;8(12):1154–64.
6. Von Woedtke T, Haese K, Heinze J, Oloff C, Stieber M, Julich WD. Sporicidal efficacy of hydrogen peroxide aerosol. Pharmazie. 2004;59(3):207–11.
7. Bekeschus S, Kolata J, Winterbourn C, Kramer A, Turner R, Weltmann KD, Broker B, Masur K. Hydrogen peroxide: a central player in physical plasma-induced oxidative stress in human blood cells. Free Radic Res. 2014;48(5):542–9.
8. Bundscherer L, Nagel S, Hasse S, Tresp H, Wende K, Walther R, Reuter S, Weltmann KD, Masur K, Lindequist U. Non-thermal plasma treatment induces MAPK signaling in human monocytes. Open Chem. 2015;13(1):606–13.
9. Haertel B, Volkmann F, von Woedtke T, Lindequist U. Differential sensitivity of lymphocyte subpopulations to non-thermal atmospheric-pressure plasma. Immunobiology. 2012;217(6):628–33.
10. Barton A, Hasse S, Bundscherer L, Wende K, Weltmann K, Lindequist U, Masur K. Growth factors and cytokines are regulated by non-thermal atmospheric pressure plasma. Exp Dermatol. 2014;23(3):E7.
11. Niethammer P, Grabher C, Look AT, Mitchison TJ. A tissue-scale gradient of hydrogen peroxide mediates rapid wound detection in zebrafish. Nature. 2009;459(7249):996–9.
12. Loo AE, Wong YT, Ho R, Wasser M, Du T, Ng WT, Halliwell B. Effects of hydrogen peroxide on wound healing in mice in relation to oxidative damage. PLoS One. 2012;7(11):e49215.
13. Barekzi N, Laroussi M. Effects of low temperature plasmas on cancer cells. Plasma Process Polym. 2013;10(12):1039–50.
14. Hori M, Laroussi M, Masur K, Ikehara Y. Plasma processes and cancer—special topical cluster of the 2nd IWPCT meeting. Plasma Process Polym. 2015;12(12):1336–7.
15. Keidar M, Shashurin A, Volotskova O, Stepp MA, Srinivasan P, Sandler A, Trink B. Cold atmospheric plasma in cancer therapy. Phys Plasmas. 2013;20(5):057101–8.
16. Nagendra Kumar K, Neha K, Booki M, Ki Hong C, Young June H, Vandana M, Alexander F, Eun Ha C. Cytotoxic macrophage-released tumour necrosis factor-alpha (TNF- α ) as a killing mechanism for cancer cell death after cold plasma activation. J Phys D Appl Phys. 2016;49(8):084001.

# Cancer Immunology 24

Sander Bekeschus, Jean-Michel Pouvesle,
Alexander Fridman, and Vandana Miller

## 24.1 Introduction

Immunity tips the balance between health and disease [1]. This is well established for infectious diseases caused by viruses and bacteria [2]. If such pathogens evade or overwhelm the immune system, infection manifests as illness. The current view about many etiologies of cancer follows a similar logic. While cancer results from mutations in oncogenes, tumor suppressor genes, or other genes that maintain genetic stability, the mutated cells also have to overcome the immune surveillance and control to successfully establish malignancy [3]. This is concluded from the observation that immunosuppressed individuals have a much higher incidence of cancers than the average population [4]. The immune system is capable of detecting and removing non-infected but chronically diseased, stressed, and/or mutated cells [5].

On the other hand, manifesting cancers develop strategies to evade immune responses, both innate and adaptive, in multiple ways [6]. Accordingly, interfering with these manipulations is a valid therapeutic strategy and has recently become the major aim in oncology [7]. This is the field of cancer immunology. Mechanisms at work are complex, and this book chapter attempts to provide a basic background on that topic before addressing the potential role of the novel physical therapy of cold plasma in oncological context.

S. Bekeschus (✉)
Leibniz-Institute for Plasma Science and Technology, ZIK Plasmatis, Greifswald, Germany
e-mail: sander.bekeschus@inp-greifswald.de

J.-M. Pouvesle
GREMI UMR-6606 CNRS, Université d'Orléans, Orleans, France

A. Fridman • V. Miller
Nyheim Plasma Institute, Drexel University, Camden, NJ, USA



H.-R. Metelmann et al. (eds.), *Comprehensive Clinical Plasma Medicine*,
https://doi.org/10.1007/978-3-319-67627-2_24

**By spatiotemporal decision-making of attack, the immune system is key in etiology, progression, and outcome of infection, cancer, and disease.**

## 24.2 Cancer Immunology and Immunogenic Cell Death

The three classical pillars of cancer treatment are surgery, radiotherapy (RT), and chemotherapy (CT). Since about a decade, immunotherapy has emerged as a fourth pillar. This fourth concept acknowledges the power of the immune system in eradicating cancer. It has long been observed in RT that localized treatment on one specific tumor site decreased tumor burden at other, untreated sites on occasion [8]. The term "abscopal effect" describing remote effects was coined in 1953 to describe such an effect [9]. Today, it is known that under certain circumstances the body generates an antitumor immune response that culminates in the production of tumor-specific cytotoxic T lymphocytes that actively and selectively kill cancer cells [10]. Tumor-specificity is added to the system because malignant cells differ from non-malignant cells often in one or several ways: overexpression of protein with otherwise low abundance, expression of embryo-fetal proteins related to ontology but not present in the developed host, and/or germline mutations leading to altered proteins unique to tumor cells [11]. The question is, how can this process be targeted to be selective against cancers, and what are the events necessary to mount an immune response directed against structures of the altered self? An added complexity in the conventional treatments is the toxicity toward immune cells (Table 24.1) [12–15]. On the one hand, the eradication of immunosuppressive cells may be beneficial but there is also collateral damage of cells that may actively control tumor progression, thus forcing them to rely largely on the direct cytotoxic effects of these modalities. This in itself acts as an immunosuppressant due to massive release of tumor antigens in the microenvironment [16].

Two classical pathways of cell death are described to induce either tolerogenic (apoptosis) or immunogenic (necrosis) sequelae [17]. This view was challenged by a series of elegant experiments providing evidence that apoptosis in itself may be either tolerogenic or immunogenic with many facets in between [18]. This

**Table 24.1** Immunosuppressive effects of cancer therapies

| Treatment | Immune function | Reference |
|---|---|---|
| Irradiation | Lymphopenia | [12] |
| Steroids | Impaired DC differentiation or activation and NK-cell function, suppression of inflammation, T cell function | [13] |
| Surgery | Resection of lymph nodes | [14] |
| Chemotherapy | Lymphopenia | [15] |

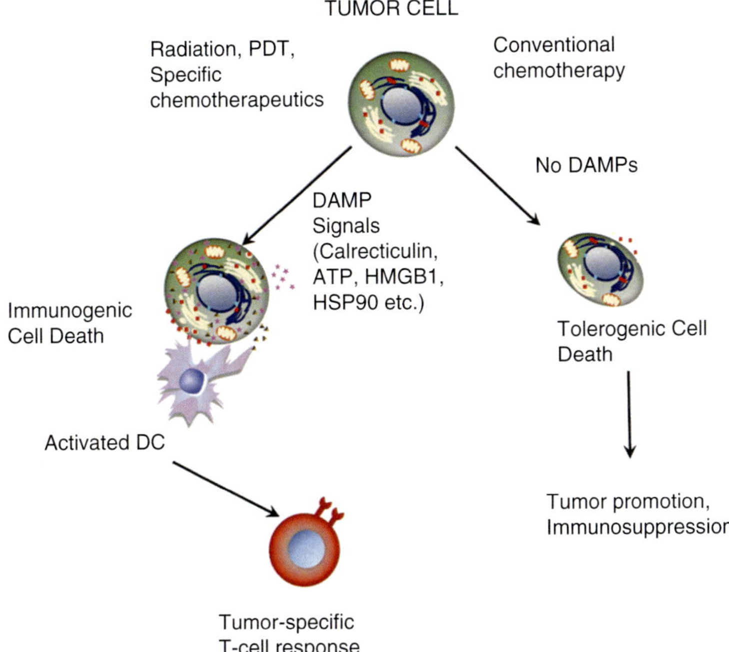


**Fig. 24.1** Immunogenic vs. tolerogenic cell death and its consequences

immunological outcome of dying cancer cells is determined by their recognition and phagocytosis by professional antigen presenting cells [19]. Immunogenicity of dying cancer cells is linked to the concurrent release of the so-called damage-associated molecular patterns (DAMPs) [20]. The molecules act as danger signals to alert immune cells, regardless of the mode of cell death. If a tumor cell is phagocytosed by a professional antigen-presenting cell, for example dendritic cells, it will be these context molecules determining whether the phagocyte will become activated or not. If activating ligands are present, dendritic cells will mature, and (cross-) present small fragments of tumor cells (peptides) to T lymphocytes [21]. Lymphocytes having a matching T cell receptor and receiving additional stimuli will then clonally expand, migrate to the periphery, and target all tumor cells bearing that cognate antigen throughout the body. If these DAMPs are not emitted, then a tolerogenic response occurs which supports tumor growth and suppresses antitumor immunity (Fig. 24.1) [22].

In the final analysis, two decisions guide antitumor immune response: (1) it is the context of cell death that matters, not the mode, and (2) larger differences in the tumor cell protein profile are thought to enhance its distingue from non-cancerous cells, adding specificity to the immune response [23].

**In immunogenic cell death (ICD), a damaging incident causes a body cell's death to be perceived as an endogenous danger signal (sterile inflammation). Together with different co-stimulatory molecular events, this elicits a cellular (T cells) and humoral (B cells) immune response, highly specific towards proteins and/or peptides present on or released by the initially damaged cell.**

## 24.3 Systemic Immune Responses with Physical Cancer Treatments

Some chemotherapeutics exhibit strong ICD responses in tumor cells [24]. The idea of using a physical therapy to vaccinate the host against cancer cells thus may seem exotic at first glance [25]. However, cold plasma seamlessly aligns with traditional as well as new physical treatment modalities in oncotherapy [26]. With many cancer treatments, radiotherapy has been the standard of care for several decades now. Highly focused radiation is sent into the tumor, destroying cells locally, and thereby releasing immunogenic molecules [27]. This leads to "sterile" inflammation, and an immune response after radiotherapy has been found in several irradiated patients either with or without combinational chemotherapy [28]. Another physical modality, electrochemotherapy (ECT), employs microsecond-pulsed electrical fields locally at the tumor site following the local administration of low, non-effective dose of a chemotherapeutic. The advantage is that ECT avoids drug side effects usually seen with higher concentrations, and induces an antitumor immune response, though only in specific settings [29]. ECT uses medically certified pulse generators, and its efficacy was proven in large-scale clinical trials [30]. Currently, it is primarily being used in skin and breast cancer in the palliative setting [31, 32]. An additional physico-chemical treatment modality for cancer is photodynamic therapy (PDT) and has recently gained interest in dermato-oncology [33]. Here, a lipophilic photosensitizer, linked to targeting molecules is dispensed to the (tumor) tissue [34]. When the area is exposed to light of a specific wavelength to energize the photosensitizer, it produces reactive oxygen and nitrogen species intracellularly, only in the targeted cells. Similar to ECT, PDT has been investigated for decades, and standardized and approved equipment and photosensitizers are available for different indications in dermatology [35]. PDT causes tumor cell death, and elicits antitumor immune responses in preclinical models of cancer [36–38]. In a similar fashion, hyperthermia is proposed to enhance the immunogenicity of tumors [39]. Locally applied, it facilitates the release of heat-shock proteins, a class of proteins known to be important in ICD [40]. Recently, high hydrostatic pressure was shown to induce ICD in tumor cells [41]. It was proposed that this procedure could be used to kill autologous tumor cells ex vivo in an immuno-stimulatory manner before feeding them to donor-derived dendritic cells [42]. When re-injected into the patient, the antigen-loaded dendritic cells would successfully elicit tumor-specific T cell responses leading to killing of tumor cells [43].

All five mentioned physical therapies are ICD inducers—and they fully or partially involve generation of reactive oxygen and nitrogen species. Cold plasmas generate a plethora of such reactive species [44–46], and it seems not too farfetched to assume that plasma may establish antitumor immunity in a similar fashion. In fact, an important advantage of non-equilibrium plasma with respect to the other approaches is its mutiparametric controllability and tenability. It may therefore not only act as ICD trigger but at the same time facilitate stimulating effects on leukocytes involved at generating immune responses. Electric fields and plasma poration have been observed with some plasma sources, suggesting a possible synergy with reactive species effects.

**Physical treatment modalities are equally potent ICD inducers with fewer systemic side effects compared to chemotherapeutics in cancer therapy.**

## 24.4 Plasma-Induced Immunogenic Cell Death (PICD): Current Tracks and Future Roads

Immunity is an important endogenous weapon fighting cancer. Cancer cell death needs to be immunogenic in order to elicit immune responses. Immunogenic cell death is observed in response to chemotherapy as well as physical therapies. Cold plasma is a physical therapy, and accumulating evidence indicates that it could become a crucial part of the cancer immunotherapy armament. Plasma treatment induced protein expression associated with an enhanced immunogenicity in leukemia cells [47]. Plasma-killed tumor cells express calreticulin, ATP, and stress of endoplasmic reticulum, all hallmarks of ICD [48, 49]. This enhances macrophage-assisted tumor cellkilling in vitro [50], primarily via soluble antitumor-factors released by the phagocytes [51]. Similar factors were found in immune cell-rich fractions of animals benefiting from plasma oncotherapy [52]. This corroborates our own data, extending on tumor-specific T cell responses in animals with plasma-treated tumors.

**Cold Physical Plasma elicits immunogenic cell death in vitro and in vivo.**

Plasma has distinct effects on isolated immune cell populations. It activates macrophages for increased migratory activity [53]. Plasma also elicits extracellular trap formation in human neutrophils [54]. Ex vivo, myeloid cells such as neutrophils and monocytes/macrophages are much less prone to plasma-induced cytotoxic effects compared to lymphocytes [55–57]. Among several T lymphocyte subpopulations, a specific memory T cell type important in tumor eradication proved to be most robust upon plasma treatment [58]. Yet, on a relative scale, lymphocytic cells seem much more sensitive to plasma treatment compared to scaffold and tumor cells [59]. Thus, plasma treatment may not only stimulate tumor-associated myeloid cells but also specifically select for lymphocyte subtypes in the tumor microenvironment.

**Immune cell viability and functions are differentially affected by cold plasmas.**

At present, four key fields are subject to current or future investigation for plasma technology in cancer immunology (Fig. 24.2). Immunogenic cell death and its associated generation of tumor-toxic T cells seems by far the most promising approach several groups in the field are following currently [60]. Second, research also focusses on the direct stimulatory effects of plasmas on leukocytes. This included, for example, the possibility to use plasmas for shifting the phenotype of tumor-promoting macrophages towards a more pro-inflammatory differentiation state. The third and so-far untouched field deals with removing the immunosuppression that tumors frequently utilize to dampen immune response at and around the tumor site. Finally, plasma treatment may be used to kill patient-derived cancer cells, before feeding these cells to autologous dendritic cells. Upon tumor cell phagocytosis, these dendritic cells are added back to the patient to aid in generation of tumor-specific cytotoxic T cells. Generally, this approach is under heavy investigation for many years now, with ambiguous success [61–63]. Since it became clear that ex vivo killed cancer cells should be of high immunogenicity, approaches have been refined recently [64].

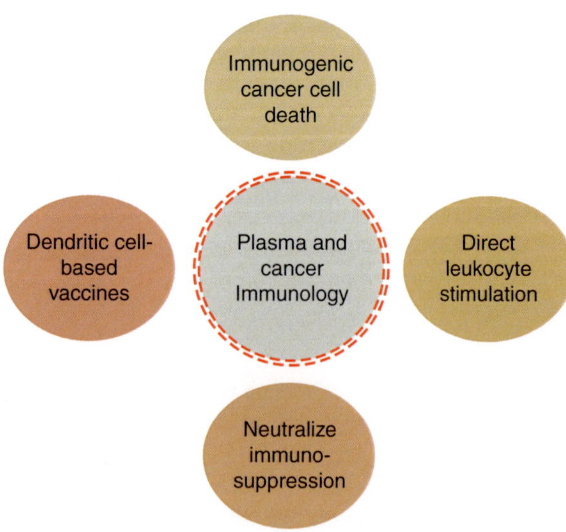


**Fig. 24.2** Relevant and promising topics in the field of cold physical plasma oncotherapy and cancer immunology

Plasmas likely will not eradicate large tumor masses by themselves but a combinatorial therapeutic regime with conventional chemotherapy, radiation, or even surgery seems plausible. With current devices and treatment approaches, tumors that are easily accessible, as on the body surfaces, are the obvious targets. For deeper tumors, ICD is a necessity for durable responses; otherwise, plasma is not competitive with existing therapies. Selectivity of therapies for cancer has always been a problem. They are invariably associated with collateral damage leading to acute and chronic toxicities that interfere with patient compliance. This is because of a combination of mode of action of these agents and the route of delivery. Plasma is likely to face similar challenges but they are not expected to be a major hurdle to its adoption. An advantage of plasma is the ability to operate the devices at different energy delivery settings for the induction of ICD or for direct ablation of the tumor cells. If used in conjunction with other treatment modalities, it could provide selectivity through use of sub therapeutic "doses" of multiple agents targeting the same pathway. Regardless of the details of plasma application, the field is part of larger fields working for many decades on cancer-related issues (Fig. 24.3). With plasma

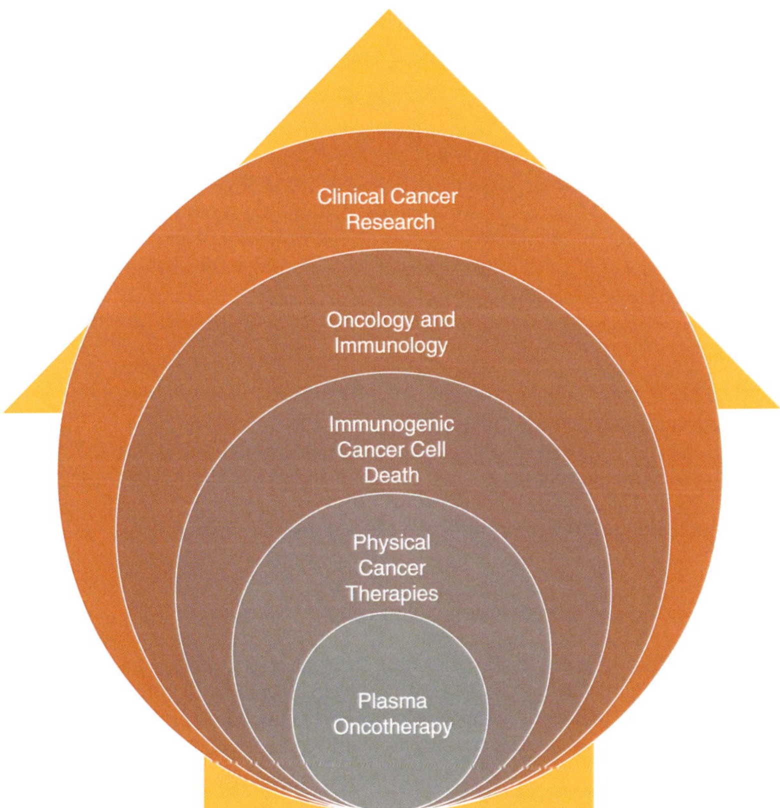


**Fig. 24.3** The research field of cold plasma oncotherapy within the framework of research concepts in clinically relevant tumor therapies

oncotherapy, we are embedded within the physical treatment modalities eliciting immunogenic cell cancer death. This field is part of the research fields of oncology and immunology in general. These research communities are embedded within the framework of clinical cancer research, which includes several other aspects in patient care, such as nursing, palliation, and cancer prevention. This is important to keep in mind to understand the hurdles and chances of new therapies such as plasma in clinical therapies.

## References

1. Kramer A, Bekeschus S, Broker BM, Schleibinger H, Razavi B, Assadian O. Maintaining health by balancing microbial exposure and prevention of infection: the hygiene hypothesis versus the hypothesis of early immune challenge. J Hosp Infect. 2013;83(Suppl 1):S29–34.
2. Leliefeld PH, Wessels CM, Leenen LP, Koenderman L, Pillay J. The role of neutrophils in immune dysfunction during severe inflammation. Crit Care. 2016;20(1):73.
3. Zitvogel L, Tesniere A, Kroemer G. Cancer despite immunosurveillance: Immunoselection and immunosubversion. Nat Rev Immunol. 2006;6(10):715–27.
4. Penn I, Starzl TE. Malignant tumors arising de novo in immunosuppressed organ transplant recipients. Transplantation. 1972;14(4):407–17.
5. Raulet DH, Guerra N. Oncogenic stress sensed by the immune system: role of natural killer cell receptors. Nat Rev Immunol. 2009;9(8):568–80.
6. Abdollahi A, Folkman J. Evading tumor evasion: current concepts and perspectives of anti-angiogenic cancer therapy. Drug Resist Updat. 2010;13(1–2):16–28.
7. Vinay DS, Ryan EP, Pawelec G, Talib WH, Stagg J, Elkord E, Lichtor T, Decker WK, Whelan RL, Kumara HM, Signori E, Honoki K, Georgakilas AG, Amin A, Helferich WG, Boosani CS, Guha G, Ciriolo MR, Chen S, Mohammed SI, Azmi AS, Keith WN, Bilsland A, Bhakta D, Halicka D, Fujii H, Aquilano K, Ashraf SS, Nowsheen S, Yang X, Choi BK, Kwon BS. Immune evasion in cancer: mechanistic basis and therapeutic strategies. Semin Cancer Biol. 2015;35(Suppl):S185–98.
8. Ehlers G, Fridman M. Abscopal effect of radiation in papillary adenocarcinoma. Br J Radiol. 1973;46(543):220–2.
9. Mole RH. Whole body irradiation; radiobiology or medicine? Br J Radiol. 1953;26(305):234–41.
10. Schirrmacher V. Cancer-reactive memory t cells from bone marrow: spontaneous induction and therapeutic potential (review). Int J Oncol. 2015;47(6):2005–16.
11. Kroemer G, Galluzzi L, Kepp O, Zitvogel L. Immunogenic cell death in cancer therapy. Annu Rev Immunol. 2013;31:51–72.
12. Claude L, Perol D, Ray-Coquard I, Petit T, Blay JY, Carrie C, Bachelot T. Lymphopenia: a new independent prognostic factor for survival in patients treated with whole brain radiotherapy for brain metastases from breast carcinoma. Radiother Oncol. 2005;76(3):334–9.
13. Galon J, Franchimont D, Hiroi N, Frey G, Boettner A, Ehrhart-Bornstein M, O'Shea JJ, Chrousos GP, Bornstein SR. Gene profiling reveals unknown enhancing and suppressive actions of glucocorticoids on immune cells. FASEB J. 2002;16(1):61–71.
14. Panici PB, Maggioni A, Hacker N, Landoni F, Ackermann S, Campagnutta E, Tamussino K, Winter R, Pellegrino A, Greggi S, Angioli R, Manci N, Scambia G, Dell'Anna T, Fossati R, Floriani I, Rossi RS, Grassi R, Favalli G, Raspagliesi F, Giannarelli D, Martella L, Mangioni C. Systematic aortic and pelvic lymphadenectomy versus resection of bulky nodes only in optimally debulked advanced ovarian cancer: a randomized clinical trial. J Natl Cancer Inst. 2005;97(8):560–6.
15. Weiner HL, Cohen JA. Treatment of multiple sclerosis with cyclophosphamide: critical review of clinical and immunologic effects. Mult Scler. 2002;8(2):142–54.

16. Fraser JM, Janicki CN, Raveney BJ, Morgan DJ. Abortive activation precedes functional deletion of cd8+ t cells following encounter with self-antigens expressed by resting b cells in vivo. Immunology. 2006;119(1):126–33.
17. Wyllie AH. Cell death: a new classification separating apoptosis from necrosis. In: Bowen ID, Lockshin RA, editors. Cell death in biology and pathology. Dordrecht: Springer; 1981. p. 9–34.
18. Green DR, Ferguson T, Zitvogel L, Kroemer G. Immunogenic and tolerogenic cell death. Nat Rev Immunol. 2009;9(5):353–63.
19. Garg AD, Romano E, Rufo N, Agostinis P. Immunogenic versus tolerogenic phagocytosis during anticancer therapy: mechanisms and clinical translation. Cell Death Differ. 2016;23(6):938–51.
20. Garg AD, Dudek AM, Agostinis P. Cancer immunogenicity, danger signals, and damps: what, when, and how? Biofactors. 2013;39(4):355–67.
21. Fehres CM, Unger WW, Garcia-Vallejo JJ, van Kooyk Y. Understanding the biology of antigen cross-presentation for the design of vaccines against cancer. Front Immunol. 2014;5:149.
22. Garg AD, Martin S, Golab J, Agostinis P. Danger signalling during cancer cell death: origins, plasticity and regulation. Cell Death Differ. 2014;21(1):26–38.
23. Schumacher TN, Schreiber RD. Neoantigens in cancer immunotherapy. Science. 2015;348(6230):69–74.
24. Obeid M, Tesniere A, Ghiringhelli F, Fimia GM, Apetoh L, Perfettini JL, Castedo M, Mignot G, Panaretakis T, Casares N, Metivier D, Larochette N, van Endert P, Ciccosanti F, Piacentini M, Zitvogel L, Kroemer G. Calreticulin exposure dictates the immunogenicity of cancer cell death. Nat Med. 2007;13(1):54–61.
25. Adkins I, Fucikova J, Garg AD, Agostinis P, Spisek R. Physical modalities inducing immunogenic tumor cell death for cancer immunotherapy. Oncoimmunology. 2014;3(12):e968434.
26. Galluzzi L, Buque A, Kepp O, Zitvogel L, Kroemer G. Immunogenic cell death in cancer and infectious disease. Nat Rev Immunol. 2017;17(2):97–111.
27. Reynders K, Illidge T, Siva S, Chang JY, De Ruysscher D. The abscopal effect of local radiotherapy: using immunotherapy to make a rare event clinically relevant. Cancer Treat Rev. 2015;41(6):503–10.
28. Golden EB, Apetoh L. Radiotherapy and immunogenic cell death. Semin Radiat Oncol. 2015;25(1):11–7.
29. Kamensek U, Kos S, Sersa G. Adjuvant immunotherapy as a tool to boost effectiveness of electrochemotherapy. Handbook of electroporation. 2016. p. 1–16.
30. Mir LM, Gehl J, Sersa G, Collins CG, Garbay JR, Billard V, Geertsen PF, Rudolf Z, O'Sullivan GC, Marty M. Standard operating procedures of the electrochemotherapy: instructions for the use of bleomycin or cisplatin administered either systemically or locally and electric pulses delivered by the cliniporator (tm) by means of invasive or non-invasive electrodes. EJC Suppl. 2006;4(11):14–25.
31. Matthiessen LW, Johannesen HH, Hendel HW, Moss T, Kamby C, Gehl J. Electrochemotherapy for large cutaneous recurrence of breast cancer: a phase ii clinical trial. Acta Oncol. 2012;51(6):713–21.
32. Snoj M, Matthiessen LW. Electrochemotherapy of cutaneous metastases. Handbook of electroporation. 2016. p. 1–14.
33. Griffin LL, Lear JT. Photodynamic therapy and non-melanoma skin cancer. Cancers (Basel). 2016;8(10).
34. DeRosa MC, Crutchley RJ. Photosensitized singlet oxygen and its applications. Coord Chem Rev. 2002;233:351–71.
35. Mallidi S, Anbil S, Bulin AL, Obaid G, Ichikawa M, Hasan T. Beyond the barriers of light penetration: strategies, perspectives and possibilities for photodynamic therapy. Theranostics. 2016;6(13):2458–87.
36. Duan X, Chan C, Guo N, Han W, Weichselbaum RR, Lin W. Photodynamic therapy mediated by nontoxic core-shell nanoparticles synergizes with immune checkpoint blockade

to elicit antitumor immunity and antimetastatic effect on breast cancer. J Am Chem Soc. 2016;138(51):16686–95.
37. Maeding N, Verwanger T, Krammer B. Boosting tumor-specific immunity using pdt. Cancers (Basel). 2016;8(10)
38. Tanaka M, Kataoka H, Yano S, Sawada T, Akashi H, Inoue M, Suzuki S, Inagaki Y, Hayashi N, Nishie H, Shimura T, Mizoshita T, Mori Y, Kubota E, Tanida S, Takahashi S, Joh T. Immunogenic cell death due to a new photodynamic therapy (pdt) with glycoconjugated chlorin (g-chlorin). Oncotarget. 2016;7(30):47242–51.
39. Frey B, Weiss EM, Rubner Y, Wunderlich R, Ott OJ, Sauer R, Fietkau R, Gaipl US. Old and new facts about hyperthermia-induced modulations of the immune system. Int J Hyperthermia. 2012;28(6):528–42.
40. Larson N, Gormley A, Frazier N, Ghandehari H. Synergistic enhancement of cancer therapy using a combination of heat shock protein targeted hpma copolymer-drug conjugates and gold nanorod induced hyperthermia. J Control Release. 2013;170(1):41–50.
41. Fucikova J, Moserova I, Truxova I, Hermanova I, Vancurova I, Partlova S, Fialova A, Sojka L, Cartron PF, Houska M, Rob L, Bartunkova J, Spisek R. High hydrostatic pressure induces immunogenic cell death in human tumor cells. Int J Cancer. 2014;135(5):1165–77.
42. Moserova I, Truxova I, Garg AD, Tomala J, Agostinis P, Cartron PF, Vosahlikova S, Kovar M, Spisek R, Fucikova J. Caspase-2 and oxidative stress underlie the immunogenic potential of high hydrostatic pressure-induced cancer cell death. Oncoimmunology. 2017;6(1):e1258505.
43. Vandenberk L, Belmans J, Van Woensel M, Riva M, Van Gool SW. Exploiting the immunogenic potential of cancer cells for improved dendritic cell vaccines. Front Immunol. 2015;6:663.
44. Schmidt-Bleker A, Bansemer R, Reuter S, Weltmann K-D. How to produce an nox-instead of ox-based chemistry with a cold atmospheric plasma jet. Plasma Process Polym. 2016;13(11):1120–7.
45. Jablonowski H, von Woedtke T. Research on plasma medicine-relevant plasma–liquid interaction: what happened in the past five years? Clin Plasma Med. 2015;3(2):42–52.
46. Dunnbier M, Schmidt-Bleker A, Winter J, Wolfram M, Hippler R, Weltmann KD, Reuter S. Ambient air particle transport into the effluent of a cold atmospheric-pressure argon plasma jet investigated by molecular beam mass spectrometry. J Phys D. 2013;46(43):435203.
47. Bekeschus S, Wende K, Hefny MM, Rodder K, Jablonowski H, Schmidt A, Woedtke TV, Weltmann KD, Benedikt J. Oxygen atoms are critical in rendering thp-1 leukaemia cells susceptible to cold physical plasma-induced apoptosis. Sci Rep. 2017;7(1):2791.
48. Lin A, Truong B, Patel S, Kaushik N, Choi EH, Fridman G, Fridman A, Miller V. Nanosecond-pulsed dbd plasma-generated reactive oxygen species trigger immunogenic cell death in a549 lung carcinoma cells through intracellular oxidative stress. Int J Mol Sci. 2017;18(5)
49. Bekeschus S, Roder K, Fregin B, Otto O, Lippert M, Weltmann KD, Wende K, Schmidt A, Gandhirajan RK. Toxicity and immunogenicity in murine melanoma following exposure to physical plasma-derived oxidants. Oxidative Med Cell Longev. 2017;2017:4396467.
50. Lin A, Truong B, Pappas A, Kirifides L, Oubarri A, Chen S, Lin S, Dobrynin D, Fridman G, Fridman A, Sang N, Miller V. Uniform nanosecond pulsed dielectric barrier discharge plasma enhances anti-tumor effects by induction of immunogenic cell death in tumors and stimulation of macrophages. Plasma Process Polym. 2015;12(12):1392–9.
51. Kaushik NK, Kaushik N, Min B, Choi KH, Hong YJ, Miller V, Fridman A, Choi EH. Cytotoxic macrophage-released tumour necrosis factor-alpha (tnf-alpha) as a killing mechanism for cancer cell death after cold plasma activation. J Phys D. 2016;49(8):084001.
52. Kazue M, Kenta Y, Yuki S, Taketoshi A, Ryo O. Anti-tumor immune response induced by nanosecond pulsed streamer discharge in mice. J Phys D. 2017;50(12):12LT01.
53. Miller V, Lin A, Fridman G, Dobrynin D, Fridman A. Plasma stimulation of migration of macrophages. Plasma Process Polym. 2014;11(12):1193–7.
54. Bekeschus S, Winterbourn CC, Kolata J, Masur K, Hasse S, Broker BM, Parker HA. Neutrophil extracellular trap formation is elicited in response to cold physical plasma. J Leukoc Biol. 2016;100(4):791–9.

55. Bekeschus S, Kolata J, Muller A, Kramer A, Weltmann K-D, Broker B, Masur K. Differential viability of eight human blood mononuclear cell subpopulations after plasma treatment. Plasma Med. 2013;3(1–2):1–13.
56. Bundscherer L, Bekeschus S, Tresp H, Hasse S, Reuter S, Weltmann K-D, Lindequist U, Masur K. Viability of human blood leucocytes compared with their respective cell lines after plasma treatment. Plasma Med. 2013;3(1–2):71–80.
57. Bekeschus S, Iseni S, Reuter S, Masur K, Weltmann K-D. Nitrogen shielding of an argon plasma jet and its effects on human immune cells. IEEE Trans Plasma Sci. 2015;43(3):776–81.
58. Bekeschus S, Rödder K, Schmidt A, Stope MB, von Woedtke T, Miller V, Fridman A, Weltmann K-D, Masur K, Metelmann H-R, Wende K, Hasse S. Cold physical plasma selects for specific t helper cell subsets with distinct cells surface markers in a caspase-dependent and nf-κb-independent manner. Plasma Process Polym. 2016;13(12):1144–50.
59. Wende K, Reuter S, von Woedtke T, Weltmann KD, Masur K. Redox-based assay for assessment of biological impact of plasma treatment. Plasma Process Polym. 2014;11(7):655–63.
60. Miller V, Lin A, Fridman A. Why target immune cells for plasma treatment of cancer. Plasma Chem Plasma Process. 2016;36(1):259–68.
61. Garg AD, Vandenberk L, Koks C, Verschuere T, Boon L, Van Gool SW, Agostinis P. Dendritic cell vaccines based on immunogenic cell death elicit danger signals and t cell-driven rejection of high-grade glioma. Sci Transl Med. 2016;8(328):328ra327.
62. Kyte JA, Mu L, Aamdal S, Kvalheim G, Dueland S, Hauser M, Gullestad HP, Ryder T, Lislerud K, Hammerstad H, Gaudernack G. Phase i/ii trial of melanoma therapy with dendritic cells transfected with autologous tumor-mrna. Cancer Gene Ther. 2006;13(10):905–18.
63. Vandenberk L, Garg AD, Verschuere T, Koks C, Belmans J, Beullens M, Agostinis P, De Vleeschouwer S, Van Gool SW. Irradiation of necrotic cancer cells, employed for pulsing dendritic cells (dcs), potentiates dc vaccine-induced antitumor immunity against high-grade glioma. Oncoimmunology. 2016;5(2):e1083669.
64. Garg AD, Coulie PG, Van den Eynde BJ, Agostinis P. Integrating next-generation dendritic cell vaccines into the current cancer immunotherapy landscape. Trends Immunol. 2017;38:577–93.

# Perspectives in Ophthalmology 25

Emilio Martines, Helena Reitberger, Catherine Chow, Paola Brun, Matteo Zuin, and Thomas A. Fuchsluger

## 25.1 Infections of the Cornea and Vision Loss

The ocular surface is continuously exposed to microorganisms that can cause or aggravate infections like bacterial conjunctivitis and keratitis. Risk, type and frequency of these infections are dependent on geographic region an on medical supplies. In particular, the bacterial keratitis is considered an ocular emergency that requires immediate and appropriate treatment to limit corneal morbidity and vision loss. Factors resulting in increased infection risk mainly are ocular trauma, previous corneal surgery and contact lens wear. Certain microbes such as staphylococcal species (spp.), *Pseudomonas aeruginosa* and *Streptococcus pneumoniae* are more likely to cause bacterial keratitis. Moreover, of all possible viral and fungal infections, the vast majority is caused by *Herpes simplex* virus and *Aspergillus* and *Candida* spp. [1–3]. Initial therapy for keratitis involves topical e.g., fluoroquinolones or topical broad-spectrum, fortified antibiotics. However, the emergence of bacterial resistance to topical antibiotics and antifungal drugs compromises an effective healing and is exacerbated by the need for prolonged therapeutic treatment [4]. Insufficient treatment results on permanent corneal scars requiring

E. Martines • M. Zuin
Istituto Gas Ionizzati del CNR and Consorzio RFX Padova, Padova, Italy

H. Reitberger • T. A. Fuchsluger (✉)
Department of Ophthalmology, Friedrich-Alexander-University Erlangen-Nuremberg, University Hospital Erlangen, Erlangen, Germany
e-mail: thomas.fuchsluger@uk-erlangen.de

C. Chow
St. Joseph Stift Hospital, Bremen, Germany

P. Brun
Unit of Microbiology, Department of Molecular Medicine, University of Padova, Padova, Italy



H.-R. Metelmann et al. (eds.), *Comprehensive Clinical Plasma Medicine*,
https://doi.org/10.1007/978-3-319-67627-2_25

transplantation of a donor cornea, or persistent epithelial defect with corneal thinning in acute surgical intervention. For these reasons, novel, immediate therapeutic strategies that are irrespective of the type of infection are an unmet need in ophthalmology and a breakthrough in the treatment of infectious corneal diseases.

In this context, the therapeutic application of disinfecting non-thermal atmospheric plasma (so-called "cold plasma") could open a new treatment strategy. Here, a primary requirement is the safety of the treated corneal area, which must be safeguarded with respect to thermal effects and the risk of electrical shock. In order to meet the last requirement, the approach of using an indirect plasma treatment, with no direct contact of the plasma with the treated surface, has been adopted. In this article, we will present two different cold plasma setups: (1) using helium gas (Martines et al.), (2) using argon gas (Fuchsluger et al.)

## 25.2 Chances of Cold Plasma-Based Treatment for Reducing the Infectious Microbial Load

Martines et al. developed a plasma source [5, 6] in which a helium plasma is generated by a high voltage (of the order of 1 $kV_{pp}$) at radiofrequency (around 5 MHz). This is applied between two parallel brass grids serving as electrodes. The grids close the ends of two coaxial tubes, the innermost of which carries a helium flow of the order of 2 L/min. The high voltage is applied to the inner grid, whereas the outer one, which closes a tube of conducting material, is grounded. In this way the outer part of the device is fully grounded, granting an adequate level of electrical safety, even in case of accidental contact with the treated surface. The helium plasma produced between the two grids contains traces of air coming from outside the source, and this drives the production of reactive oxygen and nitrogen species. These species, together with the helium excited metastable states formed in the plasma, are responsible of the observed biological effects. On the other hand, no charged species can reach the treated surface, due to the very fast recombination time: however, this does not prevent the disinfectant effect. The typical distance between the outer grid and the treated substrate in tests is around 1 mm.

Fuchsluger et al. worked with argon based cold plasma to treat corneal infections. The plasma pen kINPen MED M12150063 by neoplas tools GmbH, Greifswald, Germany, is optimized for a gas flow of 5 L/min. The optimal distance of plasma pen tip to the sample was 5 cm, the duration of treatment between 30 s and 1 min.

Challenge tests performed *in vitro* based on the international standard ISO 14729 have shown the effectiveness of the helium plasma treatment in reducing microbial load of Gram-positive and Gram-negative bacteria and fungi. As reported in Fig. 25.1, microbial inactivation followed a double exponential decay, with a fast phase lasting around 2 min for Gram-positive bacteria and around 1 min for Gram-negative ones. During the fast phase, the logarithmic reduction factor RF = log(initial CFU/mL)—log(final CFU/mL) was around 4 in Gram-positive bacteria and around 3 in Gram-negative ones. Overall, a 2-min treatment appeared to be sufficient to exceed the RF = 3 value recommended by ISO 14729. A 5-min treatment allows to reach RF = 5. The antimicrobial potential of different plasma sources is confirmed by several past and recently published articles indicating the enormous potential of cold atmospheric plasma in disinfection of surfaces [7], prevention of hospital-acquired infections [8], decontamination of food [9]. Interestingly, as reported in Fig. 25.1, bacteria resistant to conventional antibiotics (i.e., methicillin-resistant [MR] *S. aureus* and vancomycin resistant [VR] *E. coli*) were inactivated by the plasma treatment at the same rate of non-antibiotic resistant bacteria. These results

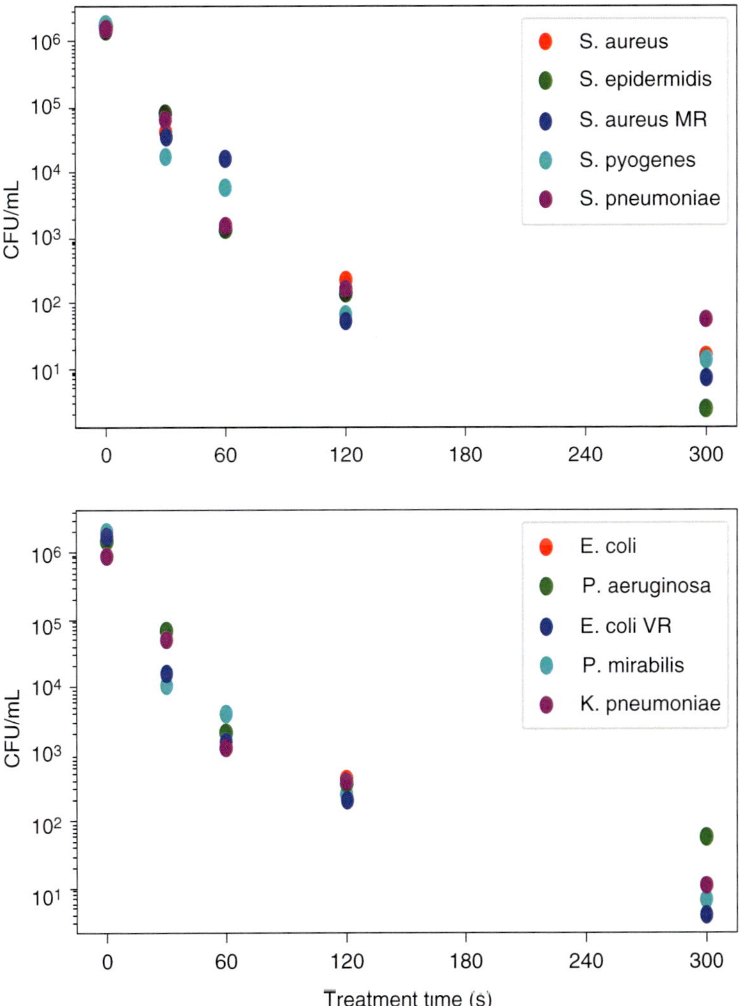


**Fig. 25.1** Microorganism survival as a function of plasma treatment duration, for Gram positive (top) and Gram negative (bottom) bacteria. The points at 0 s represent the untreated controls. Each point is the mean of four independent experiments

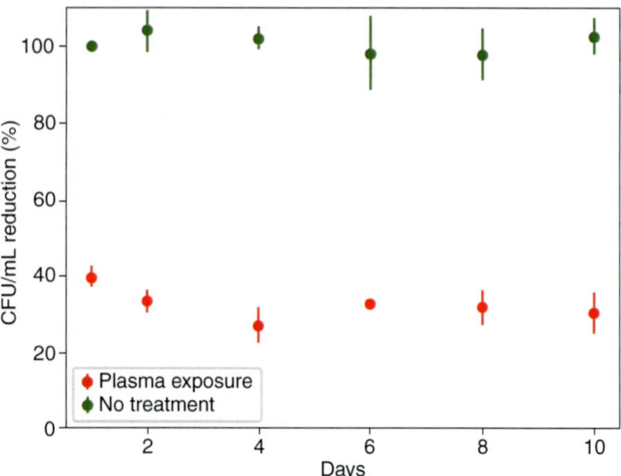


**Fig. 25.2** Reduction of *S. aureus* following 1-min plasma treatment in the different days of the experiment looking for resistance development (in red). The green point refer to the untreated control

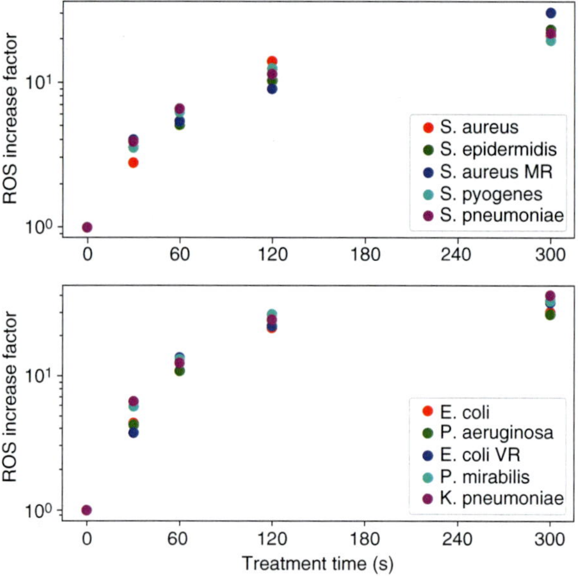


**Fig. 25.3** Increase factor of intracellular ROS in Gram positive (top) and Gram negative (bottom) bacteria after the plasma treatment. The increase factor is evaluated with respect to the control case

were comparable when using argon instead of helium-based cold plasma. Moreover, as shown in Fig. 25.2, repeated helium plasma treatments (once a day for 10 days, 1 min plasma treatment) did not reduce bactericidal effect in *S. aureus,* thus ruling out the possibility of resistance to plasma antimicrobial effects.

For both Gram-positive and Gram-negative bacteria, formation of reactive oxygen species inside the bacterial cells were well correlated with, and most likely accounts for, the disinfectant effects of plasma [10]. This was shown in Fig. 25.3, where the increase factor in intracellular ROS following the helium plasma treatment, as measured by a fluorescent probe, was plotted as a function of treatment

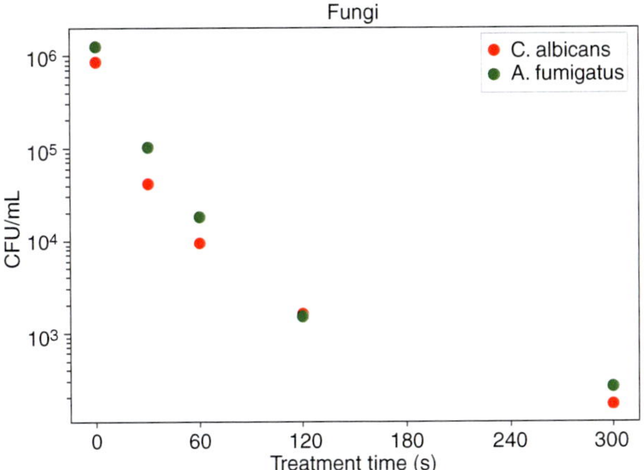


**Fig. 25.4** Microorganism survival as a function of plasma treatment duration, for two different fungi responsible for keratitis. The points at 0 s represent the untreated controls. Each point is the mean of four independent experiments

time. It was possible to see that ROS enhancements by factor ≤40 for Gram-positive and ≤30 for Gram-negative bacteria were achieved with a 5-min treatment. As reported in Fig. 25.4, the helium plasma treatment was also effective in deactivating *C. albicans* and *A. fumigatus*, fungi involved in 5% of infectious keratitis [3]. In this case the transition from fast to slow exponential decay was not readily seen from the data, but could be located in the range of treatment times spanning from 1 to 2 min. Overall, a reduction factor exceeding 3 could be obtained for both fungal species, with treatment times of around 3 min. Concerning other ocular pathogen types, Heaselgrave and colleagues suggested the use of plasma also against protozoan pathogens, demonstrating the inactivation of trophozoites and cysts of *Acanthamoeba polyphaga* [11]. The antiviral effect of plasma is more difficult to achieve. Mature forms of viral particles which are involved in diffusion of infections, are usually not affected by direct plasma exposure [10] but easily inhibited when replicating inside the host cells [12, 13]. Indeed, during replication the reactive oxygen species induced by the plasma treatment in infected host cells most likely destroy uncoated viruses, thus preventing the release of new viral particles.

## 25.3 Laboratory Experiments in Human Corneas

To prove the effectiveness of the described plasma treatment for corneal infections, the penetration depth on corneal tissue of helium plasma-induced effects was investigated. As already described, plasma caused generation of reactive oxygen species (ROS) in living matter. Therefore, in this experiment human cornea unsuitable for surgical transplantation was loaded with cell-permeant 2′,7′-dichlorodihydrofluorescein diacetate ($H_2$DCFDA) non-fluorescent probe converted to highly fluorescent DCF upon oxidation. Following 2-min treatment with plasma, the cornea was fixed, cut to obtain serial sections of 8 μm thickness separated by 40 μm layers and then visualized at the confocal microscopy. As reported in Fig. 25.5, ROS the related fluorescent signal is evident not only in the epithelial layer but also in most of the

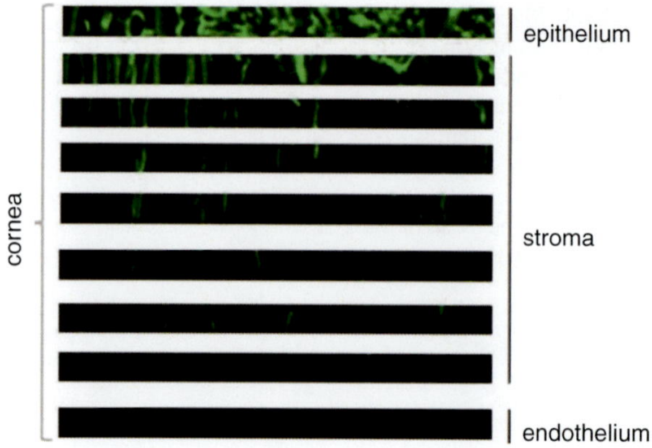

**Fig. 25.5** Penetration of the plasma treatment effect, as detected by the fluorescence caused by the formation of intracellular ROS, inside the cornea. The figure displays fluorescence in ten slices of 8 μm thickness, separated one from the other by 40 μm

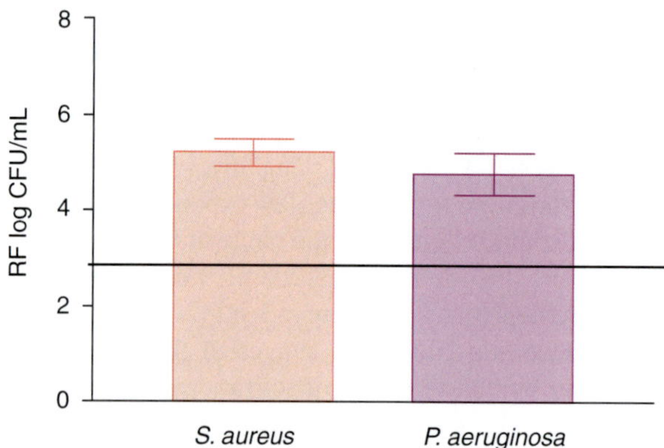


**Fig. 25.6** Logarithm of the reduction factor after 5-min plasma treatment in ex vivo human corneas infected with two different bacteria. Each value is the mean of three independent experiments

stroma, against the intuitive understanding that the plasma treatment is only superficial. Taking into account that pathogens penetrate in the cornea for about one third in depth [3], the plasma treatment has the potential to penetrate in the tissue and to reach also invasive pathogens. It is worth mentioning that, since the penetration of the fluorescent probe in the deeper layers of the cornea is unknown, the obtained result likely underestimates the actual penetration of the plasma effect. A second experiment was performed in order to test the effectiveness of the plasma disinfectant properties in a situation more similar to the actual one. Corneas were *ex vivo* infected and incubated for 16 h at 37 °C to allow for bacterial penetration, colonization, and growth. Corneas were then treated for 2 min with helium plasma and finally minced to collect also invasive microbes. As reported in Fig. 25.6, the plasma treatment significantly decreased the survival of bacteria recovered from infected tissues, thus confirming also *ex vivo* the previously reported disinfectant effects.

The ROS generated by the plasma treatment have mild and transient effects in conjunctival fibroblasts and keratocytes [10]. As other laboratories have already demonstrated [14, 15], short-term plasma treatment does not affect viability of eukaryotic cells even if mechanisms of cell proliferation and damage occur simultaneously and balance one with the other following the intracellular ROS generation mediated by plasma treatment [16, 17]. In our experiments, cells cultured from human conjunctiva or cornea were treated with helium plasma for 2 or 5 min and cell viability was analyzed by the MTT test. One hour after a 2-min plasma treatment, the cell viability was not significantly reduced when compared to untreated cells, while a significant reduction of viability was observed following a 5-min treatment. However, the viability of cells treated for 2 or 5 min significantly increased after 24 h of culture [10].

A transient accumulation of 8-oxo-2′-deoxyguanosine (8-OHdG) was observed in cultured cells following plasma treatment [10] without important induction of thymine dimers. The formation of pyrimidine dimers (thymine or cytosine dimers or thymine-cytosine heterodimers) consequent to UV irradiation can impair DNA replication and transcription. We evaluated the presence of thymine dimers (TD) in the nuclei of cells exposed to helium plasma using the system developed by Al-Adhami et al. [18], with some modifications ([10]): corneal specimens were stained with anti-TD mAb and counterstained with Hoechst to evidence nucleic DNA. Positive controls were prepared by exposing the tissue sections to 8 J/cm$^2$ UV rays having a wavelength of 254 nm for 10 min; negative controls were slides not incubated with the anti-TD antibody. All slides were analyzed by fluorescence microscopy. As shown in Fig. 25.7, nuclei of cells exposed to the plasma source for up to 5 min did not show TD signals. In fact, anti-TD antibodies and Hoechst staining co-localized in the nuclei of UV-irradiated cells, whereas only Hoechst staining was evident and localized in the nuclei of plasma-treated tissues. Finally, to assess the lack of negative effects of plasma, treated human corneas were analyzed for

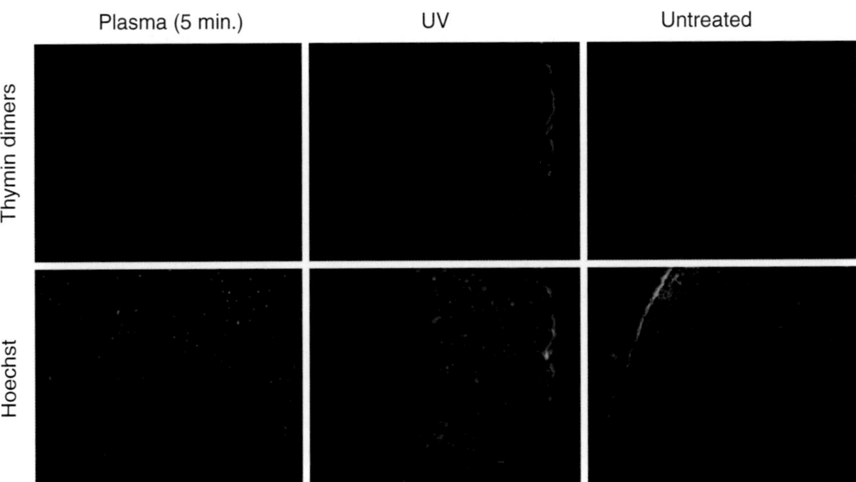


**Fig. 25.7** Thymine dimers formation (red) in the nuclei (blue) of corneal tissue treated with the plasma source for 5 min (left), treated with 254 nm UV light (center) as positive control and untreated (right) as negative control

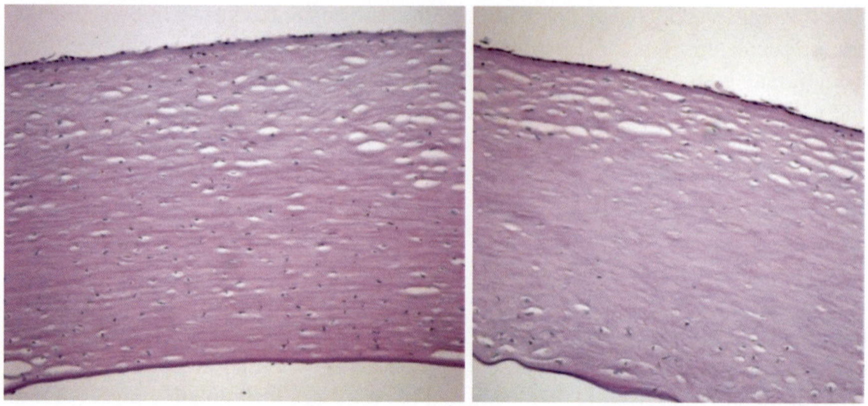

**Fig. 25.8** Corneal tissue morphology after 5-min plasma treatment (left) and control (right) at 100 magnification

morphological changes. Tissues were embedded in paraffin, cut into 5 μm sections, and stained with hematoxylin and eosin. As evident in Fig. 25.8, the plasma treatment did not induce significant morphological changes in the corneal stroma.

## 25.4 From Bench to Bedside: Treatment of Corneal Infections with Argon-Based Cold Plasma in Patients

Argon-based cold-plasma treatment of microbes in the dish and on ex vivo corneal tissue resulted in very comparable results as application of helium-based cold plasma. As next step, corneal infections and ulcerations were treated in patients refractive to conventional therapies.

Figure 25.9 shows a 71 year-old patient with severe Staphylococcus aureus-induced corneal ulcer and massive intraocular infection (hypopyon). Vision was considerably reduced, intraocular pressure elevated. The ulceration did not respond well over 5 days. Neither to intensive local, nor to intravitreal and to systemic broad-spectrum antibiotic treatment. The patient therefore received on day 5 after admission a 30 s treatment, 90° angle to the corneal surface with a "plasma tip to cornea" distance of 5 mm. The patient rapidly recovered without recurrence after the first plasma treatments. The 6 months follow-up showed a healed corneal surface with a merely small corneal scar. Visual acuity had recovered from hand movements at admission to 0,6 and the last follow-up visit.

In conclusion, the proposed indirect plasma treatment appears to be a promising tool for the development of a new painless treatment of infectious keratitis with short duration application [19]. Hopefully, in a short time a plasma-based device could become a routinely used tool in the ophthalmology patient service and surgery room, where it could also be applied in the pre- and post-surgery phase as a standard tool for tissue disinfection.

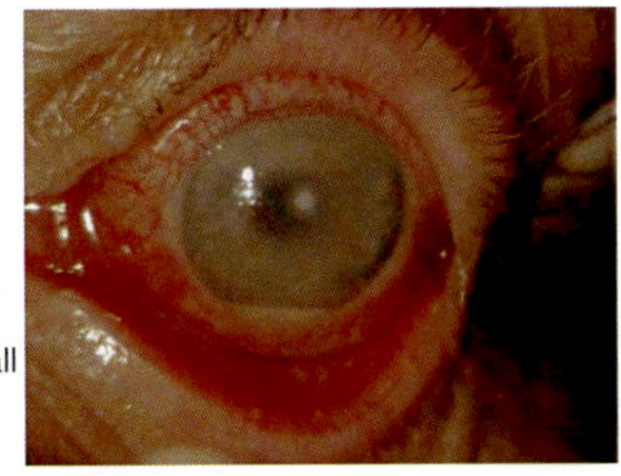

1. At admission:
Central ulcer with massive intraocular infection
*visual acuity: hand movements*

4. 6 weeks after admission, end of plasma treatment:
Central ulcer healed to small small stromal scar,
no intraocular infection
*visual acuity: 0,6*

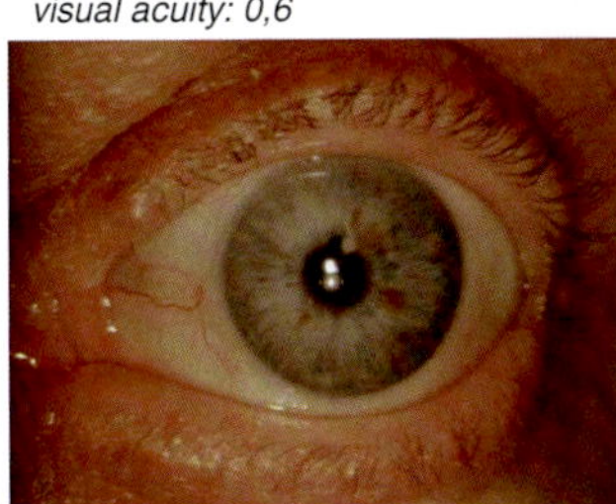

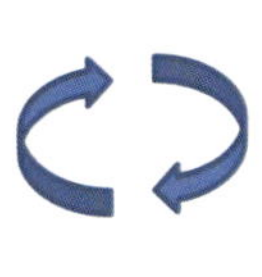

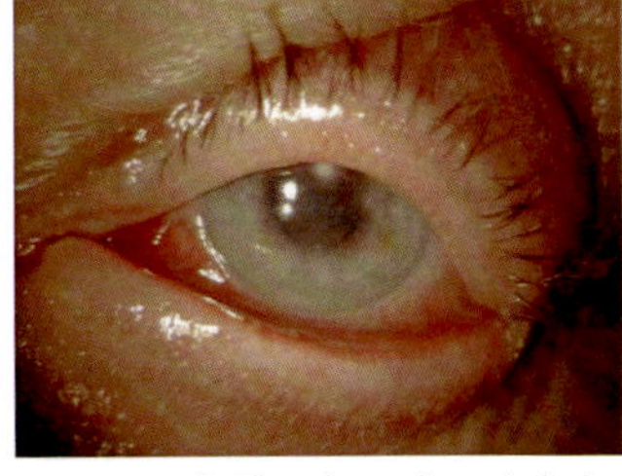

2. Five days after admission, 1st plasma treatment:
Central ulcer unchanged, less intraocular infection
*visual acuity: counting fingers*

3. 17 days after admission, 4th plasma treatment:
Central ulcer healed to small epithelial (superior) defect,
no intraocular infection
*visual acuity: 0,4*

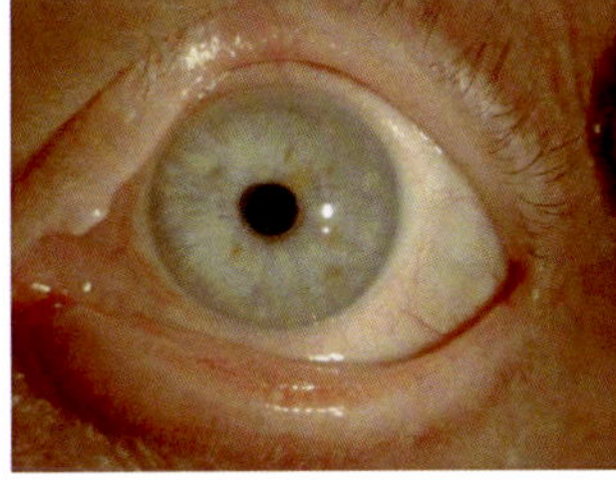

**Fig. 25.9** Plasma treatment of a corneal ulceration associated with massive intraocular infection. (**1**) At admission: Central ulcer with massive intraocular infection. *Visual acuity: hand movements*. (**2**) Five days after admission, first plasma treatment: Central ulcer unchanged, less intraocular infection. *Visual acuity: counting fingers*. (**3**) Seventeen days after admission, fourth plasma treatment: Central ulcer healed to small epithelial (superior) defect, no intraocular infection. *Visual acuity: 0,4*. (**4**) Six weeks after admission, end of plasma treatment: Central ulcer healed to small stromal scar, no intraocular infection. *Visual acuity: 0,6*

## References


1. Neumann M, Sjostrand J. Central microbial keratitis in a Swedish city population. Acta Ophthalmol. 1993;71:160–4.
2. Thomas PA, Geraldine P. Infectious keratitis. Curr Opin Infect Dis. 2007;20:129–41.
3. Zimmerman AB, Nixon AD, Rueff EM. Contact lens associated microbial keratitis: practical considerations for the optometrist. Clin Optom. 2016;8:1–12.
4. Grundmann H, Aires de Sousa M, Boyce J, Tiemersma E. Emergence and resurgence of meticillin-resistant *Staphylococcus aureus* as a public-health threat. Lancet. 2006;368:874–85.
5. Leonardi A, Deligianni V, Martines E, Zuin M, Cavazzana R, Serianni G, Spolaore M. Plasma device for treating living tissues, PCT patent n. WO 2009/043925. Published on 9 Apr 2009.
6. Martines E, Zuin M, Cavazzana R, Gazza E, Serianni G, Spagnolo S, Spolaore M, Leonardi A, Deligianni V, Brun P, Aragona M, Brun P. A new plasma source for sterilization of living tissues. New J Phys. 2009;11:115014.

7. O'Connor N, Cahill O, Daniels S, Galvin S, Humphreys H. Cold atmospheric pressure plasma and decontamination. Can it contribute to preventing hospital-acquired infections? J Hosp Infect. 2014;88:59–65.
8. Cahill OJ, Claro T, O'Connor N, Cafolla AA, Stevens NT, Daniels S, Humphreys H. Cold air plasma to decontaminate inanimate surfaces of the hospital environment. Appl Environ Microbiol. 2014;80:2004–10.
9. Aboubakr HA, Williams P, Gangal U, Youssef MM, El-Sohaimy SA, Bruggeman PJ, Goyal SM. Virucidal effect of cold atmospheric gaseous plasma on feline calicivirus, a surrogate for human norovirus. Appl Environ Microbiol. 2015;81:3612–22.
10. Brun P, Brun P, Vono M, Venier P, Tarricone E, Deligianni V, Martines E, Zuin M, Spagnolo S, Cavazzana R, Cardin R, Castagliuolo I, Valerio AL, Leonardi A. Disinfection of ocular cells and tissues by atmospheric-pressure cold plasma. PLoS One. 2012;7:e33245.
11. Heaselgrave W, Shama G, Andrew PW, Kong MG. Inactivation of Acanthamoeba spp. and other ocular pathogens by application of cold atmospheric gas plasma. Appl Environ Microbiol. 2016;82:3143–8.
12. Alekseev O, Donovan K, Limonnik V, Azizkhan-Clifford J. Nonthermal dielectric barrier discharge (DBD) plasma suppresses herpes simplex virus type 1 (HSV-1) replication in corneal epithelium. Transl Vis Sci Technol. 2014;3:2.
13. Volotskova O, Dubrovsky L, Keidar M, Bukrinsky M. Cold atmospheric plasma inhibits HIV-1 replication in macrophages by targeting both the virus and the cells. PLoS One. 2016;11:e0165322.
14. Hasse S, Duong Tran T, Hahn O, Kindler S, Metelmann HR, von Woedtke T, Masur K. Induction of proliferation of basal epidermal keratinocytes by cold atmospheric-pressure plasma. Clin Exp Dermatol. 2016;41:202–9.
15. Wende K, Straßenburg S, Haertel B, Harms M, Holtz S, Barton A, Masur K, von Woedtke T, Lindequist U. Atmospheric pressure plasma jet treatment evokes transient oxidative stress in HaCaT keratinocytes and influences cell physiology. Cell Biol Int. 2014;38:412–25.
16. Brun P, Pathak S, Castagliuolo I, Palù G, Brun P, Zuin M, Cavazzana R, Martines E. Helium generated cold plasma finely regulates activation of human fibroblast-like primary cells. PLoS One. 2014;9:e104397.
17. Rosani U, Tarricone E, Venier P, Brun P, Deligianni V, Zuin M, Martines E, Leonardi A, Brun P. Atmospheric-pressure cold plasma induces transcriptional changes in ex vivo human corneas. PLoS One. 2015;10:e0133173.
18. Al-Adhami BH, Nichols RAB, Kusel JR, O'Grady J, Smith HV. Detection of UV-induced thymine dimmers in individual Cryptosporidium parvum and Cryptosporidium hominis oocysts by immunofluorescence microscopy. Appl Environ Microbiol. 2007;73:947–55.
19. Martines E, Brun P, Brun P, Cavazzana R, Deligianni V, Leonardi A, Tarricon E, Zuin M. Towards a plasma treatment of corneal infections. Clin Plasma Med. 2013;**1**:17–24.

# Plasma Activated Medium

# 26

Hiromasa Tanaka and Masaru Hori

## 26.1 Plasma Activated Medium

The emerging field of plasma medical science combines plasma science and medical science. Medical applications of non-thermal atmospheric pressure plasma have been studied for several decades [1–7]. Indirect treatments with plasma have attracted a great deal of attention because they have broadened the ways that plasma can be applied to medicine beyond direct applications. Indirect treatments include two major approaches: plasma immunotherapy and plasma activated medium (PAM). Plasma can activate the immune system to kill cancer cells [8–11], and plasma can activate the medium to kill cancer cells [7, 12–20]. Thus, plasma directly affects not only cells/tissues, but also the cell/tissue microenvironment.

This chapter introduces PAM and its applications. It is essential to understand the interactions between plasma and liquids to understand PAM's effects and capabilities. Many researchers are discovering anti-tumor factors in PAM based on plasma chemistry and molecular cell biology. The applications of PAM are expanding from cancer therapy to treatment of age-related macular degeneration (AMD) and regenerative medicine.

## 26.2 Chemistry in Plasma Activated Medium

The interaction between plasma and liquids is an important topic in plasma medical science. Figure 26.1 depicts reaction products from plasma inputs to physiological outputs in gas phase, liquid phase, and the intracellular domain [7]. Plasma consists of electrons, ions, radicals, and light such as ultra violet (UV) and

H. Tanaka (✉) • M. Hori
Nagoya University, Nagoya, Japan
e-mail: htanaka@plasma.engg.nagoya-u.ac.jp



H.-R. Metelmann et al. (eds.), *Comprehensive Clinical Plasma Medicine*,
https://doi.org/10.1007/978-3-319-67627-2_26

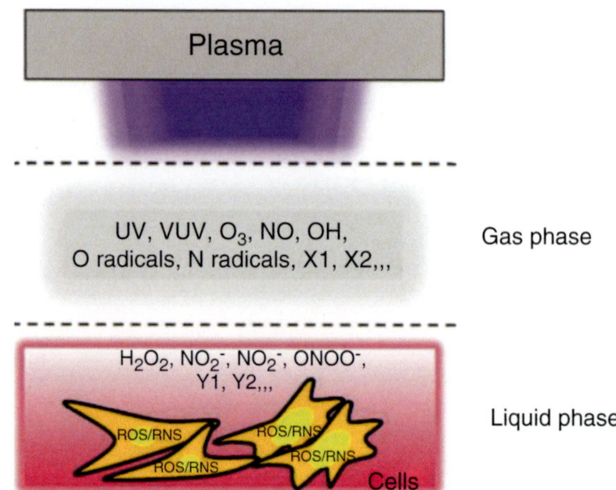


**Fig. 26.1** Plasma inputs to physiological outputs. The plasma-cell/tissue system consists of multiple inputs from plasma and complex biological signaling networks. Reactive species in gas phase and liquid phase generated by plasma interact with cells, which leads to the induction of intracellular ROS and RNS. These processes lead to physiological outputs, such as apoptosis, morphological changes, and altered proliferation (reproduced from Tanaka et al. 2014)

vacuum ultra violet (VUV). Reactive species are generated through interactions between plasma and nitrogen, oxygen, and moisture in the air. The reactive species react with liquids to produce hydrogen peroxide, nitrite and nitrate ions, which then interact with cells to produce reactive oxygen species (ROS) and reactive nitrogen species (RNS). In response, several intracellular signaling pathways are activated or deactivated driving various physiological outputs, such as apoptosis and morphological changes.

Hydrogen peroxide, nitrite and nitrate ions are general reaction products generated through interactions between plasma and liquids, and are not dependent on the characteristics of the solutions. Plasma also interacts with the constituents of solutions to produce specific reaction products. Recent studies have revealed that both specific factors and general factors are important for producing some physiological outputs, including apoptosis of cancer cells [20].

PAM was originally produced using culture media such as Dulbecco's Modified Eagle Medium (DMEM) and Roswell Park Memorial Institute Medium (RPMI) [12, 13]. These media contains about 30 components, including inorganic salts, amino acids, vitamins, and glucose. These factors are activated by plasma, and the reaction products can positively or negatively regulate signaling networks involved in various physiological outputs.

Ringer's solutions, such as Ringer's lactate solution (which contains sodium chloride, potassium chloride, calcium chloride, and L-sodium lactate), acetic acid Ringer's solution (which contains sodium chloride, potassium chloride, calcium chloride, and sodium acetate), and bicarbonate Ringer's solution (which contains

**Table 26.1** Components of Ringer's solutions

| Components (g/L) | Ringer's lactate solution | Acetate acid Ringer's solution | Bicarbonate Ringer's solution |
|---|---|---|---|
| NaCl | 6.0 | 6.0 | 5.8 |
| KCl | 0.30 | 0.30 | 0.30 |
| $CaCl_2 \cdot 2H_2O$ | 0.20 | 0.10 | 0.11 |
| L-sodium lactate | 3.1 | – | – |
| $C_2H_3NaO_2 \cdot 2H_2O$ | – | 3.80 | – |
| $MgCl_2$ | – | – | 0.20 |
| $NaHCO_3$ | – | – | 2.35 |
| Sodium citrate•$2H_2O$ | – | – | 0.20 |

sodium chloride, potassium chloride, calcium chloride, magnesium chloride, sodium citrate, and sodium hydrogen carbonate) are simple isotonic solutions that have the same osmolality as body fluids (Table 26.1).

Since Ringer's solutions have fewer components than cell culture media, systematic combinatorial experiments are possible, and various plasma activated Ringer's lactate solutions were synthesized to elucidate which components are responsible for the anti-tumor effects of plasma activated Ringer's lactate solution (PAL) (Fig. 26.2, [19]). The results of these experiments revealed that L-sodium lactate is an anti-tumor factor, while sodium chloride, potassium chloride, and calcium chloride are not anti-tumor factors in Ringer's lactate solution treated with plasma.

## 26.3 Cancer Therapy Using Plasma Activated Medium

Since the first report of selective PAM mediated killing of glioblastoma cells [12], PAM mediated anti-tumor effects have been demonstrated for various other cancer cell types. Peritoneal metastases of cancers generally imply a poor prognosis, and PAM has been tested in this scenario. *In vitro* and *in vivo* experiments showed that PAM exhibited anti-tumor effects on anti-cancer drug resistant ovarian cancers [13], ovarian clear-cell carcinoma [21], gastric cancers [15, 22], and pancreatic cancers [16]. PAM mediated anti-tumor effects have also been demonstrated for non-small cell lung carcinoma cells [23], liver cancer cells, breast cancer cells, neuroblastoma cells [24], and urinary bladder squamous cell carcinoma cells [25].

Animal studies are essential to address the clinical applications of PAM. The anti-tumor effects of PAM treatment were investigated in a mouse xenograft model in which ovarian cancer cells [13] or pancreatic cancer cells [16] were injected subcutaneously. Figure 26.3 shows the experimental results using mice bearing NOS2 (parental ovarian cancer cells) and NOS2-TR (paclitaxel resistant ovarian cancer cells) xenografts. PAM significantly reduced the growth of both NOS2 and NOS2-TR tumors, and no significant adverse effects were observed.

**a**

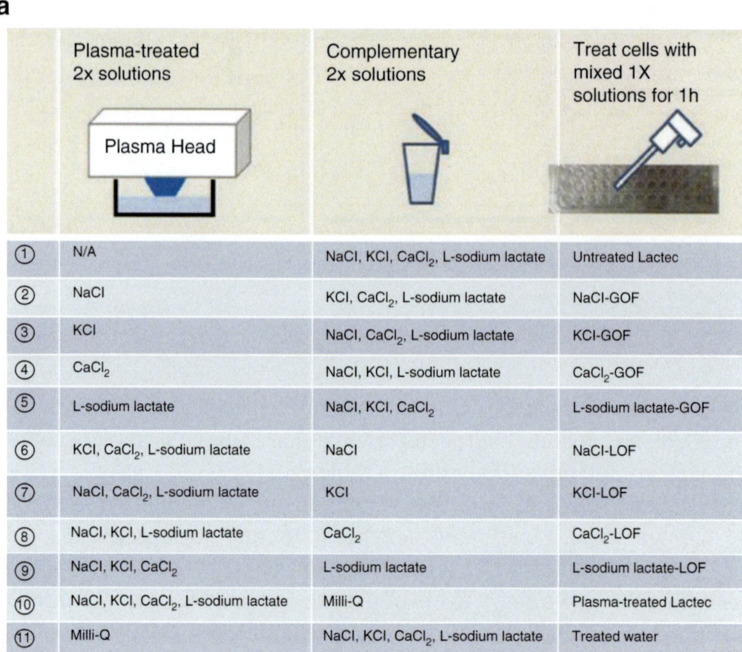

| | Plasma-treated 2x solutions | Complementary 2x solutions | Treat cells with mixed 1X solutions for 1h |
|---|---|---|---|
| ① | N/A | NaCl, KCl, $CaCl_2$, L-sodium lactate | Untreated Lactec |
| ② | NaCl | KCl, $CaCl_2$, L-sodium lactate | NaCl-GOF |
| ③ | KCl | NaCl, $CaCl_2$, L-sodium lactate | KCl-GOF |
| ④ | $CaCl_2$ | NaCl, KCl, L-sodium lactate | $CaCl_2$-GOF |
| ⑤ | L-sodium lactate | NaCl, KCl, $CaCl_2$ | L-sodium lactate-GOF |
| ⑥ | KCl, $CaCl_2$, L-sodium lactate | NaCl | NaCl-LOF |
| ⑦ | NaCl, $CaCl_2$, L-sodium lactate | KCl | KCl-LOF |
| ⑧ | NaCl, KCl, L-sodium lactate | $CaCl_2$ | $CaCl_2$-LOF |
| ⑨ | NaCl, KCl, $CaCl_2$ | L-sodium lactate | L-sodium lactate-LOF |
| ⑩ | NaCl, KCl, $CaCl_2$, L-sodium lactate | Milli-Q | Plasma-treated Lactec |
| ⑪ | Milli-Q | NaCl, KCl, $CaCl_2$, L-sodium lactate | Treated water |



**b**

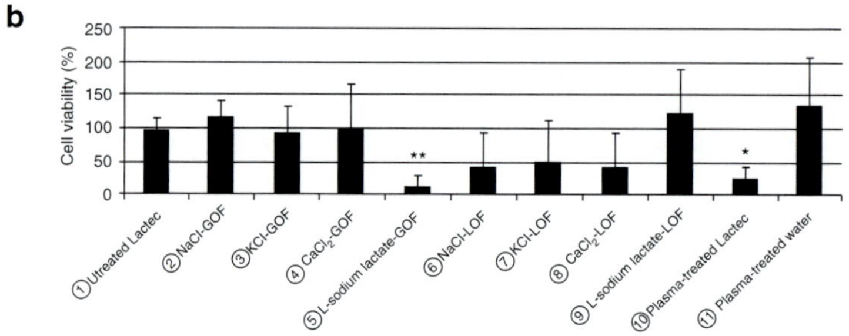


**Fig. 26.2** Identification of components in PAL with anti-tumor effects. (**a**) Schematic of experiments for identifying the anti-tumor components in Ringer's lactate solution induced by plasma irradiation. Each doubly concentrated NaCl, KCl, $CaCl_2$ and L-sodium lactate solution was treated with plasma for 2 min and then mixed with the complementary doubly concentrated solutions. These solutions are referred to as NaCl-GOF, KCl-GOF, $CaCl_2$-GOF and L-sodium lactate-GOF (②–⑤). Each doubly concentrated solution lacking NaCl (KCl + $CaCl_2$+ L-sodium lactate), KCl (NaCl + $CaCl_2$+ L-sodium lactate), $CaCl_2$ (NaCl + KCl + L-sodium lactate) or L-sodium lactate (NaCl + KCl + $CaCl_2$) was treated with plasma for 2 min, and mixed with the complementary doubly concentrated solutions. These solutions are referred to as NaCl-LOF, KCl-LOF, $CaCl_2$-LOF and L-sodium lactate-LOF (⑥–⑨). Doubly concentrated Ringer's lactate solution was treated with plasma and mixed with the same volume of Milli-Q water (⑩), and vice versa (⑪). (**b**) 10,000 U251SP cells were seeded in 200 μL medium in a 96-well plate. On the following day, the media in the 96-well plate were replaced with 200 μL of the solutions described in (**a**). After 1 h, these solutions were replaced with 200 μL culture medium. On the following day, cell viability was measured by the MTS assay and calculated as a percentage of surviving cells relative to control. Data are mean ± SEM. $^*P < 0.05$, $^{**}P < 0.01$ versus control (reproduced from Tanaka et al. 2016)

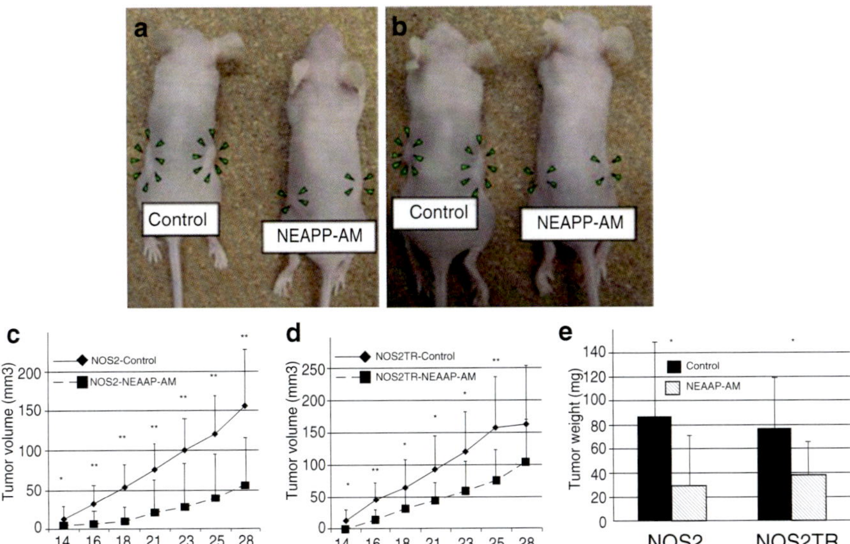


**Fig. 26.3** Anti-tumor effects of PAM (NEAPP-AM) in mice carrying anti-cancer drug resistant ovarian cancer cells. (**a**, **b**) Macroscopic observation of nude mice bearing subcutaneous NOS2 (**a**) and NOS2TR (**b**) tumors on both flanks. Mice were implanted with NOS2 and NOS2TR cells and then treated by local administration of 0.4 mL medium alone or NEAPP-AM into both sides of the mice three times a week. All mice were sacrificed at 29 days after implantation. Green arrowheads indicate tumor formation. (**c**, **d**) Time-dependent changes in tumor volume in xenograft models are shown, medium alone (diamonds) or NEAPP-AM (squares). Each point on the line graph represents the mean tumor volume ($mm^3$) for each group on a particular day after implantation, and the bars represent SD. $^*P < 0.05$, $^{**}P < 0.01$ versus control (reproduced from Utsumi et al. 2013)

PAM was also evaluated *in vivo* using a peritoneal metastasis mouse model of gastric cancer [22] (Fig. 26.4). Enhanced green fluorescent protein-tagged GCIY (GCIY-EGFP) gastric cancer cells [26] were used for monitoring the growth of the peritoneally disseminated gastric cancer cells. PAM treatment inhibited the formation of peritoneal metastases, and adverse effects were not observed within the experimental period. These results suggest PAM is a promising novel therapeutic strategy for peritoneal metastasis.

Understanding the modes of action of PAM is important for addressing PAM's potential therapeutic applications in medicine. Several mechanisms have been proposed to explain the anti-tumor effects of PAM.

A glioblastoma cell line that has a *phosphatase and tension homolog* (*PTEN*) mutation and *epidermal growth factor receptor* (*EGFR*) mutation that constitutively activate both the phosphoinositide 3-kinase (PI3K)-AKT signaling pathway [27] and Rat sarcoma (RAS)—Mitogen-activated Protein Kinase (MAPK) signaling pathway [28], which are involved in survival and proliferation signaling networks and essential for cell growth and inhibiting apoptosis. PAM downregulated both PI3K-AKT and RAS-MAPK signaling in a glioblastoma cell line [12, 14]. These results suggest that PAM induces apoptosis by downregulating survival and proliferation signaling networks (Fig. 26.5, [7]).

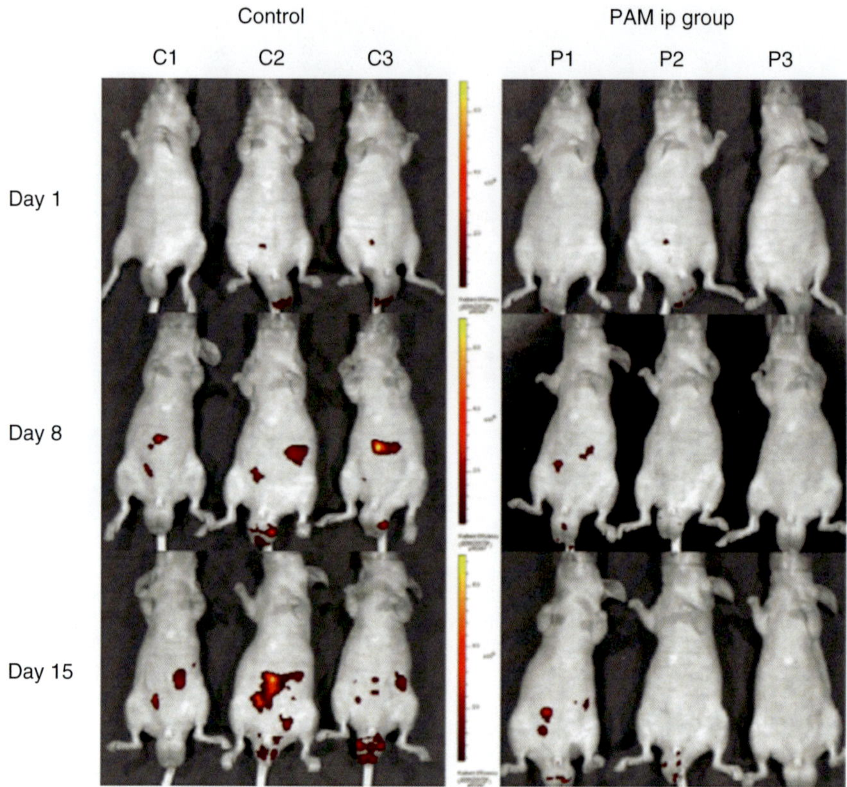


**Fig. 26.4** Intraperitoneal administration of PAM in a peritoneal dissemination mouse model. The efficacy and feasibility of administering PAM intraperitoneally was investigated using GCIY-EGFP gastric cancer cells. *In vivo* imaging was performed, and epifluorescent images in the dorsal position were acquired every 7 days (reproduced from Takeda et al. 2016)

## 26.4 Possible Applications of Plasma Activated Medium

PAM is being considered not only for cancer therapy but also for the treatment of age-related macular degeneration (AMD, [29]). Choroidal neovascularization (CNV) is the creation of new blood vessels in the choroid layer of the eye, a common occurrence in AMD. CNV in a mouse eye was created by laser. PAM reduced the laser-CNV (Fig. 26.6, [29]), and did not induce retinal toxicity.

PAM may have applications for regenerative medicine where it is important to selectively eliminate undifferentiated stem cells from differentiated cells. It was

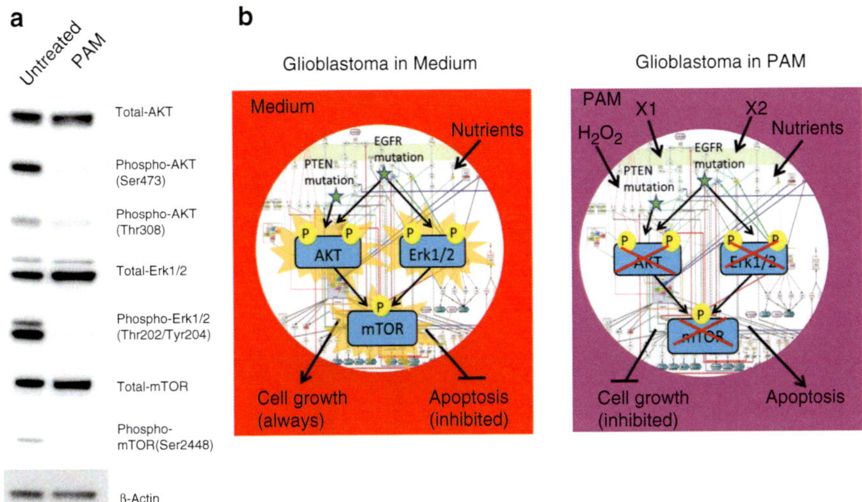


**Fig. 26.5** Intracellular molecular mechanisms of anti-tumor effects of PAM on glioblastoma cell lines. PAM downregulated survival and proliferation signaling networks in glioblastoma brain tumor cells. (**a**) Western Blot analyses of survival and proliferation signaling molecules. Activities of AKT kinase, ERK kinase, and mTOR kinase that are hub molecules of survival and proliferation signaling networks were downregulated by PAM. (**b**) Molecular mechanisms underlying the induction of apoptosis in PAM-treated glioblastoma (reproduced from Tanaka et al. 2014)

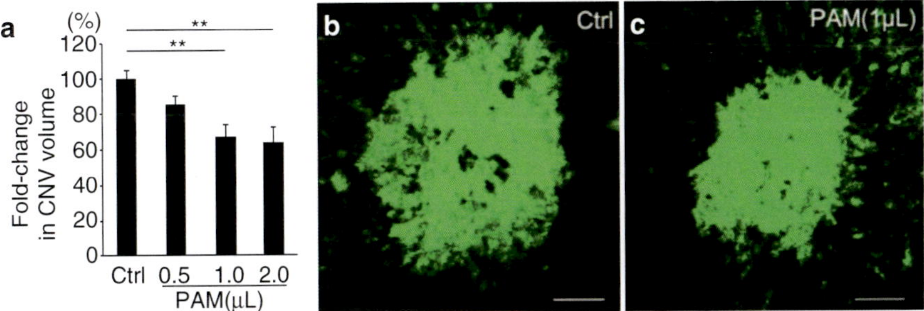


**Fig. 26.6** PAM reduced CNV volume *in vivo*. (**a**) The volumes of laser-CNV in eyes injected with 1.0 μL or 2.0 mL PAM was reduced by 33% (P = 0.0035) and 36% (P = 0.0049), respectively, compared with control (Ctrl) eyes. (**b**, **c**) Representative images of laser-CNV in control eye (**b**) and 1 μL PAM-injected eyes (**c**). Scale bar = 50 μm, **P < 0.01 (reproduced from Ye et al. 2015)

shown that undifferentiated human induced pluripotent stem cells (hiPSCs) were more sensitive to PAM than differentiated normal human dermal fibroblasts (NHDFs, Fig. 26.7) and hiPSC-derived differentiated cells [30]. These results suggest that PAM is a promising tool in regenerative medicine.

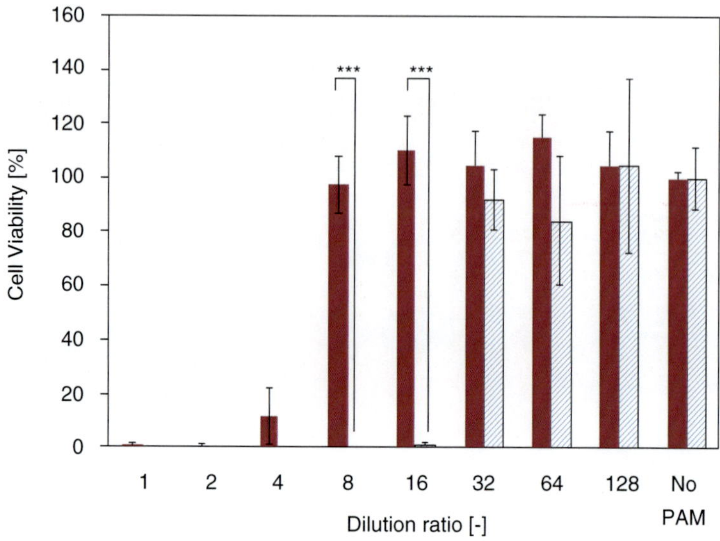


**Fig. 26.7** Quantitative effects of PAM on undifferentiated hiPSCs and differentiated NHDFs. PAM was diluted to an optimal concentration with fresh medium and was added to each well (n = 3). After 24 h, cell viabilities (%) were evaluated. Red bars denote NHDFs, and blue shaded bars denote hiPSCs. The means ± SD of three experiments are shown; ***$p < 0.005$ (reproduced from Matsumoto et al. 2016)

## 26.5 Future Perspectives for PAM

PAM was originally developed as a novel cancer therapy. However, potential applications have expanded to include the treatment of AMD and roles in regenerative medicine. In the future, the applications of PAM are likely to broaden further. However, for PAM to achieve its full biomedical potential further research is required to understand in detail the modes of action of the physiological outputs induced by novel plasma activated solutions as well as the complex interactions between plasma and liquids.

## References

1. von Woedtke T, Metelmann HR, Weltmann KD. Clinical plasma medicine: state and perspectives of in vivo application of cold atmospheric plasma. Contrib Plasma Phys. 2014;54:104–17.
2. Weltmann KD, Kindel E, Brandenburg R, Meyer C, Bussiahn R, Wilke C, von Woedtke T. Atmospheric pressure plasma jet for medical therapy: plasma parameters and risk estimation. Contrib Plasma Phys. 2009;49:631–40.
3. Fridman G, Friedman G, Gutsol A, Shekhter AB, Vasilets VN, Fridman A. Applied plasma medicine. Plasma Process Polym. 2008;5:503–33.
4. Laroussi M. From killing bacteria to destroying cancer cells: 20 years of plasma medicine. Plasma Process Polym. 2014;11:1138–41.

5. Kong MG, Kroesen G, Morfill G, Nosenko T, Shimizu T, van Dijk J, Zimmermann JL. Plasma medicine: an introductory review. New J Phys. 2009;11:115012.
6. Isbary G, Shimizu T, Li YF, Stolz W, Thomas HM, Morfill GE, Zimmermann JL. Cold atmospheric plasma devices for medical issues. Expert Rev Med Devices. 2013;10:367–77.
7. Tanaka H, Mizuno M, Ishikawa K, Takeda K, Nakamura K, Utsumi F, Kajiyama H, Kano H, Okazaki Y, Toyokuni S, Maruyama S, Kikkawa F, Hori M. Plasma medical science for cancer therapy: toward cancer therapy using nonthermal atmospheric pressure plasma. IEEE Trans Plasma Sci. 2014;42:3760–4.
8. Miller V, Lin A, Fridman G, Dobrynin D, Fridman A. Plasma stimulation of migration of macrophages. Plasma Process Polym. 2014;11:1193–7.
9. Miller V, Lin A, Kako F, Gabunia K, Kelemen S, Brettschneider J, Fridman G, Fridman A, Autieri M. Microsecond-pulsed dielectric barrier discharge plasma stimulation of tissue macrophages for treatment of peripheral vascular disease. Phys Plasmas. 2015;22:122005.
10. Lin A, Truong B, Pappas A, Kirifides L, Oubarri A, Chen SY, Lin SJ, Dobrynin D, Fridman G, Fridman A, Sang N, Miller V. Uniform nanosecond pulsed dielectric barrier discharge plasma enhances anti-tumor effects by induction of immunogenic cell death in tumors and stimulation of macrophages. Plasma Process Polym. 2015;12:1392–9.
11. Miller V, Lin A, Fridman A. Why target immune cells for plasma treatment of cancer. Plasma Chem Plasma Process. 2016;36:259–68.
12. Tanaka H, Mizuno M, Ishikawa K, Nakamura K, Kajiyama H, Kano H, Kikkawa F, Hori M. Plasma-activated medium selectively kills glioblastoma brain tumor cells by down-regulating a survival signaling molecule, AKT kinase, plasma. Medicine. 2013;1:265–77.
13. Utsumi F, Kajiyama H, Nakamura K, Tanaka H, Mizuno M, Ishikawa K, Kondo H, Kano H, Hori M, Kikkawa F. Effect of indirect nonequilibrium atmospheric pressure plasma on anti-proliferative activity against chronic chemo-resistant ovarian cancer cells in vitro and in vivo. PLoS One. 2013;8:e81576.
14. Tanaka H, Mizuno M, Ishikawa K, Nakamura K, Utsumi F, Kajiyama H, Kano H, Maruyama S, Kikkawa F, Hori M. Cell survival and proliferation signaling pathways are downregulated by plasma-activated medium in glioblastoma brain tumor cells, plasma. Medicine. 2014;2:207–20.
15. Torii K, Yamada S, Nakamura K, Tanaka H, Kajiyama H, Tanahashi K, Iwata N, Kanda M, Kobayashi D, Tanaka C, Fujii T, Nakayama G, Koike M, Sugimoto H, Nomoto S, Natsume A, Fujiwara M, Mizuno M, Hori M, Saya H, Kodera Y. Effectiveness of plasma treatment on gastric cancer cells. Gastric Cancer. 2014;18:635–43.
16. Hattori N, Yamada S, Torii K, Takeda S, Nakamura K, Tanaka H, Kajiyama H, Kanda M, Fujii T, Nakayama G, Sugimoto H, Koike M, Nomoto S, Fujiwara M, Mizuno M, Hori M, Kodera Y. Effectiveness of plasma treatment on pancreatic cancer cells. Int J Oncol. 2015;47:1655–62.
17. Tanaka H, Mizuno M, Ishikawa K, Kondo H, Takeda K, Hashizume H, Nakamura K, Utsumi F, Kajiyama H, Kano H, Okazaki Y, Toyokuni S, Akiyama S, Maruyama S, Yamada S, Kodera Y, Kaneko H, Terasaki H, Hara H, Adachi T, Iida M, Yajima I, Kato M, Kikkawa F, Hori M. Plasma with high electron density and plasma-activated medium for cancer treatment. Clin Plasma Med. 2015;3:72–6.
18. Tanaka H, Mizuno M, Toyokuni S, Maruyama S, Kodera Y, Terasaki H, Adachi T, Kato M, Kikkawa F, Hori M. Cancer therapy using non-thermal atmospheric pressure plasma with ultra-high electron density. Phys Plasmas. 2015;22:122003.
19. Tanaka H, Nakamura K, Mizuno M, Ishikawa K, Takeda K, Kajiyama H, Utsumi F, Kikkawa F, Hori M. Non-thermal atmospheric pressure plasma activates lactate in Ringer's solution for anti-tumor effects. Sci Rep. 2016;6:36282.
20. Tanaka H, Ishikawa K, Mizuno M, Toyokuni S, Kajiyama H, Kikkawa F, Metelmann HR, Hori M. State of the art in medical applications using non-thermal atmospheric pressure plasma. Rev Mod Plasma Phys. 2017;1:3.
21. Utsumi F, Kajiyama H, Nakamura K, Tanaka H, Hori M, Kikkawa F. Selective cytotoxicity of indirect nonequilibrium atmospheric pressure plasma against ovarian clear cell carcinoma. Springerplus. 2014;3:398.

22. Takeda S, Yamada S, Hattori N, Nakamura K, Tanaka H, Kajiyama H, Kanda M, Kobayashi D, Tanaka C, Fujii T, Fujiwara M, Mizuno M, Hori M, Kodera Y. Intraperitoneal administration of plasma-activated medium: proposal of a novel treatment option for peritoneal metastasis from gastric cancer. Ann Surg Oncol. 2017;24:1188–94.
23. Adachi T, Tanaka H, Nonomura S, Hara H, Kondo SI, Hori M. Plasma-activated medium induces A549 cell injury via a spiral apoptotic cascade involving the mitochondrial-nuclear network. Free Radic Biol Med. 2014;79C:28–44.
24. Hara H, Taniguchi M, Kobayashi M, Kamiya T, Adachi T. Plasma-activated medium-induced intracellular zinc liberation causes death of SH-SY5Y cells. Arch Biochem Biophys. 2015;584:51–60.
25. Mohades S, Laroussi M, Sears J, Barekzi N, Razavi H. Evaluation of the effects of a plasma activated medium on cancer cells. Phys Plasmas. 2015;22:122001.
26. Ohashi N, Kodera Y, Nakanishi H, Yokoyama H, Fujiwara M, Koike M, Hibi K, Nakao A, Tatematsu M. Efficacy of intraperitoneal chemotherapy with paclitaxel targeting peritoneal micrometastasis as revealed by GFP-tagged human gastric cancer cell lines in nude mice. Int J Oncol. 2005;27:637–44.
27. Yuan TL, Cantley LC. PI3K pathway alterations in cancer: variations on a theme. Oncogene. 2008;27:5497–510.
28. Dhillon AS, Hagan S, Rath O, Kolch W. MAP kinase signalling pathways in cancer. Oncogene. 2007;26:3279–90.
29. Ye F, Kaneko H, Nagasaka Y, Ijima R, Nakamura K, Nagaya M, Takayama K, Kajiyama H, Senga T, Tanaka H, Mizuno M, Kikkawa F, Hori M, Terasaki H. Plasma-activated medium suppresses choroidal neovascularization in mice: a new therapeutic concept for age-related macular degeneration. Sci Rep. 2015;5:7705.
30. Matsumoto R, Shimizu K, Nagashima T, Tanaka H, Mizuno M, Kikkawa F, Hori M, Honda H. Plasma-activated medium selectively eliminates undifferentiated human induced pluripotent stem cells. Regen Ther. 2016;5:55–63.

# Enhancement of the Penetration of Topically Applied Substances by Tissue-Tolerable Plasma

27

J. Lademann, H. Richter, A. Kramer, and O. Lademann

## 27.1 Introduction

In dermatology, ointments and lotions are widely used for the treatment of skin diseases [1–3]. However, the cutaneous barrier prevents large amounts of active substances from reaching the target structures, even in the case of inflammatory processes [4, 5]. This also applies for steroids, which are among the active drugs most frequently used in dermatology. No more than 1% of the steroid concentration finally overcomes the skin barrier [6]. Therefore, various physical techniques were developed to increase the penetration of topically applied permeabilizing agents [7, 8]. By applying any of these methods part of the skin barrier is disturbed, thus enabling an enhanced penetration. Irrespective of this development, the penetration efficacy of topically applied substances through the skin barrier remains a problem. Consequently, a systemic administration of drugs is preferred in many cases [9]. However, this involves other risks, such as drug metabolism-related changes, increased toxicity and allergies.

J. Lademann (✉) • H. Richter
Charité-Universitätsmedizin Berlin, Freie Universität Berlin, Humboldt-Universität zu Berlin, Berlin, Germany

Department of Dermatology, Center of Experimental and Applied Cutaneous Physiology (CCP), Berlin Institute of Health, Berlin, Germany
e-mail: juergen.lademann@charite.de

A. Kramer
Institute of Hygiene and Environmental Medicine, University Medicine Greifswald, Greifswald, Germany

O. Lademann
Clinic of Anesthesiology and Intensive Therapy, University Medicine Rostock, Rostock, Germany



H.-R. Metelmann et al. (eds.), *Comprehensive Clinical Plasma Medicine*,
https://doi.org/10.1007/978-3-319-67627-2_27

This chapter elucidates how the penetration of topically applied substances through the skin barrier can be strongly enhanced using tissue-tolerable plasma (TTP).

## 27.2 Materials and Methods

For the investigations, a plasma jet (KinPen09, neoplas tools GmbH Greifswald, Germany) was used. Externally resembling a big pen, this instrument accommodates an electrode system that generates the plasma. The plasma is blown out of the electrode system via an argon flow that produces a plasma torch of about 10 mm in length. The KinPen09 is shown in Fig. 27.1. The thin plasma beam is clearly visible. This plasma beam is expanded on the skin as illustrated in Fig. 27.2.

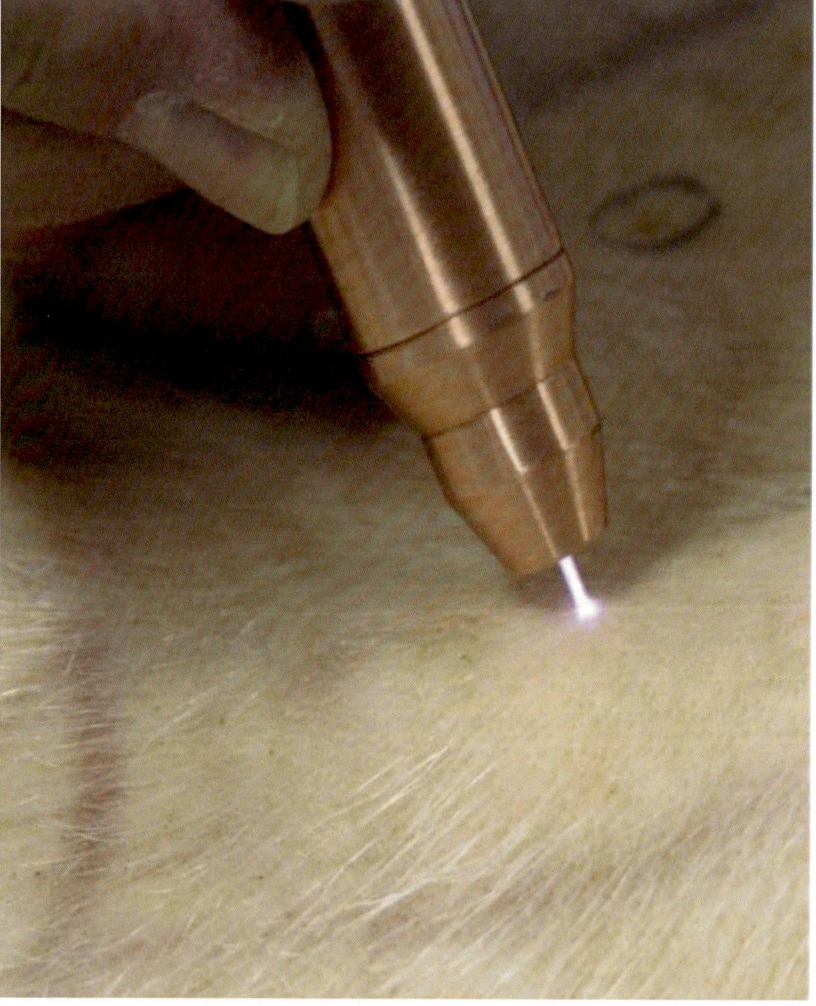

**Fig. 27.1** Photo of the KinPen09 plasma jet

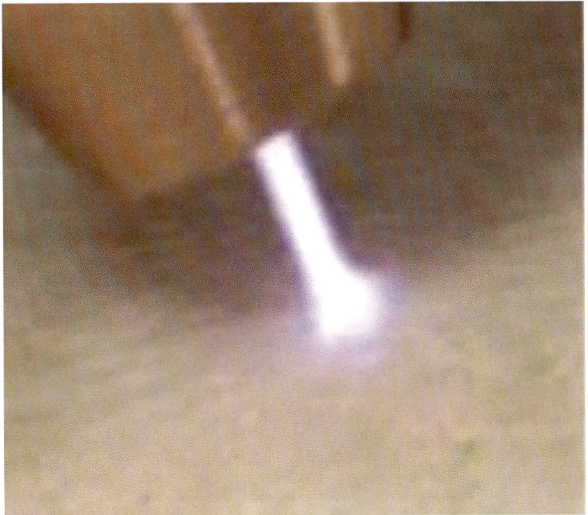

**Fig. 27.2** The plasma beam is expanded on the skin surface

The investigations were carried out on porcine ear skin which is a good model for human skin [10]. Additionally, experiments on healthy volunteers aged between 25 and 42 years have been carried out. Approval for the experiments were obtained from the Berlin Ethics Committee.

## 27.3 Results and Discussion

Plasma systems are mainly used for wound healing. The plasma treatment proved successful even for healing of chronic wounds [11]. Usually, the plasma beam is moved over the skin surface at a velocity between 6 and 10 mm/s. By laser scanning microscopic (LSM) investigations it could be demonstrated, that the skin surface was not damaged at this velocity [12]. Figure 27.3 represents a typical LSM image of a skin surface area treated with plasma at 10 mm/s. The structure of the corneocytes is intact, thermal damages are not detectable. Biopsies taken from deeper layers of the skin did not reveal any changes, neither. When the plasma beam is moved over the skin surface at a velocity of 2 mm/s, the situation is different. At this unphysiological traversing velocity the lipid structures in the uppermost two or three cellular layers of the corneocytes get fused as shown in Fig. 27.4. But even at this low traversing velocity no thermal damage was detectable in the deeper layers of the skin.

The action principle of the plasma in wound healing is based on a slight temperature increase, a determined dose of UV light emitted by the plasma, electrical signals based on the distribution of ions and electric fields and mainly a high concentration of free radicals induced in the skin by the plasma treatment [13].

First investigations on the plasma-tissue interaction were performed on porcine ear model skin at the Center of Experimental and Applied Cutaneous Physiology within the Department of Dermatology, Venerology and Allergology. Laser

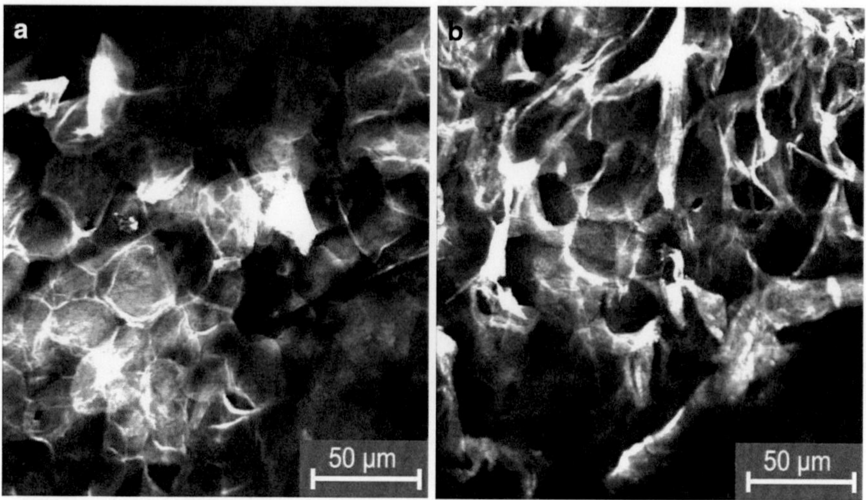


**Fig. 27.3** LSM image of a skin surface area treated with plasma at 10 mm/s [12]

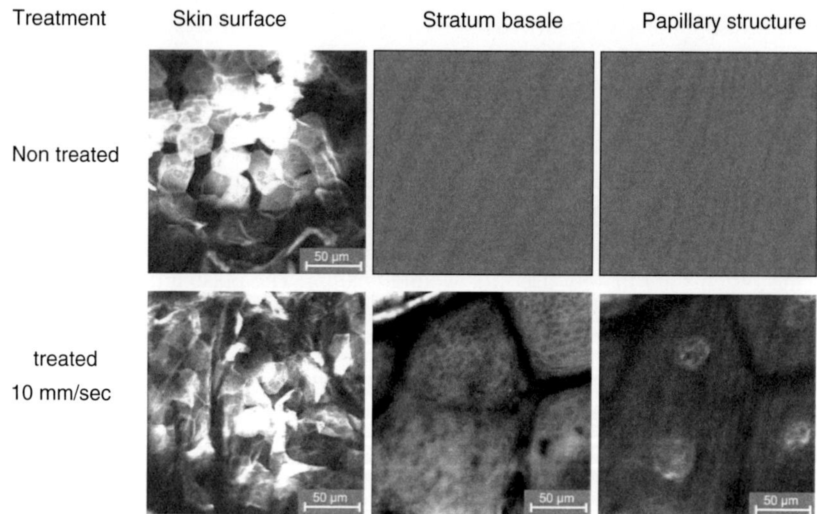


**Fig. 27.4** Fluorescence signals of the applied formulation in different depths of the skin, depending on the plasma application with a velocity of 10 mm/s [14]

scanning microscopy was applied to investigate the integrity of the skin surface subsequent to plasma therapy. For this purpose, the fluorescent dye sodium fluorescein was applied to the skin surface. The fluorescence signal served to obtain an intense representation of the skin surface. When the fluorescent dye is applied to the skin surface, it can be clearly recognized there, as depicted in Fig. 27.5. There are no fluorescence signals detected in the deeper skin layers, e.g., in the stratum basale

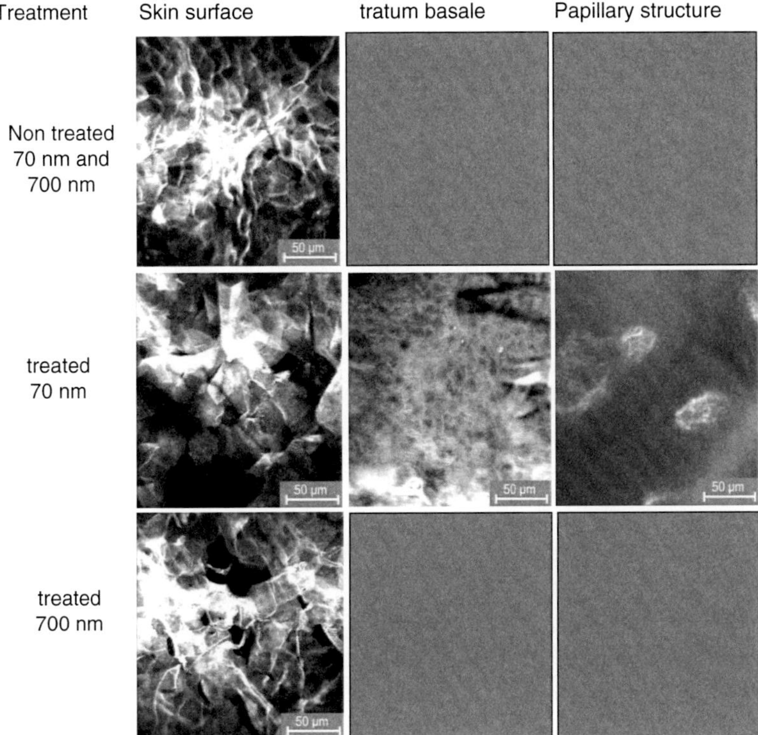


**Fig. 27.5** Fluorescence signals of the applied formulation with nanoparticles with a diameter of 70 and 700 nm in different depths of the skin without and with plasma application [14]

or in the region of the papillary structure [14], which indicates that the dye failed to pass the skin barrier. However and rather surprisingly, intensive fluorescence signals can also be detected in the deeper skin layers following the plasma treatment at a velocity of 10 mm/s [14]. This is represented in Fig. 27.4.

Consequently, the plasma-tissue interaction must provoke a disturbance of the skin barrier that permits large amounts of topically applied substances to be delivered into the deeper skin layers. Thus, beyond wound healing, the plasma technology may provide completely new applications in the field of dermatology and pharmacy.

The excellent penetration ability of topically applied substances under the action of plasma led to the question whether nor not bacteria and fungi can be transported through the skin barrier under these conditions. The size of bacteria is normally 1–10 µm in diameter [15], whereas fungi can even be as large as 200 µm [16].

In order to answer this question fluorescent particles of 70 and 700 nm, respectively, in diameter were used. Then, the penetration enhancement experiment was repeated. The nanoparticles were applied to the skin surface and their distribution on the skin and in the deeper skin layers was analyzed by laser scanning microscopy. Again it was found that without any plasma treatment the particles remained on the skin surface [14]. However, after the plasma treatment, the particles of 70 nm in diameter were detectable at high concentrations both in the stratum basale and in the papillary structure. The particles of 700 nm in size remained on the skin surface; no fluorescence signals could be detected in the deeper skin layers [14].

Consequently, a barrier disturbed by plasma is only permeable for particles of about 70 nm in size, whereas particles of ≥700 nm do no penetrate. This ensures that the plasma-tissue interaction is unable to stimulate the penetration of bacteria and fungi. In addition, it can be supposed that bacteria and fungi are destroyed by the interaction with the plasma.

After the hints for influencing the skin barrier in vitro by TTP with the probable consequence of increased skin penetration and the confirmation of penetration enhancement on porcine ear skin, this technology was now to be tested in vivo on humans. In the first experiments, the fluorescent dye sodium fluorescein was again topically applied to the skin. As in the case of the porcine ear skin, the fluorescent dye could only be detected on the skin surface but not in the deeper layers of the tissue, unless the skin was treated with plasma. In the second phase of the in vivo experiments on humans, the fluorescent dye was not applied to the skin before, but subsequent to the plasma treatment. This decision was taken to avoid an interaction between the plasma and the fluorescent dye. If active drugs are used, a plasma-chemical reaction could occur that changes the active substance. Such effects are well-known from plasma chemistry. The subsequent investigations by laser scanning microscopy demonstrated, however, that in the deeper skin layers, i.e., in the stratum basale and in the region of the papillary structure, no fluorescence signals were detectable. This means that the skin barrier regenerated very quickly so that the fluorescent dye that was applied to the skin after the plasma treatment had no time to penetrate. No matter how quickly the fluorescent dye was applied to the skin surface after the plasma treatment, the result had always been the same. This called for a method permitting substances to be applied to the skin before the plasma treatment, at the same time guaranteeing that the respective substance undergoes no structural changes during the plasma treatment.

In a next phase, nanocontainers were developed which remained unchanged by the plasma [17]. These containers shall be filled with active substances in the future. The containers will withstand the plasma treatment without being damaged. They will be transported into deeper skin layers where they have to release their drug. The selection of a suitable trigger mechanism for drug release is currently a hot topic of research.

If these research activities can be successfully implemented, the plasma technology will not only be suitable for wound healing but also for stimulating the penetration of topically applied substances, thus opening up new applications in pharmacology and dermatology.

## References

1. Lichterfeld A, Hauss A, Surber C, Peters T, Blume-Peytavi U, Kottner J. Evidence-based skin care: a systematic literature review and the development of a basic skin care algorithm. J Wound Ostomy Continence Nurs. 2015;42(5):501–24.
2. Fowler JE, Woolery-Lloyd H, Waldorf H, Saini R. Innovations in natural ingredients and their use in skin care. J Drugs Dermatol. 2010;9(6):S72–81.
3. Rosenkrantz W. Practical applications of topical therapy for allergic, infectious, and seborrheic disorders. Clin Tech Small Anim Pract. 2006;21(3):106–16.
4. Richters RJ, Falcone D, Uzunbajakava NE, Varghese B, Caspers PJ, Puppels GJ, van Erp PE, van de Kerkhof PC. Sensitive skin: assessment of the skin barrier using confocal raman microspectroscopy. Skin Pharmacol Physiol. 2017;30(1):1–12.
5. Nielsen JB, Benfeldt E, Holmgaard R. Penetration through the skin barrier. Curr Probl Dermatol. 2016;49:9.
6. Maibach HI, Feldman RJ. Occlusive dressing for the nose and ears. Arch Dermatol. 1966;93(4):465.
7. Choi WI, Lee JH, Kim JY, Kim JC, Kim YH, Tae G. Efficient skin permeation of soluble proteins via flexible and functional nano-carrier. J Control Release. 2012;157(2):272–8.
8. Zhang H, Zhai Y, Yang X, Zhai G. Breaking the skin barrier: achievements and future directions. Curr Pharm Des. 2015;21(20):2713–24.
9. Goldberg EP, Hadba AR, Almond BA, Marotta JS. Intratumoral cancer chemotherapy and immunotherapy: opportunities for nonsystemic preoperative drug delivery. J Pharm Pharmacol. 2002;54(2):159–80.
10. Jacobi U, Kaiser M, Toll R, Mangelsdorf S, Audring H, Otberg N, et al. Porcine ear skin: an in vitro model for human skin. Skin Res Technol. 2007;13(1):19–24.
11. Ulrich C, Kluschke F, Patzelt A, Vandersee S, Czaika VA, Richter H, et al. Clinical use of cold atmospheric pressure argon plasma in chronic leg ulcers: a pilot study. J Wound Care. 2015;24(5):196. 8–200, 2–3.
12. Lademann O, Kramer A, Richter H, Patzelt A, Meinke MC, Czaika V, et al. Skin disinfection by plasma-tissue interaction: comparison of the effectivity of tissue-tolerable plasma and a standard antiseptic. Skin Pharmacol Physiol. 2011;24(5):284–8.
13. Lademann J, Richter H, Alborova A, Humme D, Patzelt A, Kramer A, et al. Risk assessment of the application of a plasma jet in dermatology. J Biomed Opt. 2009;14(5):054025.
14. Lademann O, Richter H, Meinke MC, Patzelt A, Kramer A, Hinz P, et al. Drug delivery through the skin barrier enhanced by treatment with tissue-tolerable plasma. Exp Dermatol. 2011;20(6):488–90.
15. Wijenayake AU, Abayasekara CL, Pitawala HM, Bandara BM. Antimicrobial potential of two traditional herbometallic drugs against certain pathogenic microbial species. BMC Complement Altern Med. 2016;16:365.
16. Jain C, Das S, Ramachandran VG, Saha R, Bhattacharya SN, Dar S. Malassezia yeast and cytokine gene polymorphism in atopic dermatitis. J Clin Diagn Res. 2017;11(3):DC01–DC5.
17. Lademann J, Patzelt A, Richter H, Lademann O, Baier G, Breucker L, et al. Nanocapsules for drug delivery through the skin barrier by tissue-tolerable plasma. Laser Phys Lett. 2013;10(8).

# 28 Designing Clinical Studies in Wound Healing

Tobias Zahn

## 28.1 Introduction

Wound healing as an indication for new treatments is sometimes referred to as a graveyard for product development. Indeed, in particular for pharmaceutical developments, failed developments abound and dampen the interest of pharmaceutical companies and investors to fund projects in this space.

Physical plasma has generated much interest and shows promise as a new therapeutic option for wounds, as demonstrated by a growing list of publications of completed clinical studies.

Wounds vary, and patient's healing capacities differ, many different treatment modalities are available and are used—these and other factors present challenges in designing clinical studies that are specific to wound healing studies. This essay aims to reflect on some of these challenges and to describe approaches that have been successfully used to address them. And while a good study design has no influence on the efficacy or safety of the investigational product or procedure, it supports the collection of high quality data enabling conclusions that build evidence for the investigated therapy.

T. Zahn
3R Pharma Consulting GmbH, Dobel, Germany
e-mail: tobias.zahn@3rpc.com



H.-R. Metelmann et al. (eds.), *Comprehensive Clinical Plasma Medicine*,
https://doi.org/10.1007/978-3-319-67627-2_28

## 28.2 Practical Considerations in Planning a Clinical Study

Over the years, pharmaceutical regulators have developed a detailed set of internationally respected rules to guide drug development. They are available from the International Council for Harmonisation of Technical Requirements for Pharmaceuticals for Human Use, better known under its acronym ICH.[1] As the name implies these guidelines do not apply to medical devices and medical procedures and some are very specific to pharmaceuticals or individual indications, nevertheless some of the guidelines provide a very useful framework that can (and needs to) be adapted to the needs of any clinical study. In particular the ICH E6 guideline 'Good Clinical Practice' and ICH E3 guideline 'Clinical Trial Reports' should be mentioned here.

Another important source of guidance and support can be the local clinical study competence centers present at many medical research centers and university hospitals as well as institutional review boards and ethics committees. Early communication with them is usually encouraged.

**Structure of an ICH Clinical Study Protocol**[2]

1. General Information (Study title, names and contacts of responsible persons)
2. Background information (state of knowledge on the investigational therapy)
3. Study Objectives and Purpose
4. Study Design (endpoints, measures to avoid bias such as randomization and blinding)
5. Selection and Withdrawal of Study Participants (eligibility criteria, withdrawal criteria)
6. Treatment of Study Participants (mode of administration, schedule)
7. Assessment of Efficacy
8. Assessment of Safety
9. Statistics
10. Direct Access to Source Data/Documents
11. Quality Control and Quality Assurance
12. Ethics
13. Data Handling and Record Keeping
14. Financing and Insurance
15. Publication Policy
16. Supplements

[1] www.ich.org.

[2] ICH E6 (R2) guideline section 6.

The *clinical study protocol* describes in detail the planned study. In designing a clinical study and writing a clinical study protocol, decisions have to be taken on many details. The writing of a clinical study report or a publication of the results will occur much later, often several years later—at which point it will prove difficult to remember the reasons and justifications for certain details of the study design. Therefore in parallel to the writing of a clinical study protocol (from first draft to later versions) a separate *design rationale document* should be created that documents the rationale for each individual decision. This will greatly facilitate not only the writing of responses to regulatory queries, of study reports and publications but in addition provide a very useful training document for new study team members. For smaller studies, such rationales may be included directly in the study protocol—for larger studies with several sites and investigators it would make the study protocol unwieldy and a leaner document will be appreciated by team members conducting the clinical study.

No matter how small or large a study, quality control and quality assurance measures are of great importance to ensure validity of the study data. The 2016 update to the ICH E6 guideline (R2) emphasizes quality assurance. A *risk analysis* should be conducted before study initiation (and reviewed and updated regularly). Areas identified to pose risks in particular for patient safety and for data integrity can then be prioritized and specific quality assurance measures employed to ensure an early identification of any occurred deviations. Since certain risks are likely to be already addressed by measures of the protocol, a design rationale document may again prove a useful tool as it can be reviewed to identify and qualify risks.

## 28.3 Challenges in Wound Healing Studies and Design Considerations for Prospective Clinical Wound Healing Studies

"Each wound is different"—this often stated notion highlights a particular challenge for clinical studies since insights are sought that apply to more than a single patient and can be generalized to a broader population. Several patients and wounds need to be pooled in a clinical study. In the end, the definitions of the wound type and of inclusion and exclusion criteria aim to convincingly accomplish the meaning of the opposite notion: "A wound is a wound is a wound…".

All the more it is of great importance to control *confounding factors* that would potentially skew the study results. For the purpose of a clinical study the type of wound studied needs to be clearly defined to allow a precise selection of study participants. Beyond the type of wound (e.g., chronic venous ulcer, partial thickness burn) other potentially confounding factors need to be considered that influence wound healing, such as wound size, wound depth, wound age, wound status (infections!), body weight, substance abuse, disease backgrounds (e.g., diabetes), or medications (e.g., corticosteroids). To provide an example with rather narrowly defined eligibility criteria, a study investigating scarring could be conducted in surgically closed wounds of patients within an age range of 35–65 years who underwent thyroidectomy within the last 4 days, a body mass index ranging from 20 to 25, and excluding patients with a history of diabetes, substance abuse, patients using systemic corticosteroids. It will depend on the specific research question how narrow the definition of eligibility criteria needs to be. E.g., for an initial efficacy study of a new method narrowly defined criteria for a homogeneous patient and wound sample can be advantageous while for other questions a broader definition may be more appropriate. Also, the benefits of reducing and controlling confounding factors by use of very narrowly defined eligibility criteria need to be balanced against the feasibility to conduct the study and to identify and recruit a sufficient number of such narrowly defined patients.

Wound healing is a prolonged process encompassing several phases from inflammation to tissue regeneration (granulation and reepithelialisation) to scar maturation. A treatment benefit can apply to various stages and aspects of wound healing, e.g., clearance of a wound infection, time to wound closure or scar quality (e.g., pruritus, skin pliability or pigmentation). This illustrates that the goal of most wound healing studies to demonstrate an 'improvement of wound healing' is too generic. A useful *study endpoint* definition needs to be much more specific and quantifiable.

For endpoint definitions and other study design aspects a guidance document of the US FDA can be consulted [1]. Many aspects discussed in this guidance for development of therapies for chronic cutaneous ulcers and burn wounds are also applicable to other wound types. For superficial partial thickness burns (and other single skin wounds healing by secondary intention) that achieve reepithelialisation and wound closure within a couple of weeks, time to wound closure is recommended as endpoint. For diabetic foot ulcers (and other chronic wounds) it is instead recommended to determine the proportion of wounds that achieve wound closure at a predefined time point (e.g., after 120 days of study treatment).

*Randomized controlled trials* (RCTs) are considered gold standard for clinical studies, and this is often used with the understanding of a parallel group double-blind placebo-controlled study design in which both investigator and patient are unaware which patients receive the active treatment and which the control treatment. Naturally this is often not easy to accomplish or even impossible in surgical disciplines and presents a particular challenge for many wound therapies including physical plasma.

A possible solution to achieving a blinded evaluation is the use of a second investigator as blinded assessor who is unaware to the treatment—i.e., one investigator applying the treatment in an open, unblinded fashion, and a second investigator assessing the wound independently of the first investigator [2]. Obviously it will require close attention in the planning and conduct of the study to avoid any unintentional unblinding, e.g., from skin markings, from communication with the patient, or from other study team members. Another option for an *observer-blinded assessment* is the use of a photo-based blinded evaluation. This is much easier to conduct in a securely blinded fashion—the disadvantage being that a photo-based

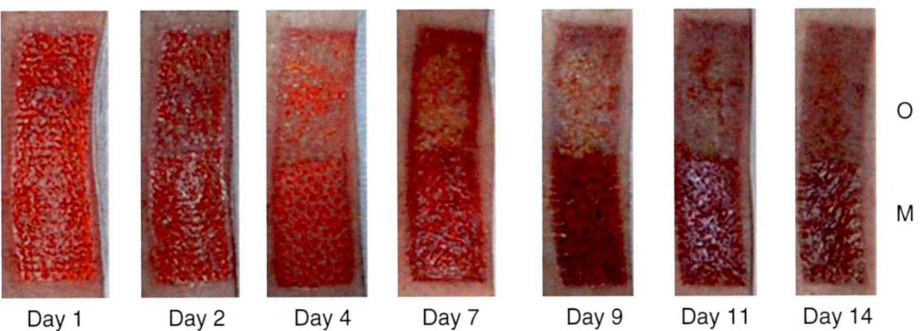


**Fig. 28.1** Intra-individual comparison of two topical treatments (here: Episalvan® gel + Mepilex® wound dressing [O] vs. Mepilex® wound dressing alone [M]) in a split-thickness skin graft donor site wound. From [6]

assessment provides much less information to the assessor compared to the direct assessment of a wound. Nevertheless, photo-based evaluation is a reliable method to determine wound closure, and use of several assessors instead of a single one can further improve quality of assessments [3, 4].

In a study design that uses open (unblinded) treatment by the investigator the randomization process has to be particularly strict and manipulation-proof to ensure that the investigator has no influence to the treatment allocation.

Consider using an *intra-individual study design* in which treatments are compared simultaneously in two wound halves (or two matching wounds) in the same patient (see Fig. 28.1 for an example). For a local topical treatment such as physical plasma this may be the most efficient study design for many research questions. It elegantly controls for confounding factors that determine an individual patient's healing capacity as both study treatment and control treatment are compared against each other in the same patient-individual background [5–7]. Consequently sample size estimates will be lower as natural background variation in wound healing is avoided. Even single-digit patient numbers can provide very convincing results in such a study design [8]. A disadvantage however is that the overall impact of a therapy on a patient may not be measurable in such a study, e.g., questions related to quality of life or differences in health care resource utilization (e.g., days hospitalized).

**Prerequisites for Using Intra-Individual Comparison in a Study Design**
- Local effect (no systemic effect)
- Restricted local application (no spreading to other wound area, no cross-contamination by active or control treatment)

If a simultaneous intra-individual treatment comparison is not feasible, for chronic or recurring wounds a sequential design may be a suitable alternative that similarly benefits from the avoidance of [9].

*Standard of care* is typically poorly defined in wound therapy. Wound care is dominated by a large number of available products and procedures, and consensus is mostly limited to general recommendations such as wound cleansing and clearing of infections (in case of contaminated or chronic wounds) and the provision of a moist wound healing environment to support the endogenous healing process. However, for a meaningful study result it is necessary to precisely define a uniform study procedure to apply the study and control treatments that is in line with a standard of care that is agreeable to a majority of experts in the field. Choice of a control treatment that is not well known will make it difficult to put the study results into a broader context. Similarly, choice of a well established but no longer considered state-of-the-art treatment will make it difficult to interpret a study result (e.g., silver sulfadiazine cream has a long history of control treatment in studies with partial thickness wounds such as grade 2 burns which led to the demonstration that silver sulfadiazine cream slows down wound healing [10]—therefore newly planned studies investigating time to wound closure should use different comparators because demonstration of accelerated healing vs. silver sulfadiazine cream would be the expected outcome anyhow).

The large variety of products and protocols used in wound treatment combined with the variety in wound types and few available *natural history* studies present a challenge in estimating the baseline result of a control treatment. Such uncertainty about the baseline treatment effect makes sample size estimates less reliable. Conservative planning of a study will increase the sample size. Such an increase may be so substantial that it may be useful to conduct a pre-study first to generate more reliable data for the natural disease progression and/or efficacy of a standard of care control treatment (which may be addressable by a retrospective study). Another approach is to plan for an *interim analysis* that will evaluate treatment success after a predefined smaller number of patients has been treated—the results of this interim analysis may lead to adaptation of the sample size in the ongoing study [6]. In order to achieve the same level of statistical significance, an interim analysis comes with a prize in that a higher level of significance has to be reached than the customary level of $p = 0.05$ (two-sided). Nevertheless this may be a small prize to pay in case of limited data on the expected success rate of the control therapy or on the effect size of the active therapy. Detailed discussions with a biostatistician are in any case strongly recommended.

Chronic wounds by definition require prolonged treatment, and treatment is typically provided in an out-patient setting with relatively little control of the study team over the actual care at the patient's home.[3] In particular in such settings *patient adherence* and proper administration of the study treatment present a challenge. This can be addressed to some degree by patient education and more visits and patient interactions than would be required for efficacy or safety evaluation (e.g., additional patient visits early after initiation of treatment, nurse visits to patients' homes, or phone calls).

[3]This applies also to frequently recurring wounds in blistering diseases, e.g., epidermolysis bullosa.

In the context of chronic wounds it is important to note that enrolment into the study and the additional attention received from the study team by itself may lead to an improvement of the wound. Patients in a standard of care treatment arm may be more compliant and diligent with their therapy. And the use of placebo creams may have a beneficial effect as a result of regular and frequent application of an emollient. Many examples exist of studies in which the success rate of the control treatment was much higher than initially expected, increasing the hurdle for an active treatment to demonstrate benefit over the control treatment in a clinical study setting.

A possible remedy here is to use a run-in phase before initiation of treatment with the study medication, e.g., [11]. Patients will be enrolled into the study and for the first weeks all be treated with the control treatment. Patients that show substantial improvement during the run-in phase, who apparently benefit from the control treatment, can then be excluded from the study before randomization into the study treatment arms.

Before embarking on larger studies, the close observation and careful documentation of *initial case studies* is very powerful to develop rich hypotheses to test in a larger trial. Collection of detailed data not only on time to wound closure but also additional parameters related to quality and functionality of the regenerated skin (e.g., redness, pigmentation, pliability, trans-epidermal water loss), possibly combined with analysis of gene and protein expression from skin biopsies can provide a comprehensive and detailed picture on the wound healing progression in treated areas. Such detailed understanding of treatment effects in a small number of patients and wounds compared to standard of care treated wounds enable to delineate the specific effects of the study treatment or its different doses or modes of application. Such detailed description and understanding is required for a well informed decision on the study procedures and endpoints in a study protocol for a larger trial that subsequently investigates efficacy and safety in a larger patient cohort.

**Conclusion**

Despite—or because of—the challenges in conducting clinical studies in wound healing, it is a worthwhile and rewarding task to generate new medical evidence in this area that affects the lives of millions of people. Wound treatment will benefit from new medical evidence generated for physical plasma as well as for other both experimental and established wound treatments. The following recommendations are intended as a summary to guide your clinical study design process:

*Keep it simple!*

A single clearly defined research question enables a lean study design. It is tempting to add a large number of analyses and read-outs, after all it takes considerable amount and effort to recruit patients into a study and we want to make the most of this opportunity. But consider the toll on patients (e.g., number of visits, skin biopsies, long questionnaires or diaries) that may hamper patient willingness to participate in a study. And consider as well the availability of resources to plan, collect and analyse all these data that after all are only secondary to your primary research question.

Unless required for the specific research question avoid conducting studies in vulnerable patient populations, e.g., children or patients in an emergency situation—informed consent, ethics committee approval and patient recruitment are much more difficult. Keep the number of languages, countries and sites involved to a minimum—and in case it is necessary to involve multiple sites, countries and languages plan for generous project management capacity.

*Keep it real!*

Know your resources and aim accordingly. But don't compromise on study quality and avoid underpowered studies—they are a waste of time and resources! Use standard procedures and treatment protocols to make the study results most meaningful for clinical practice. Focus on a research question for which the available resources allow the generation of high quality data.

*Plan thoroughly and detailed!*

We all want to get started with patient treatments in our clinical studies as quickly as possible. However, detailed planning and thorough preparation pays off during conduct and read-out of a study. Search the literature and discuss your study design with experts in the field. A thorough planning process sometimes seems tedious, yet it is key to design studies that are smooth to conduct for study teams and patients and that generate data of high quality—and such quality is paramount to create solid medical evidence.

Every clinical study requires considerable time and effort as well as commitment by patients and study team members. Be creative and diligent with your study designs—and make these efforts count to advance wound healing!

## References

1. Guidance for industry: chronic cutaneous ulcer and burn wounds—developing products for treatment. In: Services USDoHaH, editor. 2006.
2. Ottomann C, Stojadinovic A, Lavin PT, Gannon FH, Heggeness MH, Thiele R, et al. Prospective randomized phase II Trial of accelerated reepithelialization of superficial second-degree burn wounds using extracorporeal shock wave therapy. Ann Surg. 2012;255(1):23–9.
3. Rennekampff H-O, Fimmers R, Metelmann H-R, Schumann H, Tenenhaus M. Reliability of photographic analysis of wound epithelialization assessed in human skin graft donor sites and epidermolysis bullosa wounds. Trials. 2015;16:235.
4. Bloemen MCT, Boekema BKHL, Vlig M, van Zuijlen PPM, Middelkoop E. Digital image analysis versus clinical assessment of wound epithelialization: a validation study. Burns. 2012;38(4):501–5.
5. Barret JP, Podmelle F, Lipovy B, Rennekampff HO, Schumann H, Schwieger-Briel A, et al. Accelerated re-epithelialization of partial-thickness skin wounds by a topical betulin gel: results of a randomized phase III clinical trials program. Burns. 2017;43(6):1284–94.
6. Metelmann HR, Brandner JM, Schumann H, Bross F, Fimmers R, Bottger K, et al. Accelerated reepithelialization by triterpenes: proof of concept in the healing of surgical skin lesions. Skin Pharmacol Physiol. 2015;28(1):1–11.
7. Heinlin J, Zimmermann JL, Zeman F, Bunk W, Isbary G, Landthaler M, et al. Randomized placebo-controlled human pilot study of cold atmospheric argon plasma on skin graft donor sites. Wound Repair Regen. 2013;21(6):800–7.

8. Woodley DT, Cogan J, Hou Y, Lyu C, Marinkovich MP, Keene D, et al. Gentamicin induces functional type VII collagen in recessive dystrophic epidermolysis bullosa patients. J Clin Invest. 2017;127(8):3028–38.
9. Wally V, Kitzmueller S, Lagler F, Moder A, Hitzl W, Wolkersdorfer M, et al. Topical diacerein for epidermolysis bullosa: a randomized controlled pilot study. Orphanet J Rare Dis. 2013;8:69.
10. Wasiak J, Cleland H, Campbell F, Spinks A. Dressings for superficial and partial thickness burns. Cochrane Database Syst Rev. 2013;(3):Cd002106.
11. Gibbons GW, Orgill DP, Serena TE, Novoung A, O'Connell JB, Li WW, et al. A prospective, randomized, controlled trial comparing the effects of noncontact, low-frequency ultrasound to standard care in healing venous leg ulcers. Ostomy Wound Manage. 2015;61(1):16–29.

**Dr. Tobias Zahn** trained as cell biologist at Witten/Herdecke University (Germany) and the University of Colorado Health Sciences Center. Following 4 years at The Boston Consulting Group he joined Birken AG (now an Amryt Pharma company) where was responsible for the phase III clinical study program in partial thickness wounds and the marketing authorization application for Episalvan® wound gel. In 2016, Episalvan® became the first medicine authorized by the European Commission for treatment of partial thickness wounds. Since 2017 Dr. Zahn consults on clinical study planning and regulatory proceedings at 3R Pharma Consulting Gmbh (www.3rpc.com).

# Part IV

# Practical Aspects

# The Baltic Sea Region as One Test and Development Site for Cold Atmospheric Plasma (CAP) Devices

**29**

Jaanus Pikani, Hans-Robert Metelmann, Frank Graage, and Peter Frank

## 29.1 The Market Drive of Cold Atmospheric Plasma Devices

### 29.1.1 MedTech an Expanding Sector

Significant demographic shifts with ageing populations and the rise in chronic diseases and comorbidities is a major driver of the healthcare sector throughout the Baltic Sea Region (BSR).

Every segment within the health sector is currently expanding to meet demand [1].

Medical technology is poised to become one of the next industries to break out of emerging markets and play on the global stage. Compared with other industries, MedTech has been a late bloomer in emerging markets [2].

Demand for health care is growing rapidly in emerging markets, a function of rising household incomes, increased discretionary spending, and aging populations. Governments are also investing heavily in health care to combat chronic and critical illnesses.

### 29.1.2 Positive Outlook for CAP Devices

Plasma medicine means the direct application of cold atmospheric plasma (CAP) on or in the human body for therapeutic purposes [3].

First CAP sources are now CE-certified as medical devices which are the main precondition to start the introduction of plasma medicine into clinical reality. Plasma application in dentistry and, above all, CAP use for cancer treatment is becoming more and more important research fields in plasma medicine.

J. Pikani • H.-R. Metelmann • F. Graage • P. Frank (✉)
ScanBalt fmba, Copenhagen, Denmark
e-mail: pf@scanbalt.org



H.-R. Metelmann et al. (eds.), *Comprehensive Clinical Plasma Medicine*,
https://doi.org/10.1007/978-3-319-67627-2_29

The ultimate physical and technical objective is to design easily-controllable plasma devices specifically adapted to different demands (indications) in medical therapy.

No market reports appears publicly available specific for CAP devices but the general outlook for the BSR health care sector and the global market situation for MedTech support the introduction of the devices provided they are cost efficient, have equal or better therapeutic effects and are safe.

## 29.2 Barriers for Development and Introduction of CAP Devices

### 29.2.1 Create a BSR CAP Snapshot

In BSR as in the EU as such a fragmented system of research and innovation may indicate weak internal links and a too low level of cooperation between actors.

Moreover, weak transnational and trans-sectoral coordination of the whole innovation chain is impeding the translation of innovative ideas from research to market readiness, obstructing development of innovative ideas by SMEs and slowing down diffusion and adoption of innovative products and services [4].

There is no reason to believe this should be different for an emerging field like plasma medicine and the development of CAP devices.

So a focus may be to establish an effective Baltic Sea Region trans-national innovation chain within plasma medicine and CAP device development.

However, this requires a snapshot of the main public and private stakeholders which is not yet available, therefore it would be crucial to create a BSR plasma medicine and CAP device stakeholder overview.

### 29.2.2 Facilitate Industry Access to the Clinical Environment

Critically, in seeking to be modern, responsible and sustainable health care systems, health care providers should [5]:

1. be encouraged to become co-producers of health innovation through participation in regional and cross-border value chains and 'living labs' with industry and research facilities
2. be open to new and affordable innovative products e.g. CAP devices. The issue here is not the cost of new innovative products and the changes to service provision they enable. It is if their adoption reduces the demand for and the costs of acute and long-term services especially.

This is important because public expenditure on health care will jump from the present 8–12% of GDP to >14% in 2030 and continue to grow after that.

### 29.2.3 Public-Private Collaboration and Living Labs

This necessitates collaboration with industry (especially SMEs) and enhances focus on commercialization of innovative ideas from "bench to bedside" and vice versa.

However, there are significant cultural differences between the public and the private sectors. Also, public procurement procedures make it hard for SMEs with new and perhaps more effective and affordable innovative products to enter foreign markets.

Fundamentally, there is lack of efficient support structures for companies involved in health care innovation, though good examples can be found.

A target for BSR collaboration on plasma medicine and CAP device development could thus be to facilitate access to health infrastructures for start-ups and SMEs promoting commercialization based on excellent client validation opportunities, hands-on feedback and input for product development.

Co-creation and experimental testing of products in real-life are key aspects of Living Labs, which thereby help and support companies to rapidly commercialize and scale up their innovations and products to the global markets.

But Living Lab infrastructures mostly serve only locally or regionally and their access to clients is often critically low. Therefore it would be an advantage to link together regional living labs which may serve for plasma medicine and CAP device development.

### 29.2.4 Bringing CAP Devices to Patient Use

Commercialization and bringing innovative solutions to hospitals is difficult and encompasses many obstacles before reaching the patient.

For example nine pre-conditions were identified in ScanBalt BioRegion [6]:

- attract funding in the form of business angels, venture capital or investment firms
- evaluate the feasibility of the idea
- find clinical partners and communicating customer benefits
- go through quality assurance and clinical trials
- find strong management and attracting competent people
- have regional triple helix clusters and networks
- be informed about procurement rules and processes
- stay competitive in the procurement process
- have opportunities for additional training within these fields.

These are tasks which with advantage could be assisted by a macro-regional network collaboration and would be another important cornerstone in addition to linking together Living Labs in order to promote a macro-regional innovation chain.

## 29.3 Coordination of Funding Sources for Plasma Medicine and CAP Device Development

### 29.3.1 Macro-Regional Collaboration and Investments

In general Macro-regional concepts and regional clustering may assist to [7]:

- Promote the health economy
- Address grand societal needs and challenges with collaborative measures
- Reduce disparities between the levels of development between regions
- Mobilize growth potential to achieve economic, social and territorial cohesion
- Enhance investments in knowledge
- Increase networking and coordination between main stakeholders
- Improve framework conditions
- Reduce fragmentation
- Avoid unnecessary duplication
- Promote smart specialization
- Mobilize regional and national investments

Macro-regional collaboration has shown the capacity to mobilize regional and national investments which otherwise would not have been available for trans-national collaboration based on a common vision and strategy for the macro-region [8].

### 29.3.2 Coordination Between Funding Sources

In addition macro-regional collaboration has shown the capacity to coordinate regional and national investments with various EU funding sources like regional development funds and research funds.

An example here is ScanBalt which with the common aim of the Baltic Sea Region as one test and development site for health care products and services [9] has been able to direct regional investments coupled with ERFI and research funds towards this aim.

**Conclusions**

Plasma medicine and CAP device development are in the author's opinion in a position to benefit from a macro-regional collaboration in the Baltic Sea Region.

Such a collaboration is a lever to bridge gaps in the innovation chain, increase investments and coordinate between funding sources in the pursuit of a common goal.

This goal could be the Baltic Sea Region as a globally leading hub for plasma medicine research and for CAP device development.

ScanBalt BioRegion may be a model to be applied for the collaboration.

## References


1. ScanBalt. The health economy in the Baltic Sea Region: challenges and opportunities. 2013. http://scanbalt.org/files/graphics/Illustrations/BSR%20Health%20Economy.pdf.
2. Dora S, Khanna D, Luo Y, Poon L, Schweizer C. 2017. MedTech may be emerging markets next new thing. https://www.bcg.com/publications/2017/globalization-medical-devices-technology-medtech-may-be-emerging-markets-next-new-thing.aspx.
3. Weltmann K-D, von Woedtke TH. Plasma medicine—current state of research and medical application. Plasma Phys Control Fusion. 2016;59(1).
4. ScanBalt. EU framework programme and the role of macro-regions. 2011. http://scanbalt.org/wp-content/uploads/2016/04/ScanBalt-PositionPaper-FP-8-Role-of-Macro-regions.pdf.
5. EU Council. Towards modern, responsive and sustainable health systems. 2011. https://www.consilium.europa.eu/uedocs/cms_data/docs/pressdata/en/lsa/122395.pdf.
6. Kuura G, Edgar B. Major challenges for SME-s to be commercially successful. 2011. http://scanbalt.org/projects/finalised+projects/bshr+healthport/reports.
7. HealthPort. The health economy in the Baltic Sea Region: challenges and opportunities. 2013. http://scanbalt.org/files/graphics/Illustrations/BSR%20Health%20Economy.pdf.
8. DanuBalt. Macro-regional development and the health economy: practical experiences, models and concepts for macro-regional collaboration between regions and clusters. 2016. http://scanbalt.org/wp-content/uploads/2016/04/Macro-Regional-Development-May-2016.pdf.
9. Bielawski et al. The Baltic Sea region as one test site for development of health care products and services. 2015. http://scanbalt.org/baltic-sea-region-one-test-site-development-health-care-products-services/.

# Safe and Effective Plasma Treatment by Structured Education

# 30

Hans-Robert Metelmann, Stefan Hammes, Kristina Hartwig, Thomas von Woedtke, Tran Thi Trung Chien, and Ajay Rana

H.-R. Metelmann, MD, DDS, PhD, DALM, FEBOMFS (✉)
Department of Oral and Maxillofacial Surgery/Plastic Surgery, University Medicine Greifswald, Greifswald, Germany

National Center of Plasma Medicine, Berlin, Germany

Deutsche Dermatologische Lasergesellschaft e.V., Konz, Germany
e-mail: metelman@uni-greifswald.de

S. Hammes
Department of Oral and Maxillofacial Surgery/Plastic Surgery, University Medicine Greifswald, Greifswald, Germany

Laser Clinic Karlsruhe, Karlsruhe, Germany

National Center of Plasma Medicine, Berlin, Germany

Deutsche Dermatologische Lasergesellschaft e.V., Konz, Germany

K. Hartwig
Department of Oral and Maxillofacial Surgery/Plastic Surgery, University Medicine Greifswald, Greifswald, Germany

Office of Diploma of Aesthetic Laser Medicine, University Medicine Greifswald, Greifswald, Germany

T. von Woedtke
Leibniz Institute for Plasma Science and Technology, Greifswald, Germany

National Center of Plasma Medicine, Berlin, Germany

Leibniz Institute for Plasma Science and Technology (INP Greifswald) and University Medicine Greifswald, Institute for Hygiene and Environmental Medicine, Greifswald, Germany
e-mail: woedtke@inp-greifswald.de

T. T. T. Chien
Hoa Lam-Shangri-La, Ho Chi Minh City, Vietnam

A. Rana
Department of Oral and Maxillofacial Surgery/Plastic Surgery, University Medicine Greifswald, Greifswald, Germany

Institute of Laser and Aesthetic Medicine (ILAMED), New Delhi, India

National Center of Plasma Medicine, Berlin, Germany


H.-R. Metelmann et al. (eds.), *Comprehensive Clinical Plasma Medicine*,
https://doi.org/10.1007/978-3-319-67627-2_30

## 30.1 Introduction

Plasma medicine and aesthetic laser medicine belong together, as two options of photonic treatment i.e. chronic wounds, infected skin and contaminated ulcerations are some of the worst complications in aesthetic laser medicine. Furthermore, treating these complications or preventing them in case of risk is the main indication for plasma medicine and the on-label-use of the devices at present.

Photonic therapy requires the adequate training of doctors and nurses so that they may use laser and plasma technology in an effective and non-hazardous manner. The standardization and structuring of the training programs and education provides the most effective approach to consistent and reliable good quality in treatment and quality management [1]. Since 1999, the *Diploma of Aesthetic Laser Medicine (D.A.L.M.)*, (http://www.laserstudium.eu), has been the main university degree in this highly specialized field with a multicenter international teaching program. The programme remains independent from manufacturers and is based at Greifswald University in cooperation with the Deutsche Dermatologische Lasergesellschaft (DDL) in Germany and Institute of Laser & Aesthetic Medicine (ILAMED) as an offshore campus in India for the English speaking countries. The D.A.L.M. degree is suitable and permitted for public announcement through the practice sign of the holder; thereby attesting of his/her expertise and experience in the field.

With the introduction of licensed plasma medical devices in 2013, the curriculum has been revamped and extended in 2016. The plasma medicine supplement comprises hands-on activities, as well as a research oriented part, either (1) included into the current curriculum or (2) as a supplement for holders of the D.A.L.M. degree or (3) independently from the standard degree program, because plasma medicine is not a form of treatment solely restricted to aesthetic laser medicine, but a research subject of its own for scientists, as well as a practical subject for nurses.

The extended *Diploma of Aesthetic Laser Medicine and Plasma Medicine,* representing the full range of today's photonic therapy options, is certified by Greifswald University at an academic degree level; providing an integrated, multidiscipline approach with learning objectives based on innovation and high quality research. The plasma medicine supplement was initiated by the same institutions who initiated the well-established D.A.L.M. program, and more recently, the National Centre of Plasma Medicine (NZPM) in Germany. Moreover, there exists a *Certificate of Esteem in Plasma Medicine* for doctors who do not wish to cover the full scope of aesthetic laser medicine, but completed and focused on the plasma medicine supplement.

These degrees and certificates are open only to licensed doctors. However scientists committed to plasma research and nurses involved in plasma treatment are encouraged to attend the lectures of the plasma medicine supplement too. They may receive a document attesting of their qualified participation by the National Center of Plasma Medicine, upon request; to make their newly gained expertise known.

## 30.2 Diploma in Aesthetic Laser Medicine (D.A.L.M.)

The curriculum of D.A.L.M. covers the full range of laser medicine in aesthetic medicine and surgery: from laser technology, laser physics, laser-tissue interactions, laser safety; to medical humanities, research, practical management aspects and detailed hands-on-clinical application. All subjects of education and training requirements are assembled in a scientific and practice-oriented study program that forms the basis of the lectures, training units and the final exam. Licensed doctors (MD) are enrolled as guest student at the University of Greifswald individually, and set up themselves a relevant study program by enrolling for lectures and practical trainings of their own choice. HAMMES has performed a scientific investigation of the educational effectiveness of the D.A.L.M. program. According to the results of his research; the program is a combination of lectures, training sessions, self-study and in-depth scientific foundation which lasts 18–24 months and is organized in three pillars of studies [2].

### 30.2.1 Dies Academicus (Lecture Units)

The foundational lectures are offered at the monthly *Dies academicus*. The *Dies* takes the form of an all-day seminar with successive inputs by all lecturers, taking place at the facility of the responsible lecturer, i.e. in alternating locations. A complete *Dies* program comprises the eight certificates received upon completion of eight seminars that cover all areas of laser medicine.

### 30.2.2 Hospitationes (Training Units)

The basic hands-on-training units take place at the *Hospitationes* in the Institutes of the lecturers. The main tenets of the training program are: observation, assistance, independent treatment with assistance and independent treatment under supervision.

The full *Hospitationes* program comprises eight certificates of attendance that cover all areas of laser medicine in clinical practice.

### 30.2.3 Studium Generale (Self-Study)

Self-study by participating to additional lectures, scientific and technical meetings and continuing education courses outside the regular study program is mandatory. Initially, visiting reputed conferences also serves to orientate the student within the subject area. A minimum of five certificates of attendance of meetings and international conferences document self-study in laser medicine.

### 30.2.4 Colloquium (Exam)

The Examination Board finalizes this 3-pillar-study program. It is performed as a panel discussion as per the regulations for the conduct of examinations enacted by the Federal Ministry of Education. The exams take place at Greifswald University (mainly for German speaking students) or on behalf of and supervised by Greifswald University at ILAMED, in New Delhi (India) (mainly for English speaking students). The exam comprises of the presentation of the candidate's diploma thesis, of an empirical discussion of at least five cases treated under the responsibility of the candidate, and of a demonstration of knowledge and practical abilities in the whole range of aesthetic laser medicine.

The *Diploma of Aesthetic Laser Medicine (D.A.L.M.)* provides the evidence of a doctor's qualification in aesthetic laser medicine.

## 30.3 Diploma in Aesthetic Laser and Plasma Medicine

Licensed doctors interested in applying plasma clinically and having already completed the D.A.L.M. degree or having begun the program; should be encouraged to apply for the added curriculum in plasma medicine. The intention of such university-based education and manufacturer-independent courses is to make the doctor's use of plasma devices effective and non-hazardous for patients [3]. The additional program to the regular D.A.L.M. curriculum focuses on plasma technology, plasma physics, plasma biology, plasma immunology, plasma tissue interactions, plasma safety and clinical plasma medicine in all its practical and research aspects.

### 30.3.1 Plasma Medicine Supplement

The special study program part concerning plasma medicine is based upon participation to

- two seminars of *Dies academicus* with a focus on plasma medicine sciences and research,
- two hands-on-training courses like *Hospitationes*, putting an emphasis upon bed-side training,
- two conferences featuring plasma medicine research as *Studium generale*, for example at the meetings of the National Center of Plasma Medicine (NZPM) in Germany, at the conferences of the International Society of Plasma Medicine (ICPM) or at the annual International Workshop on Plasma for Cancer Treatment in (IWPTC) , and finally
- presentation and discussion at the *Colloquium* of the board examination of two fully documented cases of plasma treatment or of one scientific paper in the field of plasma medicine, prepared for publication in a peer-reviewed journal like *Clinical Plasma Medicine*.

The *Diploma of Aesthetic Laser and Plasma Medicine* is giving evidence of a doctor's qualification in aesthetic laser medicine as well as in plasma medicine.

## 30.4 Certificate of Esteem in Plasma Medicine

Licensed doctors (M.D., D.D.S.) not involved in aesthetic laser medicine but interested to become qualified in the safe and effective use of plasma medicine may consider education and hands-on training in plasma medicine independently from the D.A.L.M. degree. They are invited to participate to the courses of the plasma medicine supplement without enrollment at Greifswald University but at the National Center of Plasma Medicine. Participants having successfully completed the full program of the plasma medicine supplement as presented above shall receive a *Certificate of Esteem in Plasma Medicine* by the National Center of Plasma Medicine, which will give evidence of a doctor's qualification in plasma medicine.

Scientists with non-medical background involved or active in the field of plasma medicine research, in randomized clinical trials, as members of the editorial board or as reviewers in relevant journals, and mainly interested in learning about the doctor's view in clinical plasma medicine, are very much welcome. They may proceed to their own selection of seminars and participate at the clinical courses in German or in English. The same goes for nurses practicing in the field of wound care management. They do not need to enroll at Greifswald University, but at the National Center of Plasma Medicine, if they would like to receive an official certificate of qualified participation by this institution.

Plasma medicine is rapidly developing, and the study program of plasma medicine supplement has to keep up with the latest scientific advances in this discipline. Scientists are warmly invited to join the faculty of the plasma medicine supplement as lecturers; and qualified nurses, as practical teachers. The faculty of the plasma medicine supplement consists of lecturers covering the complete field of this very innovative kind of photonic treatment, from basic research and engineering, to clinical treatment. The plasma medicine supplement study program is committed to excellence in the scientific and medical community and is globally oriented, setting new standards of education in plasma medicine.

## 30.5 Under-Graduate Education in Plasma Medicine

Separately from the extended D.A.L.M. program reserved for post-graduate specialization of doctors, professional information of scientists, and training of nurses, there is an under-graduate lecture course "Introduction into Plasma Medicine" offered at Greifswald University Medicine. This program (in German language) is the first of its kind in medical schools and dental schools internationally and it is particularly directed to under graduate students of medicine and dentistry as well as human biology. The curriculum is consisting of a series of one-hour-lectures weekly within one semester held by the professorship for plasma medicine, which was appointed in 2011.

The current agenda of the lecture course includes the following main topics:

Introduction: What is plasma?
Atmospheric pressure plasma sources; devices
Clinical plasma medicine: current applications
Wound healing
Cancer treatment
Mechanisms of biological plasma effects
Risk consideration
Outlook
Further development of plasma devices
Further fields of application: dentistry; plasma-treated liquids

With the edition of the first textbook on plasma medicine in 2016 [4] appropriate teaching material is available for students' self-studies. By this lecture series, the students receive the opportunity to meet and learn about the new field of plasma medicine during their regular studies in medical school and dental school. Starting with this facultative lecture the students' academic education in plasma medicine will be further developed during the next years. The aim is to establish plasma medicine as compulsory elective subject of the regular curriculum of medical and dental students.

## References

1. Metelmann HR, Waite PD, Hammes S. Quality standards in aesthetic medicine. In: Raulin C, Karsai S, editors. Laser and IPL technology in dermatology and aesthetic medicine. Berlin: Springer; 2011. p. 377–81.
2. Hammes S. Qualitätssicherung in der ästhetischen Medizin durch universitäre Weiterbildung: Diploma in Aesthetic Laser Medicine. Heidelberg: Springer; 2011.
3. Hammes S, Metelmann HR, Westermann U. Qualitätsmanagement durch postgraduale Weiterbildung. In: Metelmann HR, von Woedtke T, Weltmann KD, editors. Plasmamedizin. Heidelberg: Springer; 2016. p. 201–7.
4. Metelmann HR, von Woedtke T, Weltmann KD, editors. Plasma Medizin. Kaltplasma in der medizinischen Anwendung. Berlin: Springer; 2016.

# Training Wound Nurses in Plasma Medicine

# 31

Stefanie Kirschner, Bedriska Bethke, Anne Kirschner, Silke Brückner, and Birgit Gostomski

## 31.1 Starting Situation

*Keyset: Plasma-supported outpatient wound care is one approach to provide optimal care and treatment for patients with chronic wounds at home.*

That the population is ageing and that diseases are consequently increasing can be confirmed statistically [1]. The prevalence of leg and foot ulcers—one of the most common chronic wounds—also increases with age. This correlation has been observed around in the world in many studies [2]. The number of patients with chronic wounds will continue to rise around the world in coming years. In developed countries, it is estimated that 1–2% of the population will develop a chronic wound at some point in their lives [3]. In 2015 there were about two million people suffering from chronic open wounds in Germany and this trend is rising ([4], p. 3). One reason for this development is the measurable increase in diseases with an associated risk of chronic wounds such as diabetes.

In Germany a lack of continuity and quality in the treatment of chronic wounds has been identified and these deficiencies often delay or impede wound healing. This situation is particularly stressful for the patients because, in addition to the physical impairments (e.g. pain), chronic wounds are also associated with reduced independence and social interaction. The healthcare system is also heavily burdened by supposedly cost-effective therapeutic techniques which, however, often involve high nursing costs but a lack of successful outcomes [5, 6]. According to the German Network for Quality Development in Nursing (Deutsches Netzwerk für Qualitätsentwicklung in der Pflege, DNQP) patients

S. Kirschner (✉) • A. Kirschner
Vocational Education Cente Müritz, Waren, Germany
e-mail: stefanie.kirschner@rbb-mueritz.de

B. Bethke • S. Brückner • B. Gostomski
Department of Health, Nursing and Administration, University of Applied Sciences Neubrandenburg, Neubrandenburg, Germany


H.-R. Metelmann et al. (eds.), *Comprehensive Clinical Plasma Medicine*,
https://doi.org/10.1007/978-3-319-67627-2_31

with chronic wounds should ideally be treated in their own homes because care based on the acute care model is not indicated for chronic wounds. The acute care model is not compatible with either the chronic nature of the disease nor with the daily needs of patients [7, 8]. However, statistics indicate that in Germany very few patients with a chronic wound are treated at home (0.4% of patients with diabetic foot syndrome and 1.7% of patients with a leg ulcer) ([9], cited from [7]). Most patients receive hospital-based treatment (Heyer 2016). The reason for this lies in both the lack of multi-professional outpatient teams and a failure to negotiate care interfaces. Plasma-supported outpatient wound care is one approach to provide optimal care and treatment for patients with chronic wounds at home. This would help to prevent hospitalisations and readmissions. Particularly in rural areas where wound care for patients by specialists may become increasingly difficult to realise [10], outpatient-based cold plasma devices—operated by specialist nursing personnel—are a reliable, more feasible, patient-guided and cost-effective treatment option. Creating a close cooperation between doctors and nursing personnel in the plasma-supported wound healing process can considerably improve wound management for those affected because providing local wound care requires medical and nursing expertise that is adapted to the particular stage of the wound and that is based on comprehensive diagnostics. To ensure that there is a rapid and close collaboration between specialist nursing personnel and doctors in rural areas, mobile information and communication technology will become increasingly important in outpatient plasma-supported wound care. Mobile information and communication technologies enable fast and high quality exchange of information between remotely located doctors and specialist nursing personnel. This procedure promises to deliver positive outcomes regarding the quality of the treatment and patient safety while avoiding additional hospitalisation and saving time and costs. This is achieved by rapidly confirming diagnoses and agreeing on a joint treatment appropriate for the current wound status. Complications in wound healing can thus be promptly identified and countermeasures initiated through quick and easy access to medical and nursing expertise.

The positive medical effects of plasma-supported wound care have already been considered in the previous chapters and will therefore not be revisited in this article. It is much more the role of the specialist nurse—as a second important figure in the plasma-supported wound care process—that will be considered more closely here.

## 31.2 The Role of Nursing in Plasma-Supported Wound Care

*Keyset: Nursing personnel can be responsible for implementation in the wound management process.*

Wound care is defined as a physician-directed task in Germany. Since October 2013 this task may be delegated to nursing personnel.[1] Accordingly, initial wound care is carried out by a doctor (responsibility for the diagnosis). The doctor must then decide if and to whom he or she will delegate the ongoing care of the patient's wound. The doctor is therefore responsible for the duties of selecting, initiating and monitoring wound care [11].

Nursing personnel can be responsible for implementation in the wound management process. They are then responsible for wound management and must provide high quality and effective treatment of the wound. In future, delegation of wound management by a doctor to nursing personnel could be supplemented or replaced by substitution. The tasks carried out by nursing personnel in wound care would then range from assessment to planning of interventions to be applied to implementation of the therapy plan (wound management) [12].

## 31.3 Duties of the Nursing Personnel

*Keyset: The expert standard forms the foundation for nursing wound care in Germany.*

In 2009 the German Network for Quality Development in Nursing [13] published the expert standard 'Nursing of individuals with chronic wounds', which according to section 113a of the German Social Code XI is binding for all approved nursing facilities in Germany. The expert standard makes a critical contribution to the transfer of scientifically verified research findings to nursing practice to ensure and develop quality in nursing and thus forms the foundation for nursing wound care in Germany [9].

According to its objectives, the following duties are fundamental for nurses in wound care and thus also in plasma-supported wound care:

- determining the individual's disease awareness as well as the wound- and therapy-related limitations of the patient,
- supporting health-related self-care, quality of life and well-being of the patient,
- wound management,
- coordinating inter- and intraprofessional wound care as well as
- supporting wound healing and preventing recurrences ([7], p. 19; [14], p. 392).

[1] This can be consulted in the 'Agreement about delegation of medical services to non-medical personnel in contractual outpatient care as defined by section 28, paragraph 1, page 3 of the German Social Code (SGB V)'.

**Table 31.1** Action levels in wound care by nursing personnel ([7], p. 21ff.; [15], p. 219 ff.)

| Action level | Duties of the nurse |
|---|---|
| Assessment | As part of the patient's nursing history, the nurse determines and documents aspects of the illness, his or her individual disease awareness, wound- and therapy-related limitations in self-care and quality of life, medical wound diagnosis and options for health-related self-care |
| Action plan | Together with the patient and his or her relatives, the nurse plans individual and routine measures with the involvement of other professional groups. The action plan includes details about stresses associated with the wound, treatment and routine tasks as well as limitations of the patient and details about proper and ongoing wound care, prevention of recurrences and avoidance of any further harm |
| Coordination of the actions | On the basis of the action plan, the nurse coordinates the professional groups involved in the care process, incorporating the patient and his or her relatives. The nurse bears responsibility here for implementing hygienic and correct wound care and ongoing implementation of the action plan. The nurse maintains ongoing documentation that is intended to ensure the transparency and traceability of the care process |
| Education | The nurse informs, advises, trains and guides the patient and his or her relatives about how to deal with the chronic disease and about any measures necessary for wound healing. The nurse provides information about the cause of the wound, proper diet, individually adapted skin care, selection of clothing and shoes, smoking cessation, handling symptoms such as pain, wound odour and wound exudate as well as other support options |
| Evaluation | The nurse assesses the healing progress and reviews the efficacy of the measures carried out |

The expert standard 'Nursing individuals with chronic wounds' indicates which structural, process and outcome quality must be given to achieve these objectives and considers risk analysis/assessment, the required competencies, action plan, education and evaluation (Table 31.1) ([7], p. 21).

## 31.4 Competencies Required to Implement Plasma-Supported Wound Care

*Keyset: The subject matter related to specific and complex wound care approaches such as plasma-supported wound care generally requires more extensive competencies.*

A new and innovative approach for treating chronic wounds is plasma-supported wound treatment, a technique that requires specific competencies of the nursing personnel for its application. Nursing personnel have already acquired the initial basic knowledge of wound care during their training in vocational college. The subject matter related to specific and complex wound care approaches such as plasma-supported wound care generally requires more extensive competencies that can only be taught as part of continuing education programs.

**Table 31.2** Basic modules for the continuing education program for 'Specialist nursing personnel in plasma-supported wound care'

| Module name | Module unit |
|---|---|
| **Basic module I** Apply professionalprinciples | • Ethical thinking and action<br>• Theory-based nursing<br>• Incorporation of the health and disease model<br>• Economic considerations in healthcare |
| **Basic module II** Initiate and design developments | • Learning<br>• Planning and designing instruction processes<br>• QM—Design work processes in complex situations<br>• Work in projects |

The expert standard 'Nursing of individuals with chronic wounds' should therefore form the foundation of continuing education programs to teach competencies in plasma-supported wound care. The 'DKG recommendation on nursing continuing education' guideline published by the German Hospital Federation on 29 September 2015 should be taken into account when designing a relevant continuing education program. The guideline includes recommendations and directions for how such a continuing education program should be designed to comply with the current state of knowledge in nursing, medicine and related disciplines. This guideline includes concrete procedures for determining entry requirements and the duration, form and structure of the continuing education program as well as assessment procedures [16, 17].

According to section 7 of the DKG recommendation, a continuing education program should be made up of basic modules and specialist modules [16, 17].

Basic modules act as connective elements between nursing education and the specific requirements of those participating in the continuing education program. They form the basis of proper and skilled behaviour in the professional context and are precisely defined by the German Hospital Federation (Table 31.2) [16, 17].

Specialist modules describe the specific technical tasks of the nursing personnel. The structure of the specialist modules outlined here for a possible continuing education program for 'Specialist nursing personnel in plasma-supported wound care' is based on the 'DKG recommendation for nursing continuing education' but the contents are determined by the expert standard 'Nursing of individuals with chronic wounds' as well as the specific knowledge that is required for the preparation, implementation and follow-up of plasma-supported wound care [16, 17]. The link between the basic modules and the specialist modules must ensure that nursing personnel acquire the relevant competencies for high-quality, effective and efficient plasma-supported wound care.

An initial design for possible specialist modules for a continuing education program for 'Specialist nursing personnel in plasma-supported wound care' could look as follows:

### 31.4.1 Specialist Module I

#### 31.4.1.1 Principles of the Wound Care Process

- Pathophysiology
- Assessment of the wound status and the course of wound healing, documentation
- Therapy measures and their influence on quality of life and social participation
- Prophylaxis and prevention of recurrence
- Experience of illness and nursing-related issues for those affected
- Integration of the patient's disease awareness into the nursing and care process
- Self-care and the necessary competencies for those affected
- Legal principles (delegation, occupational health and safety, hygiene)
- Implementation of the expert standard in practice

### 31.4.2 Specialist Module II

#### 31.4.2.1 Action Levels in the Expert Standard

**Assessment**

- Incorporation of the patient and his or her relatives in the care process
- The use of standardised evaluation tools to assess the treatment need

Action plan

- Documentation with differentiated information on the limitations, anxieties, knowledge, self-care options and deficits of the patient and wound diagnosis with detailed information on the current wound situation
- Planning of individual and routine measures
- Description and documentation of various interventions and measures for wound treatment
- Guidelines of the Association of Scientific Medical Societies (Arbeitsgemeinschaft Wissenschaftlicher Medizinischer Fachgesellschaften, AWMF)

**Coordination of the measures**

- Coordination of the care process
- Outpatient and inpatient care and case management
- Organisation of the network in the area of wound care

**Education**

- Informing, advising, training and guiding the patient and his or her relatives
- Cooperation, coordination and communication with appreciation of interprofessional relationships
- Advising those professional groups and management that are involved

**Evaluation**

- Assessing the healing progress and the efficacy of the measures carried out
- Initiating any necessary changes in the action plan

### 31.4.3 Specialist Module III

#### 31.4.3.1 Implementation of Plasma-Supported Wound Care

- Advantages of plasma-supported wound care
- Methods and techniques for specific wound diseases
- Planning, preparation
- Implementation
- Post-processing and follow-up care
- Effect, side effects, complications, emergency management

#### 31.4.3.2 Advantages of Plasma-Supported Wound Care Carried out by Nursing Personnel

*Keyset: The inclusion of nurse's in the plasma-supported wound care process offers advantages for all persons involved in the process.*

The use of plasma medicine in the care of chronic wounds is still in its infancy in Germany. Nursing is also just starting to take advantage of this new field and to develop specific nursing duties. Nurses are therefore included in the plasma-supported wound care process along with the doctors and the patients and their involvement is associated with advantages for the doctor and the patient as well as the nurses themselves.

Advantages from the nurse's perspective

- New areas of activity may increase the interest young people have in the nursing profession. Delegation of the plasma-supported wound care process to nursing personnel can therefore contribute to increasing the attractiveness of the profession.
- An increase in expertise can be expected. Plasma-supported wound care is a new and innovative approach, the use of which requires specific competencies of the nursing personnel which are acquired in appropriate continuing education programs.

Advantages from the patient's perspective

- Plasma-supported wound care is a highly specialised and individual treatment procedure that can be administered by nursing personnel outside inpatient infra-structure in the patient's home.
- A close cooperation between doctors and nursing personnel within plasma-supported wound care enables comprehensive, rapid and more effective treat-

ment of the patient because medical and nursing expertise go hand in hand and treatment steps can be discussed at any time.
- The plasma devices are small and easily transported. It is therefore possible to care for the patient at home which ensures ongoing treatment and care. This is particularly important for immobile patients who are not able to regularly visit the hospital or medical practice for wound care.

Advantages from the doctor's perspective

- Comprehensive and regular wound monitoring and documentation can be expected. As part of the patient's nursing history, the nurse determines and documents aspects of the illness, his or her individual disease awareness, wound- and therapy-related limitations in self-care and quality of life, medical wound diagnosis and options for health-related self-care. ([7], p. 21; [14], p. 219).
- Nurses generally have more intense contact with the patient which enables them to address and eliminate any worries, anxieties and problems that arise in relation to the (wound) treatment.

## References

1. Statistisches Bundesamt. Statistisches Jahrbuch Deutschland und International. 2016. https://www.destatis.de/DE/Publikationen/StatistischesJahrbuch/StatistischesJahrbuch2016.pdf?__blob=publicationFile. Accessed 1 July 2017.
2. Heyer A. Versorgungsepidemiologie des Ulcus cruris in Deutschland Erkrankungshäufigkeit, Versorgungsqualität und Prädiktoren der Wundheilung. Wiesbaden: Springer Fachmedien; 2016.
3. Krister Järbrink, Gao Ni, Henrik Sönnergren, Artur Schmidtchen, Caroline Pang, Ram Bajpai, Josip Car, (2016) Prevalence and incidence of chronic wounds and related complications: a protocol for a systematic review. Systematic Reviews 5 (1).
4. BVMed—Bundesverband Medizintechnologie e. VEinsatz von hydroaktiven Wundauflagen. Informationsbroschüre Wirtschaftlichkeit und Gesundheitspolitik. 2015. https://www.google.de/#q=Ausgaben+des+Gesundheitssystems+f%C3%BCr+WundversorguWu. Accessed 6 Jul 2016.
5. RKI—Robert Koch Institut. 2008. https://www.rki.de/DE/Content/Infekt/EpidBull/Archiv/2008/Ausgaben/41_08.pdf?__blob=publicationFile. Accessed 7 May 2016.
6. Schmidt M et al. Pharm. Ztg. Online. 2011. http://www.pharmazeutische-zeitung.de/index.php?id=37747. Accessed 7 May 2016.
7. DNQP—Deutsches Netzwerk für Qualitätsentwicklung in der Pflege. 2015. Expertenstandard Pflege von Menschen mit chronischen Wunden. Osnabrück.
8. Schmidt S. Expertenstandards in der Pflege—eine Gebrauchsanleitung. Berlin: Springer; 2016.
9. MDS—Medizinischer Dienst des Spitzenverbandes Bund der Krankenkasse. Expertenstandards nach § 113 a SGB XI. 2016. https://www.mds-ev.de/themen/pflegequalitaet/expertenstandards.html. Accessed 27 Apr 2017.
10. Kopetsch, T. - Bundesärztekammer und Kassenärztliche Bundesvereinigung. Dem deutschen Gesundheitswesen gehen die Ärzte aus! Studie zur Altersstruktur-und Arztzahlentwicklung. 2010. https://www.aerztekammer-bw.de/40presse/05aerztestatistik/20.pdf Accessed 8 July 2016.

11. Kassenärztliche Bundesvereinigung. GKV-Spitzenverband. 2015. http://www.kbv.de/media/sp/24_Delegation.pdf. Accessed 7 May 2016.
12. GBA—Gemeinsamer Bundesausschuss. Richtlinie nach § 63 Abs. 3c SGB V des Gemeinsamen Bundesausschusses über die Festlegung ärztlicher Tätigkeiten zur Übertragung auf Berufsangehörige der Alten- und Krankenpflege zur selbständigen Ausübung von Heilkunde im Rahmen von Modellvorhaben nach § 63 Abs. 3c SGB V. 2012. https://www.g-ba.de/downloads/62-492-600/2011-10-20_RL-63Abs3c.pdf. Accessed 29 Apr 2016.
13. DNQP—Deutschen Netzwerk für Qualitätsentwicklung in der Pflege. 2009. https://www.kritische-ereignisse.de/tl_files/akel/Auszug_DNQP-Expertenstandard_Chronische_Wunden.pdf. Accessed 7 May 2016.
14. Döbele M, Becker U, Philbert-Hasucha S. Wundmanagement. In: Döbele M, Becker U Ambulante Pflege von A bis Z. Berlin: Springer; 2016. S. 392.
15. Protz K. Moderne Wundversorgung. München: Urban & Fischer; 2016. S. 192 ff.
16. DKG—Deutsche Krankenhausgesellschaft. DKG-Empfehlung zur pflegerischen Weiterbildung. 2015. http://www.dkgev.de/dkg.php/cat/314/aid/14004/title/Empfehlung_mit_Erlaeuterungen_und_Materialien. Accessed 13 Jan 2016.
17. DKG—Deutsche Krankenhausgesellschaft. Erläuterungen zur modularen DKG-Empfehlung vom 29.09.2015 für die Weiterbildung in den pflegerischen Fachgebieten. 2015. http://www.dkgev.de/dkg.php/cat/314/aid/14004/title/Empfehlung_mit_Erlaeuterungen_und_Materialien. Accessed 13 Jan 2016.

# Part V

# Scientifically Based Plasma Medical Devices Available on the Market

# kINPen MED®

# 32

Renate Schönebeck

## 32.1 Development

In the 1960s, the first cold atmospheric pressure plasmas (CAP) suitable for the modification and decontamination of plastics in an industrial application were generated In the 1990s, the coincidence of an increasing development of bacterial resistance to antibiotics and the refinement of these plasma sources suggested a closer research into the potential suitability for the decontamination of the human skin. The renowned *Leibniz Institute for Plasma Science and Technology e.V. (INP Greifswald)*—which at that time had already assumed a leading role in low temperature plasma research—took on this task by Weltmann et al. [1, 2], Weltmann and von Woedtke [3], Bekeschus et al. [4] and started to work on the development of suitable plasma sources within the framework of a large interdisciplinary research project (Campus PlasmaMed) including partners from medicine and industry. The project result was the prototype of the kINPen® MED device, which was further developed to marketability in cooperation with *neoplas tools GmbH*, Greifswald, Germany, who obtained medical device approval for the device in 2013 as the first CE-certified atmospheric pressure plasma jet.

The kINPen® MED is a cold atmospheric pressure argon plasma jet for superficial treatment of wounds that are hard to heal and human skin illnesses caused by certain pathogens. The cold physical plasma generated by the kINPen® MED has an effect on microorganisms such as bacteria, viruses or fungi, including multi-drug resistant pathogens, and accelerates the initial healing of the wound.

The plasma jet applies a physical cold plasma with a temperature of ca. 37°C to the wound. Surfaces with a more complex structure, recesses, cavities and even hair follicles are easy to reach and can be treated evenly. The inert gas argon that is used for plasma generation guarantees a consistent and stable atmosphere around the generated plasma jet, and thus a high and consistent treatment quality.

R. Schönebeck
Neoplas Tools GmbH, Greifswald, Germany
e-mail: Renate.schoenebeck@neoplas-tools.eu



H.-R. Metelmann et al. (eds.), *Comprehensive Clinical Plasma Medicine*,
https://doi.org/10.1007/978-3-319-67627-2_32

## 32.2 About the Device

The kINPen® MED plasma device consists of a base unit which is attached firmly to a handpiece that creates the plasma jet (Fig. 32.1).

It creates a high electrical voltage (2–3 kV) by employing a high-frequency generator (1 MHz) using a stainless-steel electrode inside a ceramic capillary. The device's operating gas, argon, flows through the ceramic capillary. Due to high-frequency discharge, the gas that is flowing between the electrodes is converted into a physical plasma and pushed out of the device as a jet (Fig. 32.2) thanks to the feeding of the gas.

During treatment, the plasma jet is traced over the skin area that is in need of treatment at a distance that is kept by a spacer (Fig. 32.3). The skin areas that are being treated should be covered as evenly as possible, at a moderate speed of around 5 mm/s.

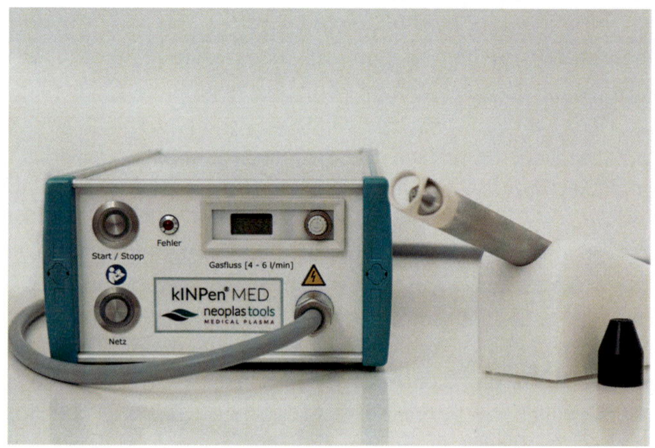


**Fig. 32.1** Base unit with handpiece, spacer, tray and protective cap

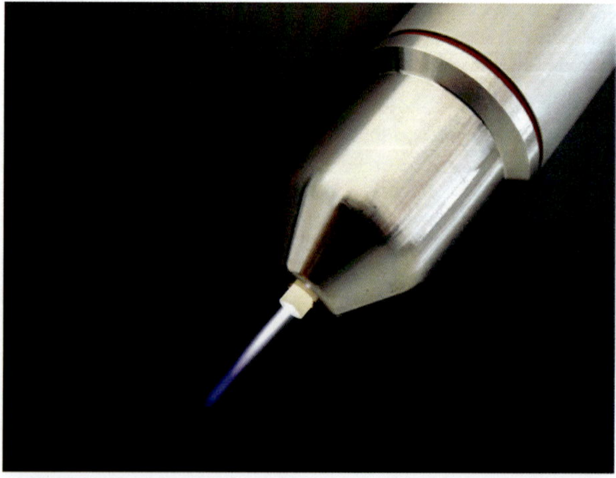

**Fig. 32.2** Device head with jet

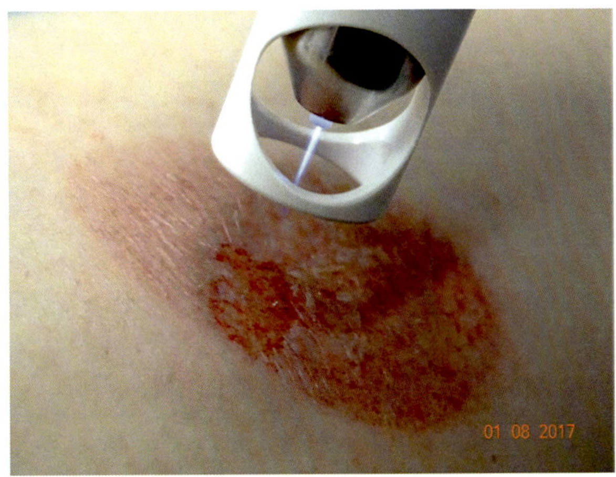


**Fig. 32.3** Treatment of a burn wound

The kINPen® MED's plasma has a treatment field of approximately 1 $cm^2$. The intensity of the treatment is controlled by the length of treatment and, in order to achieve the best possible effect, should amount to roughly 30–60 $s/cm^2$ per treatment area.

The beneficial effects are created by the "cocktail" of excited types of gas present in plasma, as well as low radiation in UV-light conditions, an electromagnetic field, a short-term rise in temperature and the creation of free radicals. These physical effects, which are already being used individually for therapeutic purposes in medicine, are combined synergistically. The skin surface that comes in contact with the jet profits from the antimicrobial, antimycotic or antiviral effect and cellular proliferation is enhanced.

The plasma is produced in the same place as it is used and it is kept stable. It can work quickly, variably and without making direct contact with the surface and, thanks to the jet procedure, can even access the smallest of cavities (Fig. 32.4), which are hard to reach or not suitable for treatment with antiseptics.

The therapy is used as a supplement to standard wound management. The application can be performed in one-day to three-day intervals as long as there are no side effects. The duration of the cold plasma therapy depends on the individual wound condition and the treatment frequency.

Prior to the plasma treatment necrotic wounds have to undergo debridement. The plasma treatment should be performed before topical medication to avoid undesired interactions with antiseptics.

The device is easy to use, it only has a power switch and an on/off button to start the flow of gas and can display error messages on the display (Fig. 32.5).

The attending doctor can therefore delegate its use easily. Operator satisfaction is high, because the area that is in need of treatment can be treated precisely with the handpiece and the tracing of the handpiece is similar to how scalpels are used.

For flexible use in a practice or hospital, *neoplas-tools GmbH* offers a hospital transport trolley to which the device and the gas cylinder are fixed (Fig. 32.6). The trolley also offers storage space for other materials that may be required during the treatment, turning it into a full-featured treatment unit that can be moved flexibly to the patient's side.

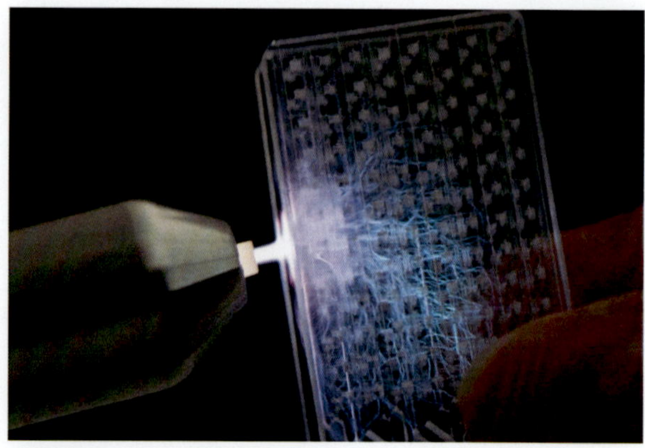

**Fig. 32.4** Illustration of the hiatus penetration properties

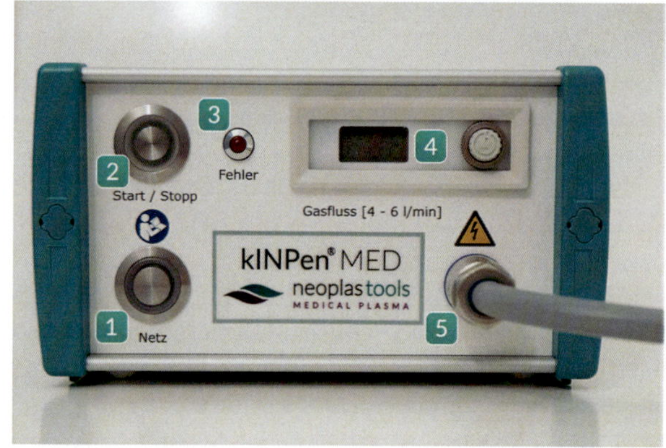


**Fig. 32.5** Base unit with 1 power switch, 2 start/stop key, 3 error display (LED), 4 gas flow control 5 supply tube for the handpiece

The satisfaction and compliance of the patients is also high. Mostly, positive changes to the area being treated can be seen very quickly, which is very motivating, especially for patients that have often experienced years of painful suffering without improvement under other therapies. The treatment itself is not, or in a few cases, only very minimally, painful. In some cases, permanent pain is reduced considerably after treatment or disappears completely. Patients with itchy skin conditions report a reduction or complete disappearance of itchiness, in some cases it did not reappear after the first treatment.

## 32.3 Decontamination with the kINPen® MED

Although highly efficient antiseptics, antibiotics and a number of treatment methods are available, the successful treatment of chronic wounds continues to constitute a significant problem for both patients and the healthcare system. It is particularly problematic that

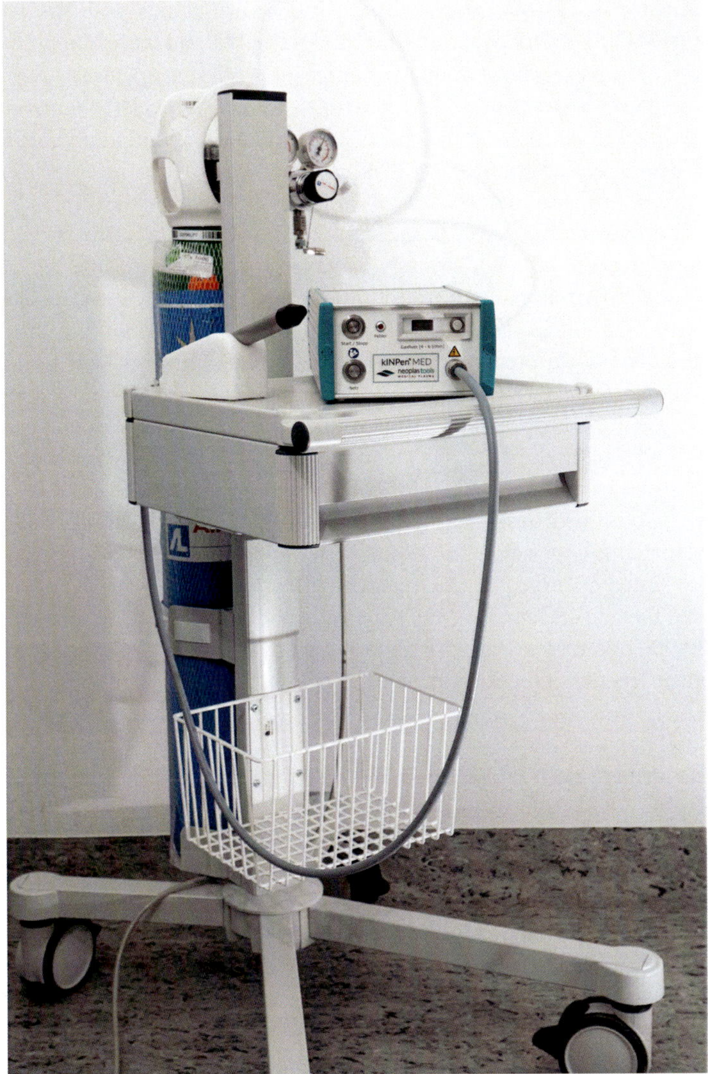


**Fig. 32.6** Treatment unit on the transport trolley

(a) chronic wounds are very often populated with partly multi-drug resistant microorganisms, which slow down or stop the healing of the wound and
(b) the wounds show a weak inflammatory profile which generally has a negative influence on the division of skin cells and on the wound closure.

The clinical and preclinical data of the past years show that treatment with the kINPen® MED can have a positive effect on the healing of the wound, after the wound has been decontaminated successfully.

Daeschlein et al. [5, 6] carried out *in vitro* investigations with the preceding model of the kINPen® MED, the Plasmajet kINPen 09, and were able to prove the inactivation of 105 examined wound infections (11 different species).

In a comparative study on the effect of plasma on skin cells, Wende et al. [7] proved that the kINPen 09 and the approved medical device, kINPen® MED, show the same level of effectiveness.

Finally, in a further *ex vivo* examination of 13 different species, including most of multi-drug resistant species, Daeschlein et al. [5] were able to prove that the microorganisms were killed or severely damaged by physical plasma.

The positive *in vitro* results were followed up *in vivo*. Between December 2014 and October 2015, for instance, an overall population of 42 patients with (partially long-term) ulcers of different origin was treated with the kINPen® MED at the hospital *Klinikum Altenburger Land*, Altenburg, Germany. All cases included were considered "beyond therapy", i.e. all standard therapies including vascular sanitation, state-of-the-art wound dressing or vacuum therapy did not lead to any healing progress. Treated with kINPen® MED, MRSA sanitation occurred in 90% of patients, verified by triple smear test. During the follow-up period 22 wounds healed completely, 18 patients experienced a considerable reduction of the wound surface, and the therapy failed in two cases (no treatment effect).

Between the market launch of the plasma jet and mid-2017 an estimated number of min. 30,000 treatments were performed on patients with a large variety of wound healing disorders and infectious diseases.

## 32.4 Acceleration of Wound Healing with the kINPen® MED

Kramer et al. [8] found in an *in vitro* investigation that there was an increased rate of proliferation on human cells that were treated with plasma immediately after they were removed, when compared to the untreated control. They also observed the remission of chronic wounds after 3–24 weeks in four dogs and two cats, who were treated with the kINPen 09 because of chronic wounds and partly due to the failure of other therapies. The plasma treatment was sometimes carried out in addition to treatment with antiseptics and was applied twice a week on average. They summarised that plasma treatment supports wound healing.

Barton et al. [9] eventually determined that treatment with plasma leads to an increased production of growth factors for the new creation of vessels, and immune hormones for the communication with cells in the immune system; which are both important for healing wounds.

These and further results from investigations into the effects of physical plasma on cells paved the way for systematically proving the speeding up of wound healing in an animal trial. However, there are no animal models with chronic wounds and therefore it is difficult or hardly possible to investigate improved healing on living animals (*in vivo*). It was, however, possible to slow down wound healing on the ears of hairless mice [10]. Using this as a basis, at the end of 2014, an animal study with 77 mice was started at the Leibniz Institute for Plasma Science and Technology

(INP), in cooperation with University Medicine Rostock (Department of Experimental Surgery), whose aim was to examine the effects of plasma treatment on the wound healing process [11]. The treatments were carried out precisely on the surface of the wound, which had an average area of 0.5 $cm^2$ (±0.2 $cm^2$). The results show that after 14 days, the wound surface on the ears of mice treated with plasma (20 s) was approximately 40% smaller when compared to the surface of the untreated control.

Recent images taken with a hyperspectral camera by *Diaspective Vision GmbH*, Pepelow, Germany (Fig. 32.7) provide convincing evidence of a component that considerably supports accelerated wound healing. The images taken prior to, directly after, and 10 min after the plasma treatment clearly show that both the hemoglobin level and the oxygen supply increase significantly after a plasma application with the kINPen ®MED device. Moreover, this does not only apply to the superficial area directly reached by the plasma, but also to the skin layers up to a depth of ca. 8 mm.

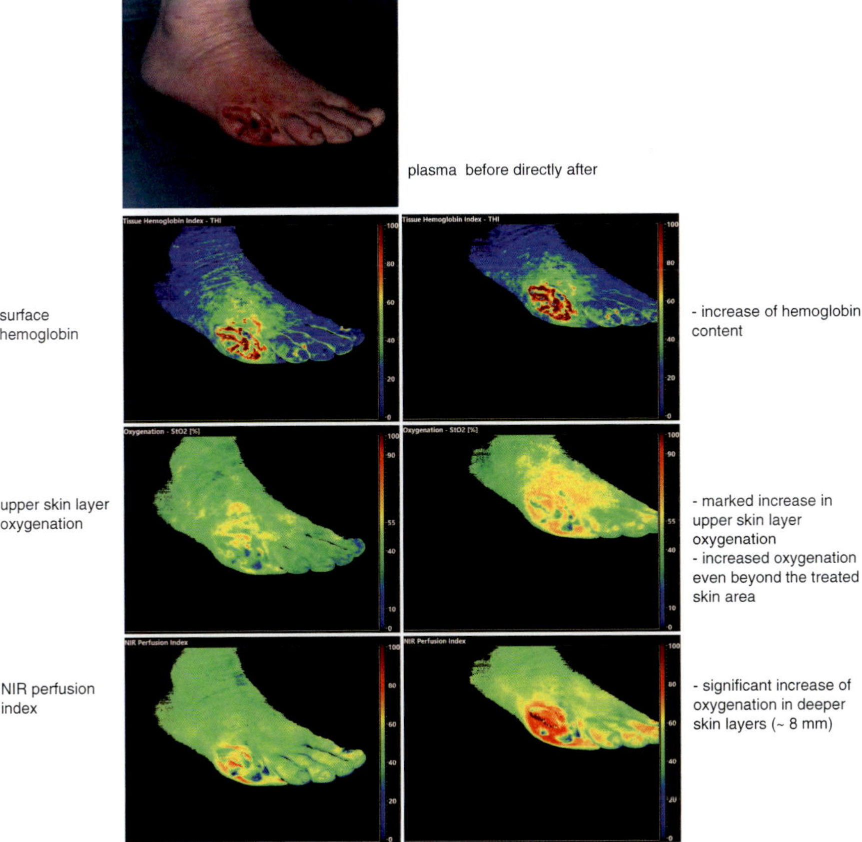


**Fig. 32.7** Hyperspectral analysis image of microcirculation changes in a diabetic foot (Printed with the kind permission of Dr. Kai Masur)

## 32.5 Positive Effects and Features of the kINPen® MED Therapy

- supports wound healing
- anti-bacterial and anti-inflammatory effect, deactivates multi-resistant pathogens
- wide range of indications for acute and chronic wounds
- painless non-invasive procedure that does not require anesthesia
- precise application even in recesses and cavities
- easy handling
- can be delegated by the attending physician
- no side effects or formation of resistances observed

## 32.6 Outlook and Further Developments

*neoplas tools GmbH* is in continuous and close cooperation with hospitals, universities and research institutions. It initiates and supports studies and observational studies, and is refining the device on the basis of information gathered in medical practice.

One result of this close cooperation is the development of an exchangeable head for the kINPen® MED, which is anticipated to be available from early 2018. With this new version, the user will be able to exchange and autoclave the device head. This ensures that the device can be used safely and without any problems even during operations in an operating room.

In addition *neoplas tools GmbH* is working on the development of a special device for applications in dentistry based on a prototype investigated and constructed by *Leibniz-Institute for Plasma Science and Technology e.V., INP Greifswald*, Germany. First results of plasma applications in the oral cavity obtained by the hospital *Charité*—Universitätsmedizin Berlin, Germany, provide highly promising indications of treatment options for root caries, mycoses, mouth ulcers, jaw bone necrosis and wound healing disorders. The development of a special dental pen is connected with the hope of supplying an effective instrument for the adjuvant treatment of periodontitis and periimplantitis [12–14]).

In order to extend the study situation concerning medical plasma applications of the kINPen®MED device, a placebo-controlled study with the title "Kaltplasmatherapie zur Beschleunigung der Wundheilung bei oberflächlichen, infizierten chronischen Wunden bei diabetischem Fußsyndrom" (Cold plasma therapy for the acceleration of healing of superficial and infected chronic wounds in the presence of diabetic foot syndrome) is currently being conducted by the diabetes centres in Bad Oeynhausen and Karlsburg, Germany. Apart from this a joint application for ethical approval of the plasma treatment of actinic keratosis has been filed together with the University of Mainz. The results of both studies are expected for the end of 2018.

**Table 32.1** Successfully tested fields of application of the kINPen® MED, in accordance with the current licence

| Indications | Therapy until now |
|---|---|
| Ulcers of all kinds of aetiology | |
| Acne vulgaris | Diverse, can be very lengthy |
| Rosacea + rhinophyma (common inflamed reddening and bulbous reddened swelling of the nose) | Cosmetics, antibiotics in severe cases, operative laser treatment |
| Herpes genitalis, recidivans and all other herpes | Aciclovir, development of resistance |
| Eczema/Lichen simplex chronicus (severely itchy, chronic skin condition) | Cortisone |
| Verrucae, warts | Different types of therapy such as cryotherapy, lasers, incisions etc. |
| Tinea pedis, athlete's foot, onychomycosis (often very hard to treat) | Treatment with creams and tablets (side effects) |
| Molluscum contagiosum | Various therapies, for children often under use of anaesthetics |
| Wound dehiscence | |
| Oral mycoses | |

Within the framework of her doctoral thesis supervised by Prof. Dr. Thomas Fuchsluger, Helena Reitberger investigated the effect of plasma on eye cells at the Universitätsaugenklinik Erlangen (university eye clinic in Erlangen, Germany). Her results demonstrated that there is no damage, i.e. that neither apoptosis nor any oxydative stress was triggered during a 0.5 to 2-min treatment with the kINPen®MED. Based on these results, four patients with infected corneal ulcers have so far been treated with the device with highly promising results within the framework of individual healing efforts at a hospital in Bremen, Germany. The publication of these cases is scheduled for the end of 2017.

## 32.7 Successfully Treated Indications

According to the current licence, the kINP®MED is meant to be used for treating chronic wounds and pathogen-caused illnesses of the skin and skin appendages (Table 32.1).

## References

1. Weltmann KD, von Woedtke T, Brandenburg R, Ehlbeck J. Biomedical applications of atmospheric pressure plasma. Chem List. 2008;102:1450–1.
2. Weltmann KD, Kindel E, Brandenburg R, Meyer C, Bussiahn R, Wilke C, von Woedtke T. Atmospheric pressure plasma jet for medical therapy: plasma parameters and risk estimation. Contrib Plasma Phys. 2009;49:631.
3. Weltmann KD, von Woedtke T. Basic requirements for plasma sources in medicine. Eur Phys J Appl Phys. 2011;55:13804.

4. Bekeschus S, Schmidt A, Weltmann KD, von Woedtke T. The plasma jet kINPen—a powerful tool for wound healing. Clin Plasma Med. 2016;4:19–28.
5. Daeschlein G, Scholz S, Ahmed R, von Woedtke T, Haase H, Niggemeier M, Kindel E, Brandenburg R, Weltmann KD, Juenger M. Skin decontamination by low-temperature atmospheric pressure plasma jet and dielectric barrier discharge plasma. J Hosp Infect. 2012;81:177–83.
6. Daeschlein G, Napp M, von Podwils S, Lutze S, Emmert S, Lange A, Klare I, Haase H, Gümbel D, von Woedtke T, Jünger M. In vitro susceptibility of multidrug resistant skin and wound pathogens against low-temperature atmospheric pressure plasma jet (appj) and dielectric barrier discharge plasma (dbd). Plasma Process Polym. 2014;11:175–83.
7. Wende K, Reuter S, von Woedtke T, Weltmann KD, Masur K. Redox-based assay for assessment of biological impact of plasma treatment. Plasma Process Polym. 2014;11:655–63.
8. Kramer A, Lademann J, Bender CP, Sckell A, Hartmann B, Münch S. Suitability of tissue tolerable plasma (TTP) for the management of chronic wounds. Clin Plasma Med. 2013;1:11–8.
9. Barton A, Wende K, Bundscherer L, Hasse S, Schmidt A, Bekeschus S, Weltmann KD, Lindquist U, Masur K. Nonthermal plasma increases expression of wound healing in a keratinocyte cell line. Plasma Med. 2013;3:125–36.
10. Barker JH, Kjolseth D, Kim M, Frank J, Bondar I, Uhl E, Kamler M, Messmer K, Tobin GR, Weiner LJ. The hairless mouse ear: an in vivo model for studying wound neovascularization. Wound Repair Regen. 1994;2:138–43.
11. Schmidt A, Bekeschus S, Wende K, Vollmar B, von Woedtke T. Cold plasma jet accelerates wound healing in a murine model of full—thickness skin. Exp Dermatol. 2017;26:156–62.
12. Abu-Sirhan S, Hertel M, Preissner S, Wirtz HC, Herbst SR, Pierdzioch P, Raguse JD, Hartwig S. Bactericidal efficacy of cold plasma in processed bone. A new approach for adjuvant therapy of medication-related osteonecrosis of the jaw? Clin Plasma Med. 2016;4:9–13.
13. Herbst SR, Hertel M, Ballout H, Pierdzioch P, Weltmann K-D, Wirtz HC, Abu-Sirhan S, Kostka E, Paris S, Preissner S. Bactericidal efficacy of cold plasma at different depths of infected root canals in vitro. Open Dent J. 2015;9:486–91.
14. Preissner S, Kastner I, Schütte E, Hartwig S, Schmidt-Westhausen AM, Paris S, Preissner R, Hertel M. Adjuvant antifungal therapy using tissue tolerable plasma on oral mucosa and removable dentures in oral candidiasis patients: a randomised double-blinded split-mouth pilot study. Mycoses. 2016;59:467–75.

# PlasmaDerm® - Based on di_CAP Technology

# 33

Dirk Wandke

## 33.1 Introduction

The use of physical plasma under atmospheric pressure has been established in daily use in surgery for tissue dissection and sclerotherapy for many years [1]. When used as intended, the respective medical devices can be classified as medically safe. These devices are usually based on the principle of the plasma jet, i.e. an inert gas is fed to the devices and is forced out of a nozzle after the plasma is ignited and a spot is applied to the site to be treated. However, this single-spot application limits the use of the devices for the treatment of larger surfaces, which is usually needed for wound care.

The use of direct cold atmospheric pressure plasma in wound treatment is a novel, innovative concept; there are numerous potential uses both after surgical procedures and for chronic wounds. The patented PlasmaDerm® di_CAP technology allows faster direct treatment of larger areas and also combines a number of well-known effects whose advantages are evident, especially the combination of effective deep stimulation of microcirculation to increase oxygen saturation and the significant reduction of bacteria, including many antibiotic-resistant pathogens. PlasmaDerm® thus activates wound healing in all phases. The device fulfils an "unmet need", especially due to its simplicity of use. The patented di_CAP (direct cold atmospheric plasma) technology has already received acclaim from many sides for its innovative nature.

The PlasmaDerm®-di_CAP technology is an application form that allows treatment of a large area while also having a flexible design that means it can be adapted to any topology of the treatment area.

D. Wandke
CINOGY GmbH Plasma Technology for Health, Duderstadt, Germany
e-mail: dirk.wandke@cinogy.de



H.-R. Metelmann et al. (eds.), *Comprehensive Clinical Plasma Medicine*,
https://doi.org/10.1007/978-3-319-67627-2_33

Treatment areas of dozens up to a hundred square centimetres are possible. Another advantage of the PlasmaDerm® di_CAP technology is that no additional gas needs to be added because the plasma is formed directly from the ambient air. This also expands the indications for use to include outpatient treatment, as no replacement or transport of gas bottles is required.

PlasmaDerm®, which is classified as a Class IIa medical device, and the associated sterile spacer have been declared in conformity with EU Council Directive 93/42/EEC.

## 33.2 Device Technology

The generation of plasma in the PlasmaDerm® di_CAP technology is based on the concept of dielectric barrier discharge. For this, the plasma is generated between two electrodes under atmospheric pressure; at least one of the two electrodes is completely covered by an electrical insulating material. The purpose is to limit current flow, among other things. Figure 33.1 shows a schematic representation of this method.

In the PlasmaDerm® di_CAP technology, the area of skin or wound to be treated functions as a counter electrode. The advantage of this is that the plasma is generated or applied directly to the area to be treated. This is illustrated in Fig. 33.2.

The PlasmaDerm® device consists of a control unit about the size of a laptop in combination with a hand-held unit approx. 2 cm in diameter and approx. 20 cm long. The hand-held unit has a connector for the sterile spacer intended for single use. Ease of handling and mobile use are ensured by the implementation of a one-button technique. Only the customary power supply of 100–240 V is required for use. After switching on the PlasmaDerm® device and attaching the sterile spacer, treatment can begin.

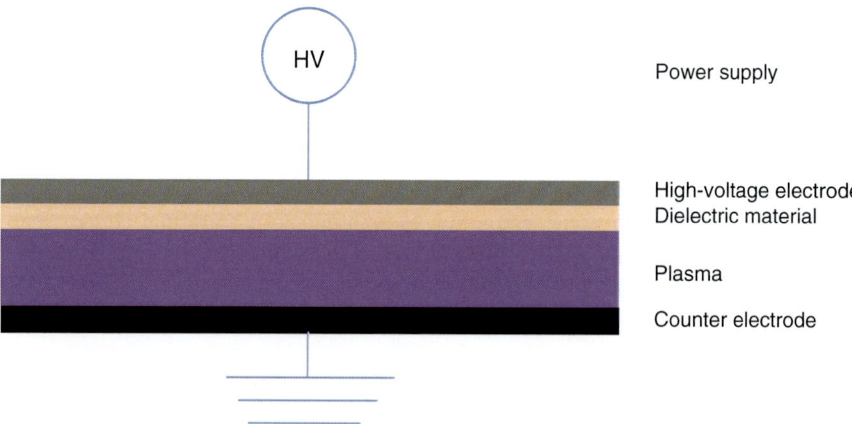


**Fig. 33.1** Schematic representation of a dielectric barrier discharge

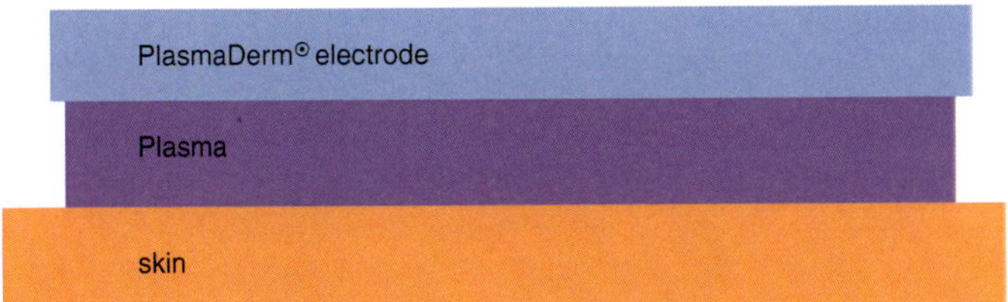


**Fig. 33.2** Schematic representation of PlasmaDerm® on the surface of the skin

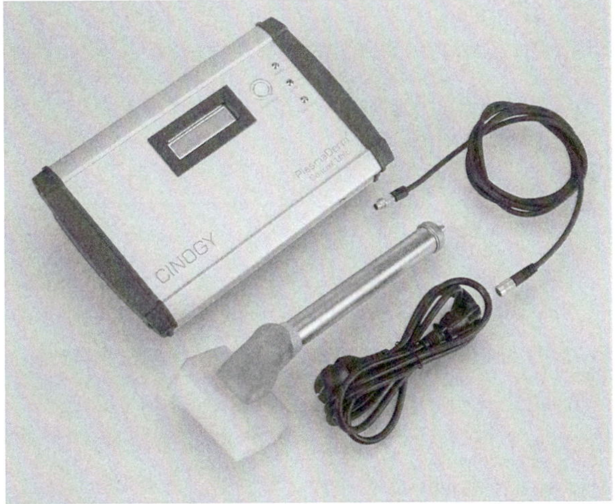


**Fig. 33.3** PlasmaDerm® control unit and hand-held unit

Due to the single-use spacer, there is no risk of cross-contamination. No time-consuming and expensive sterilisation is needed. After a preset time of 90s, the device automatically switches off plasma generation. Treatment can be continued after pressing the ON button again. There are no other technical features of the device that need to be considered. Figure 33.3 shows the PlasmaDerm® control unit and the hand-held unit. Figure 33.4 shows the flexible PlasmaDerm® spacer.

## 33.3 Mode of Action

The effectiveness of the direct cold plasma generated by the PlasmaDerm® device is due to the combination of a therapeutically relevant electrical field, low-level radiation in the useful UV-A and UV-B wavelength range, and activated gas particles (molecules) from the ambient air. PlasmaDerm® therapy thus for the first time combines a number of well-known, therapeutically effective components for a synergistic effect.

The electrical field used in PlasmaDerm® therapy ensures deep stimulation of the skin or wound treated. This deep stimulation has a long-lasting effect, reflected in the increased microcirculation in the area of skin treated. Stimulating microcirculation improves the oxygen supply to the wound.

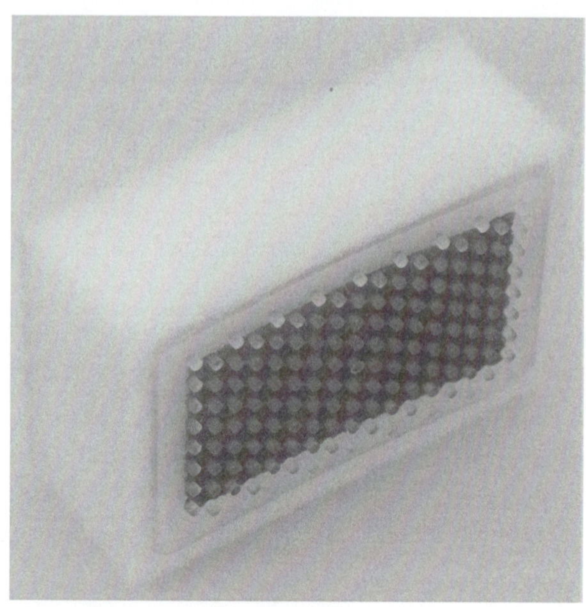

**Fig. 33.4** PlasmaDerm® FLEX9060 spacer

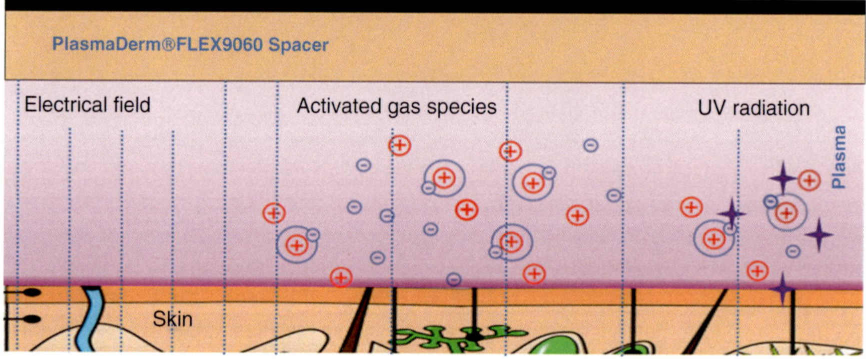


**Fig. 33.5** Schematic representation of the mode of action for PlasmaDerm®

PlasmaDerm® has a reliable topical anti-bacterial effect and is effective even against problematic antibiotic-resistant bacteria such as methicillin-resistant Staphylococcus aureus (MRSA).

A schematic representation of the mode of action is shown in Fig. 33.5.

## 33.4 Use and Treatment Recommendation

The non-invasive PlasmaDerm® therapy treatment can be optimally integrated as one step when changing dressings. The one-button technique makes it easy to use. Due to the broad range of effect, treatment is indicated in all phases of wound healing.

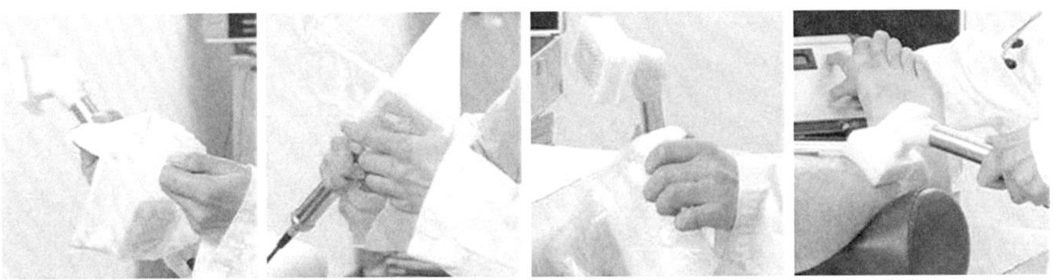

**Fig. 33.6** Easy to use: Unwrap the PlasmaDerm®FLEX9060 spacer, attach it to the hand-held unit, place the spacer on the area of skin to be treated, and start the 90-s treatment with the one-button technique

The sterile PlasmaDerm® spacer is applied to the skin or wound and the area is treated with direct cold plasma. Depending on the size of the area to be treated, one of the different versions of the PlasmaDerm® spacer can be selected to ensure the even, simultaneous treatment of the entire area of skin or wound in one session. A characteristic discharge sound indicates correct plasma generation. Depending on the healing phase, PlasmaDerm® treatment should be applied up to once a day for optimal results. Application is quick and easy. The recommended duration is 90s per $cm^2$ of skin. Due to optimisation of the technical settings, PlasmaDerm® can be operated in a one-button technique. PlasmaDerm® has an intentionally simple, partially automatic operating concept so it can also be applied by nursing staff after they have been instructed in its use.

No additional hygiene measures are required except disinfection of the hand-held unit and control unit with a disinfectant wipe.

Figure 33.6 shows the simple application of PlasmaDerm® treatment.

## 33.5 Indications

The primary indications for PlasmaDerm® treatment are wound healing disorders occurring after operations, e.g. surgical procedures. The healing properties of PlasmaDerm® can also be used for wound healing disorders caused by other conditions, e.g. venous and arterial ulcers, pressure ulcers, or diabetic foot syndrome. The deep stimulation of the electrical field and the associated stimulation of microcirculation result in the improved supply of oxygen and nutrients to wound tissue. In the wound bed, the topical plasma components effectively reduce bacteria.

## 33.6 Application Safety

The devices of the PlasmaDerm® product range generate histocompatible plasma with gas temperatures at body temperature ($T \leq 40°C$) on the treatment area. Figure 33.7 shows the generation of histocompatible plasma on a finger.

**Fig. 33.7** Histocompatible plasma over a skin surface

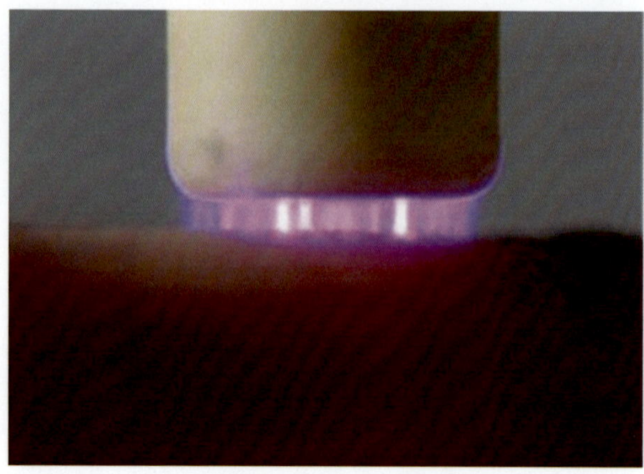

In the conformity assessment procedure, all potential risks were identified and all required tests for patient and user safety were conducted and assessed in a risk management procedure. Applicable national and international standards and requirements and the latest research data were and are adhered to.

With the declaration of conformity based on EU Council Directive 93/42/EEC, CINOGY GmbH, the legal manufacturer of the PlasmaDerm® product range, guarantees the highest safety standards for patients and users. Safety is enhanced by the implementation of a complete quality management system based on DIN EN ISO 13485, which covers all cycles of the PlasmaDerm® products from development and production to service.

The safety and tolerability of PlasmaDerm® has been proven in clinical studies and in daily practice with approx. 20,000 applications up to now.

## 33.7 Studies

The antimicrobial properties have been proven in various in vitro and in vivo studies. It has also been shown that treatment with histocompatible physical plasma is tolerated with no problems [2–4]. In vitro tests have proven its potent effectiveness against all relevant skin and wound bacteria and clinically relevant fungi [3, 5]. Additionally, no clinically relevant differences were found under in vivo conditions when used against multidrug resistant pathogens compared with their non-multidrug resistant variants [6–8].

A randomised, two-armed, controlled clinical trial based on DIN EN ISO 14155 at the Goettingen University Hospital proved safety for patients and users, antimicrobial effectiveness on chronic ulcerous wounds, and practicability [9, 10].

The improvement of microcirculation with PlasmaDerm® treatment was proven in a prospective cohort study with 20 + 20 healthy patients in whom oxygen saturation increased significantly by 24% in the application area on the forearm after PlasmaDerm® therapy [11, 12].

Not yet published studies, test series, case reports, and approx. 20,000 applications in daily practice confirm the observed results.

## 33.8 Brief Summary of PlasmaDerm® Treatment

The greatest advantage of the PlasmaDerm® di_CAP technology is that it combines the mechanisms of different treatment methods. UV-, ozone-, and electrotherapy are already available. However, with the PlasmaDerm® treatment, a better effect is achieved in a shorter time. PlasmaDerm® treatment reduces the number of bacteria on the surface of the skin and wound while simultaneously increasing microcirculation in tissue. These are decisive factors for better wound healing.

- Increases blood flow
- Reduce bacteria without leading to resistance
- Effective against antibiotic-resistant bacteria
- Non-allergenic
- Non-invasive, painless treatment
- Easy, time-saving application

## References


1. Zenker M. Argon plasma coagulation. GMS Krankenhygiene Interdiszip. 2008;3(1.) Doc15. Published online 2008/11/03.
2. Daeschlein G, Scholz S, Ahmed R, von Woedtke T, Haase H, Niggemeier M, Kindel E, Brandenburg R, Weltmann KD, Juenger M. Skin decontamination by low-temperature atmospheric pressure plasma jet and dielectric barrier discharge plasma. J Hosp Infect. 2012;81(3):177–83.
3. Daeschlein G, Scholz S, Ahmed R, Majumdar A, von Woedtke T, Haase H, Niggemeier M, Kindel E, Brandenburg R, Weltmann KD, Jünger M. Cold plasma is well-tolerated and does not disturb skin barrier or reduce skin moisture. JDDG. 2012;10(7):509–15.
4. Rajasekaran P, Opländer C, Hoffmeister D, Bibinov N, Suschek CV, Wandke D, Awakowicz P. Characterization of dielectric barrier discharge (DBD) on mouse and histological evaluation of the plasma-treated tissue. Plasma Process Polym. 2011;8:246–55.
5. Daeschlein G, von Woedtke T, Kindel E, Brandenburg R, Weltmann KD, Jünger M. Antibacterial activity of atmospheric pressure plasma jet (APPJ) against relevant wound pathogens in vitro on simulated wound environment. Plasma Process Polym. 2009;6:224–30.
6. Daeschlein G, Scholz S, Arnold A, von Podewils S, Haase H, Emmert S, von Woedtke T, Weltmann KD, Jünger M. In vitro susceptibility of important skin and wound pathogens against low temperature atmospheric pressure plasma jet (APPJ) and dielectric barrier discharge plasma (DBD). Plasma Process Polym. 2012;9:380–9.
7. Daeschlein G, Scholz S, von Podewils S, Arnold A, Klare I, Haase H, Emmert S, von Woedtke T, Jünger M. Cold plasma—a new antimicrobial treatment tool against multidrug resistant pathogens. In: Mendez-Vilas A, editor. Worldwide research efforts in the fighting against microbial pathogens—from basic research to technological developments. Boca Raton: Brown Walker Press; 2013. p. 110–3.
8. Daeschlein G, Napp M, von Podewils S, Lutze S, Emmert S, Lange A, Klare I, Haase H, Gümbel D, von Woedtke T, Jünger M. In vitro susceptibility of multidrug resistant skin and

wound pathogens against low temperature atmospheric pressure plasma jet (APPJ) and dielectric barrier discharge plasma (DBD). Plasma Process Polym. 2014;11:175–83.

9. Brehmer F, Haenssle HA, Daeschlein G, Ahmed R, Pfeiffer S, Görlitz A, Simon D, Schön MP, Wandke D, Emmert S. Alleviation of chronic venous leg ulcers with a hand-held dielectric barrier discharge plasma generator (PlasmaDerm® VU-2010): results of a monocentric, two-armed, open, prospective, randomized and controlled trial (NCT01415622). JEADV. 2016;29:148–55.
10. Emmert S, Brehmer F, Hänßle H, Helmke A, Mertens N, Ahmed R, Simon D, Wandke W, Maus-Friedrichs W, Daeschlein G, Schön MP, Viöl W. Atmospheric pressure plasma in dermatology: Ulcus treatment and much more. Clin Plasma Med. 2013; Epub 2013 Jan 2. https://doi.org/10.1016/j.cpme.2012.11.002.
11. Kisch T, Schleusser S, Helmke MKL, Wenzel ET, Hasemann B, Mailaender P, Kraemer R. The repetitive use of non-thermal dielectric barrier discharge plasma boosts cutaneous microcirculatory effects. Microvasc Res. 2016;106:8–13.
12. Kisch T, Helmke A, Schleusser S, Song J, Liodaki E, Stang FH, Mailaender P, Kraemer R. Improvement of cutaneous microcirculation by cold atmospheric plasma (CAP): results of a controlled, prospective cohort study. Microvasc Res. 2016;104:55–62.

# MicroPlaSter and SteriPlas

# 34

F. Herbst, J. van Schalkwyk, and M. McGovern

## 34.1 Medical Device Path to CE Marking

To obtain CE marking for the SteriPlas, Adtec Europe Ltd. used the MDD Annex IX and MEDDEV 2.4/1 approach which currently is still the easiest route to decision-making and documentation.

Adtec decided that the device could be used as:

1. active (Fig. 34.1)
   (a) Rule 9, therapeutic device to administer energy → possible, but this is not the main function and the energy blocking design stops most radiation.
   (b) Rule 11, administer medicines & other substances to the body → unlikely that any substance is absorbed by the body
2. non-invasive (Fig. 34.2)
   (a) Rule 1, does not contact patient or only contact intact skin → unlikely that parts will only come into contact with intact skin
   (b) Rule 4, in contact with injured skin, intended to manage wound environment → most likely explanation of the essential function of the SteriPlas

F. Herbst • J. van Schalkwyk • M. McGovern (✉)
Adtec Europe Ltd, Hounslow, UK
e-mail: francois@adtec.eu.com; juan@adtec.eu.com; mary@adtec.eu.com



H.-R. Metelmann et al. (eds.), *Comprehensive Clinical Plasma Medicine*,
https://doi.org/10.1007/978-3-319-67627-2_34

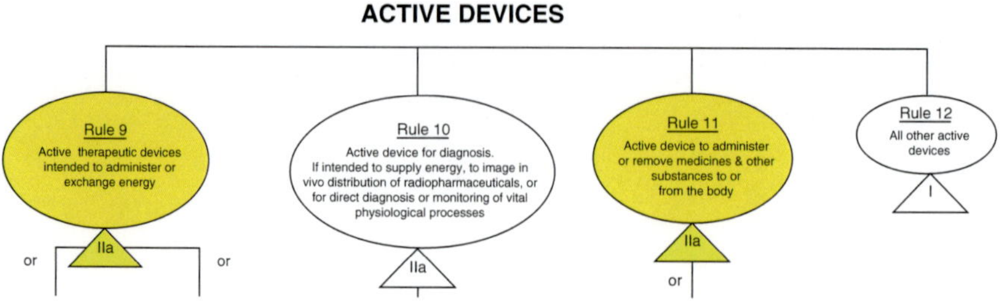


Fig. 34.1 Active device rules (MEDDEV 2.4/1)

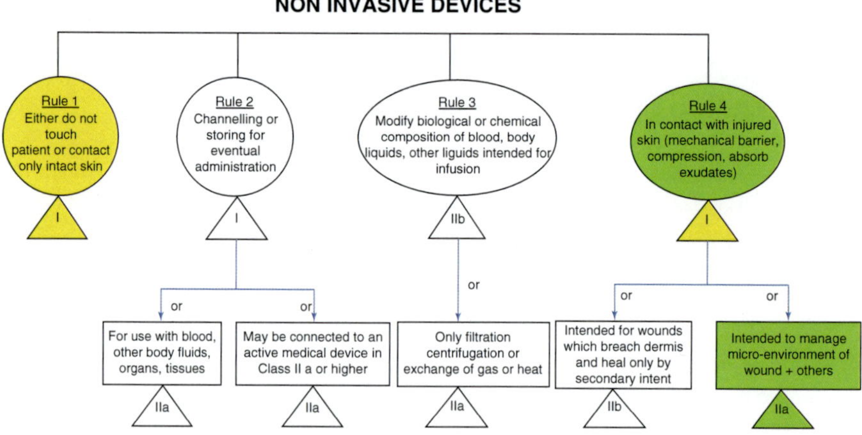


Fig. 34.2 Non-invasive device rules (MEDDEV 2.4/1)

## 34.2 Classification of MicroPlaSter/SteriPlas Medical Device—Class IIa

The devices generate plasma under atmospheric pressure conditions using argon as working gas. The plasma is an ionized gas that acts on the microbes inactivating them without affecting the normal mammalian skin cells in proximity to the plasma treatment area. The plasma acts by treating the microbes in the microenvironment of the wound/infection and is non-invasive to the body. From clinical trials and years of experience, it was concluded that the SteriPlas would be used to manage wound environments and Adtec's quality management system would be tailored to support this. The most appropriate rule that applied was deemed Rule 4, therefor defining the device as Class IIa.

## 34.3 Quality System

As ADTEC Europe limited design, manufacture and support our device, we choose to qualify the device under 93/42/EEC Annex II.

**Table 34.1** Quality system as per Annex II of 93/42/EEC

| Annex | Conformity assessment | Class | Quality system requirements | Design requirements | Notify body assesses conformity |
|---|---|---|---|---|---|
| II | Full quality assurance system by notified body to ISO 13485 | IIa | Full quality system<br>Quality objectives and business organization<br>Design monitoring and verification<br>Manufacturing stage inspection and quality assurance techniques<br>Final inspection | Design procedure<br>Risk assessment<br>Safety test<br>EMC<br>Validation | On-site QMS audit (requirements referred to in Annex II Section 3.2) and technical documentation (Technical File) review |

As per Annex II (Table 34.1).

For Adtec to qualify this system and sell it as a Medical Device, we did the following steps:

- Implement a Quality Management System under ISO 13485
- Design the product using EN 60601
- Full risk assessment under ISO 14791
- Ensure at all the Essential Requirements of the MDD are met

In this document, we are looking into the design process of CE qualifying this unit—complying with safety and EMC tests at an accredited Test House.

## 34.4 Product Safety

All medical devices should be designed by using the safety regulation in EN 60601. IEC 60601 is a series of technical standards for the safety and effectiveness of medical electrical equipment, published by the International Electrotechnical Commission.

All devices have to comply with EN 60601-1. Depends of the function the device, your device will apply with different families under the group.

To ensure the product safety Adtec non thermal plasma device have qualified under the following:

**BS EN 60601-1 ed. 3.1 Medical electrical equipment—Part 1: General requirements for basic safety and essential performance.**

A full safety test needs to be performed by a Test House.

**IEC 60601-1-2:2014 Medical electrical equipment—Part 1–2: General requirements for basic safety and essential performance—Collateral standard: Electromagnetic compatibility—Requirements and tests.**

A full EMC test needs to be performed by a Test House.

**BS EN 62304:2006 + A1:2015—Medical device software. Software life-cycle processes.**

A software assessment needs to be performed.

**BS EN 62366-1:2015—Medical devices. Application of usability engineering to medical devices.**

A usability file needs to be created using the above standard.

## 34.5 Risk Assessment

Adtec did a full risk assessment under ISO 14971 to ensure that the device is safe for the user and patient.

Data from the clinical trial, design process, Safety and EMC testing have been used to verify and check the data.

All the data from clinical trial and research have been used as an input for the new device. Adtec did extensive tests regarding UV and Ozone gasses in the clinical trial.

This assessment have been reviewed constantly while the products are in the field to ensure that the product is always safe.

## 34.6 Technical File

For best practice guidelines on technical files, there are some guideline documents worth reading.

NBOG BPG 2009-4 provides guidance on Notified Body's Tasks of Technical Documentation Assessment and details the scope and requirements of Notified body guidelines. NB-MED/2.5.1-5 provides more detailed requirements for Technical Documentation.

For Adtec SteriPlas, we used the guideline document from our Notified Body. Essentially everything related to the device is included.

Basic outline of Technical File topics:

- Description of the Device, variants, accessories and intended use of the device
- Instructions for use and relevant service and installation manuals
- Device, packaging and shipping labels
- Company information, functions and responsibilities regarding the device
- Device classification and rationale for decision as per MDD/MEDDEV
- Declaration if medicine, blood, tissue or any such derivatives used in the device
- Constructional data including drawings, BOMs, production tests, inspection details
- Declaration of conformity draft, to be signed when device is approved for CE
- Essential requirements checklist as in Annex I of the MDD
- Other directives that apply to the device like RoHS, Machinery etc.
- Biocompatibility of materials used that come into contact with patients, see ISO 10993-1
- Risk management Plan, Analysis and Report for the device as per ISO 14971
- Clinical Evaluation Report and Data provided per Annex X
- Defined lifetime for the device and how it was determined
- Harmonised standards used to achieve conformity
- Test data gained through safety, EMC and performance tests

- Product performance data that shows the product meets its intended specifications
- Transport, storage and packaging specifications and conditions
- Sterility state that is achieved and the validation thereof
- Sales literature that states medical claims, intended use, features
- Quality Management System process overview
- Vigilance/post market surveillance system as required by the MDD Annex II and V
- Mechanism for informing the notified body when there are significant changes

Adtec stores all technical data digitally and manages it through an index system. Part of the Technical File is the Quality Management System processes. This is to demonstrate that processes such as design and manufacturing can sustain the quality of the device and thus ensure the Essential Performance is upheld.

Technical files are updated as changes occur so it is vital to keep up to date with documentation. Notified bodies will review certain areas of Technical Files annually to comply with MDD requirements.

## 34.7 Medical Devices

### 34.7.1 Product Description

The following devices fall within the ADTEC Healthcare plasma devices (see Figs. 34.3 and 34.4):

- MicroPlaSter—ARPP-MS-02
- SteriPlas—ARPP-SP-01

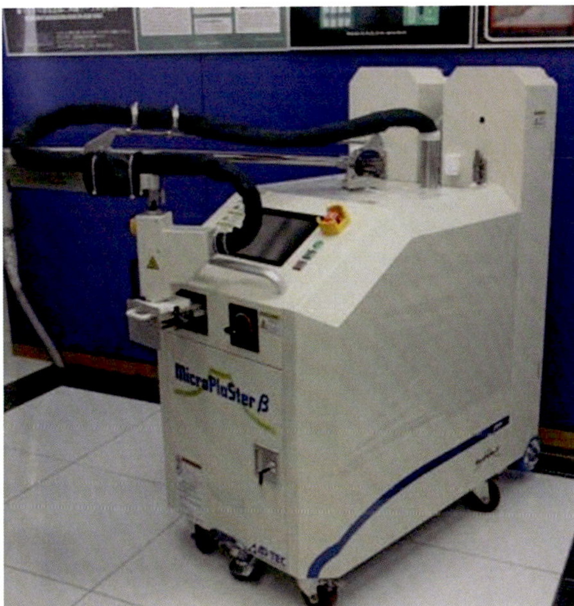


**Fig. 34.3** MicroPlaSter—ARPP-MS-02

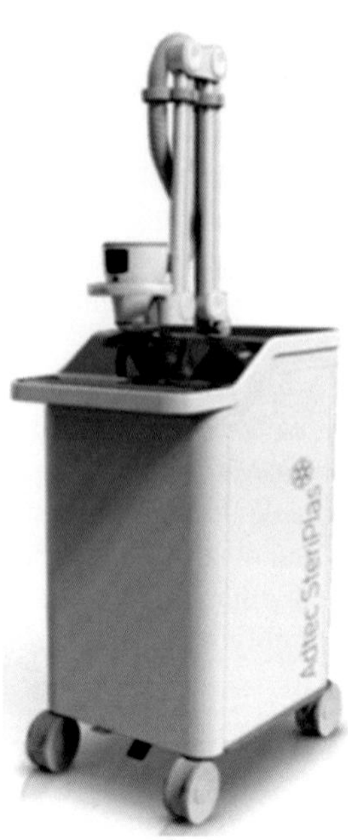


**Fig. 34.4** SteriPlas—ARPP-SP-01

The ARPP-SP-01 is a new product in the MicroPlaSter family. The ARPP-SP-01 (SteriPlas) is the next generation of the ARPP-MS-02. (MicroPlaSter). The Plasma generating device used in the treatment head is exactly the same in the MicroPlaSter and SteriPlas.

The clinical efficacy and results are therefore the same in the MicroPlaSter and SteriPlas and we are using the data from the MicroPlaSter Clinical report to justify the clinical evidence of the SteriPlas.

## 34.8 Mechanical Overview

### 34.8.1 Specification—Main Unit (Table 34.2)

**Table 34.2** Specification comparison between Adtec MicroPlaSter and SteriPlas

| Name | MicroPlaSter | SteriPlas |
|---|---|---|
| Model | ARPP-MS-02 | ARPP-SP-01 |
| Plasma gas temperature | ≤40 ° at a distance of 20 mm from the plasma torch head | ≤40 °C (104 °F) at a distance of 20 mm from the plasma torch grid |
| Operating time | 20 s–9.5 min/time | 20 s–9.5 min plasma on time |
| Plasma gas | Argon, purity ≥99.95% | Argon, minimum purity 99.95% |
| Gas flow rate/ pressure | Mass flow controller for Ar: 0.5–10 SLM ≤0.4 Mpa | Mass flow controller for Ar: 0.5–10 SLM ≤0.4 Mpa |
| Gas cylinders | (Germany) Argon Cylinder Type: 10 L (U.K.) Argon Cylinder Type: X | SMC KK4P-06E, Mating part: KK4S-06H |

**Table 34.2** (Continued)

| Name | MicroPlaSter | SteriPlas |
|---|---|---|
| Duty Cycle | After plasma off, the torch needs 1 min to cool down before changing SCC | After plasma off, wait 1 min before changing Sensor Module ARPP-SP-02 |
| Input | AC23 0 V 1φ, 50/60 Hz | 110 V/220 V–50/60 Hz (Class I) |
| Power consumption | 2.3 kVA | 1.5 kVA |
| Main body dimensions | W700 × D1200 × H2000(m) | W563 × D821 × H1943 mm |
| Arm operation range dimensions | L1360(mm) × H750(mm) × R120° | L1635 × H650 mm × ±60° |
| Operating temp range | 10 °C–30 °C | 10–30 °C (50–86 °F) |
| Operating humidity range | 10–80% relative | 10–80% RH |
| Weight incl. gas | 280 kg | 150 kg (330 lbs) |

### 34.8.2 Applied Parts Specifications (Table 34.3)

**Table 34.3** Applied parts comparison between Adtec MicroPlaSter and SteriPlas

| Name | Surface contact clip (SCC) | SteriPlas sensor module (SSM) |
|---|---|---|
| Model | ARPP-SCC-01 | ARPP-SP-02 |
| Type | B | B |
| Usage | Single use | Single use |
| Material | Polypropylene (PP) | Nylon (polyamide) |
| Temperature | ≤40° C at a distance of 20mm from the plasma torch grid | ≤40° C at a distance of 20mm from the plasma torch grid |

## 34.9 Instructions for Use

The SteriPlas product is a non-thermal plasma-generating device for antimicrobial use in the treatment of wounds, ulcers and infections on the external surface of the body. The controlled neutral plasma is effective in wound management; it positively influences wound healing by reducing microbial load and modifying the wound microenvironment.

The intended use of the device is as a treatment to be administered in a hospital or clinic usually as general care. The treatment can be administered to inpatients and outpatients and to any external region of the body except the eyes.

# DIN SPEC 91315: A First Attempt to Implement Mandatory Test Protocols for the Characterization of Plasma Medical Devices

# 35

Veronika Hahn, Ronny Brandenburg, and Thomas von Woedtke

The different applications of physical plasma in medicine - described in the previous chapters - lead to a demand for experimental data to ensure the provision of effective and safe plasma sources without unwanted side effects. Although, the requirements for the development and improvement of plasma devices are known in general, the characterization of special needs for medical purposes are yet to be defined. The plasma devices differ in the kind of plasma source and the working conditions employed, such as water content of the gas, type and amplitude of high voltage, and feed gas composition. Thus, a control and monitoring, and thereby a comparability of different cold atmospheric plasma (CAP) devices based on technical parameters is not yet possible. Therefore, it is recommended that a mandatory set of parameters be defined. They should be characterized to determine the efficacy of newly developed plasma devices.

This catalog DIN SPEC 91315:2014–06 [1] comprises the general requirements for plasma sources in medicine. (The DIN SPEC 91315 is the basis for the whole chapter and for this reason has not been referenced until now.)

A selected group of experts developed the DIN SPEC 91315 according to the PAS (Publicly Available Specification) procedure during workshops between 2012 and 2014. The DIN SPEC 91315 is not yet part of the DIN standards but is, to our knowledge, the first compilation of protocols for the characterization of plasma sources for medical purposes. However, it must be highlighted that for the licensing of plasma sources as medical devices, all mandatory standards like the DIN EN

V. Hahn (✉) • R. Brandenburg
Leibniz Institute for Plasma Science and Technology (INP Greifswald), Greifswald, Germany
e-mail: veronika.hahn@inp-greifswald.de; brandenburg@inp-greifswald.de

T. von Woedtke
Leibniz Institute for Plasma Science and Technology (INP Greifswald)
and University Medicine Greifswald, Institute for Hygiene and Environmental Medicine, Greifswald, Germany
e-mail: woedtke@inp-greifswald.de



H.-R. Metelmann et al. (eds.), *Comprehensive Clinical Plasma Medicine*,
https://doi.org/10.1007/978-3-319-67627-2_35

60601–1 [2], IEC 60479–1 [3], and relevant laws have to be observed. Moreover, in the DIN SPEC 91315, no limit values are defined because the assessment of the different parameters strongly depends on the intended effect and application of the plasma device. The test procedures recommended by the DIN SPEC 91315 are specifically adapted for atmospheric-pressure plasma applications to provide a representative set of parameters for basic characterization of plasma sources for medical applications. At best, this testing can be regarded as a preliminary stage to achieve the prerequisites for licensing.

The test protocols of the DIN SPEC 91315 comprise physical evaluation criteria such as temperature, radiation (optical emission) or gas emission as well as criteria concerning biological effects such as antimicrobial properties or impact on the vitality of human cells. The detection of chemical species like nitrite, nitrate and hydrogen peroxide, along with the determination of the pH value, are also recommended for further elucidation of complex plasma effects that are mainly mediated by liquid phases. Uncomplicated and reproducible test protocols provide an easy way to characterize the plasma sources and are also accessible to small companies without large research divisions. If possible, test methods prescribed in other standards are included.

The first plasma source characterized completely by the DIN SPEC 91315 was the atmospheric-pressure plasma jet kINPen® Med (neoplas tools GmbH, Greifswald, Germany; [4]), which is licensed as a medical device. This kINPen® Med and a surface dielectric barrier discharge were previously tested for their antimicrobial properties according to the DIN SPEC 91315 [5].

The experiments related to DIN SPEC 91315 should be carried out under conditions that are estimated for the eventual application, which could be humidity or the distance between plasma and target. Furthermore, the reproducibility of the experimental data has to be ensured. Thus, at least two replicates (N = 3) are mandatory. The plasma sources differ in most cases in their geometry and operation parameters. The measurement procedures must therefore be adapted according to the respective source geometry, regardless of the parameter determined.

Different **physical evaluation criteria** are recommended for the estimation of the efficacy of the plasma source; one of them is the ***gas temperature***. Thus, for jet plasma it is necessary to measure the temperature from the discharge opening to the end of the visible plasma effluent being applied to the biological sample.

The gas temperature, in particular, is important for medical applications. The aim in medicine is the local treatment of skin or tissue zones without impairment of the surrounding tissue. A high local temperature caused by plasma increases the risk of heating and, as a consequence, coagulation without healing.

The ***thermal output*** (given in watts) can be determined by calorimetry with a suitable substrate such as copper. This is an additional parameter to characterize the heat impact on the target in the course of plasma treatment.

The ***optical emission*** should also be measured. Thus, the photon emission (electromagnetic radiation) can be determined by optical emission spectroscopy according to DIN 51008-2 [6] from 200 to 900 nm (UV and VIS-region). The calibration of the spectrometer in relation to the relative spectral position and the absolute spectral sensitivity is important before the respective measurements. Moreover, optical emission spectroscopy in the UV/VIS range allows the detection of emitting chemical species in the plasma, and this method is therefore useful for obtaining general information about the plasma composition.

UV radiation is well known to cause skin cancer such as melanoma [7]. Furthermore, the non-melanocytic skin cancers basal cell and squamous cell carcinoma can also result from UV radiation [8–11]. Due to the mostly repeated or continuously application of a plasma source on the skin, radiation safety should be ensured. For the measurement of ultraviolet radiation, a suitable spectrometer for UV-A (320–400 nm), UV-B (280–320 nm), and UV-C (200–280 nm) is required.

The determination of the ***gas composition*** should be performed according to DIN EN ISO 12100 [12]. Such tests are focused on the detection of generated harmful or toxic species such as nitrogen dioxide or ozone, which have to be expected at a varying extent when plasma devices are used in an atmospheric air environment. Gas emission can be measured by commercially available gas analysis systems with suitable sensitivity (at least down to ppm level) whereby the determination should be performed in different solid angles simulating the intended device position in medical practice.

The different kinds of ***current flows*** such as the patient leakage current can be determined as proposed in DIN EN 60601-1 [2] and DIN EN 60601-2-57 [13]. The leakage current measurement must be performed with a defined conductive surface. On the one hand, the leakage current avoids impairment of the patient, and on the other, the impact of electrical fields on the target can be part of the complex biological interaction between plasma and living tissue. Therefore, mean electrical current is an important measure to estimate the biological impact of a given plasma source.

The **biological evaluation criteria** comprise the determination of the ***effect on microorganisms*** in course of the plasma treatment (*in vitro*). For these tests four bacteria *Staphylococcus aureus* DSM 799/ATCC 6538, *Staphylococcus epidermidis* DSM 20044/ATCC 14990, *Escherichia coli* K-12 DSM 11250/NCTC 10538, *Pseudomonas aeruginosa* DSM 50071/ATCC 10145, and the yeast *Candida albicans* DSM 1386/ATCC 10321 can be used. Two test methods are introduced for the determination of the antimicrobial activity of the respective plasma source *in vitro*. The first method is performed in a liquid medium, and the second on a wet solid medium.

For the experiments with the liquid medium, the microorganism suspension is treated time-dependently with plasma, with subsequent determination of the total viable count. For the tests on the wet solid medium, agar plates are inoculated with the respective microorganism. Then, localized spot-like CAP treatment without moving the plasma device is carried out. After incubation of the plates, the growth inhibition zones (defined as circular area without visible growth of the tested microorganism, and named in accordance with agar disc diffusion assay) are measured.

Antimicrobial testing is a useful and easy way to estimate biological effectiveness in general. The use of microorganism suspensions (liquid medium) provides basic information on the bulk of the efficacy of the plasma mediated by the liquid environment. Using the inhibition zone assay on wet agar surfaces, in addition to the general determination of the antimicrobial plasma effect, the area of effectiveness of a given plasma source can be depicted and is strongly dependent on its geometry.

Experiments with the kINPen® Med and a surface dielectric barrier discharge have shown, amongst others, that more reproducible results can be gained with microorganisms in the stationary phase compared to cells in the exponential growth phase [5]. Thus, the DIN SPEC 91315 test protocols recommend the utilization of microorganisms in the stationary phase.

Beyond the effect of plasma on microorganisms, *in vitro* ***vitality tests of eukaryotic cell cultures*** are an additional part of the DIN SPEC. The test protocol includes the utilization of the immortalized skin fibroblast cell line GM00637.

Potential cytotoxic effects are determined by MTT- [3-(4,5-dimethylthiazol-2-yl)-2,5-diphenyl-2H-tetrazolium bromide] or MTS-tests [3-(4,5-dimethylthiazol-2-yl)-5-(3-carboxymethoxyphenyl)-2-(4-sulfophenyl)-2H–tetrazolium], which are commercially available. The basis of these tests is the metabolism of the tetrazolium salt to formazan by vital cells. Thus, the measurement of the extinction enables a statement about the part of the vital and non-vital cells.

The ***detection of chemical species*** is important to evaluate the extent of the formation of reactive nitrogen and/or oxygen species because it is well known that biological plasma effects are mainly mediated via liquid phases. Hydrogen peroxide ($H_2O_2$) is representative for the generation of reactive oxygen species (ROS), whereas nitrite and nitrate are representatives for the generation of reactive nitrogen species (RNS, RONS). The pH-value represents the reactive (biological) environment [14]. Even if these substances themselves and their generation in the liquid environment of cells are not mainly responsible for biological plasma effects, they can serve as indicators for complex reaction changes as a consequence of plasma-liquid interactions. Their varying appearance in liquids after plasma treatment may be part of the characterization of a plasma source. They may allow basic conclusions on the main reactive processes induced by the respective plasma source, as well as initial indications of its biological activity.

The tests can be carried out using commercially available kits, and the respective reaction products can be detected spectrophotometrically. Therefore, measurements are created for a punctual treatment of the water surface i.e., without moving the device. Nitrite is detected by the reaction with *N*-(1-naphthyl)ethylenediamine dihydrochloride forming a red azo dye (DIN EN 26777) [15]. Nitrate reacts with 2,6-dimethylphenol (DMP) to become 2,6-dimethyl-4-nitrophenol (DIN 38405-9) [16]. Hydrogen peroxide reacts with titanyl sulfate to form a complex (DIN 38409-15) [17]. Chromatographic analyses are also possible for the evaluation of reactive species such as ion chromatography for the detection of nitrate and nitrite.

The evaluation of the pH-value can be ascertained using an instrument according to DIN EN ISO 10523 [18]. The pH-value should be measured after the respective times needed for the inactivation of microorganisms. The determination of the pH-value should take place 5 min after plasma treatment.

With the results of the tests following DIN SPEC 91315 [1], a set of parameters is available to characterize the performance of medical plasma sources. It contains data from a huge number of experiments, showing that different plasma devices can induce similar biological effects. On the one hand, monitoring and control of such effects by physical plasma parameters (e.g., the electron density and electron temperature) is currently very difficult to achieve [19]. Thus, any comparison and characterization of plasma sources has to be attributed to biological effects. On the other hand, biological plasma effects are determined by physical and chemical parameters as well as the surrounding conditions. Therefore, the combination of physical, biological and chemical tests recommended by the DIN SPEC 91315 is a first attempt to find a way for standard characterization of plasma sources intended for medical application. This evaluates their effectiveness as well as improving safety for users (investigators, patients, and therapists). Eventually, such standardization will also improve the transfer of experimental results into industrial development of medical devices for plasma medicine.

The DIN SPEC 91315 as a first step in this direction should be improved and complemented further by the whole plasma community in order to develop a nationally and internationally mandatory standard for plasma medical devices.

## References

1. DIN SPEC 91315:2014-06. General requirements for plasma sources in medicine. DIN Deutsches Institut für Normung e.V. Berlin: Beuth; 2014 (in German).
2. DIN EN 60601-1; VDE 0750-1:2013-12, Medical electrical equipment—Part 1: General requirements for basic safety and essential performance (IEC 60601-1:2005 + Cor.: 2006 + Cor.: 2007 + A1:2012); German version EN 60601-1:2006 + Cor.: 2010 + A1:2013. DIN Deutsches Institut für Normung e.V. Berlin: Beuth; 2013 (in German).
3. DIN IEC/TS 60479-1:2007-05; VDE V 0140-479-1:2007-05, Effects of current on human beings and livestock—Part 1: General aspects (IEC/TS 60479–1:2005 + Corrigendum October 2006), DIN Deutsches Institut für Normung e.V. Berlin: Beuth; 2007 (in German).
4. Mann MS, Tiede R, Gavenis K, Daeschlein G, Bussiahn R, Weltmann K-D, Emmert S, von Woedtke T, Ahmed R. Introduction to DIN-specification 91315 based on the characterization of the plasma jet kINPen® MED. Clin Plasma Med. 2016;4:35–45.
5. Mann MS, Schnabel U, Weihe T, Weltmann K-D, von Woedtke T. A reference technique to compare the antimicrobial properties of atmospheric pressure plasma sources. Plasma Med. 2015;5(1):27–47.
6. DIN 51008-2, Optical Emission Spectrometry (OES)—Part 2: Terms for flame and plasma systems. DIN Deutsches Institut für Normung e.V. Berlin: Beuth 2001 (in German).
7. Ribero S, Glass D, Bataille V. Genetic epidemiology of melanoma. Eur J Dermatol 2016;26(4):335-339.
8. Goldberg LH. Basal cell carcinoma. Lancet. 1996;347:663–7.
9. Armstrong BK, Kricker A. The epidemiology of UV induced skin cancer. J Photochem Photobiol B. 2001;63:8–18.
10. Kennedy C, Bajdik CD, Willemze R, de Gruijl FR, Bavinck JNB. The Influence of painful sunburns and lifetime sun exposure on the risk of actinic keratoses, seborrheic warts, melanocytic nevi, atypical nevi, and skin cancer. J Invest Dermatol. 2003;120(6):1087–93.
11. Goldenberg G. Treatment considerations in actinic keratosis. JEADV. 2017;31(2):12–6.
12. DIN EN ISO 12100:2011-03. Safety of machinery—General principles for design—Risk assessment and risk reduction (ISO 12100:2010); German version EN ISO 12100:2010. Berlin: DIN Deutsches Institut für Normung e.V. Berlin: Beuth; 2011.
13. DIN EN 60601-2-57; VDE 0750-2-57:2011-11, Medical electrical equipment—Part 2–57: Particular requirements for the basic safety and essential performance of non-laser light source equipment intended for therapeutic, diagnostic, monitoring and cosmetic/aesthetic use (IEC 60601-2-57:2011); German version EN 60601-2-57:2011. DIN Deutsches Institut für Normung e.V. Berlin: Beuth; 2011 (in German).

14. Jablonowski H, von Woedtke T. Research on plasma medicine-relevant plasma-liquid interaction: what happened in the past five years? Clin Plasma Med. 2015;3:42–52.
15. DIN EN 26777, Water quality; determination of nitrite; molecular absorption spectrometric method (ISO 6777:1984); German version EN 26777:1993. DIN Deutsches Institut für Normung e.V. Berlin: Beuth; 1993.
16. DIN 38405-9 German standard methods for examination of water, waste water and sludge—Anions (group D)—Part 9: Spectrometric determination of nitrate (D 9). DIN Deutsches Institut für Normung e.V. Berlin: Beuth; 2011 (in German).
17. DIN 38409-15, German standard methods for the examination of water, waste water and sludge; general measures of effects and substances (group H); determination of hydrogen peroxide and its adducts (H 15). DIN Deutsches Institut für Normung e.V. Berlin: Beuth; 1987 (in German).
18. DIN EN ISO 10523, Water quality—Determination of pH (ISO 10523:2008); German version EN ISO 10523:2012. DIN Deutsches Institut für Normung e.V. Berlin: Beuth; 2012.
19. Bruggeman P, Brandenburg R. Atmospheric pressure discharge filaments and micro-plasmas: physics, chemistry and diagnostics. J Phys D Appl Phy. 2013;46:464001. (28pp).

# Index





H.-R. Metelmann et al. (eds.), *Comprehensive Clinical Plasma Medicine*,
https://doi.org/10.1007/978-3-319-67627-2

**D**

**R**

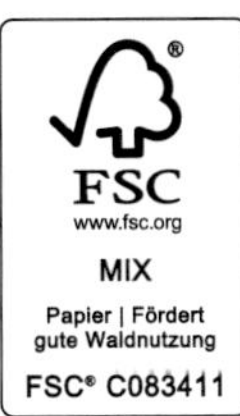


Zeitfracht Medien GmbH
Ferdinand-Jühlke-Straße 7
99095 Erfurt, Deutschland
produktsicherheit@kolibri360.de